**NURSE'S
5-MINUTE
CLINICAL
CONSULT**

Signs &
Symptoms

Wolters Kluwer | Lippincott Williams & Wilkins
Health

Philadelphia • Baltimore • New York • London
Buenos Aires • Hong Kong • Sydney • Tokyo

STAFF

Executive Publisher
Judith A. Schilling McCann, RN, MSN

Editorial Director
H. Nancy Holmes

Clinical Director
Joan M. Robinson, RN, MSN

Art Director
Elaine Kasmer

Editorial Project Manager
Ann E. Houska

Clinical Manager
Collette Bishop Hendler, RN, BS, CCRN

Clinical Project Managers
Janet S. Rader Clark, RN, BSN;
Kathryn Henry, RN, BSN, CCRC

Editors
Jennifer D. Kowalak, Julie Munden

Clinical Editors
Anita Lockhart, RN, MSN;
Carol A. Saunderson, RN, BA, BS

Copy Editors
Leslie Dworkin, Jeannine Fielding,
Linda Hager, Laura M. Healy,
Marna Poole, Joysa Winter

Designer
Jan Greenberg

Digital Composition Services
Diane Paluba (manager), Joyce Rossi Biletz,
Donna S. Morris

Manufacturing
Beth J. Welsh

Editorial Assistants
Karen J. Kirk, Jeri O'Shea, Linda K. Ruhf

Indexer
Barbara Hodgson

The clinical treatments described and recommended in this publication are based on research and consultation with nursing, medical, and legal authorities. To the best of our knowledge, these procedures reflect currently accepted practice. Nevertheless, they can't be considered absolute and universal recommendations. For individual applications, all recommendations must be considered in light of the patient's clinical condition and, before administration of new or infrequently used drugs, in light of the latest package-insert information. The authors and publisher disclaim any responsibility for any adverse effects resulting from the suggested procedures, from any undetected errors, or from the reader's misunderstanding of the text.

5MCCSS010807

Library of Congress

Nurse's 5-minute clinical consult. Signs and symptoms.
        p. ; cm.
    Includes bibliographical references and index.
    1. Nursing assessment—Handbooks, manuals, etc. 2. Nursing diagnosis—Handbooks, manuals, etc. 3. Symptoms—Handbooks, manuals, etc. I. Lippincott Williams & Wilkins. II. Title: Nurse's five-minute clinical consult. Signs and symptoms. III. Title: Signs and symptoms.
    [DNLM: 1. Nursing Assessment—methods—Handbooks. 2. Clinical Medicine—Handbooks. WY 49 N972953 2008]
    RT48.N78 2008
    616.07'5—dc22
ISBN-13: 978-1-58255-703-8 (alk. paper)
ISBN-10: 1-58255-703-9 (alk. paper)   2007018759

Contents

Contributors and consultants

Helen Ballestas, RN, MSN, CRRN, PhD(C)
Faculty—Nursing Department
New York Institute of Technology
Old Westbury

Sharon Lee Conner, RN, BSN, CMSRN
Clinical Educator
Integris Health
Oklahoma City

Marsha L. Conroy, RN, BA, BSN, MSN, APN
Nurse Educator
Cuyahoga Community College
Indiana Wesleyan University
Cleveland

Laurie Donaghy, RN, CEN
Staff Nurse
Frankford Hospital
Philadelphia

Marianne Ellis, RN, CCRN
Staff Nurse, Critical Care
Bayonne Medical Center
Bayonne, N.J.

Matt Freeman CNP, MPH
Nurse Practitioner/Clinical Instructor
Ohio State University College of Nursing
Columbus

Shirley Lyon Garcia, RN, BSN
Nursing Program Director, PNE
McDowell Technical Community College
Marion, N.C.

Kenneth Hazell, PhD(C), MSN, ARNP
Nursing Program Director
Keiser University
Fort Lauderdale, Fla.

Fiona Johnson, RN, MSN, CCRN
Clinical Education Specialist
Memorial Health University Medical
   Center
Savannah, Ga.

Christine Kennedy, MSN, RN
Specialty Clinic Nurse
VA Connecticut Healthcare Systems
West Haven

Alexis Puglia, RN
Staff Nurse
Chestnut Hill Hospital
Philadelphia

Donna Ratcliff, RN, BSN
Med/Surg Nurse Educator
North Oakland Medical Centers
Pontiac, Mich.

Marguerite Sheipe, MSN, CRNP
Family Nurse Practitioner
Healthlink Medical Center
Southampton, Pa.

Alexander John Siomko, MSN, RN, BC, CRNP, APRN, BC
Staff Nurse
Methodist Hospital Division
Thomas Jefferson University Hospital
Philadelphia

Signs & Symptoms

Abdominal distention

OVERVIEW

- Increased abdominal girth from increased intra-abdominal pressure
- Occurs when increased fluid and gas can't pass freely through the GI tract
- Can be mild or severe, localized or diffuse, and gradual or sudden

 ACTION STAT! *Quickly check for signs of hypovolemia, difficulty breathing, or severe abdominal pain. Ask about recent accidents and observe for signs of trauma and peritoneal bleeding, such as Cullen's sign (ecchymosis around the umbilicus) or Turner's sign (ecchymosis over the flanks). Auscultate all abdominal quadrants and gently palpate the abdomen for rigidity. If you detect rigidity along with abnormal bowel sounds, and the patient complains of pain, begin emergency interventions. Place the patient in the supine position, give oxygen, and insert an I.V. catheter. Insert a nasogastric tube to relieve acute intraluminal distention and get the patient ready for surgery.*

HISTORY

- Ask about onset and duration.
- Obtain a medical history, noting GI or biliary disorders, chronic constipation, abdominal surgery, and recent accidents.

PHYSICAL ASSESSMENT

- Observe the recumbent patient for abdominal asymmetry and contour.
- Check for localized distention, which may cause a sensation of pressure, fullness, or tenderness.
- Assess for generalized distention, which may cause bloating, heart pounding, and difficulty breathing when lying flat or breathing deeply.
- Inspect for tense, glistening skin and bulging flanks, which may indicate ascites. (See *Detecting ascites*.)
- Observe for everted or inverted umbilicus.
- Inspect the abdomen for signs of incisional, inguinal, or femoral hernia.
- Auscultate for bowel sounds, abdominal rubs, and bruits.
- Percuss and palpate the abdomen.
- Prepare the patient for pelvic or genital examination.
- Obtain vital signs, abdominal girth, and weight.

CAUSES

MEDICAL
Abdominal cancer
- Generalized distention may occur when advanced cancer (ovarian, hepatic, or pancreatic) produces ascites.
- Other signs and symptoms are severe abdominal pain, anorexia, jaundice, GI hemorrhage, dyspepsia, weight loss, abdominal mass, and muscle weakness and atrophy.

TOP TECHNIQUE

Detecting ascites

To differentiate ascites from other causes of abdominal distention, check for shifting dullness, fluid wave, and puddle sign, as described here.

SHIFTING DULLNESS
Step 1. With the patient in a supine position, percuss from the umbilicus outward to the flank, as shown. Draw a line on the patient's skin to mark the change from tympany to dullness.

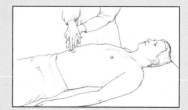

Step 2. Turn the patient onto his side. (Note that this positioning causes ascitic fluid to shift.) Percuss again and mark the change from tympany to dullness. A difference between these lines can indicate ascites.

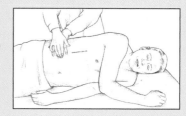

FLUID WAVE
Have another person press deeply into the patient's midline to prevent vibration from traveling along the abdominal wall. Place one of your palms on one of the patient's flanks. Strike the opposite flank with your other hand. If you feel the blow in the opposite palm, ascitic fluid is present.

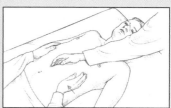

PUDDLE SIGN
Position the patient on his elbows and knees, which causes ascitic fluid to pool in the most dependent part of the abdomen. Percuss the abdomen from the flank to the midline. The percussion note becomes louder at the edge of the puddle, or the ascitic pool.

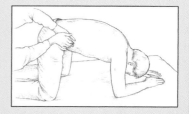

Abdominal trauma

- Acute and dramatic distention may occur with brisk internal bleeding.
- Other signs and symptoms include abdominal rigidity with guarding, decreased or absent bowel sounds, vomiting, tenderness, abdominal bruising, pain over the trauma site or scapula, and, if blood loss is significant, hypovolemic shock.

Bladder distention

- In mild bladder distention, there's slight dullness on percussion above the symphysis pubis.
- In severe bladder distention, there's a palpable, rounded suprapubic mass.

Cirrhosis

- Ascites causes distention.
- Umbilical eversion and *caput medusae* (dilated veins around the umbilicus) are common.
- Other signs and symptoms include vague abdominal pain, hepatomegaly, fever, anorexia, nausea, vomiting, constipation or diarrhea, bleeding tendencies, severe pruritus, palmar erythema, spider angiomas, leg edema, and jaundice (a late sign).

Heart failure

- In severe cardiovascular impairment, ascites occurs.
- Signs and symptoms include peripheral edema, jugular vein distention, dyspnea, and tachycardia.
- Other signs and symptoms include hepatomegaly, nausea, vomiting, productive cough, crackles, cool extremities, cyanotic nail beds, nocturia, exercise intolerance, nocturnal wheezing, diastolic hypertension, and cardiomegaly.

Irritable bowel syndrome

- Periodic intestinal spasms may cause intermittent, localized distention; lower abdominal pain or cramping
- Other signs and symptoms include diarrhea that may alternate with constipation or normal bowel function; nausea; dyspepsia; straining or urgency at defecation; feeling of incomplete evacuation; and small, mucus-streaked stools.

Large-bowel obstruction

- A life-threatening disorder in which abdominal distention occurs.
- Constipation precedes distention.
- Other signs and symptoms include tympany, high-pitched bowel sounds, and sudden colicky lower abdominal pain.
- Late signs include fecal vomiting and diminished peristaltic waves.

Mesenteric artery occlusion, acute

- In this life-threatening disorder, abdominal distention usually occurs several hours after the sudden onset of severe, colicky periumbilical pain and rapid or forceful bowel evacuation.
- Pain becomes constant and diffuse.
- Other signs and symptoms include severe abdominal tenderness with rigidity, absent bowel sounds, vomiting, diarrhea, and constipation.
- Late signs and symptoms include fever and signs of shock.

Nephrotic syndrome

- Ascites cause distention.

Ovarian cysts

- Lower abdominal distention is accompanied by umbilical eversion.
- Lower abdominal pain and a palpable mass may be present.

Paralytic ileus

- Generalized distention occurs with a tympanic percussion note.
- Bowel sounds may be absent or hypoactive.
- Other signs and symptoms include vomiting and severe constipation or flatus with small, frequent stools.

Peritonitis

- Abdominal distention occurs with sudden and severe abdominal pain that worsens with movement.
- Rebound tenderness and abdominal rigidity may be present.
- Other signs and symptoms are hypoactive or absent bowel sounds, fever, chills, nausea, vomiting, and signs of shock (with significant blood loss).

Small-bowel obstruction

- In this life-threatening disorder, abdominal distention is most pronounced during late obstruction, especially in the distal small bowel.
- Bowel sounds may be hypoactive or hyperactive, with tympany.
- Other signs and symptoms are colicky periumbilical pain, constipation, nausea, vomiting, drowsiness, malaise, dehydration, and hypovolemic shock.

Toxic megacolon, acute

- In this life-threatening disorder, dramatic distention gradually occurs.
- Bowel sounds may be diminished or absent.
- Other signs and symptoms are abdominal pain and rebound tenderness, fever, tachycardia, and dehydration.

NURSING CONSIDERATIONS

- Place the patient on his left side to help flatus escape.
- If the patient has ascites, elevate the head of the bed to ease breathing.
- Give the patient pain medication, as ordered and needed.
- Prepare the patient for tests.

PEDIATRIC POINTERS

- Distention may be hard to observe.
- In children, ascites, congenital GI malformations, overeating, and constipation are causes.
- In neonates, abdominal distention caused by ascites usually results from GI or urinary perforation; in older children, from heart failure, cirrhosis, or nephrosis.

PATIENT TEACHING

- Teach the patient to breath slowly to relieve abdominal distention.
- Emphasize the importance of oral hygiene to prevent dry mouth.
- Explain fluid and diet restrictions.

Abdominal mass

OVERVIEW

- Manifests as localized swelling in one abdominal quadrant
- May signify an enlarged organ, a neoplasm, an abscess, a vascular defect, or a fecal mass

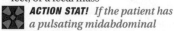 **ACTION STAT!** *If the patient has a pulsating midabdominal mass and severe abdominal or back pain, suspect an abdominal aneurysm. Quickly take vital signs. Withhold food and fluids until the patient is examined. Administer oxygen, and start an I.V. infusion. Look for signs of shock, which occurs with significant blood loss.*

HISTORY

- If the mass is painful, ask if the pain is constant or occurs only with palpation and if it's localized or generalized.
- Ask if the mass has changed size or location.
- Obtain a medical history, noting GI disorders.
- Ask the patient if he's experienced such symptoms as constipation, diarrhea, rectal bleeding, abnormally colored stools, vomiting, and changes in appetite.
- Ask women to describe their menstrual cycles, noting any abnormalities.

PHYSICAL ASSESSMENT

- Auscultate first, listening for bruits or rubs.
- Percuss the mass, noting the sound.
- Lightly palpate and then deeply palpate the abdomen, assessing painful or suspicious areas last.
- Estimate the size of the mass and determine its shape and consistency.
- Note whether the mass is palpable in supine and sidelying positions.
- Determine if the mass moves with your hand or in response to respiration.

- Note the contour and consistency of the mass.

CAUSES

MEDICAL
Abdominal aortic aneurysm
- A life-threatening disorder, it produces severe upper abdominal pain or, less often, lower back or dull abdominal pain if rupture occurs.
- The condition may persist for years, producing only a pulsating periumbilical mass with a systolic bruit over the aorta.
- Other signs and symptoms of rupture include mottled skin below the waist, absent femoral and pedal pulses, lower blood pressure in the legs than in the arms, mild to moderate tenderness with guarding, abdominal rigidity, and shock (with significant blood loss).

Bladder distention
- A smooth, rounded, fluctuant suprapubic mass develops.
- With extreme distention, the mass may extend to the umbilicus.
- Severe suprapubic pain and urinary frequency may also develop.

Cholecystitis
- Deep palpation below the liver border may reveal a smooth, firm, sausage-shaped mass; with acute inflammation, however, the gallbladder may be too tender to be palpated.
- The condition may produce severe right-upper-quadrant pain that may radiate to the right shoulder, chest or back; abdominal rigidity and tenderness; fever; pallor; diaphoresis; anorexia; nausea; and vomiting.
- Attacks typically occur 1 to 6 hours after meals.
- Murphy's sign — inspiratory arrest brought on while palpating the right upper quadrant when the patient takes a deep breath — is common.

Cholelithiasis
- A painless, smooth, and sausage-shaped mass develops in the right upper quadrant.

- Passage of a calculus through the bile duct or cystic duct may cause severe right-upper-quadrant pain that radiates to the epigastrium, back, or shoulder blades.
- Other signs and symptoms include anorexia, nausea, vomiting, chills, diaphoresis, restlessness, low-grade fever, jaundice (if common bile duct is obstructed), intolerance to fatty foods, and indigestion.

Colon cancer
- If present in the right colon, a right-lower-quadrant mass may occur with occult bleeding and anemia and abdominal aching, pressure, or dull cramps.
- Other signs and symptoms of right colon cancer include weakness, fatigue, exertional dyspnea, vertigo, and, with intestinal obstruction, obstipation and vomiting.
- If present in the left colon, a palpable left-lower-quadrant mass produces rectal bleeding and pressure, intermittent abdominal fullness or cramping, and pain relief with defecation.
- Late signs of left colon cancer include obstipation; diarrhea; or pencil-shaped, grossly bloody, or mucus-streaked stools.

Crohn's disease
- Tender, sausage-shaped masses are usually palpable in the right lower quadrant and, at times, in the left lower quadrant.
- Colicky right-lower-quadrant pain and diarrhea are common.
- Other signs and symptoms include fever; anorexia; weight loss; hyperactive bowel sounds; nausea; abdominal tenderness with guarding; and perirectal, skin, or vaginal fistulas.

Diverticulitis
- A left-lower-quadrant mass that's usually tender, firm, and fixed may develop.
- Other signs and symptoms may include intermittent abdominal pain that's relieved by defecating or passing flatus, alternating diarrhea and constipation, nausea, low-grade

fever, and a distended and tympanic abdomen.

Gallbladder cancer
- A moderately tender, irregular mass may develop in the right upper quadrant.
- Chronic, progressively severe epigastric or right-upper-quadrant pain that may radiate to the right shoulder occurs.
- Other signs and symptoms include nausea, vomiting, anorexia, weight loss, jaundice and, at times, hepatomegaly.

Gastric cancer
- An epigastric mass may develop.
- Early findings include chronic dyspepsia and epigastric discomfort.
- Late findings include weight loss, feeling of fullness, fatigue and, occasionally, coffee-ground vomitus or melena.

Hepatic cancer
- A tender, nodular mass in the right upper quadrant or right epigastric area develops.
- Pain is aggravated by jolting.
- Other signs and symptoms include weight loss, weakness, anorexia, nausea, fever, dependent edema, jaundice, ascites, and a bruit or hum (if the tumor is large).

Hepatomegaly
- A firm, blunt, irregular mass may be present in the epigastric region or below the right costal margin.
- Other signs and symptoms include ascites, right-upper-quadrant pain and tenderness, anorexia, nausea, vomiting, leg edema, jaundice, palmar erythema, spider angiomas, gynecomastia, testicular atrophy, and splenomegaly.

Hydronephrosis
- A smooth, boggy mass is detected in one or both flanks.
- Severe colicky renal pain or dull flank pain radiates to the groin, vulva, or testes.
- Other signs and symptoms include hematuria, pyuria, dysuria, alternat-

ing oliguria and polyuria, nocturia, accelerated hypertension, nausea, and vomiting.

Ovarian cyst
- A smooth, rounded, fluctuant mass may develop in the suprapubic region.
- Mild pelvic discomfort, lower back pain, menstrual irregularities, and hirsutism may occur with large or multiple cysts.
- Abdominal tenderness, distention, and rigidity may occur with twisted or ruptured cysts.

Pancreatic abscess
- Occasionally, a palpable epigastric mass may develop, with accompanying pain and tenderness.
- Other signs and symptoms include nausea, vomiting, diarrhea, tachycardia, hypotension, and an abrupt rise in temperature (although it may also rise steadily).

Renal cell cancer
- A smooth, firm, nontender mass develops near the affected kidney.
- Dull, constant abdominal or flank pain and hematuria occur.
- Other signs and symptoms include elevated blood pressure, fever, and urine retention; and in late stages, cachexia, nausea, vomiting, and leg edema.

Splenomegaly
- The spleen is palpable in the left upper quadrant.
- Other signs and symptoms include a feeling of abdominal fullness, left-upper-quadrant pain and tenderness, splenic rub, splenic bruits, and low-grade fever.

Uterine leiomyomas (fibroids)
- A round, multinodular mass may develop in the suprapubic region.
- Other signs and symptoms may include menorrhagia, a feeling of heaviness in the abdomen; back pain; constipation; urinary frequency and urgency; and edema and varicosities of the leg.

NURSING CONSIDERATIONS
- Offer emotional support to the patient and his family.
- Position the patient comfortably.
- Give drugs for pain or anxiety, as needed.
- If bowel obstruction occurs, watch for indications of peritonitis and shock.

PEDIATRIC POINTERS
- In neonates, most abdominal masses result from renal disorders.
- In older infants and children, abdominal masses are usually caused by enlarged organs.
- Other common causes include Wilms' tumor, neuroblastoma, intussusception, volvulus, Hirschsprung's disease (congenital megacolon), pyloric stenosis, and abdominal abscess.

GERIATRIC POINTERS
- Ultrasonography is used to evaluate a prominent midepigastric mass in thin, elderly patients.

PATIENT TEACHING
- Explain any diagnostic tests that are needed.
- Discuss underlying condition and treatment options.

Abdominal pain

- Arises from the abdominopelvic viscera, the parietal peritoneum, or the capsules of the liver, kidney, or spleen (see *Abdominal pain: Types and locations*)
- May be acute or chronic and diffuse or localized
- Visceral pain: develops slowly into a deep, dull, aching pain that's poorly localized in the epigastric, periumbilical, or lower midabdominal region
- Somatic (parietal, peritoneal) pain: produces a sharp, more intense, and well-localized discomfort that rapidly follows the insult and is aggravated by coughing
- Sharp, well-localized, referred pain: felt in skin or deeper tissues

ACTION STAT! *If the patient is experiencing sudden and severe abdominal pain, quickly take his vital signs and palpate pulses below the waist. Be alert for signs of hypovolemic shock. Start an I.V. line. If the skin is mottled below the waist with a pulsating epigastric mass or rebound tenderness and rigidity, the patient may need emergency surgery.*

HISTORY

- Obtain a medical history, noting previous abdominal pain; substance abuse; vascular, GI, genitourinary, or reproductive disorders; and menstrual patterns and changes.
- Ask the patient to describe the pain and to rate it on a scale of 0 to10. (See *Assessing abdominal pain.*)
- Ask the patient if he's had appetite changes, increased flatulence, constipation, diarrhea, bowel movement changes, urinary frequency and urgency, and painful urination.

PHYSICAL ASSESSMENT

- Take the patient's vital signs.
- Assess skin turgor and mucous membranes.
- Inspect the patient's abdomen for distention or visible peristaltic waves and measure his abdomen.
- Auscultate for bowel sounds and characterize their motility.
- Percuss all abdominal quadrants.
- Palpate the entire abdomen for masses, rigidity, and tenderness.
- Check for costovertebral angle tenderness, abdominal tenderness with guarding, and rebound tenderness.

CAUSES

MEDICAL
Abdominal aortic aneurysm, dissecting
- This life-threatening disorder is characterized initially by dull lower abdominal, lower back, or severe chest pain.
- Constant upper abdominal pain may worsen when the patient lies down and subside when the patient leans forward or sits up.
- A pulsating epigastric mass may be palpated before rupture.
- Other signs and symptoms include mottled skin and absent pulses below the waist, lower blood pressure

Abdominal pain: Types and locations

AFFECTED ORGAN	VISCERAL PAIN	PARIETAL PAIN	REFERRED PAIN
Appendix	Periumbilical area	Right lower quadrant	Right lower quadrant
Distal colon	Hypogastrium and left flank for descending colon	Over affected area	Left lower quadrant and back (rare)
Gallbladder	Middle epigastrium	Right upper quadrant	Right subscapular area
Ovaries, fallopian tubes, and uterus	Hypogastrium and groin	Over affected area	Inner thighs
Pancreas	Middle epigastrium and left upper quadrant	Middle epigastrium and left upper quadrant	Back and left shoulder
Proximal colon	Periumbilical area and right flank for ascending colon	Over affected site	Right lower quadrant and back (rare)
Small intestine	Periumbilical area	Over affected site	Midback (rare)
Stomach	Middle epigastrium	Middle epigastrium and left upper quadrant	Shoulders
Ureters	Costovertebral angle	Over affected site	Groin: scrotum in men, labia in women (rare)

Assessing abdominal pain

If your patient complains of abdominal pain, ask him to describe the type of pain he's experiencing and how and when it started. This table will help you assess the patient's pain and determine the possible causes.

TYPE OF PAIN	POSSIBLE CAUSE
Burning	Peptic ulcer, gastroesophageal reflux disease
Cramping	Biliary colic, irritable bowel syndrome, diarrhea, constipation, flatulence
Severe cramping	Appendicitis, Crohn's disease, diverticulitis
Stabbing	Pancreatitis, cholecystitis

in the legs than in the arms, abdominal tenderness with guarding, abdominal rigidity, and signs of shock.

Adrenal crisis
◆ Severe abdominal pain appears early.
◆ Other signs and symptoms include nausea, vomiting, dehydration, profound weakness, anorexia, and fever.
◆ Late signs and symptoms include progressive loss of consciousness; signs and symptoms of shock; and increased motor activity, which may progress to delirium or seizures.

Anthrax, GI
◆ Early signs and symptoms include loss of appetite, nausea, vomiting, and fever.
◆ Late signs and symptoms include abdominal pain, severe bloody diarrhea, and hematemesis.

Appendicitis
◆ In this life-threatening disorder, the pain initially occurs in the epigastric or umbilical region and then localizes in the right lower quadrant.
◆ Pain is accompanied by abdominal rigidity, tenderness, and rebound tenderness.
◆ Other signs and symptoms include anorexia, nausea, and vomiting.
◆ Late signs and symptoms include malaise, constipation (or diarrhea), low-grade fever, and tachycardia.

Cholecystitis
◆ Severe right-upper-quadrant pain may be sudden or gradual over several hours, usually after meals.
◆ Pain may radiate to right shoulder, chest, or back.
◆ Palpating the right upper quadrant while the patient takes a deep breath causes inspiratory arrest.
◆ Other signs and symptoms include anorexia, nausea, vomiting, fever, abdominal rigidity, tenderness, pallor, and diaphoresis.

Cholelithiasis
◆ Sudden, severe, and paroxysmal pain in the right upper quadrant may radiate to the epigastrium, back, or shoulder blades.

◆ Other signs and symptoms include anorexia, nausea, vomiting, diaphoresis, restlessness, abdominal tenderness with guarding, fatty food intolerance, and indigestion.

Cirrhosis
◆ A dull abdominal aching occurs early in the disorder with accompanying anorexia, indigestion, nausea, vomiting, constipation, or diarrhea.
◆ The pain worsens in the right upper quadrant when the patient sits up or leans forward
◆ Other signs and symptoms include fever, ascites, leg edema, weight gain, hepatomegaly, jaundice, severe pruritus, bleeding tendencies, palmar erythema, and spider angiomas.

Crohn's disease
◆ Acute attacks result in severe cramping pain in lower abdomen.
◆ Weeks or months of milder cramping pain typically precede an attack.
◆ Pain may be relieved by defecation.
◆ Chronic signs and symptoms include right-lower-quadrant pain, with diarrhea, steatorrhea, and weight loss.
◆ Other signs and symptoms include hyperactive bowel sounds, dehydration, weight loss, fever, abdominal tenderness with guarding, and a palpable mass in a lower quadrant.

Cystitis
◆ Abdominal pain and tenderness are usually suprapubic.
◆ Other signs and symptoms include malaise, flank pain, low back pain, nausea, vomiting, urinary frequency and urgency, nocturia, dysuria, fever, and chills.

Diverticulitis
◆ Intermittent, diffuse left-lower-quadrant pain occurs in mild cases.
◆ The pain may worsen with eating but is relieved by passing stool or gas.
◆ Rupture causes severe left-lower-quadrant pain, abdominal rigidity and, possibly, signs and symptoms of shock and sepsis.
◆ Other signs and symptoms include nausea, constipation or diarrhea, low-grade fever, and a palpable ab-

dominal mass that's usually tender, firm, and fixed.

Duodenal ulcer
◆ Pain is localized and steady, gnawing, burning, aching, or hungerlike.
◆ Pain occurs 2 to 4 hours after a meal and may cause nocturnal awakening.
◆ Pain may be high in the midepigastrium and slightly off-center (usually on the right).
◆ Other symptoms include changes in bowel habits and heartburn or retrosternal burning.

Ectopic pregnancy
◆ Pain occurs in lower abdomen and may be sharp, dull, or cramping, and constant or intermittent.
◆ Fallopian tube rupture causes sharp lower abdominal pain, which may radiate to shoulders and neck; signs of shock may also occur.
◆ Other signs and symptoms include vaginal bleeding, nausea, vomiting, urinary frequency, a tender adnexal mass, and a 1- to 2-month history of amenorrhea.

Endometriosis
◆ Constant, severe pain in the lower abdomen usually begins 5 to 7 days before the start of menses.
◆ Pain may be aggravated by defecation.
◆ Other symptoms include constipation, abdominal tenderness, dysmenorrhea, dyspareunia, and deep sacral pain.

Escherichia coli *0157:H7* infection
◆ Abdominal cramping, watery or bloody diarrhea, nausea, vomiting, and fever occur after eating contaminated foods.
◆ Hemolytic uremia may occur in children younger than age 5 and in elderly patients, possibly leading to acute renal failure.

Gastric ulcer
◆ Diffuse, gnawing, burning pain in the left upper quadrant or epigastric area occurs 1 to 2 hours after meals.
◆ Pain may be relieved by ingesting food or antacids.

(continued)

- Vague bloating and nausea after meals, weight change, anorexia, and GI bleeding may also occur.

Gastritis
- The onset of pain is rapid, ranging from mild epigastric discomfort to burning in the left upper quadrant.
- Other signs and symptoms may include belching, fever, malaise, anorexia, nausea, bloody or coffee-ground emesis, and melena.

Gastroenteritis
- Cramping or colicky pain originates in the left upper quadrant and then radiates or migrates to the other quadrants.
- Pain is accompanied by diarrhea, hyperactive bowel sounds, headache, myalgia, nausea, and vomiting.

Heart failure
- Right-upper-quadrant pain is common.
- Signs and symptoms include jugular vein distention, dyspnea, tachycardia, and peripheral edema.
- Other signs and symptoms include nausea, vomiting, ascites, productive cough, crackles, cool extremities, and cyanotic nail beds.

Hepatitis
- Liver enlargement causes discomfort or dull pain and tenderness in the right upper quadrant.
- Other signs and symptoms include dark urine, clay-colored stools, nausea, vomiting, anorexia, jaundice, malaise, and pruritus.

Herpes zoster
- Abdominal and chest pain may occur in the areas served by the nerves affected by the infection.
- Pain, tenderness, fever, and erythematous papules (which rapidly evolve into vesicles) also occur.

Intestinal obstruction
- This life-threatening disorder produces short episodes of intense, colicky, cramping pain.
- Accompanying signs and symptoms include abdominal distention, tenderness, and guarding; visible peristaltic waves; high-pitched, tinkling, or hyperactive sounds near the obstruction and hypoactive or absent sounds distally; obstipation; pain-induced agitation; and hypovolemic shock (late sign).
- In jejunal and duodenal obstruction, nausea and bilious vomiting occur early.
- In distal obstruction, nausea and vomiting are commonly feculent.
- Bowel sounds are absent in complete obstruction.

Irritable bowel syndrome
- Lower abdominal cramping or pain is aggravated by ingestion of coarse or raw foods.
- Pain may be alleviated by defecation or passage of flatus.
- Stress, anxiety, and emotional lability intensify the symptoms.
- Other signs and symptoms include abdominal tenderness, diarrhea alternating with constipation or normal bowel function, small stools with visible mucus, dyspepsia, nausea, and abdominal distention with a feeling of incomplete evacuation.

Mesenteric artery ischemia
- Sudden, severe abdominal pain develops after 2 or 3 days of colicky periumbilical pain and diarrhea.
- Condition tends to occur in patients older than age 50 with chronic heart failure, cardiac arrhythmia, cardiovascular infarct, or hypotension.
- Initially, the abdomen is soft and tender with decreased bowel sounds.
- Other signs and symptoms include vomiting, anorexia, alternating periods of diarrhea and constipation and, in late stages, extreme abdominal tenderness with rigidity, tachycardia, tachypnea, absent bowel sounds, and cool, clammy, skin.

Ovarian cyst
- Torsion or hemorrhage causes pain and tenderness in the right or left lower quadrant.
- Standing or stooping causes severe sharp pain.

- The pain becomes brief and intermittent if torsion self-corrects or dull and diffuse if it doesn't.
- Other signs and symptoms include slight fever, mild nausea and vomiting, palpable abdominal mass, amenorrhea, and abdominal distention.

Pancreatitis
- In acute pancreatitis (a life-threatening disorder), fulminating, continuous upper abdominal pain may radiate to both flanks and to the back.
- In chronic pancreatitis, severe left-upper-quadrant or epigastric pain radiates to the back.
- Early findings include abdominal tenderness, nausea, vomiting, fever, pallor, tachycardia, abdominal rigidity, rebound tenderness, and hypoactive bowel sounds.
- Turner's sign (ecchymosis of the abdomen or flank) or Cullen's sign (a bluish tinge around the umbilicus) signals hemorrhagic pancreatitis.
- Jaundice may occur as a late sign.

Pelvic inflammatory disease
- Pain occurs in the right or left lower quadrant.
- Extent of pain ranges from vague discomfort to deep, severe, and progressive pain.
- Metrorrhagia may precede or accompany the onset of pain.
- Other signs and symptoms include abdominal tenderness, palpable abdominal or pelvic mass, fever, chills, nausea, vomiting, urinary discomfort, and abnormal vaginal bleeding or purulent vaginal discharge.

Perforated ulcer
- A life-threatening disorder, sudden, severe, and prostrating epigastric pain may radiate through the abdomen to the back or to the right shoulder.
- Other signs and symptoms include abdominal rigidity, tenderness with guarding, generalized rebound tenderness, absent bowel sounds, grunting and shallow respirations, fever, tachycardia, hypotension, and syncope.

Peritonitis
◆ A life-threatening disorder, sudden and severe pain can be diffuse or localized.
◆ Movement worsens the pain.
◆ Other signs and symptoms include fever; chills; nausea; vomiting; hypoactive or absent bowel sounds; abdominal tenderness, distention, and rigidity; rebound tenderness and guarding; hyperalgesia; tachycardia; hypotension; tachypnea; and psoas and obturator signs.

Prostatitis
◆ Vague abdominal pain or discomfort may develop in the lower abdomen, groin, perineum, or rectum.
◆ Scrotal pain, penile pain, and pain on ejaculation may occur in chronic cases.
◆ Other signs and symptoms include dysuria, urinary frequency and urgency, fever, chills, low back pain, myalgia, arthralgia, and nocturia.

Pyelonephritis, acute
◆ Progressive lower quadrant pain in one or both sides, flank pain, and costovertebral tenderness occur.
◆ Pain may radiate to the lower midabdomen or the groin.
◆ Other signs and symptoms include abdominal and back tenderness, high fever, shaking chills, nausea, vomiting, and urinary frequency and urgency.

Renal calculi
◆ Depending on the location of calculi, severe abdominal or back pain may occur.
◆ The classic symptom is severe, colicky pain that travels from the costovertebral angle to the flank, suprapubic region, and external genitalia.
◆ Other signs and symptoms include pain-induced agitation, nausea, vomiting, abdominal distention, fever, chills, hypertension, and urinary urgency.

Sickle cell crisis
◆ Sudden, severe abdominal pain may accompany chest, back, hand, or foot pain.

◆ Other signs and symptoms include weakness, aching joints, dyspnea, and scleral jaundice.

Smallpox (variola major)
◆ Early findings include abdominal pain, high fever, malaise, prostration, severe headache, and backache.
◆ A maculopapular rash develops at the same time on the mucosa of the mouth, pharynx, face, and forearms and spreads to the trunk and legs.

Splenic infarction
◆ Sudden, severe pain in the left upper quadrant and chest that may worsen during inspiration.
◆ Pain radiates to the left shoulder with splinting of the left diaphragm, abdominal guarding, and, occasionally, a splenic rub.

Ulcerative colitis
◆ Vague abdominal discomfort leads to cramping lower abdominal pain.
◆ Pain may become steady and diffuse, increasing with movement and coughing.
◆ Recurrent and possibly severe diarrhea with blood, pus, and mucus may relieve pain.
◆ Other signs and symptoms include a soft, extremely tender abdomen; high-pitched, infrequent bowel sounds; nausea; vomiting; anorexia; weight loss; and mild, intermittent fever.

OTHER
Drugs
◆ Salicylates and nonsteroidal anti-inflammatory drugs commonly cause burning and gnawing pain in the left upper quadrant or epigastric area.

Abdominal trauma
◆ Generalized or localized abdominal pain occurs with abdominal tenderness, vomiting, and ecchymoses on the abdomen.
◆ Hemorrhage into the peritoneal cavity causes abdominal rigidity.
◆ Bowel sounds are decreased or absent.
◆ Hypovolemic shock may occur.

NURSING CONSIDERATIONS
◆ Have the patient lie in a supine position with his knees slightly flexed.
◆ Monitor the patient for such life-threatening findings as tachycardia, hypotension, clammy skin, abdominal rigidity, rebound tenderness, changes in the pain's location or intensity, or sudden relief from pain.
◆ Withhold food and fluids.
◆ Prepare for I.V. infusion and insertion of a nasogastric or other intestinal tube.
◆ Peritoneal lavage or abdominal paracentesis may be required.

PEDIATRIC POINTERS
◆ Disorders can cause different signs in children than in adults.
◆ Because children have difficulty describing abdominal pain, pay attention to nonverbal cues.
◆ A child's complaint of abdominal pain may reflect an emotional need such as a wish to avoid school or to gain adult attention.

GERIATRIC POINTERS
◆ Advanced age may decrease signs and symptoms of acute abdominal disease.

PATIENT TEACHING
◆ Explain the diagnostic tests the patient will need.
◆ Explain which foods and fluids the patient should avoid.
◆ Tell the patient to report any changes in bowel habits.
◆ Instruct the patient how to position himself to alleviate symptoms.

Abdominal rigidity

OVERVIEW

- Also known as *abdominal muscle spasm* or *involuntary guarding*
- Involves abnormal muscle tension or inflexibility of the abdomen
- May be voluntary (from fear or nervousness) or involuntary (reflecting potentially life-threatening peritoneal irritation or inflammation (see *Recognizing voluntary rigidity*)
- Involuntary rigidity: most common in GI disorders but also in pulmonary or vascular disorders and from the effects of insect toxins

ACTION STAT! *Quickly take the patient's vital signs. Give oxygen and insert an I.V. line for fluid and blood replacement. Anticipate the need for drugs to support blood pressure. Insert nasogastric tube to relieve abdominal distention. Prepare the patient for catheterization, and monitor intake and output of fluids. Because surgery may be necessary, prepare the patient for laboratory tests and X-rays.*

HISTORY

- Ask about the onset of abdominal rigidity.
- Ask if abdominal pain is present and when it began.
- Determine the location of rigidity (localized or generalized).
- Ask about aggravating and alleviating factors, such as position changes, coughing, vomiting, elimination, and walking.

PHYSICAL ASSESSMENT

- Inspect the abdomen for peristaltic waves.
- Check for a visibly distended bowel loop.
- Auscultate for bowel sounds.
- Perform light palpation to locate the rigidity and to determine its severity.
- Check for signs of dehydration, such as poor skin turgor and dry mucous membranes.

CAUSES

MEDICAL

Abdominal aortic aneurysm, dissecting

- In this life-threatening disorder, mild to moderate abdominal rigidity occurs.
- Constant upper abdominal pain may radiate to the lower back.
- A pulsating mass may be present in the epigastrium with a systolic bruit over the aorta before rupture; after rupture, the mass stops pulsating.
- Significant blood loss causes signs of shock (tachycardia, tachypnea, and cool and clammy skin).
- Other signs and symptoms include mottled skin and absent pulses below the waist, lower blood pressure in the legs than in the arms, and mild to moderate tenderness with guarding.

Mesenteric artery ischemia

- Sudden, severe abdominal pain and rigidity occur in the central or periumbilical region after 2 to 3 days of

 TOP TECHNIQUE

Recognizing voluntary rigidity

Distinguishing voluntary from involuntary abdominal rigidity is a must for accurate assessment. Review this comparison so that you can quickly tell the two apart.

VOLUNTARY RIGIDITY

- Usually symmetrical
- More rigid on inspiration (expiration causes muscle relaxation)
- Eased by relaxation techniques, such as positioning the patient comfortably and talking to him in a calm, soothing manner
- Painless when the patient sits up using his abdominal muscles alone

INVOLUNTARY RIGIDITY

- Usually asymmetrical
- Equally rigid on inspiration and expiration
- Unaffected by relaxation techniques
- Painful when the patient sits up using his abdominal muscles alone

persistent, low-grade abdominal pain and diarrhea.
- Rigidity is accompanied by severe abdominal tenderness, fever, vomiting, anorexia, diarrhea, constipation, and signs of shock.

Peritonitis
- Rigidity is localized or generalized depending on the cause of peritonitis.
- Other signs and symptoms include abdominal tenderness and distention, rebound tenderness, guarding, hyperalgesia, hypoactive or absent bowel sounds, nausea, vomiting, fever, chills, tachycardia, tachypnea, and hypotension.

OTHER
Insect toxins
- Rigidity usually accompanies generalized, cramping abdominal pain.
- Other signs and symptoms include low-grade fever, nausea, vomiting, tremors, burning sensations in the hands and feet, increased salivation, hypertension, paresis, and hyperactive reflexes.

NURSING CONSIDERATIONS

- Monitor the patient closely for signs of shock.
- Position the patient in a supine position with knees slightly flexed.
- Withhold analgesics until a tentative diagnosis has been made.
- Withhold food and fluids.
- Administer an I.V. antibiotic as prescribed.
- Prepare for diagnostic tests which may include blood, urine, and stool studies; chest and abdominal X-rays; computed tomography; magnetic resonance imaging; gastroscopy; and colonoscopy.

PEDIATRIC POINTERS
- Voluntary rigidity may be difficult to distinguish from involuntary rigidity if associated pain makes the child restless, tense, or apprehensive.
- It may stem from gastric perforation, hypertrophic pyloric stenosis, duodenal obstruction, meconium ileus, intussusception, cystic fibrosis, celiac disease, and appendicitis.
- When involuntary rigidity is suspected, monitor the patient for early signs of dehydration and shock, which can rapidly become life-threatening.

GERIATRIC POINTERS
- Advanced age and impaired cognition decrease pain perception and intensity.
- Weakening of abdominal muscles with aging means less muscle spasms and decreased rigidity.

PATIENT TEACHING

- Explain about the diagnostic tests or surgery the patient will need.
- Instruct the patient on measures to take to reduce anxiety.

Accessory muscle use

◆ Stabilizes the thorax during respiration when breathing requires extra effort (see *Accessory muscles: Locations and functions*)

◆ May indicate acute respiratory distress, diaphragmatic weakness, fatigue, or chronic respiratory disease

ACTION STAT! *Look for signs of acute respiratory distress. Quickly auscultate for abnormal, diminished, or absent breath sounds. Check for airway obstruction and attempt to restore airway patency. Begin suctioning and manual or mechanical ventilation. Assess oxygen saturation using pulse oximetry, and administer oxygen. You may need to use a high flow rate initially, but be attentive to the patient's respiratory drive. (Too much oxygen may decrease respiratory drive.) If the patient has chronic obstructive pulmonary disease, use a low flow rate for mild exacerbations. Start an I.V. line.*

HISTORY

◆ Ask about the onset, duration, and severity of signs and symptoms.

◆ Obtain a medical and family history, noting any respiratory, cardiac, and infectious disorders.

◆ Ask about recent trauma, pulmonary function testing, or respiratory therapy.

◆ Ask the patient if he smokes and if his line of work exposes him to occupational hazards.

PHYSICAL ASSESSMENT

◆ Perform a detailed chest assessment, noting abnormal respiratory rate, pattern, or depth.

◆ Assess skin color, temperature, and turgor.

◆ Check for clubbing of the fingers.

CAUSES

MEDICAL

Acute respiratory distress syndrome

◆ In this life-threatening disorder, accessory muscle use increases in response to hypoxia.

◆ Intercostal, supracostal, and sternal retractions occur on inspiration.

◆ Grunting occurs on expiration.

◆ Other signs and symptoms include tachypnea, dyspnea, diaphoresis, diffuse crackles, anxiety, tachycardia, mental sluggishness, and a cough with pink, frothy sputum.

Airway obstruction

◆ This life-threatening disorder is characterized by inspiratory stridor.

◆ Accessory muscle use increases.

◆ Other signs and symptoms include dyspnea, tachypnea, gasping, wheezing, coughing, intercostal retractions, cyanosis, and tachycardia.

Amyotrophic lateral sclerosis

◆ Motor neuron disease causes progressive muscle atrophy.

◆ Accessory muscle use increases as disorder affects the diaphragm.

◆ Associated signs and symptoms include fasciculations, muscle atrophy and weakness, spasticity, incoordination, and hyperactive deep tendon reflexes.

◆ Other signs and symptoms include impaired speech; difficulty chewing, swallowing, and breathing; choking; and excessive drooling.

Asthma

◆ Accessory muscle use increases during acute attacks.

◆ Severe dyspnea, tachypnea, wheezing, cough, nasal flaring, cyanosis,

---

Accessory muscles: Locations and functions

Physical exertion and pulmonary disease usually increase the work of breathing, taxing the diaphragm and external intercostal muscles. When this happens, accessory muscles provide the extra effort needed to maintain respirations. The scalene, sternocleidomastoid, and trapezius muscles assist with inspiration, whereas the upper chest, sternum, internal intercostal, and abdominal muscles assist with expiration.

In inspiration, the scalene muscles elevate, fix, and expand the upper chest. The sternocleidomastoid muscles raise the sternum, expanding the chest's anteroposterior and longitudinal dimensions. The pectoralis major muscles elevate the chest, increasing its anteroposterior size, and the trapezius muscles raise the thoracic cage.

With expiration, the internal intercostals depress the ribs, decreasing the chest size. The abdominal muscles pull the lower chest down, depress the lower ribs, and compress the abdominal contents—all of which exert pressure on the chest.

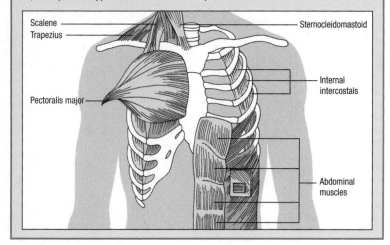

Scalene
Trapezius
Sternocleidomastoid
Internal intercostals
Pectoralis major
Abdominal muscles

tachycardia, diaphoresis, and apprehension occur.
- Auscultation reveals faint or absent breath sounds, inspiratory and expiratory wheezing, and coarse rhonchi.

Chronic bronchitis
- Productive cough and exertional dyspnea precede accessory muscle use.
- Other signs and symptoms include wheezing, barrel chest, clubbing of the fingers, cyanosis, and edema.

Emphysema
- Increased accessory muscle use occurs with progressive exertional dyspnea and a minimally productive cough.
- Auscultation reveals decreased breath sounds and distant heart sounds.
- Other signs and symptoms include pursed-lip breathing, tachypnea, peripheral cyanosis, anorexia, weight loss, malaise, barrel chest, and clubbing of the fingers.

Pneumonia
- Increased accessory muscle use is accompanied by a sudden high fever with chills.
- Other signs and symptoms include chest pain, productive cough, dyspnea, tachypnea, and tachycardia.

Pulmonary edema
- Increased accessory muscle use is accompanied by dyspnea, tachypnea, orthopnea, crepitant crackles, wheezing, and a cough with pink, frothy sputum.
- Other signs and symptoms include sudden restlessness; tachycardia; ventricular gallop; and cool, clammy, cyanotic skin.

Pulmonary embolism
- This life-threatening disorder may cause increased accessory muscle use.
- Common symptoms include sudden dyspnea, tachycardia, and pleuritic or substernal chest pain.
- Other signs and symptoms include restlessness, anxiety, tachycardia,

productive cough, hemoptysis, and cyanosis.

Spinal cord injury
- Injury to cervical vertebrae C3 to C5 affects the upper respiratory muscles and diaphragm, causing increased accessory muscle use.
- Other signs and symptoms include unilateral or bilateral Babinski's reflex; hyperactive deep tendon reflexes; spasticity; and variable or total loss of pain and temperature sensation, proprioception, and motor function.

Thoracic injury
- Increased accessory muscle use may occur depending on the type and extent of injury.
- Other signs and symptoms include an obvious chest wound or bruising, chest pain, dyspnea, and shock (with significant blood loss).

NURSING CONSIDERATIONS

- If the patient is alert, elevate the head of the bed to ease his breathing.
- Encourage the patient to get plenty of rest.
- Encourage the patient to drink plenty of fluids to liquefy secretions, unless he's on fluid restriction.
- Administer oxygen.
- Prepare the patient for diagnostic tests, such as pulmonary function studies, chest X-ray, lung scans, arterial blood gas analysis, and sputum culture.

PEDIATRIC POINTERS
- Upper airway obstruction usually produces respiratory distress and increased accessory muscle use.
- Disorders associated with airway obstruction include acute epiglottitis, croup, pertussis, cystic fibrosis, and asthma.
- Suprasternal, intercostal, or abdominal retractions indicate accessory muscle use.
- Respiratory distress can rapidly progress to respiratory failure be-

cause a child's accessory muscles tire sooner than those of an adult.

GERIATRIC POINTERS
- Because of age-related loss of elasticity in the rib cage, accessory muscle use may be part of an older person's normal breathing pattern.

PATIENT TEACHING

- Teach the patient relaxation techniques to reduce his apprehension.
- Provide resources for quitting smoking, as appropriate.
- Explain measures to prevent infection.
- Explain prescribed drugs and how to take them.
- Provide instruction on pursed-lip, diaphragmatic breathing to ease the work of breathing for patients with chronic lung disorders.
- Teach the patient coughing and deep-breathing exercises to keep airways clear.

Agitation

- Refers to a state of hyperarousal, increased tension, and irritability
- Can lead to confusion, hyperactivity, and overt hostility
- Can arise gradually or suddenly and last for minutes or months

HISTORY

- Determine the severity of the agitation, including the approximate number and quality of agitation-induced behaviors.
- Obtain a history, including the patient's diet and known allergies.
- Ask about past or present illnesses, trauma, stress, and sleep patterns.
- Question the patient about drug and alcohol use.

PHYSICAL ASSESSMENT

- Check for signs of drug abuse.
- Obtain baseline vital signs and neurologic status.

CAUSES

MEDICAL

Affective disturbance

- Agitation may occur in depressed and manic phases and in personality disorders.
- Psychomotor agitation may involve an inability to sit still, hand-wringing, pacing, and irritability.

Alcohol withdrawal syndrome

- Mild to severe agitation occurs along with hyperactivity, tremors, and anxiety.
- Severe agitation accompanies hallucinations, insomnia, diaphoresis, and depressed mood in alcohol withdrawal syndrome, the potentially life-threatening stage of alcohol withdrawal.

Anxiety

- Varying degrees of agitation result.
- Other signs and symptoms include nausea, vomiting, diarrhea, cool and clammy skin, frontal headache, back pain, insomnia, and tremors.

Chronic renal failure

- Moderate to severe agitation occurs, marked especially by confusion and memory loss.
- Other signs and symptoms include nausea, vomiting, anorexia, mouth ulcers, ammonia breath odor, GI bleeding, pallor, edema, dry skin, and uremic frost.

Dementia

- Mild to severe agitation can result from many common syndromes, such as Alzheimer's disease and Huntington's disease.
- Other signs and symptoms include hypoactivity; wandering; hallucinations; aphasia; insomnia; and decreased memory, attention span, problem-solving ability, and alertness.

Drug withdrawal syndrome

- Mild to severe agitation occurs.

- Related findings vary with the drug but include anxiety, abdominal cramps, diaphoresis, and anorexia.

Hepatic encephalopathy

- Patients may experience agitation, drowsiness, stupor, fetor hepaticus (the peculiar breath odor characteristic of hepatic disease), asterixis, and hyperreflexia.
- Lethargy, aberrant behavior, and apraxia may also occur.

Hypersensitivity reaction

- Moderate to severe agitation may be the first sign.
- Urticaria, pruritus, and facial and dependent edema may occur.
- In anaphylactic shock, a potentially life-threatening hypersensitivity reaction, associated findings include the rapid onset of apprehension, urticaria or diffuse erythema, warm and moist skin, paresthesia, pruritus, edema, dyspnea, wheezing, stridor, hypotension, and tachycardia.

Hypoxemia

- Agitation starts as restlessness, then rapidly worsens.
- Other signs and symptoms include confusion, impaired judgment and motor coordination, tachycardia, tachypnea, dyspnea, and cyanosis.

Increased intracranial pressure

- Agitation precedes other early signs and symptoms, such as headache, nausea, and vomiting.
- Other signs and symptoms include respiratory changes; sluggish, nonreactive, or unequal pupils; widening pulse pressure; tachycardia; decreased level of consciousness; seizures; and motor changes.

Post–head-trauma syndrome

- Agitation is characterized by disorientation, loss of concentration, angry outbursts, and emotional lability.
- Other signs and symptoms include fatigue, wandering, and poor judgment.

OTHER

Drugs

◆ Mild to moderate agitation may occur with central nervous system stimulants.

Radiographic contrast media

◆ Agitation may occur as a hypersensitivity reaction to injected contrast medium.

Vitamin B_6 deficiency

◆ Agitation ranges from mild to severe.
◆ Other effects include seizures, peripheral paresthesia, oculogyric crisis, and dermatitis.

NURSING CONSIDERATIONS

◆ Monitor the patient's vital signs and neurologic status.
◆ Eliminate stressors that may trigger agitation.
◆ Provide adequate lighting.
◆ Maintain a calm environment.
◆ Maintain a consistent routine.
◆ Allow the patient time to sleep.
◆ Ensure a balanced diet, and provide vitamin supplements and hydration.
◆ Remain calm, nonjudgmental, and nonargumentative.
◆ Prepare the patient for diagnostic tests, such as computed tomography scanning, magnetic resonance imaging, and blood studies.

PEDIATRIC POINTERS

◆ In children, agitation accompanies the expected childhood diseases and more severe disorders—such as hyperbilirubinemia, phenylketonuria, vitamin A deficiency, hepatitis, frontal lobe syndrome, increased intracranial pressure, and lead poisoning—that can lead to brain damage.
◆ In neonates, agitation can stem from alcohol or drug withdrawal.

GERIATRIC POINTERS

◆ Environmental change or deviation from usual activities (or rituals) may provoke agitation in elderly people.

PATIENT TEACHING

◆ Provide the patient with an orientation to the unit and its procedures and routines.
◆ Explain stress-reduction measures.
◆ Provide reassurance and emotional support to the patient and his family.

Alopecia

- Hair loss (diffuse or patchy) that usually develops gradually
- Can be scarring (permanent; follicles are destroyed) or nonscarring (temporary; follicles are damaged)

HISTORY

- Ask about the onset of hair loss or thinning.
- Determine which areas of the body are affected.
- Question the patient about associated signs and symptoms, such as itching and rashes.
- Obtain a medical history
- Ask about menstrual irregularities in women and sexual dysfunction in men.
- Ask about hair care and habits.
- Check for a family history of alopecia.

PHYSICAL ASSESSMENT

- Assess the extent and pattern of scalp hair loss. (See *Recognizing four of the most common patterns of alopecia.*)
- Inspect the underlying skin for follicular openings, erythema, loss of pigment, scaling, induration, broken hair shafts, and hair regrowth.
- Examine the rest of the skin for jaundice, edema, hyperpigmentation, pallor, or duskiness. Note the size, color, texture, and location of any lesions.
- Examine nails for vertical or horizontal pitting, thickening, brittleness, or whitening.
- Palpate for lymphadenopathy, enlarged thyroid or salivary glands, and masses in the abdomen or chest.

CAUSES

MEDICAL
Alopecia areata
- Well-circumscribed patches of nonscarring scalp alopecia develop.
- Patches of alopecia are bordered by loose hairs with rough, brushlike tips on narrow, less-pigmented shafts.
- Horizontal or vertical nail pitting may occur.

Arterial insufficiency
- Patchy alopecia occurs, typically on the legs.
- Alopecia may be accompanied by thin, shiny, atrophic skin and thickened nails.
- Skin on the legs turns pale when the legs are elevated and dusky when they're dependent.
- Other signs and symptoms include weak or absent peripheral pulses, cool extremities, paresthesia, leg ulcers, and intermittent claudication.

Burns
- Scarring or keloid formation from full-thickness or third-degree burns causes permanent alopecia.

Cutaneous T-cell lymphoma
- Alopecia mucinosa may occur in the premycotic stage and may persist through the plaque and tumor stages.
- Scattered papules or plaques may occur on clothed areas, or a zebralike pattern of scaly erythema may form on the trunk.

Exfoliative dermatitis
- Loss of scalp and body hair is preceded by several weeks of generalized scaling and erythema.
- Other signs and symptoms include nail loss, pruritus, malaise, fever, weight loss, lymphadenopathy, and gynecomastia.

Fungal infections
- Tinea capitis produces irregular balding areas, scaling, and erythematous lesions.
- Broken scalp hairs surround the balding areas.
- Classic ring-shaped appearance occurs as lesions enlarge and the centers heal.
- Pruritus and thick, whitish nails may occur.

Hodgkin's disease
- Permanent alopecia may occur if lymphoma infiltrates the scalp.
- Alopecia may be accompanied by edema, pruritus, and hyperpigmentation.

Hypopituitarism
- In women, sparse or absent pubic and axillary hair, infertility, and breast atrophy occur.

Recognizing four of the most common patterns of alopecia

Distinctive patterns of alopecia result from different causes. The illustrations below show four of the most common patterns.

Tinea capitis, a fungal infection, produces irregular bald patches with scaly, red lesions.

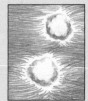

Alopecia areata causes expanding patches of nonscarring hair loss bordered by "exclamation point" hairs.

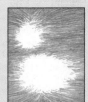

Trauma from habitual hair pulling or injudicious grooming habits may cause permanent peripheral alopecia.

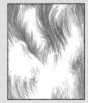

Chemotherapeutic drugs produce diffuse, yet temporary, hair loss.

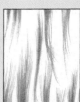

- In men, decreased facial and body hair, infertility, decreased libido, impotence, and poor muscle development occur.

Hypothyroidism
- Hair on the face, scalp, and genitals thins and becomes dull, coarse, and brittle.
- Hair loss in the outer one-third of the eyebrows occurs.
- Other signs and symptoms include fatigue; constipation; cold intolerance; weight gain; dry, flaky, inelastic skin; puffy face, hands, and feet; thick, brittle nails; slow mental function; bradycardia; menorrhagia, and myalgia.

Lupus erythematosus
- Hair becomes brittle and falls out in patches in discoid and systemic lupus.
- Broken hairs commonly appear above the forehead.
- Characteristic findings in both types of lupus include raised, red, scaling plaques with follicular plugging, telangiectasia, central atrophy, and facial plaques in a butterfly-shaped pattern.
- Rash may vary in severity from malar erythema to discoid lesions in systemic lupus.
- Systemic lupus affects multiple body systems and may produce photosensitivity, weight loss, fatigue, lymphadenopathy, arthritis, and emotional lability.

Myotonic dystrophy
- Premature baldness occurs in the adult form.
- Myotonia, the inability to relax a muscle after its contraction, is a primary sign.
- Other signs include muscle wasting and cataracts.

Sarcoidosis
- If sarcoidosis infiltrates the scalp, scarring alopecia occurs.
- Accompanying findings include fever, weight loss, fatigue, lymphadenopathy, substernal pain, cough, shortness of breath, muscle weakness, arthralgia, myalgia, cranial nerve palsies, and various lesions of the face and the oral and nasal mucosa.

Seborrheic dermatitis
- Hair loss on the scalp may occur, beginning at the vertex and frontal areas.
- Pruritus occurs along with reddened, dry skin with branlike scales that flake off easily.

Skin cancer, metastasized
- Scarring alopecia may develop slowly along with scalp induration and atrophy.
- Related findings include weight loss, fever, altered bowel habits, abdominal pain, and lymphadenopathy.

Thyrotoxicosis
- Diffuse hair loss occurs.
- Hair loss may be accentuated at the temples.
- Hair becomes fine, soft, and friable.
- Skin is uniformly flushed and thickened, marked by red, raised, pruritic patches.
- Other signs and symptoms include fine tremors, nervousness, an enlarged thyroid gland, sweating, heat intolerance, amenorrhea, palpitations, weight loss despite increased appetite, diarrhea, and exophthalmos.

OTHER
Drugs
- Chemotherapeutic drugs may cause patchy, reversible alopecia.
- Other drugs that may cause diffuse hair loss include allopurinol, antithyroid drugs, beta blockers, carbamazepine, colchicine, excessive doses of vitamin A, gentamicin, heparin, hormonal contraceptives, indomethacin, lithium, trimethadione, valproic acid, and warfarin.

Protein deficiency
- Hair becomes brittle, fine, dry, and thin, possibly with pigment changes.
- Characteristic muscle wasting may be accompanied by edema, hepatomegaly, apathy, irritability, anorexia, diarrhea, and dry and flaky skin.

Radiation therapy
- Radiation therapy produces reversible hair loss a few weeks after exposure.

NURSING CONSIDERATIONS
- A skin biopsy may be performed to determine the cause of alopecia.
- Microscopic examination of a plucked hair may aid diagnosis.
- For patients with partial baldness or alopecia areata, topical application of minoxidil (Rogaine) for several months stimulates localized hair growth.

PEDIATRIC POINTERS
- Alopecia normally occurs during the first 6 months of life.
- If the infant is always placed in the same position resulting in bald areas, advise parents to change the infant's position regularly.
- Common causes include use of chemotherapy or radiation therapy, seborrheic dermatitis, alopecia mucinosa, tinea capitis, hypopituitarism, trichotillomania, progeria, and congenital hair shaft defects.

PATIENT TEACHING
- Discuss the underlying condition.
- Explain to the patient that hair loss resulting from chemotherapy is reversible.
- Teach the patient to use gentle hair care.
- Tell the patient about head wear and hairpieces.
- Explain the importance of head protection (sunblock, hat).

Amenorrhea

- Amenorrhea: absence of menstrual flow
- Primary amenorrhea: fails to begin before age 16
- Secondary amenorrhea: begins at appropriate age but later ceases for 3 or more months in the absence of physiologic causes
- Pathologic amenorrhea: anovulation or physical obstruction to menstrual flow (see *How amenorrhea develops*)
- Anovulation: may result from hormonal imbalance, debilitating disease, stress or emotional disturbances, strenuous exercise, malnutrition, obesity, drug or hormonal treatments, or anatomic abnormalities

HISTORY

- Ask about frequency and duration of the patient's previous menses.
- Obtain the date of her last menses.
- Determine the onset and nature of menstrual pattern changes.
- Ask about related signs (breast swelling or weight changes).
- Obtain a medical history, including illnesses, use of hormonal contraceptives, exercise and eating habits, emotional state, weight changes, and stress levels.
- Obtain family medical and menstrual history.

PHYSICAL ASSESSMENT

- Observe for secondary sex characteristics and signs of virilization.
- If performing a pelvic examination, check for anatomic aberrations of the outflow tract.

CAUSES

MEDICAL
Adrenal tumor
- Amenorrhea may be accompanied by acne, thinning scalp hair, hirsutism, increased blood pressure, truncal obesity, and psychotic changes.
- Asymmetrical ovarian enlargement and rapid onset of signs of virilizing are key findings.

Adrenocortical hyperplasia
- Amenorrhea precedes characteristic cushingoid signs, such as truncal obesity, moon face, "buffalo hump," bruises, purple striae, hypertension,

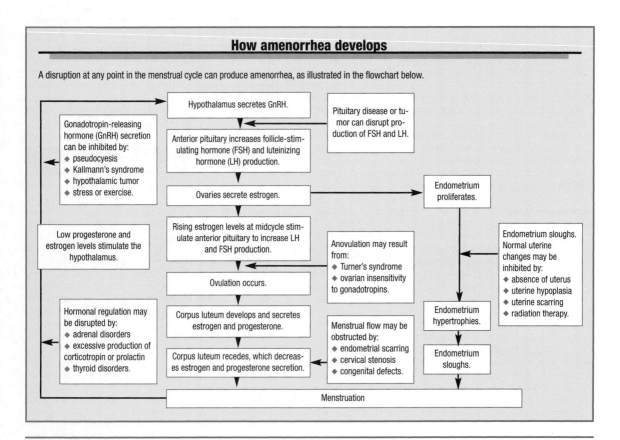

How amenorrhea develops

A disruption at any point in the menstrual cycle can produce amenorrhea, as illustrated in the flowchart below.

Hypothalamus secretes GnRH.

Gonadotropin-releasing hormone (GnRH) secretion can be inhibited by:
- pseudocyesis
- Kallmann's syndrome
- hypothalamic tumor
- stress or exercise.

Pituitary disease or tumor can disrupt production of FSH and LH.

Anterior pituitary increases follicle-stimulating hormone (FSH) and luteinizing hormone (LH) production.

Ovaries secrete estrogen.

Endometrium proliferates.

Low progesterone and estrogen levels stimulate the hypothalamus.

Rising estrogen levels at midcycle stimulate anterior pituitary to increase LH and FSH production.

Anovulation may result from:
- Turner's syndrome
- ovarian insensitivity to gonadotropins.

Endometrium sloughs. Normal uterine changes may be inhibited by:
- absence of uterus
- uterine hypoplasia
- uterine scarring
- radiation therapy.

Ovulation occurs.

Hormonal regulation may be disrupted by:
- adrenal disorders
- excessive production of corticotropin or prolactin
- thyroid disorders.

Corpus luteum develops and secretes estrogen and progesterone.

Menstrual flow may be obstructed by:
- endometrial scarring
- cervical stenosis
- congenital defects.

Endometrium hypertrophies.

Corpus luteum recedes, which decreases estrogen and progesterone secretion.

Endometrium sloughs.

Menstruation

renal calculi, psychiatric disturbances, and widened pulse pressure.
◆ Thinning scalp hair and hirsutism typically appear.

Adrenocortical hypofunction
◆ Amenorrhea, fatigue, irritability, weight loss, increased pigmentation, nausea, vomiting, and orthostatic hypotension may result.

Anorexia nervosa
◆ Primary or secondary amenorrhea may occur.
◆ Other signs and symptoms include weight loss, emaciated appearance, dry skin, compulsive behavior patterns, blotchy or sallow complexion, constipation, reduced libido, decreased pleasure in once-enjoyable activities, loss of scalp hair, lanugo (downy hair) on the face and arms, skeletal muscle atrophy, and sleep disturbances.

Congenital absence of ovaries and uterus
◆ Primary amenorrhea and absence of secondary sex characteristics occur.

Corpus luteum cysts
◆ Sudden amenorrhea may occur.
◆ Abdominal pain and breast swelling may also occur.

Hypothyroidism
◆ Amenorrhea may be primary or secondary.
◆ Early signs and symptoms include fatigue, forgetfulness, cold intolerance, weight gain, and constipation.
◆ Subsequent signs and symptoms include dry, flaky, inelastic skin; puffy face, hands, and feet; hoarseness; dry, sparse hair; thick, brittle nails; slow mental function; bradycardia; and myalgia.
◆ Other common signs and symptoms include anorexia, abdominal distention, decreased libido, ataxia, intention tremor, nystagmus, and delayed reflex relaxation time.

Pituitary infarction
◆ The postpartum patient fails to lactate and resume menses.

◆ Other signs and symptoms include headaches, visual field defects, oculomotor palsies, loss of pubic and axillary hair, and an altered level of consciousness.

Pituitary tumor
◆ Amenorrhea may be the first sign.
◆ Other findings include headache, vision disturbances, cushingoid signs, and acromegaly.

Polycystic ovarian syndrome
◆ Irregular menstrual cycles, oligomenorrhea, and secondary amenorrhea or periods of profuse bleeding may alternate with periods of amenorrhea.
◆ Other signs and symptoms include obesity, hirsutism, slight deepening of the voice, and enlarged ovaries.

Pseudoamenorrhea
◆ An anatomic anomaly obstructs menstrual flow, causing primary amenorrhea.
◆ Examination may reveal a bulging pink or blue hymen.

Testicular feminization
◆ Primary amenorrhea may indicate this form of male pseudohermaphroditism.
◆ The patient is outwardly female but genetically male, with breast and external genital development but scant or absent pubic hair.

Thyrotoxicosis
◆ Overproduction of thyroid hormone may result in amenorrhea.
◆ Classic signs and symptoms include an enlarged thyroid gland, nervousness, heat intolerance, diaphoresis, tremors, palpitations, tachycardia, dyspnea, weakness, and weight loss despite increased appetite.

Turner's syndrome
◆ Primary amenorrhea and failure to develop secondary sex characteristics may signal this syndrome.
◆ Typical features include short stature, webbing of the neck, low nuchal hairline, a broad chest with widely spaced nipples, poor breast

development, underdeveloped genitals, and edema of the legs and feet.

OTHER
Drugs
◆ Busulfan (Myleran), chlorambucil (Leukeran), injectable or implanted contraceptives, cyclophosphamide (Cytoxan), and phenothiazines may cause amenorrhea.
◆ Hormonal contraceptives may cause anovulation and amenorrhea when stopped.

Radiation therapy
◆ Irradiation of the abdomen may damage the endometrium or ovaries, causing amenorrhea.

Surgery
◆ Surgical removal of the ovaries or uterus produces amenorrhea.

NURSING CONSIDERATIONS

◆ In patients with secondary amenorrhea, rule out pregnancy before starting diagnostic testing.
◆ Provide emotional support as amenorrhea can cause severe emotional distress.

PEDIATRIC POINTERS
◆ Adolescent girls are prone to amenorrhea caused by emotional upsets stemming from school, social, or family problems.

GERIATRIC POINTERS
◆ In women older than age 50, amenorrhea usually represents the onset of menopause.

PATIENT TEACHING

◆ Explain treatment and expected outcomes.
◆ Encourage the patient to discuss her fears.
◆ Refer the patient for psychological counseling, if needed.

Amnesia

OVERVIEW

- A disturbance in or loss of memory
- Depending on the cause, may arise suddenly or slowly and may be temporary or permanent
- May be classified as partial or complete and as anterograde or retrograde
- Anterograde amnesia: memory loss for events that occurred after the onset of the causative trauma or disease
- Retrograde amnesia: memory loss for events that occurred before the onset of the causative trauma or disease
- Organic (or true) amnesia: results from temporal lobe dysfunction and characteristically spares patches of memory; common in patients with seizures or head trauma and can be an early indicator of Alzheimer's disease
- Hysterical amnesia: has a psychogenic origin and characteristically causes complete memory loss
- Treatment-induced amnesia: usually transient

HISTORY

- Gather information from the patient's family or friends.
- Ask when the amnesia first appeared and what types of things the patient is unable to remember.
- Ask if he can learn new information and how long he remembers it.
- Ask if amnesia encompasses a recent or a remote period.

PHYSICAL ASSESSMENT

- Take the patient's vital signs and assess his level of consciousness (LOC).
- Notice the patient's general appearance, behavior, mood, and train of thought.
- Test the patient's recent memory by asking him to identify and repeat three items. Retest him after 3 minutes.
- Test his intermediate memory by asking, "Who was the president before this one?" and "What was the last type of car you bought?"
- Test his remote memory with such questions as "How old are you?" and "Where were you born?"
- Check his pupils; they should be equal in size and should constrict quickly when exposed to direct light.
- Assess extraocular movements.
- Test motor function by having the patient move his arms and legs through their range of motion. Compare to the opposite limb.
- Evaluate sensory function with pinpricks on the patient's skin.

CAUSES

MEDICAL

Alzheimer's disease

- Alzheimer's disease usually begins with retrograde amnesia, which progresses slowly over many months or years to include anterograde amnesia and, eventually, severe and permanent memory loss.
- Other signs and symptoms include agitation, inability to concentrate, disregard for personal hygiene, confusion, irritability, and emotional lability.
- Later signs and symptoms include aphasia, dementia, incontinence, and muscle rigidity.

Cerebral hypoxia

- After recovery from hypoxia (brought on by such conditions as carbon monoxide poisoning or acute respiratory failure), total amnesia may occur.

- Sensory disturbances, such as numbness and tingling, may also occur.

Head trauma

- Amnesia may last for minutes, hours, or longer depending on the trauma's severity.
- Brief retrograde and longer anterograde amnesia as well as persistent amnesia about the traumatic event occur.
- Severe head trauma can cause permanent amnesia or difficulty retaining recent memories.
- Other signs and symptoms may include altered respirations and LOC; headache; dizziness; confusion; visual disturbances, such as blurred or double vision; and motor and sensory disturbances, such as hemiparesis and paresthesia, on the side of the body opposite the injury.

Herpes simplex encephalitis

- Recovery from herpes simplex encephalitis commonly leaves the patient with severe and possibly permanent amnesia.
- Other signs and symptoms include those of meningeal irritation, such as headache, fever, and altered LOC; seizures; and various motor and sensory disturbances, such as paresis, numbness, and tingling.

Hysteria

- Hysterical amnesia, a complete and long-lasting memory loss, begins and ends abruptly and is typically accompanied by confusion.

Seizures

- In temporal lobe seizures, amnesia occurs suddenly and lasts for several seconds to minutes. The patient may recall an aura or nothing at all.
- An irritable focus on the left side of the brain primarily causes amnesia for verbal memories, whereas an irritable focus on the right side of the brain causes graphic and nonverbal amnesia.
- Other signs and symptoms may include decreased LOC during the seizure, confusion, abnormal mouth

movements, and visual, olfactory, and auditory hallucinations.

Vertebrobasilar circulatory disorders
- Vertebrobasilar ischemia, infarction, embolus, or hemorrhage may cause complete amnesia that begins abruptly, lasts for several hours, and ends abruptly.
- Other signs and symptoms include dizziness, decreased LOC, ataxia, blurred or double vision, vertigo, nausea, and vomiting.

Wernicke-Korsakoff syndrome
- Retrograde and anterograde amnesia can become permanent without treatment of this thiamine (vitamin B_1) deficiency.
- Accompanying signs and symptoms include apathy, an inability to concentrate or to put events into sequence, and confabulation to fill memory gaps.
- Other signs and symptoms include diplopia, decreased LOC, headache, ataxia, and symptoms of peripheral neuropathy, such as numbness and tingling.

OTHER
Drugs
- Anterograde amnesia can be precipitated by general anesthetics, especially fentanyl, halothane, and isoflurane; barbiturates, most commonly pentobarbital; and certain benzodiazepines, especially triazolam.

Electroconvulsive therapy
- Sudden onset of retrograde or anterograde amnesia occurs with electroconvulsive therapy
- The amnesia lasts for several minutes to several hours.
- Severe, prolonged amnesia occurs with treatments given frequently over a prolonged period.

Temporal lobe surgery
- Usually performed on only one lobe, temporal lobe surgery causes brief, mild amnesia.
- Removal of both lobes results in permanent amnesia.

NURSING CONSIDERATIONS

- Prepare the patient for diagnostic tests, such as computed tomography scan, magnetic resonance imaging, EEG, or cerebral angiography.
- Provide reality orientation for the patient with retrograde amnesia, and encourage his family to help by supplying familiar photos, objects, and music.
- If the patient has severe amnesia, consider his basic needs, such as safety, elimination, and nutrition. If necessary, arrange for placement in an extended-care facility.

PEDIATRIC POINTERS
- A child who suffers from amnesia during seizures may be mistakenly labeled as "learning disabled."
- To prevent this mislabeling, stress the importance of adhering to the prescribed medication regimen, and discuss ways that the child, his parents, and his teachers can cope with amnesia.

PATIENT TEACHING

- Teach patient and family members about diagnostic tests and what to expect during the hospital stay.
- Adjust your patient-teaching techniques for the patient with anterograde amnesia because he can't acquire new information.
- Include his family in teaching sessions.
- Write down all instructions—particularly medication dosages and schedules—so the patient won't have to rely on his memory.

Analgesia

- No sensitivity to pain
- Important sign of central nervous system disease, often indicating a specific type and location of spinal cord lesion
- Occurs with loss of temperature sensation (thermoanesthesia) as sensory nerve impulses travel together in spinal cord
- May also occur with other sensory deficits—such as paresthesia, loss of proprioception and vibratory sense, and tactile anesthesia—in various disorders involving peripheral nerves, spinal cord, and brain
- Incomplete lesion of the spinal cord, if accompanied by thermoanesthesia only
- Classified as partial or total below the level of the lesion and as unilateral or bilateral, depending on the cause and level of the lesion
- Onset slow and progressive with tumor or abrupt with trauma
- May be transient and may resolve spontaneously

ACTION STAT! *Suspect spinal cord injury if the patient complains of analgesia over a large body area, accompanied by paralysis. Immobilize his spine in proper alignment, using a cervical collar and a long backboard, if possible. If a collar or backboard isn't available, place the patient in a supine position on a flat surface and place sandbags around his head, neck, and torso. Use correct technique and extreme caution when moving him to avoid worsening the spinal injury. Continuously monitor respiratory rate and rhythm, and watch for accessory muscle use because a complete lesion above the T6 level may cause diaphragmatic and intercostal muscle paralysis. Have an artificial airway and a handheld resuscitation bag available, and be prepared to start emergency resuscitation measures in case of respiratory failure.*

HISTORY

- Ask about the onset of analgesia (sudden or gradual).
- Ask if the patient had recent trauma, such as a fall, a sports injury, or an automobile accident.
- Obtain a complete medical history, noting especially any incidence of cancer in the patient or his family.

PHYSICAL ASSESSMENT

- Take vital signs and assess level of consciousness.
- Test pupillary, corneal, cough, and gag reflexes to rule out brain stem and cranial nerve involvement.
- If the patient is conscious, evaluate his speech and ability to swallow.
- If possible, observe the patient's gait and posture and assess his balance and coordination.
- Evaluate muscle tone and strength in all extremities.
- Test for other sensory deficits over all dermatomes (individual skin segments innervated by a specific spinal nerve) by applying light tactile stimulation with a tongue depressor or cotton swab.
- Perform a more thorough check of pain sensitivity, if necessary, using a pin. (See *Testing for analgesia*.)
- In each arm and leg, test vibration sense (using a tuning fork), proprioception, and superficial and deep tendon reflexes (DTRs).
- Check for increased muscle tone by extending and flexing the patient's elbows and knees as he tries to relax.

CAUSES

MEDICAL
Anterior cord syndrome
- Analgesia and thermoanesthesia occur bilaterally below the level of the lesion along with flaccid paralysis and hypoactive DTRs.

Central cord syndrome
- Analgesia and thermoanesthesia typically occur bilaterally in several dermatomes and may extend in a cape-like fashion over the arms, back, and shoulders.
- Weakness in the hands progresses to weakness and muscle spasms in the arms and shoulder girdle.
- Hyperactive DTRs and spastic weakness of the legs may develop.
- If the lesion affects the lumbar spine, hypoactive DTRs and flaccid weakness may persist in the legs.
- With brain stem involvement, additional signs and symptoms include facial analgesia and thermoanesthesia, vertigo, nystagmus, atrophy of the tongue, dysarthria, anhidrosis, dysphagia, urine retention, decreased intestinal motility, and hyperkeratosis.

Spinal cord hemisection
- Contralateral analgesia and thermoanesthesia occur below the level of the lesion.
- Loss of proprioception, spastic paralysis, and hyperactive DTRs develop ipsilaterally.
- Other signs and symptoms include urine retention with overflow incontinence.

OTHER
Drugs
- Analgesia may occur with use of a topical or local anesthetic, although numbness and tingling are more common.

NURSING CONSIDERATIONS

- Prepare the patient for spinal X-rays, and maintain spinal alignment and stability during transport to the laboratory.
- Focus your care on preventing further injury to the patient because analgesia can mask injury or developing complications.
- Prevent formation of pressure ulcers through meticulous skin care, gentle massage, use of lamb's wool pads, and frequent repositioning, especial-

ly when significant motor deficits hamper the patient's movement.

♦ Guard against scalding by testing the patient's bathwater temperature before he bathes.

♦ Provide psychological support. Help the patient and family understand and cope with diagnosis, potential disabilities, and lifestyle changes.

PEDIATRIC POINTERS

♦ Because a child may have difficulty describing analgesia, observe him carefully during the assessment for nonverbal clues to pain, such as facial expressions, crying, and retraction from stimuli.

♦ Remember that pain thresholds are high in infants, so your assessment findings may not be reliable.

♦ Test bathwater carefully for a child who is too young to test it himself.

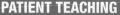

♦ Teach the patient about diagnostic tests and hospital procedures.

♦ Teach the patient about safety precautions to avoid injury to the area of his body affected by analgesia.

♦ Advise the patient to test bath water at home using a thermometer or a body part with intact sensation.

♦ Emphasize the importance of good skin care and frequent position changes to prevent pressure ulcers.

TOP TECHNIQUE

Testing for analgesia

By carefully and systematically testing the patient's sensitivity to pain, you can determine whether his nerve damage has a segmental or peripheral distribution and help locate the causative lesion.

Tell the patient to relax, and explain that you're going to lightly touch areas of his skin with a small pin. Have him close his eyes. Apply the pin firmly enough to produce pain without breaking the skin. (Practice on yourself first to learn how to apply the correct pressure.)

Starting with the patient's head and face, move down his body, pricking his skin on alternating sides. Have the patient report when he feels pain. Use the blunt end of the pin occasionally, and vary your test pattern to gauge the accuracy of his response.

Document your findings thoroughly, clearly marking areas of lost pain sensation either on a dermatome chart (shown at left) or on appropriate peripheral nerve diagrams (shown below).

DERMATONE CHART

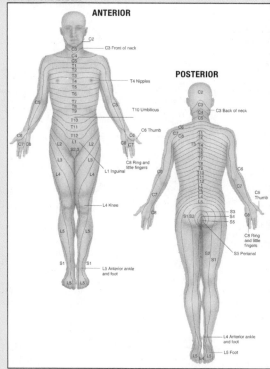

PERIPHERAL NERVES

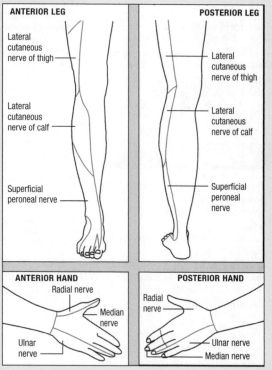

Anhidrosis

- Abnormal deficiency of sweat
- Results from neurologic and skin disorders; congenital abnormalities of sweat glands; atrophic or traumatic changes to sweat glands; and the use of certain drugs
- Classified as generalized (complete) or localized (partial)
- Generalized anhidrosis: can lead to life-threatening impairment of thermoregulation
- Anhidrosis can occur at skin surface, even if neurologic stimulation is normal (see *Eccrine dysfunction in anhidrosis*)

ACTION STAT! *If anhidrosis is suspected in a patient with hot, flushed skin, nausea, dizziness, palpitations, and substernal tightness, quickly take a rectal temperature and other vital signs and assess level of consciousness (LOC). If the rectal temperature is higher than 102.2° F (39° C) and is accompanied by tachycardia, tachypnea, altered blood pressure, and decreased LOC, suspect life-threatening anhidrotic asthenia (heatstroke). Start rapid cooling measures and give I.V. fluid replacement. Frequently check vital signs, hemodynamic status, and neurologic status until the patient's temperature drops below 102° F (38.9° C). Then place him in an air-conditioned room.*

HISTORY

- Obtain a description of previous sweating.
- Determine when onset of anhidrosis occurred.
- Question the patient about recent exposure to heat.
- Obtain a medical history, including neurologic, skin, and autoimmune disorders and systemic diseases.
- Obtain a drug history.

PHYSICAL ASSESSMENT

- Perform a neurologic assessment to detect a disorder of the central or peripheral nervous system as a cause of anhidrosis.
- Inspect skin color, texture, and turgor.
- Document appearance of skin lesions.

CAUSES

MEDICAL
Anhidrotic asthenia (heatstroke)
- A life-threatening condition, generalized anhidrosis occurs with hot, flushed skin; tachycardia; tachypnea; confusion; and seizure or loss of consciousness.
- In early stages, rectal temperature may exceed 102.2° F.
- Other signs and symptoms include severe headache and muscle cramps, which later disappear; fatigue; nausea and vomiting; dizziness; palpitations; substernal tightness; and elevated blood pressure followed by hypotension.

Burns
- Burns destroy eccrine glands, causing permanent anhidrosis in affected areas.
- Blistering, edema, and pain or loss of sensation may also occur.

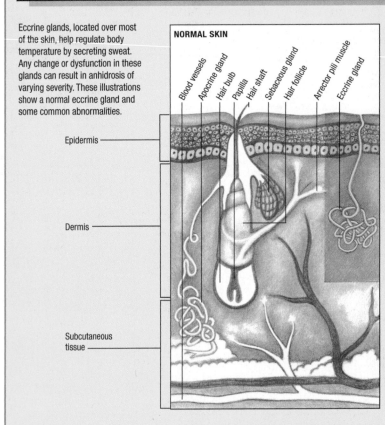

Eccrine dysfunction in anhidrosis

Eccrine glands, located over most of the skin, help regulate body temperature by secreting sweat. Any change or dysfunction in these glands can result in anhidrosis of varying severity. These illustrations show a normal eccrine gland and some common abnormalities.

NORMAL SKIN

Blood vessels · Apocrine gland · Hair bulb · Papilla · Hair shaft · Sebaceous gland · Hair follicle · Arrector pili muscle · Eccrine gland

Epidermis

Dermis

Subcutaneous tissue

Miliaria crystallina

◆ Anhidrosis and clear, tiny, fragile blisters develop under the arms and breasts.
◆ Typically occurs in a neonate and can be widespread on the body.

Miliaria profunda

◆ Localized anhidrosis occurs with compensatory facial hyperhidrosis.
◆ Whitish papules appear mostly on the trunk.
◆ If severe and extensive, miliaria profunda can progress to life-threatening anhidrotic asthenia.
◆ Other signs and symptoms include inguinal and axillary lymphadenopathy, weakness, shortness of breath, palpitations, and fever.

Miliaria rubra (prickly heat)

◆ Anhidrosis is localized.
◆ Small, erythematous papules with centrally placed blisters appear on trunk and neck.
◆ Related symptoms include paroxysmal itching and paresthesia.

Nervous system disorders

◆ Cerebral cortex and brain stem lesions may cause anhidrotic palms and soles.
◆ Peripheral neuropathy causes anhidrosis over the legs with compensatory hyperhidrosis over the head and neck.

Shy-Drager syndrome

◆ This degenerative neurologic syndrome causes ascending anhidrosis in the legs.

◆ Other signs and symptoms include severe orthostatic hypotension, loss of leg hair, decreased salivation and tearing, mydriasis, and, eventually, focal neurologic signs, such as leg tremors, incoordination, and muscle wasting.

Spinal cord lesions

◆ Anhidrosis may occur symmetrically below the level of the lesion.
◆ Compensatory hyperhidrosis occurs in adjacent areas.

OTHER
Drugs

◆ Anticholinergics, such as atropine and scopolamine, can cause generalized anhidrosis.

NURSING CONSIDERATIONS

◆ Prepare patient for tests to evaluate sweat patterns.
◆ Apply a topical agent to detect sweat on the skin, and give a systemic cholinergic to stimulate sweating, as ordered.

PEDIATRIC POINTERS

◆ In infants, common causes of anhidrosis include miliaria rubra and congenital skin disorders.
◆ Because slow development of the thermoregulatory center makes an infant, especially a premature one, anhidrotic for several weeks after birth, caution parents against overdressing their infant.

PATIENT TEACHING

◆ Advise about ways to stay cool, such as maintaining a cool environment, moving slowly during warm weather, and avoiding strenuous exercise and hot foods.
◆ Discuss with the patient the anhidrotic effects of drugs he's receiving.

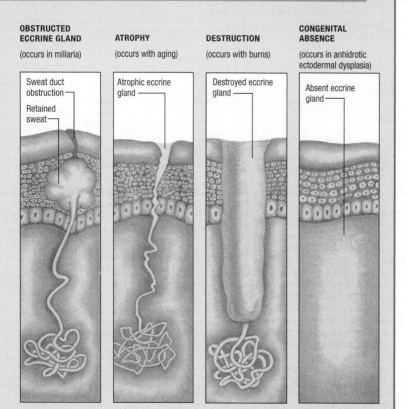

OBSTRUCTED ECCRINE GLAND
(occurs in miliaria)

Sweat duct obstruction
Retained sweat

ATROPHY
(occurs with aging)

Atrophic eccrine gland

DESTRUCTION
(occurs with burns)

Destroyed eccrine gland

CONGENITAL ABSENCE
(occurs in anhidrotic ectodermal dysplasia)

Absent eccrine gland

Anorexia

OVERVIEW

- Lack of appetite in the presence of a physiologic need for food
- Appears as a common symptom of GI and endocrine disorders
- May indicate a severe psychological disturbance
- If chronic, leads to life-threatening malnutrition

HISTORY

- Ask about weight history.
- Explore dietary and exercise habits.
- Obtain a dental history.
- Obtain a medical history, including stomach or bowel disorders and changes in bowel habits.
- Ask about alcohol and drug use.
- Explore situational or psychological causes of appetite loss.

PHYSICAL ASSESSMENT

- Take the patient's vital signs and weigh the patient.

 TOP TECHNIQUE *Weigh the patient in the same clothing and at the same time of day.*
- Perform a complete physical examination. (See *Is your patient malnourished?*)

CAUSES

MEDICAL
Acquired immunodeficiency syndrome
- Infections and Kaposi's sarcoma in the GI and respiratory tracts may lead to anorexia.
- Other signs and symptoms include fatigue, afternoon fevers, night sweats, diarrhea, cough, bleeding, lymphadenopathy, oral thrush, gingivitis, and skin disorders.

Adrenocortical hypofunction
- Anorexia may begin slowly; weight loss is gradual.
- Other common signs and symptoms include nausea and vomiting, abdominal pain, diarrhea, weakness, fatigue, malaise, vitiligo, bronze-colored skin, and purple striae.

Alcoholism
- Chronic anorexia leads to malnutrition.

- Other signs and symptoms are signs of liver damage, paresthesia, tremors, hypertension, bruising, GI bleeding, and abdominal pain.

Anorexia nervosa
- Anorexia begins insidiously, leading to life-threatening malnutrition.
- Complicated food preparation and eating rituals and avid exercise are common.
- Other signs and symptoms include cachexia; constipation; amenorrhea; dry, blotchy or sallow skin; anhedonia; decreased libido; alopecia; sleep disturbances; and distorted self-image. (See *Diagnosing anorexia nervosa.*)

Appendicitis
- Anorexia follows abrupt epigastric pain, nausea, and vomiting.
- Pain localizes in right lower quadrant (McBurney's point) and abdominal rigidity, rebound tenderness, constipation (or diarrhea), slight fever, and tachycardia develop.

Cancer
- Anorexia occurs with weight loss, weakness, apathy, and cachexia.
- Other signs and symptoms include nausea, vomiting, oral lesions, and changes in bowel habits.

Chronic renal failure
- Chronic anorexia is common and insidious.
- Other systemic signs and symptoms include nausea, vomiting, mouth ulcers, ammonia breath odor, metallic taste, GI bleeding, constipation or diarrhea, drowsiness, confusion, tremors, pallor, dry and scaly skin, pruritus, alopecia, purpuric lesions, and edema.

Cirrhosis
- Anorexia occurs early and continues throughout disease course.
- Weakness, nausea, vomiting, constipation or diarrhea, and dull abdominal pain are early signs.
- Other signs and symptoms include lethargy, slurred speech, bleeding tendencies, ascites, severe pruritus,

 TOP TECHNIQUE

Is your patient malnourished?

When assessing a patient with anorexia, be sure to check for these common signs of malnutrition.

Hair. Dull, dry, thin, fine, straight, and easily plucked; areas of lighter or darker spots and hair loss
Face. Generalized swelling, dark areas on cheeks and under eyes, lumpy or flaky skin around the nose and mouth, enlarged parotid glands
Eyes. Dull appearance; dry and either pale or red membranes; triangular, shiny gray spots on conjunctivae; red and fissured eyelid corners; bloodshot ring around cornea
Lips. Red and swollen, especially at corners
Tongue. Swollen, purple, and raw-looking, with sores or abnormal papillae
Teeth. Missing, or emerging abnormally; visible cavities or dark spots; spongy, bleeding gums

Neck. Swollen thyroid gland
Skin. Dry, flaky, swollen, and dark, with lighter or darker spots, some resembling bruises; tight and drawn, with poor skin turgor
Nails. Spoon-shaped, brittle, and ridged
Musculoskeletal system. Muscle wasting, knock-knee or bowlegs, bumps on ribs, swollen joints, musculoskeletal hemorrhages
Cardiovascular system. Tachycardia, arrhythmias, elevated blood pressure
Abdomen. Enlarged liver and spleen
Reproductive system. Decreased libido, amenorrhea
Nervous system. Irritability, confusion, paresthesia in hands and feet, loss of proprioception, decreased ankle and knee reflexes

dry skin, hepatomegaly, fetor hepaticus (breath odor with hepatic disease), jaundice, edema, gynecomastia, and right-upper-quadrant pain.

Crohn's disease
◆ Anorexia causes marked weight loss.
◆ Acute inflammatory signs and symptoms mimic those of appendicitis.
◆ Other signs and symptoms may include diarrhea, abdominal pain, fever, abdominal mass, weakness, and perianal or vaginal fistulas.

Depression
◆ Anorexia reflects anhedonia in depressive syndrome.
◆ Other signs and symptoms include poor concentration, indecisiveness, delusions, menstrual irregularities, decreased libido, insomnia or hypersomnia, fatigue, mood swings, poor self-image, and social withdrawal.

Gastritis
◆ Onset of anorexia may be sudden.
◆ Postprandial epigastric distress, with nausea, vomiting (commonly hematemesis), fever, belching, hiccups, and malaise, may occur.

Hepatitis
◆ In viral hepatitis, anorexia begins in the preicteric phase, accompanied by fatigue, malaise, headache, arthralgia, myalgia, photophobia, nausea and vomiting, fever, hepatomegaly, and lymphadenopathy.
◆ Anorexia may continue through the icteric phase, along with weight loss, dark urine, clay-colored stools, jaundice, right-upper-quadrant pain, irritability, and severe pruritus.

Hypopituitarism
◆ Anorexia usually develops slowly.
◆ Other signs and symptoms include amenorrhea; decreased libido; lethargy; cold intolerance; pale, thin, and dry skin; dry, brittle hair; and decreased temperature, blood pressure, and pulse rate.

Hypothyroidism
◆ Anorexia is usually insidious.
◆ Vague early signs and symptoms include fatigue, forgetfulness, cold intolerance, unexplained weight gain, and constipation.
◆ Subsequent signs and symptoms include decreased mental stability; dry, flaky, and inelastic skin; edema of the face, hands, and feet; ptosis; hoarseness; thick, brittle nails; coarse, broken hair; and bradycardia.

Pernicious anemia
◆ Insidious anorexia may cause considerable weight loss.
◆ Weakness; sore, burning, and pale tongue; and numbness and tingling in the extremities are the classic triad of this disorder.
◆ Other signs and symptoms include alternating constipation and diarrhea, abdominal pain, nausea and vomiting, bleeding gums, ataxia, positive Babinski's and Romberg's signs, diplopia and blurred vision, irritability, headache, malaise, and fatigue.

OTHER
Drugs
◆ Anorexia may occur with digoxin toxicity.
◆ Amphetamines, chemotherapeutic agents, sympathomimetics, and some antibiotics may also cause anorexia.

Radiation therapy
◆ Radiation treatments may cause anorexia.

Total parenteral nutrition
◆ Maintenance of glucose levels by I.V. therapy may cause anorexia.

NURSING CONSIDERATIONS
◆ Promote protein and calorie intake by providing high-calorie snacks or frequent, small meals.
◆ Take a 24-hour diet history daily.
◆ Maintain strict calorie and nutrient counts for meals because the patient may exaggerate his intake.
◆ In severe malnutrition, provide supplemental nutrition.
◆ Encourage the family to provide favorite foods to stimulate appetite.
◆ Monitor the patient for infection.

PEDIATRIC POINTERS
◆ Anorexia occurs in many illnesses but usually resolves promptly.
◆ In preadolescent or adolescent patients, be alert for subtle signs of anorexia nervosa.

PATIENT TEACHING
◆ Explain the condition, stressing the importance of proper nutrition.
◆ Instruct the patient in performing oral hygiene before meals.
◆ Teach the patient useful techniques to help manage the disorder, including establishing a target weight and maintaining a record of his progress by keeping a weight log.
◆ Encourage him to seek psychological and nutritional counseling.

Diagnosing anorexia nervosa

A diagnosis pf anorexia nervosa is made when the patient meets the following criteria as determined by the *Diagnostic and Statistical Manual of Mental Disorders*, 4th Edition, Text Revision:
◆ refusal to maintain body weight over a minimal normal weight for age and height (for instance, weight loss leading to maintenance of body weight 15% below that expected); or failure to achieve expected weight gain during a growth period, leading to a body weight 15% below that expected
◆ intense fear of gaining weight or becoming fat, despite underweight status
◆ distorted perception of body weight, size, or shape (that is, the person claims to feel fat even when emaciated or believes that one body area is too fat even when it's obviously underweight)
◆ in women, absence of at least three consecutive menses when otherwise expected to occur.

Anosmia

OVERVIEW

- Absence of a sense of smell
- Results from nasal mucosa irritation or swelling that obstructs the olfactory area (temporary)
- Occurs if the olfactory neuroepithelium or part of the olfactory nerve is destroyed (permanent)
- May be accompanied by ageusia — the loss of the sense of taste (see *Understanding the sense of smell*)

HISTORY

- Ask about the onset and duration of anosmia.
- Determine the presence or history of any other signs and symptoms, such as nasal congestion, discharge or bleeding, postnasal drip, sore throat, loss of sense of taste or appetite, and facial or eye pain.
- Obtain a history of nasal disease, allergies, or head trauma.
- Question the patient about heavy smoking, use of nose drops or nasal spray, and cocaine use.

PHYSICAL ASSESSMENT

- Inspect and palpate the nasal area for obvious injury, inflammation, deformities, and septal deviation or perforation.
- Observe the contour and color of the nasal mucosa and the size and color of the turbinates.
- Assess for nasal obstruction and discharge.
- Palpate the sinus area for tenderness and contour.
- Test olfactory nerve function (cranial nerve I) by having the patient identify common odors.

CAUSES

MEDICAL

Anterior cerebral artery occlusion

- Permanent anosmia may follow vascular damage involving the olfactory nerve.
- Other signs and symptoms include contralateral weakness and numbness, confusion, and impaired motor and sensory functions.

Degenerative brain disease

- Anosmia may occur with Alzheimer's disease, Parkinson's disease, and other degenerative central nervous system disorders.
- Other signs and symptoms include dementia, tremor, rigidity, and gait disturbance.

Understanding the sense of smell

Our noses can distinguish the odors of thousands of chemicals, thanks to a highly developed complex of sensory cells. The olfactory epithelium contains olfactory receptor cells, along with olfactory glands and sustentacular cells, both of which secrete mucus to keep the epithelial surface moist. The mucus covering the olfactory cells probably traps airborne odorous molecules, which then fit into the appropriate receptors on the cell surface. In response to this stimulus, the receptor cell then transmits an impulse along the olfactory nerve (cranial nerve I) to the olfactory area of the cortex, where it's interpreted. Any disruption along this transmission pathway, or any obstruction of the epithelial surface due to dryness or congestion, can cause anosmia.

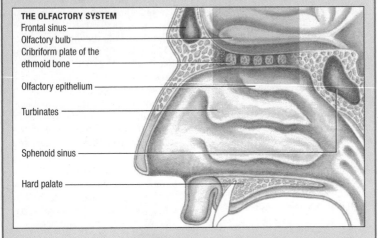

THE OLFACTORY SYSTEM
- Frontal sinus
- Olfactory bulb
- Cribriform plate of the ethmoid bone
- Olfactory epithelium
- Turbinates
- Sphenoid sinus
- Hard palate

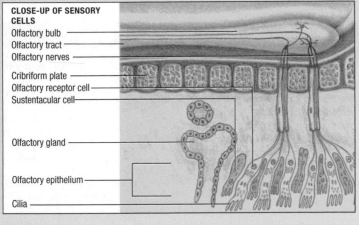

CLOSE-UP OF SENSORY CELLS
- Olfactory bulb
- Olfactory tract
- Olfactory nerves
- Cribriform plate
- Olfactory receptor cell
- Sustentacular cell
- Olfactory gland
- Olfactory epithelium
- Cilia

Head trauma

◆ Permanent anosmia may follow trauma that results in damage to the olfactory nerve.
◆ Other signs and symptoms include epistaxis, headache, nausea and vomiting, altered level of consciousness, blurred or double vision, "raccoon eyes," Battle's sign, and otorrhea.

Lead poisoning

◆ Anosmia may be permanent or temporary, depending on the extent of damage to the nasal mucosa.
◆ Other signs and symptoms include abdominal pain, weakness, headache, nausea, vomiting, constipation, wristdrop or footdrop, lead line on the gums, metallic taste, seizures, delirium, and coma.

Neoplasm (brain, nasal, or sinus)

◆ Anosmia may be permanent if a neoplasm destroys or displaces the olfactory nerve.
◆ Other signs and symptoms include unilateral or bilateral epistaxis, swelling and tenderness in the affected area, vision disturbances, decreased tearing, and elevated intracranial pressure.

Pernicious anemia

◆ May be temporary or permanent.
◆ Weakness; sore, burning, and pale tongue; and numbness and tingling in the extremities are the classic triad of this disorder.
◆ Other signs and symptoms include distortion of taste, pallor, headache, irritability, dizziness, nausea, vomiting, diarrhea, and shortness of breath.

Polyps (nasal)

◆ Temporary anosmia occurs when multiple polyps obstruct nasal cavities.
◆ Nasal obstruction may be accompanied by a sensation of fullness in the face, nasal discharge, headache, and shortness of breath.
◆ Examination reveals smooth, pale, grape-like polyp clusters.

Rhinitis

◆ Temporary anosmia occurs.
◆ In viral rhinitis, signs and symptoms include nasal congestion, sneezing, watery or purulent nasal discharge, dryness or tickling sensation in the nasopharynx, headache, low-grade fever, chills, and red, swollen nasal mucosa.
◆ In allergic rhinitis, signs and symptoms include nasal congestion, itching mucosa, thin nasal discharge, sneezing, tearing, and headache.
◆ In atrophic rhinitis, signs and symptoms include purulent, yellow-green, foul-smelling crusts on sclerotic mucous membranes; paradoxical nasal congestion in an airway that's more open than usual; thin, atrophic turbinates; and dry nasopharynx.
◆ In vasomotor rhinitis, signs and symptoms include chronic nasal congestion, watery nasal discharge, postnasal drip, sneezing, and pale nasal mucosa.

Septal fracture

◆ Anosmia is usually temporary, caused by airflow obstruction.
◆ Other signs and symptoms include septal deviation, swelling, epistaxis, hematoma, nasal congestion, and ecchymoses.

Septal hematoma

◆ Anosmia is temporary.
◆ Related signs and symptoms include epistaxis, headache, mouth breathing, and dusky red, inflamed nasal mucosa.

Sinusitis

◆ Anosmia is temporary.
◆ Other signs and symptoms include nasal congestion; sinus pain, tenderness, and swelling; severe headache; watery or purulent discharge; postnasal drip; inflamed throat and nasal mucosa; enlarged, purulent turbinates; malaise; low-grade fever; and chills.

OTHER

Drugs

◆ Anosmia may result from prolonged use of nasal decongestants, which produces rebound nasal congestion.
◆ Anosmia can also result from use of naphazoline, reserpine, amphetamines, phenothiazines, and estrogen.

Radiation therapy

◆ Radiation therapy may cause permanent anosmia.

Surgery

◆ Temporary anosmia may result from damage to the olfactory nerve or nasal mucosa during nasal or sinus surgery.
◆ Permanent anosmia accompanies a permanent tracheostomy, which disrupts nasal breathing.

NURSING CONSIDERATIONS

FOR ANOSMIA FROM NASAL CONGESTION

◆ Give a local decongestant or antihistamine.
◆ Provide a vaporizer or humidifier.
◆ Advise against excessive use of local decongestants.

FOR PERMANENT ANOSMIA

◆ Administer vitamin A orally or by injection, which may improve symptoms.

PEDIATRIC POINTERS

◆ Anosmia in children may result from nasal obstruction by a foreign body or enlarged adenoids.

PATIENT TEACHING

◆ Explain proper use of nose drops and sprays.
◆ If the patient is mouth breathing, give instruction on oral hygiene.

Anuria

OVERVIEW

- Urine output of less than 100 ml in 24 hours
- Indicates either urinary tract obstruction or acute renal failure (see *Major causes of acute renal failure*)
- Without immediate treatment, may rapidly cause uremia and other complications of urine retention

✳ ***ACTION STAT!*** *Determine if urine is forming. Prepare to catheterize the patient to relieve any lower urinary tract obstruction and to check for residual urine. If you collect more than 75 ml of urine, suspect lower urinary tract obstruction. If you collect less than 75 ml, suspect renal dysfunction or obstruction higher in the urinary tract.*

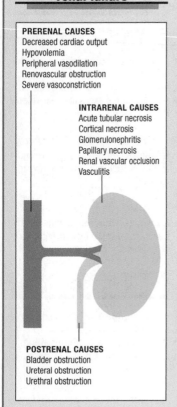

Major causes of acute renal failure

PRERENAL CAUSES
Decreased cardiac output
Hypovolemia
Peripheral vasodilation
Renovascular obstruction
Severe vasoconstriction

INTRARENAL CAUSES
Acute tubular necrosis
Cortical necrosis
Glomerulonephritis
Papillary necrosis
Renal vascular occlusion
Vasculitis

POSTRENAL CAUSES
Bladder obstruction
Ureteral obstruction
Urethral obstruction

HISTORY

- Ask about any changes in voiding pattern.
- Determine the amount of fluid normally ingested and amount ingested in last 24 to 48 hours.
- Note the time and amount of last urination.
- Ask about drug use.
- Obtain a medical history, noting previous renal or urinary tract disease, prostate problems, congenital abnormalities, and abdominal, renal, or urinary tract surgery.

PHYSICAL ASSESSMENT

- Inspect and palpate the abdomen for asymmetry, distention, or bulging.
- Inspect the flank area for edema or erythema.
- Percuss and palpate the bladder.
- Palpate the kidneys and percuss the costovertebral angle.
- Auscultate over the renal arteries for bruits. (See *Assessing for renal bruits*.)

CAUSES

MEDICAL
Acute tubular necrosis

- Anuria occurs occasionally; oliguria (diminished urine output) is more common.
- Oliguria precedes the onset of diuresis.
- Other findings reflect the underlying cause and may include signs and symptoms of hyperkalemia, uremia, and heart failure.

Glomerulonephritis, acute

- Anuria or oliguria occurs.
- Other signs and symptoms include mild fever, malaise, flank pain, gross hematuria, edema, elevated blood pressure, headache, nausea, vomiting, abdominal pain, crackles, and dyspnea.

Hemolytic-uremic syndrome

- Anuria occurs in the initial stages and lasts 1 to 10 days.
- Other signs and symptoms include vomiting, diarrhea, abdominal pain, hematemesis, melena, purpura, fever, elevated blood pressure, hepatomegaly, ecchymoses, edema, hematuria, pallor, and signs of upper respiratory tract infection.

TOP TECHNIQUE

Assessing for renal bruits

Use the bell of your stethoscope to auscultate for bruits at the sites shown in the photograph below.

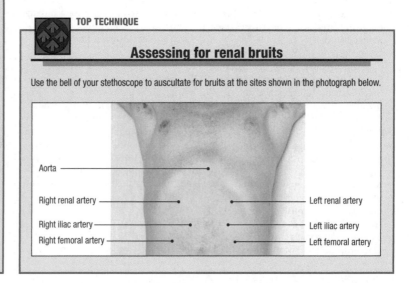

Aorta

Right renal artery — Left renal artery

Right iliac artery — Left iliac artery

Right femoral artery — Left femoral artery

Renal artery occlusion, bilateral
◆ Anuria or severe oliguria is accompanied by severe, continuous upper abdominal and flank pain; nausea and vomiting; decreased bowel sounds; fever; and diastolic hypertension.

Renal vein occlusion, bilateral
◆ Anuria sometimes develops with lower back pain, fever, flank tenderness, and hematuria.
◆ Development of pulmonary emboli, a common complication, produces sudden dyspnea, pleuritic pain, tachypnea, tachycardia, crackles, and, possibly, hemoptysis.

Urinary tract obstruction
◆ Acute or total anuria may alternate with or precede burning pain on urination, overflow incontinence or dribbling, urinary frequency and nocturia, voiding in small amounts, or altered urine stream.
◆ Other signs and symptoms include bladder distention, pain and a sensation of fullness in the lower abdomen and groin, upper abdominal and flank pain, nausea and vomiting, and signs of secondary infection.

OTHER
Diagnostic tests
◆ Contrast media can cause nephrotoxicity, producing oliguria and, rarely, anuria.

Drugs
◆ Nephrotoxic drugs that can cause anuria or oliguria include antibiotics (especially aminoglycosides), adrenergics, anesthetics, anticholinergics, ethyl alcohol, heavy metals, and organic solvents.

NURSING CONSIDERATIONS

◆ If catheterization fails to initiate urine flow, prepare the patient for diagnostic studies, such as ultrasonography, cystoscopy, retrograde pyelography, and renal scan to detect any obstruction higher in the urinary tract.
◆ If an obstruction is present, prepare the patient for surgery to remove the obstruction, and insert a nephrostomy tube or ureterostomy tube to drain the urine.
◆ Monitor vital signs and measure and record intake and output, saving urine for inspection.
◆ Restrict daily fluids to 600 ml more than the previous day's total urine output.
◆ Restrict foods and juices high in potassium and sodium.
◆ Have the patient maintain a balanced diet and control protein intake.
◆ Weigh the patient daily.

PEDIATRIC POINTERS
◆ In neonates, anuria is the absence of urine output for 24 hours.
◆ In children, anuria commonly results from loss of renal function.

GERIATRIC POINTERS
◆ Hospitalized or bedridden patients may be unable to generate pressure to void in a supine position.

PATIENT TEACHING

◆ Discuss fluids and foods the patient should avoid.
◆ Instruct the patient on nephrostomy tube or ureterostomy tube care, if needed.
◆ Discuss underlying condition and treatment plan.

Anxiety

- Nonspecific feeling of uneasiness or dread
- Mild anxiety: can cause slight physical or psychological discomfort
- Severe anxiety: can be incapacitating or even life-threatening

HISTORY

- Determine the patient's chief complaint.
- Ask about the duration of the anxiety.
- Determine precipitating or exacerbating factors.
- Obtain a medical history, including drug use.

PHYSICAL ASSESSMENT

- Perform a physical examination.
- Focus on complaints that trigger or are aggravated by anxiety.
- Assess level of consciousness (LOC) and observe behavior.

CAUSES

MEDICAL

Acute respiratory distress syndrome
- Acute anxiety occurs along with tachycardia, mental sluggishness and, in severe cases, hypotension.
- Respiratory symptoms include dyspnea, tachypnea, intercostal and suprasternal retractions, crackles, and rhonchi.

Anaphylactic shock
- Acute anxiety signals the onset of anaphylactic shock.
- Anxiety is accompanied by urticaria, angioedema, pruritus, and shortness of breath.
- Others signs and symptoms include light-headedness, hypotension, tachycardia, nasal congestion, sneezing, wheezing, dyspnea, barking cough, abdominal cramps, vomiting, diarrhea, and urinary urgency and incontinence.

Angina pectoris
- Acute anxiety may precede or follow an attack.
- Sharp, crushing substernal or anterior chest pain may radiate to the back, neck, arms, or jaw during an attack.

Asthma
- Acute anxiety occurs with dyspnea, wheezing, productive cough, accessory muscle use, hyperresonant lung fields, diminished breath sounds, coarse crackles, cyanosis, tachycardia, and diaphoresis.

Autonomic hyperreflexia
- Anxiety, severe headache, and dramatic hypertension may be early signs.
- Pallor and motor and sensory deficits occur below the level of the lesion.
- Flushing occurs above the level of the lesion.

Cardiogenic shock
- Acute anxiety is accompanied by cool, pale, clammy skin; tachycardia; weak, thready pulse; tachypnea; ventricular gallop; crackles; jugular vein distention; decreased urine output; hypotension; narrowing pulse pressure; and peripheral edema.

Chronic obstructive pulmonary disease
- Acute anxiety occurs with exertional dyspnea, cough, wheezing, crackles, hyperresonant lung fields, tachypnea, and accessory muscle use.
- Other signs include "barrel" chest, pursed-lip breathing, and finger clubbing (late in the disease).

Heart failure
- Acute anxiety is a symptom of inadequate oxygenation.
- Other signs and symptoms include restlessness, shortness of breath, tachypnea, decreased LOC, edema, crackles, ventricular gallop, hypotension, diaphoresis, and cyanosis.

Hyperthyroidism
- Acute anxiety may be an early sign.
- Classic signs and symptoms include heat intolerance, weight loss despite increased appetite, nervousness, tremor, palpitations, sweating, an enlarged thyroid gland, exophthalmos, and diarrhea.

Hyperventilation syndrome
- Anxiety, pallor, and circumoral and peripheral paresthesia occur.
- Other signs and symptoms include carpopedal spasms, chest pain, tachycardia, belching, flatus, and dizziness.

Hypochondriasis
- Mild to moderate chronic anxiety occurs.
- Patient is focused more on the belief that he has a specific serious disease than on the actual symptoms.
- Difficulty swallowing, back pain, light-headedness, and upset stomach are common complaints.

Hypoglycemia
- Mild to moderate anxiety occurs.
- Other signs and symptoms include dizziness, hunger, mild headache, palpitations, blurred vision, weakness, and diaphoresis.

Mitral valve prolapse
◆ Panic may occur.
◆ A hallmark sign of mitral valve prolapse is a midsystolic click, followed by an apical murmur.
◆ Paroxysmal palpitations with sharp, stabbing, or aching precordial pain may also occur.

Mood disorder
◆ Anxiety may be the chief complaint in the depressive or manic form.
◆ In the depressive form, the patient may exhibit dysphoria; anger; insomnia or hypersomnia; decreased libido, energy, and concentration; appetite disturbance; multiple somatic complaints; and suicidal thoughts.
◆ In the manic form, the patient may exhibit a reduced need for sleep, hyperactivity, increased energy, rapid or pressured speech and, in severe cases, paranoid ideas and other psychotic symptoms.

Myocardial infarction
◆ A life-threatening disorder, acute anxiety occurs with persistent, crushing substernal pain that may radiate.
◆ Accompanying signs and symptoms include shortness of breath, nausea, vomiting, diaphoresis, and cool, pale skin.

Obsessive-compulsive disorder
◆ Chronic anxiety occurs along with thoughts or impulses to perform ritualistic acts.
◆ Anxiety builds if the patient can't perform rituals and diminishes if he can.
◆ The patient recognizes the acts as irrational, but he can't control them.

Pheochromocytoma
◆ Acute, severe anxiety accompanies the main sign of persistent or paroxysmal hypertension due to this adrenal tumor.
◆ Common signs and symptoms include tachycardia, diaphoresis, orthostatic hypotension, tachypnea, flushing, severe headache, palpitations, nausea, vomiting, epigastric pain, and paresthesia.

Phobias
◆ Chronic anxiety occurs with persistent fear of an object, activity, or situation that results in a strong desire to avoid it.
◆ The patient recognizes the fear as irrational, but he can't suppress it.

Postconcussion syndrome
◆ Chronic anxiety or periodic attacks of acute anxiety may occur, especially in situations demanding attention, judgment, or comprehension.
◆ Other symptoms include irritability, insomnia, dizziness, and mild headache.

Posttraumatic stress disorder
◆ Chronic anxiety occurs with intrusive, vivid thoughts and memories of the traumatic event.
◆ The event is relived in dreams and nightmares.
◆ Related symptoms include insomnia, depression, and feelings of numbness and detachment.

Pulmonary edema
◆ Acute anxiety occurs along with dyspnea, orthopnea, cough with frothy sputum, tachycardia, tachypnea, crackles, ventricular gallop, hypotension, thready pulse, and cool, clammy skin.

Pulmonary embolism
◆ Hypoxia may result in acute anxiety and restlessness.
◆ Other signs and symptoms include dyspnea, tachypnea, chest pain, tachycardia, blood-tinged sputum, and low-grade fever.

Somatoform disorder
◆ Anxiety and multiple somatic complaints (that can't be explained) are severe enough to impair functioning.

OTHER
Drugs
◆ Many drugs cause anxiety, especially sympathomimetics and central nervous system stimulants.
◆ Antidepressants may cause paradoxical anxiety.

NURSING CONSIDERATIONS
◆ Provide a calm, quiet atmosphere.
◆ Stay with the patient during an acute attack.
◆ Encourage the patient to express his feelings and concerns freely.
◆ Encourage anxiety-reducing measures, such as distraction, relaxation techniques, or biofeedback.

PEDIATRIC POINTERS
◆ Anxiety usually results from painful physical illness or inadequate oxygenation.
◆ The autonomic signs of anxiety tend to be more common and dramatic in children than in adults.

GERIATRIC POINTERS
◆ Distractions from ritualistic activity may provoke anxiety or agitation.

PATIENT TEACHING
◆ Teach the patient about relaxation techniques and avoiding stressful situations.
◆ Encourage the patient's verbalization of anxiety.
◆ Help the patient to identify stressors.
◆ Help the patient better understand different coping mechanisms.
◆ Help the patient identify support systems, such as family and friends.

Aphasia (dysphasia)

OVERVIEW

- Impaired expression or comprehension of written or spoken language, caused by disease or injury to these centers of the brain (see *Where language originates*)
- May slightly impede communication or make it impossible
- May be classified as anomic, Broca's, global, or Wernicke's (see *Identifying types of aphasia*)
- Anomic aphasia: eventually resolves in more than half of patients
- Global aphasia: usually irreversible

ACTION STAT! *Look for signs and symptoms of increased intracranial pressure (ICP). If you detect increased ICP, administer mannitol I.V. to reduce cerebral edema, as ordered. Make sure emergency resuscitation equipment is on hand, and anticipate preparing the patient for emergency surgery.*

HISTORY

- Obtain a medical history, noting headaches, hypertension, seizure disorders, or drug use.
- Determine the patient's preaphasia ability to communicate and perform routine tasks.

PHYSICAL ASSESSMENT

- Perform a complete neurologic examination.
- Check for obvious signs of neurologic deficit.
- Take the patient's vital signs and assess his level of consciousness (LOC).
- Assess the patient's pupillary response, eye movements, and motor function.

CAUSES

MEDICAL

Alzheimer's disease
- Anomic aphasia may begin insidiously and then progress to severe global aphasia.
- Incontinence is a late symptom.
- Other signs and symptoms include behavioral changes, loss of memory, poor judgment, restlessness, myoclonus, and muscle rigidity.

Brain abscess
- Any type of aphasia may occur.
- Aphasia may be accompanied by hemiparesis, ataxia, facial weakness, and signs of increased ICP.

Brain tumor
- Any type of aphasia may occur.
- As the tumor enlarges, behavioral changes, memory loss, motor weakness, seizures, auditory hallucinations, visual field deficits, and increased ICP may occur.

Creutzfeldt-Jakob disease
- Aphasia with a rapidly progressive dementia occurs in this viral process.
- Other signs and symptoms may include myoclonic jerking, ataxia, vision disturbances, and paralysis.

Encephalitis
- Transient aphasia may occur.
- Early signs and symptoms include fever, headache, and vomiting.
- Other signs and symptoms include seizures, confusion, stupor or coma, hemiparesis, asymmetrical deep tendon reflexes, positive Babinski's reflex, ataxia, myoclonus, nystagmus, oculomotor palsies, and facial weakness.

Head trauma
- Sudden aphasia may occur.
- Aphasia may be transient or permanent, depending on the extent of brain damage.
- Other signs and symptoms include blurred or double vision; headache; pallor; diaphoresis; numbness and paresis; discharge, containing cere-

---

Where language originates

Aphasia reflects damage to one or more of the brain's primary language centers, which are usually located in the left hemisphere. Broca's area lies next to the region of the motor cortex that controls the muscles necessary for speech. Wernicke's area is the center of auditory, visual, and language comprehension. It lies between

Heschl's gyrus, the primary receiver of auditory stimuli, and the angular gyrus, which is between the brain's auditory and visual regions. Connecting Wernicke's and Broca's areas is a large nerve bundle, the arcuate fasciculus, that enables repetition of speech.

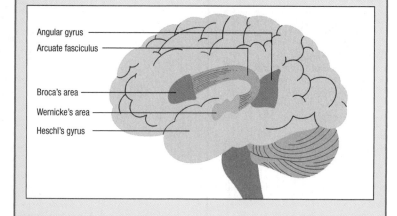

- Angular gyrus
- Arcuate fasciculus
- Broca's area
- Wernicke's area
- Heschl's gyrus

brospinal fluid from the ear or nose; altered respirations; tachycardia; behavioral changes; and increased ICP.

Seizure disorder
◆ Transient aphasia may occur if the seizures involve the language centers.

Stroke
◆ Wernicke's, Broca's, or global aphasia may occur.
◆ Other symptoms include decreased LOC, right-sided hemiparesis, homonymous hemianopsia, paresthesia, and loss of sensation.

Transient ischemic attack
◆ Sudden aphasia occurs, but resolves within 24 hours.
◆ Other symptoms include transient hemiparesis, hemianopsia, paresthesia, dizziness, and confusion.

NURSING CONSIDERATIONS

◆ Tell the patient what has happened, where he is and why, and what the date is.
◆ Expect periods of depression as the patient recognizes his disability.
◆ Help the patient communicate by providing a relaxed environment with minimal distracting stimuli.
◆ Refer to speech therapy as needed.

PEDIATRIC POINTERS
◆ Recognize that the term *childhood aphasia* is sometimes mistakenly applied to children who fail to develop normal language skills but who aren't considered mentally retarded or developmentally delayed. *Aphasia* refers solely to loss of previously developed communication skills.

◆ Brain damage associated with aphasia in children most commonly follows anoxia—the result of near drowning or airway obstruction.

GERIATRIC POINTERS
◆ Although a stroke can occur at any age or in either gender, patients are usually men older than age 65.
◆ When assessing speech in an elderly patient, make sure that his dentures and hearing aid are in place.

PATIENT TEACHING

◆ Discuss alternate means of communication.
◆ Discuss the risk reduction factors for stroke.
◆ Explain underlying condition, diagnostic tests, and treatment options.

Identifying types of aphasia

The location of the lesion as well as its accompanying signs and symptoms help to differentiate among the different types of aphasia.

TYPE	LOCATION OF LESION	SIGNS AND SYMPTOMS
Anomic aphasia	Temporal-parietal area; may extend to angular gyrus, but sometimes is poorly localized	Patient's understanding of written and spoken language is relatively unimpaired. His speech, although fluent, lacks meaningful content. Word-finding difficulty and circumlocution are characteristic. Rarely, the patient also displays paraphasias.
Broca's aphasia (expressive aphasia)	Broca's area; usually in third frontal convolution of left hemisphere	Patient's understanding of written and spoken language is relatively unimpaired, but speech is nonfluent, with evidence of word-finding difficulty, jargon, paraphasias, limited vocabulary, and simple sentence construction. He can't repeat words and phrases that are spoken to him. If Wernicke's area is intact, he recognizes speech errors, but shows frustration. He's commonly hemiparetic.
Global aphasia	Broca's area and Wernicke's area	Patient has profoundly impaired receptive and expressive ability. He can't repeat words or phrases that are spoken to him and can't follow directions. His occasional speech is marked by paraphasias or jargon.
Wernicke's aphasia (receptive aphasia)	Wernicke's area; usually in posterior or superior temporal lobe	Patient has difficulty understanding written and spoken language. He can't repeat words or phrases that are spoken to him and can't follow directions. His speech is fluent but may be rapid and rambling, with paraphasias. He has difficulty naming objects (anomia) and is unaware of speech errors.

Apnea

- Cessation of spontaneous respiration
- Occasionally temporary and self-limiting, as in Cheyne-Stokes and Biot's respirations
- In most cases, life-threatening emergency that requires immediate intervention to prevent death
- Usually results from one or more of six pathophysiologic mechanisms, each of which has numerous causes
- Most common causes: trauma, cardiac arrest, neurologic disease, aspiration of foreign objects, bronchospasm, and drug overdose (see *Causes of apnea*)

ACTION STAT! *If you detect apnea, first establish and maintain a patent airway. Place the patient in a supine position, and open his airway using the head-tilt, chin-lift technique. (Caution: If the patient has or may have a head or neck injury, use the jaw-thrust technique to prevent hyperextending the neck.) Next, quickly look, listen, and feel for spontaneous respiration; if it's absent, begin artificial ventilation until it occurs or until mechanical ventilation can be initiated.*

Because apnea may result from (or may cause) cardiac arrest, assess the patient's carotid pulse immediately after you've established a patent airway. Or, if the patient is an infant or small child, assess the brachial pulse instead. If you can't palpate a pulse, begin cardiac compression.

- Investigate the underlying cause of apnea. Ask him (or, if he's unable to answer, anyone who witnessed the episode) about the onset of apnea and events immediately preceding it.
- Take a patient history, especially noting reports of headache, chest pain, muscle weakness, sore throat, or dyspnea.
- Ask about a history of respiratory, cardiac, or neurologic disease.
- Ask about allergies and drug use.

- Inspect the head, face, neck, and trunk for soft-tissue injury, hemorrhage, or skeletal deformity.
- Don't overlook obvious clues, such as oral and nasal secretions (reflecting fluid-filled airways and alveoli) or facial soot and singed nasal hair (suggesting thermal injury to the tracheobronchial tree).
- Auscultate over all lung lobes for adventitious breath sounds, particularly crackles and rhonchi, and percuss the lung fields for increased dullness or hyperresonance.
- Auscultate the heart for murmurs, pericardial friction rub, and arrhythmias.
- Check for cyanosis, pallor, jugular vein distention, and edema.
- If appropriate, perform a neurologic assessment. Evaluate level of consciousness (LOC), orientation, and mental status; test cranial nerve and motor function, sensation, and reflexes in all extremities.

Causes of apnea

AIRWAY OBSTRUCTION

- Asthma
- Bronchospasm
- Chronic bronchitis
- Chronic obstructive pulmonary disease
- Foreign body aspiration
- Hemothorax or pneumothorax
- Mucus plug
- Obstruction by tongue or tumor
- Obstructive sleep apnea
- Secretion retention
- Tracheal or bronchial rupture

BRAIN STEM DYSFUNCTION

- Brain abscess
- Brain stem injury
- Brain tumor
- Central nervous system depressants
- Central sleep apnea
- Cerebral hemorrhage
- Cerebral infarction
- Encephalitis
- Head trauma
- Increased intracranial pressure
- Medullary or pontine hemorrhage or infarction
- Meningitis
- Transtentorial herniation

NEUROMUSCULAR FAILURE

- Amyotrophic lateral sclerosis
- Botulism
- Diphtheria
- Guillain-Barré syndrome
- Myasthenia gravis
- Phrenic nerve paralysis
- Rupture of the diaphragm
- Spinal cord injury

PARENCHYMATOUS DISEASE

- Acute respiratory distress syndrome
- Diffuse pneumonia
- Emphysema
- Near drowning
- Pulmonary edema
- Pulmonary fibrosis
- Secretion retention

PLEURAL PRESSURE GRADIENT DISRUPTION

- Flail chest
- Open chest wounds

PULMONARY CAPILLARY PERFUSION DECREASE

- Arrhythmias
- Cardiac arrest
- Myocardial infarction
- Pulmonary embolism
- Pulmonary hypertension
- Shock

MEDICAL
Airway obstruction
◆ Occlusion or compression of the trachea, central airways, or smaller airways can cause sudden apnea by blocking the patient's airflow.
◆ Acute respiratory failure may also occur.

Brain stem dysfunction
◆ Primary or secondary brain stem dysfunction can cause apnea by destroying the brain stem's ability to initiate respirations.
◆ Apnea may arise suddenly (as in trauma, hemorrhage, or infarction) or gradually (as in degenerative disease or tumor).
◆ Apnea may be preceded by decreased LOC and various motor and sensory deficits.

Neuromuscular failure
◆ Trauma or disease can disrupt the mechanics of respiration, causing sudden or gradual apnea.
◆ Associated symptoms include diaphragmatic or intercostal muscle paralysis from injury, or respiratory weakness or paralysis from acute or degenerative disease.

Parenchymatous lung disease
◆ An accumulation of fluid within the alveoli produces apnea by interfering with pulmonary gas exchange and producing acute respiratory failure.
◆ Apnea may arise suddenly, as in near drowning and acute pulmonary edema, or gradually, as in emphysema.
◆ Apnea may also be preceded by crackles and labored respirations with accessory muscle use.

Pleural pressure gradient disruption
◆ Conversion of normal negative pleural air pressure to positive pressure by chest wall injuries (such as flail chest) causes lung collapse, producing respiratory distress and, if untreated, apnea.
◆ Associated signs and symptoms include an asymmetrical chest wall and asymmetrical or paradoxical respirations.

Pulmonary capillary perfusion decrease
◆ Apnea can stem from obstructed pulmonary circulation, most commonly due to heart failure or lack of circulatory patency.
◆ It occurs suddenly in cardiac arrest, massive pulmonary embolism, and most cases of severe shock; and it occurs progressively in septic shock and pulmonary hypertension.
◆ Other signs and symptoms include hypotension, tachycardia, and edema.

Sleep-related apneas
◆ These repetitive apneas occur during sleep from airflow obstruction or brain stem dysfunction deficits.

OTHER
Drugs
◆ Central nervous system (CNS) depressants may cause hypoventilation and apnea.
◆ Benzodiazepines may cause respiratory depression and apnea when given I.V., along with other CNS depressants, to elderly or acutely ill patients.
◆ Neuromuscular blockers—such as curariform drugs and anticholinesterases—may produce sudden apnea due to respiratory muscle paralysis.

◆ Closely monitor the apneic patient's cardiac and respiratory status to prevent further apneic episodes.

PEDIATRIC POINTERS
◆ Premature neonates are especially susceptible to periodic apneic episodes because of CNS immaturity.
◆ Other common causes of apnea in infants include sepsis, intraventricular and subarachnoid hemorrhage, seizures, bronchiolitis, and sudden infant death syndrome.
◆ In toddlers and older children, the primary cause of apnea is acute airway obstruction from aspiration of foreign objects. Other causes include acute epiglottitis, croup, asthma, and systemic disorders, such as muscular dystrophy and cystic fibrosis.

GERIATRIC POINTERS
◆ In elderly patients, increased sensitivity to analgesics, sedative-hypnotics, or any combination of these drugs may produce apnea, even with normal dosage ranges.

◆ Educate the patient about safety measures related to aspiration of food or medications.
◆ Encourage cardiopulmonary resuscitation training for all adolescents and adults.
◆ Discuss underlying condition, diagnostic studies, and treatment options.

Apneustic respirations

- Characterized by prolonged, gasping inspiration, with a pause at full inspiration
- Important localizing sign of severe brain stem damage (see *Understanding apneustic respirations*)
- Must be differentiated from bradypnea and hyperpnea (disturbances in rate and depth, but not in rhythm), Cheyne-Stokes respirations (rhythmic alterations in rate and depth, followed by periods of apnea), and Biot's respirations (irregularly alternating periods of hyperpnea and apnea)

◆◆ **ACTION STAT!** *Your first priority for a patient with apneustic respirations is to ensure adequate ventilation. You'll need to insert an artificial airway and give oxygen until mechanical ventilation can begin. Next, thoroughly evaluate the patient's neurologic status, using a standardized tool such as the Glasgow Coma Scale.*

- Obtain a brief patient history from a family member, if possible, including history of recent infection or trauma.

- Perform a neurological assessment.
- Assess level of consciousness, and check vital signs.
- Continually assess and monitor the patient's neurologic and respiratory status.
- Watch for prolonged periods of apnea or signs of neurologic deterioration.
- Monitor the patient's arterial blood gas levels, or use a pulse oximetry device.

Understanding apneustic respirations

Involuntary breathing is primarily regulated by groups of neurons located in the respiratory centers in the medulla oblongata and pons. In the medulla, neurons react to impulses from the pons and other areas to regulate respiratory rate and depth. In the pons, two respiratory centers regulate respiratory rhythm by interacting with the medullary respiratory center to smooth the transition from inspiration to expiration and back.

The apneustic center in the pons stimulates inspiratory neurons in the medulla to precipitate inspiration. These inspiratory neurons, in turn, stimulate the pneumotaxic center in the pons to precipitate expiration. Destruction of neural pathways by pontine lesions disrupts normal regulation of respiratory rhythm, causing apneustic respirations.

CAUSES

MEDICAL
Pontine lesions
◆ Apneustic respirations usually result from extensive damage to the upper or lower pons due to infarction, hemorrhage, herniation, severe infection, tumor, or trauma.
◆ Typically, these respirations are accompanied by profound stupor or coma; pinpoint midline pupils; ocular bobbing (a spontaneous downward jerk, followed by a slow drift up to midline); and quadriplegia.
◆ Less common signs and symptoms include hemiplegia, with the eyes pointing toward the weak side; a positive Babinski's reflex; negative oculocephalic and oculovestibular reflexes; and, possibly, decorticate posture.

NURSING CONSIDERATIONS

◆ If appropriate, prepare the patient for such neurologic tests as EEG, computed tomography scanning, or magnetic resonance imaging.
◆ Provide emotional support to the patient and his family.

PEDIATRIC POINTERS
◆ In young children, avoid using the Glasgow Coma Scale because it requires verbal responses and assumes a certain level of language development.

PATIENT TEACHING

◆ Teach the patient and family members about the cause of apneustic respirations.
◆ Explain the rationale for diagnostic tests and hospital procedures.

Apraxia

- Inability to perform purposeful movements in the absence of significant weakness, sensory loss, poor coordination, or lack of comprehension or motivation
- Classified as ideational, ideomotor, or kinetic, or by type of impairment (see *How apraxia interferes with purposeful movement*)
- Indicative of a lesion in the cerebral hemisphere

ACTION STAT! *If signs and symptoms of increased intracranial pressure (ICP) are present, elevate the head of the bed 30 degrees and Monitor the patient for altered pupil size and reactivity, bradycardia, widened pulse pressure, and irregular respirations. Have emergency resuscitation equipment on hand, and be prepared to give mannitol I.V. to decrease cerebral edema.*

If the patient is having seizures, stay with the patient and have another nurse notify the practitioner immediately. Position the patient in a supine position, loosen tight clothing, and place a pillow or other soft object beneath his head. Avoid restraining the patient. If the patient's teeth are clenched, don't force anything into his mouth. Turn the patient's head to provide an open airway. After the seizure, reassure the patient, and orient him to time and place.

HISTORY

- Ask the patient or a family member about a history of headaches or dizziness.
- Obtain a medical history, including previous neurologic, cerebrovascular, neoplastic, or hepatic disease; atherosclerosis; or infection.

PHYSICAL ASSESSMENT

- Perform a neurologic assessment.
- Take vital signs and assess level of consciousness.
- Test the patient's motor and sensory function.
- Check deep tendon reflexes for quality and symmetry.
- Test for visual field defects.

How apraxia interferes with purposeful movement

TYPE OF APRAXIA	DESCRIPTION	EXAMINATION TECHNIQUE
Ideational apraxia	The patient can physically perform the steps required to complete a task but fails to remember the sequence in which they're performed.	Ask the patient to tie his shoelace. Typically, he'll be able to grasp the shoelace, loop it, and pull on it. However, he'll fail to remember the sequence of steps needed to tie a knot.
Ideomotor apraxia	The patient understands and can physically perform the steps required to complete the task but can't formulate a plan to carry them out.	Ask the patient to wave or cross his arms. Typically, he won't respond, but he may be able to spontaneously perform the gesture.
Kinetic apraxia	The patient understands the task and formulates a plan but fails to set the proper muscles in motion.	Ask the patient to comb his hair. Typically, he'll fail to move his arm and hand correctly to do the task. However, he'll be able to state that he needs to pick up the comb and draw it through his hair.

MEDICAL
Alzheimer's disease
◆ Gradual and irreversible ideomotor apraxia may occur.
◆ Other signs and symptoms may include amnesia, anomia, decreased attention span, apathy, aphasia, restlessness, agitation, paranoid delusions, incontinence, social withdrawal, ataxia, and tremors.

Brain abscess
◆ Apraxia occasionally results from a large brain abscess; it resolves spontaneously after the infection subsides.
◆ Depending on the location of the abscess, other signs and symptoms may include headache, fever, drowsiness, decreased metal acuity, aphasia, dysarthria, hemiparesis, hyperreflexia, incontinence, focal or generalized seizures, and ocular disturbances.

Brain tumor
◆ Apraxia may occur with or after early signs of increased ICP.
◆ Apraxia may be preceded by decreased mental acuity, headache, dizziness, and seizures.
◆ Localizing signs and symptoms of the tumor may include aphasia, dysarthria, visual field deficits, weakness, stiffness, and hyperreflexia in the extremities.

Hepatic encephalopathy
◆ Onset of constructional apraxia (the inability to copy simple drawings or patterns) is gradual and may be reversible with treatment.
◆ Early associated signs and symptoms include disorientation, amnesia, slurred speech, dysarthria, asterixis, and lethargy.
◆ Later signs and symptoms include hyperreflexia, positive Babinski's reflex, agitation, seizures, fetor hepaticus (breath odor characteristic of liver disease), stupor, and coma.

Stroke
◆ Onset of apraxia is sudden and commonly resolves spontaneously.
◆ Other signs and symptoms include headache, confusion, coma, hemiplegia, visual field deficits, aphasia, agnosia, dysarthria, and incontinence

◆ Prepare the patient for diagnostic studies such as computed tomography scanning.
◆ Because weakness, sensory deficits, confusion, and seizures may accompany apraxia, take measures to ensure the patient's safety.

PEDIATRIC POINTERS
◆ Sudden inability to perform a previously accomplished movement warrants prompt neurologic evaluation.
◆ Brain tumor is the most common cause of apraxia in children.
◆ Developmental apraxia may be caused by brain damage.

◆ Provide an explanation of apraxia.
◆ Demonstrate routine tasks.
◆ Refer the patient to physical or occupational therapy for additional retraining.

Arm pain

OVERVIEW

- Usually results from musculoskeletal disorders (see *Causes of local pain*)
- May be referred from another area
- Can be sharp or dull, burning or numbing, and shooting or penetrating

HISTORY

- Ask about history of injury.
- Determine onset, duration, and description of pain.
- Determine the location of referred pain.
- Ask about factors that aggravate or alleviate pain.
- Obtain a medical history, including current drug therapy.
- Determine whether a family history of gout or arthritis exists.

PHYSICAL ASSESSMENT

- Inspect the arm; compare it with the opposite arm for symmetry, movement, and muscle atrophy.
- Palpate for swelling, nodules, and tender areas.
- Assess circulation in both arms.
- Compare active range of motion, muscle strength, and reflexes bilaterally.
- Check responses to vibration, temperature, and pinprick.
- Examine the neck for pain, point tenderness, or muscle spasms.
- Check for arm pain when the neck is extended with the head toward the involved side.

CAUSES

MEDICAL
Angina
- Inner arm, chest, and jaw pain follows exertion.
- Pain lasts for 2 to 10 minutes and is relieved by rest or a vasodilator.
- Dyspnea, diaphoresis, and apprehension accompany pain.

Cellulitis
- Leg pain usually occurs, but arms may also be affected.
- Redness, tenderness, and edema accompany the pain.
- Other signs and symptoms may include fever, chills, tachycardia, headache, and hypotension.

Cervical nerve root compression
- If nerves supplying upper arm are affected, chronic arm and neck pain occurs.
- Pain may worsen with movement or prolonged sitting.
- Other signs and symptoms may include muscle weakness, paresthesia, and decreased reflex response.

Compartment syndrome
- The hallmark sign is severe pain with passive muscle stretching.
- Ominous findings include paralysis and absent pulse.
- Other signs and symptoms include muscle weakness, decreased reflex response, paresthesia, and edema.

Fractures
- Pain may occur at the site of injury and radiate throughout the arm.
- With a fresh fracture, the pain is intense and worsens with movement.
- Other signs and symptoms include crepitus, deformity, ecchymosis, edema, impaired distal circulation and sensation, and paresthesia.

Muscle contusion or strain
- Pain occurs in the area of injury.
- Local swelling and ecchymosis may occur.

Causes of local pain

Various disorders cause hand, wrist, elbow, or shoulder pain. In some disorders, pain may radiate from the injury site to other areas.

HAND PAIN
- Arthritis
- Buerger's disease
- Carpal tunnel syndrome
- Dupuytren's contracture
- Elbow tunnel syndrome
- Fracture
- Ganglion
- Infection
- Occlusive vascular disease
- Rediculopathy
- Raynaud's disease
- Shoulder-hand syndrome (reflex sympathetic dystrophy)
- Sprain or strain
- Thoracic outlet syndrome
- Trigger finger

WRIST PAIN
- Arthritis
- Carpal tunnel syndrome
- Fracture
- Ganglion
- Sprain or strain
- Tenosynovitis (de Quervain's disease)

ELBOW PAIN
- Arthritis
- Bursitis
- Dislocation
- Fracture
- Lateral epicondylitis (tennis elbow)
- Tendinitis
- Ulnar neuritis

SHOULDER PAIN
- Acromioclavicular separation
- Acute pancreatitis
- Adhesive capsulitis (frozen shoulder)
- Angina pectoris
- Arthritis
- Bursitis
- Cholecystitis or cholelithiasis
- Clavicle fracture
- Diaphragmatic pleurisy
- Dislocation
- Dissecting aortic aneurysm
- Gastritis
- Humeral neck fracture
- Infection
- Pancoast's syndrome
- Perforated ulcer
- Pneumothorax
- Ruptured spleen (left shoulder)
- Shoulder-hand syndrome
- Subphrenic abscess
- Tendinitis

- Mild to moderate pain occurs with movement, possibly leading to muscle weakness and atrophy.

Myocardial infarction
- A life-threatening disorder, left arm pain may occur with deep, crushing chest pain.
- Other signs and symptoms include weakness, pallor, nausea, vomiting, diaphoresis, altered blood pressure, tachycardia, dyspnea, and feelings of apprehension or impending doom.

Neoplasms of the arm
- Continuous, deep, and penetrating pain develops and worsens at night.
- Redness and swelling accompany arm pain.
- Late signs and symptoms include skin breakdown, impaired circulation, and paresthesia.

Osteomyelitis
- Vague and evanescent localized arm pain and fever occur.
- Other signs and symptoms include local tenderness, painful and restricted movement, malaise, tachycardia and, later, swelling.

NURSING CONSIDERATIONS

- Prepare the patient for diagnostic tests or X-rays.
- Monitor the patient for worsening pain, numbness, or decreased circulation distal to injury site.
- Monitor vital signs and look for tachycardia, hypotension, and diaphoresis. Take emergency actions for cardiovascular disorders (myocardial infarction).
- Apply a sling or splint to immobilize the arm.
- Make the patient comfortable by elevating the arm and applying ice.
- Clean abrasions and lacerations and apply dry, sterile dressings.

PEDIATRIC POINTERS
- Arm pain commonly results from fractures, muscle sprain, muscular dystrophy, or rheumatoid arthritis.
- If the child has a fracture or sprain, obtain a complete account of the injury; don't dismiss the possibility of child abuse.

GERIATRIC POINTERS
- Elderly patients with osteoporosis are prone to degenerative joint disease and may experience fractures from simple trauma, heavy lifting, or unexpected movements.

PATIENT TEACHING

- Explain the signs and symptoms of circulatory impairment caused by a tight cast.
- Discuss the signs and symptoms of an ischemic event.
- Discuss underlying condition, diagnostic tests, and treatments, including prescribed medications.

Asterixis (liver flap, flapping tremor)

- Also known as *liver flap* or *flapping tremor*
- Bilateral, coarse movement characterized by sudden relaxation of muscle groups holding a sustained posture
- Commonly observed in the wrists and fingers but also possible during any sustained voluntary action
- Typically signals hepatic, renal, or pulmonary disease

ACTION STAT! *Because asterixis may signal serious metabolic deterioration, quickly evaluate the patient's neurologic status and vital signs. Compare these data with his baseline, and watch carefully for acute changes. Continue to closely monitor neurologic status, vital signs, and urine output.*

Watch for signs of respiratory insufficiency, and be prepared to provide endotracheal intubation and ventilatory support. Also, be alert for complications of end-stage hepatic, renal, or pulmonary disease.

If the patient has signs of hemorrhage, prepare to insert a large-bore I.V. line for fluid and blood replacement. Position the patient flat in bed with his legs elevated 20 degrees. Begin or continue to administer oxygen.

HISTORY

- Ask about a history of hepatic or renal disease.
- If the patient has renal disease, briefly review the therapy he has received. If he's on dialysis, ask about the frequency of treatments to help gauge the disease's severity. Question a family member if the patient's level of consciousness (LOC) is significantly decreased.

PHYSICAL ASSESSMENT

- To elicit asterixis, have the patient extend his arms, dorsiflex his wrists, and spread his fingers (or do this for him, if necessary). Briefly observe him for asterixis. (See *Recognizing asterixis*.)
- If the patient has a decreased LOC but can follow verbal commands, ask him to squeeze two of your fingers. Consider rapid clutching and unclutching indications of asterixis.
- To check for asterixis in the ankle, elevate the patient's leg off the bed and dorsiflex the foot.
- If the patient can tightly close his eyes and mouth, watch for irregular

tremulous movements of the eyelids and corners of the mouth.
- If he can stick out his tongue, observe it for continuous quivering.
- If the patient has hepatic disease, assess him for early indications of hemorrhage, including restlessness, tachypnea, and cool, moist, pale skin. (If the patient is jaundiced, check for pallor in the conjunctivae and mucous membranes of the mouth.) Be aware that hypotension, oliguria, hematemesis, and melena are late signs of hemorrhage.
- If the patient is on dialysis, assess for hyperkalemia and metabolic acidosis. Look for tachycardia, nausea, diarrhea, abdominal cramps, muscle weakness, hyperreflexia, and Kussmaul's respirations.
- If the patient has pulmonary disease, check for such critical signs as labored respirations, tachypnea, accessory muscle use, and cyanosis.

CAUSES

MEDICAL
Hepatic encephalopathy
- This life-threatening disorder initially causes mild personality changes and a slight tremor.
- The tremor progresses to asterixis—a hallmark of hepatic encephalopathy—and is accompanied by lethargy, aberrant behavior, and apraxia.
- Eventually, the patient becomes stuporous and hyperventilates.
- After slipping into a coma, the patient exhibits characteristic hyperactive reflexes, positive Babinski's reflex, and fetor hepaticus.
- Other signs and symptoms include bradycardia, decreased respirations, and seizures.

Respiratory insufficiency, severe
- Characterized by life-threatening respiratory acidosis, this disorder initially produces headache, restlessness, confusion, apprehension, and decreased reflexes.

Recognizing asterixis

With asterixis, the patient's wrists and fingers are observed to "flap" because there's a brief, rapid relaxation of dorsiflexion of the wrist.

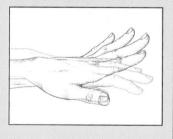

- Eventually, the patient becomes somnolent and may demonstrate asterixis before slipping into a coma.
- Hypertension may occur in early disease; hypotension, in later disease.
- Associated signs and symptoms include difficulty breathing and rapid, shallow respirations.

Uremic syndrome
- This life-threatening disorder initially causes lethargy, somnolence, confusion, disorientation, behavior changes, and irritability.
- Asterixis is accompanied by stupor, paresthesia, muscle twitching, fasciculations, and footdrop.
- Other signs and symptoms include polyuria and nocturia followed by oliguria and then anuria, elevated blood pressure, signs of heart failure and pericarditis, Kussmaul's respirations, anorexia, nausea, vomiting, diarrhea, GI bleeding, weight loss, ammonia breath odor, and metallic taste (dysgeusia).

OTHER
Drugs
- Certain drugs, such as the anticonvulsant phenytoin (Dilantin), may cause asterixis.

NURSING CONSIDERATIONS

- Provide simple comfort measures, such as allowing frequent rest periods to minimize fatigue and elevating the head of the bed to relieve dyspnea and orthopnea.
- Administer oil baths and avoid soap to relieve itching caused by jaundice and uremia.
- Provide emotional support to the patient and his family.
- If the patient is intubated or has a decreased LOC, provide enteral or parenteral nutrition.
- Closely monitor serum and urine glucose levels to evaluate hyperalimentation.
- Because the patient will probably be on bed rest, reposition him at least once every 2 hours to prevent skin breakdown.
- Observe strict hand-washing and aseptic techniques when changing dressings and caring for invasive lines because the patient's debilitated state makes him prone to infection.

PEDIATRIC POINTERS
- End-stage hepatic, renal, and pulmonary disease may also cause asterixis in children.

PATIENT TEACHING

- Explain all procedures and hospital routines to the patient and family members.
- Provide information on diagnosis, treatment, and cause of asterixis.

Ataxia

OVERVIEW

- Incoordination and irregularity of voluntary, purposeful movements
- May be acute (possibly life-threatening) or chronic
- Can be classified as cerebellar (resulting from disease of the cerebellum) or sensory (resulting from proprioception)
- Gait, trunk, limb and, possibly, speech disorders with the cerebellar form
- Gait disorders with the sensory form (see *Identifying ataxia*)

◆ **ACTION STAT!** *If ataxic movements occur suddenly, examine for signs of increased intracranial pressure and impending herniation. Determine the level of consciousness (LOC) and be alert for pupillary changes, motor weakness or paralysis, neck stiffness or pain, and vomiting. Check vital signs, especially respirations. Elevate the head of the bed. Have emergency resuscitation equip-ment readily available. Prepare the patient for computed tomography scanning or surgery.*

HISTORY

- Ask about a history of multiple sclerosis, diabetes, central nervous system infection, neoplastic disease, or stroke.
- Inquire about a family history of ataxia.
- Ask about chronic alcohol abuse or prolonged exposure to industrial toxins.
- Find out if the ataxia developed suddenly or gradually.

PHYSICAL ASSESSMENT

- Perform Romberg's test to help distinguish between cerebellar and sensory ataxia.
- Check motor strength.
- Perform complete neurologic assessment.

CAUSES

MEDICAL
Cerebellar abscess
- Limb ataxia occurs on the same side as the lesion, with gait and truncal ataxia.
- The initial symptom is headache localized behind the ear or in the occipital region.
- Other signs and symptoms include oculomotor palsy, fever, vomiting, altered level of consciousness (LOC), and coma.

Cerebellar hemorrhage
- A life-threatening disorder, ataxia is usually acute but transient; it may affect the trunk, gait, or limbs.
- Initial signs and symptoms include repeated vomiting, occipital headache, vertigo, oculomotor palsy, dysphagia, and dysarthria.
- Late symptoms, such as decreased LOC or coma, signal impending herniation.

Creutzfeldt-Jakob disease
- A viral disease affecting the nervous system
- Ataxia accompanies other neurologic signs, such as myoclonic jerking, aphasia, and rapidly progressing dementia.

Diabetic neuropathy
- Peripheral nerve damage may cause sensory ataxia.
- Other signs and symptoms include arm or leg pain, slight leg weakness, skin changes, bowel and bladder dysfunction, unsteady gait and, as neuropathy progresses, numbness in the feet.

Identifying ataxia

Ataxia may be observed in the patient's speech, in the movements of his trunk and limbs, or in his gait.

CEREBELLAR ATAXIA

With cerebellar ataxia, the patient may stagger or lurch in zigzag fashion, turn with extreme difficulty, and lose his balance when his feet are together.

GAIT ATAXIA

With gait ataxia, the patient's gait is wide based, unsteady, and irregular.

LIMB ATAXIA

With limb ataxia, the patient loses the ability to gauge distance, speed, and power of movement, resulting in poorly controlled, variable, and inaccurate voluntary movements. He may move too quickly or too slowly, or his movements may break down into component parts, giving him the appearance of a puppet or a robot. Other effects include a coarse, irregular tremor in purposeful movement (but not at rest) and reduced muscle tone.

SENSORY ATAXIA

With sensory ataxia, the patient moves abruptly and stomps or taps his feet. This occurs because he throws his feet forward and outward, and then brings them down first on the heels and then on the toes. The patient also fixes his eyes on the ground, watching his steps. However, if he can't watch them, staggering worsens. When he stands with his feet together, he sways or loses his balance.

SPEECH ATAXIA

Speech ataxia is a form of dysarthria in which the patient typically speaks slowly and stresses usually unstressed words and syllables. Speech content is unaffected.

TRUNCAL ATAXIA

Truncal ataxia is a disturbance in equilibrium in which the patient can't sit or stand without falling. Also, his head and trunk may bob and sway (titubation). If he can walk, his gait is reeling.

Diphtheria

◆ A life-threatening infection, sensory ataxia may occur within 4 to 8 weeks of the onset of symptoms.
◆ Other symptoms include fever, paresthesia, and paralysis of the limbs and, sometimes, the respiratory muscles.

Hepatocerebral degeneration

◆ Residual neurologic defects, including mild cerebellar ataxia with a wide-based and unsteady gait, occur in those who survive hepatic coma.
◆ Other signs and symptoms include altered LOC, dysarthria, rhythmic arm tremors, and choreoathetosis of the face, neck, and shoulders.

Hyperthermia

◆ If the patient survives the coma and seizures characteristic of the acute phase, cerebellar ataxia can occur.
◆ Subsequent symptoms include spastic paralysis, dementia, and slowly resolving confusion.

Metastatic cancer

◆ If cancer metastasizes to the cerebellum, gait ataxia may occur along with headache, dizziness, muscle incoordination, nystagmus, decreased LOC, nausea, and vomiting.
◆ The patient may fall toward the side of the lesion.

Multiple sclerosis

◆ Cerebellar ataxia may occur.
◆ Spinal cord involvement may cause speech and sensory ataxia.
◆ Ataxia may subside or disappear during remissions of this neurologic disorder.
◆ Other signs and symptoms include optic neuritis, optic atrophy, numbness and weakness, diplopia, dizziness, and bladder dysfunction.

Polyarteritis nodosa

◆ Sensory ataxia, abdominal and limb pain, hematuria, and elevated blood pressure may occur.
◆ Other symptoms include myalgia, headache, joint pain, and weakness.

Polyneuropathy

◆ Ataxia, severe motor weakness, muscle atrophy, and sensory loss in the limbs occur.
◆ Pain and skin changes may also occur.

Posterior fossa tumor

◆ Gait, truncal, or limb ataxia is an early sign; ataxia may worsen as the tumor enlarges.
◆ Other signs and symptoms include vomiting, headache, papilledema, vertigo, oculomotor palsy, decreased LOC, and motor and sensory impairment on the same side as the lesion.

Spinocerebellar ataxia

◆ Fatigue occurs initially, followed by stiff-legged gait ataxia.
◆ Eventually, limb ataxia, dysarthria, static tremor, nystagmus, cramps, paresthesia, and sensory deficits occur.

Stroke

◆ Infarction in the medulla, pons, or cerebellum may lead to ataxia, which may remain as a residual symptom.
◆ Worsening ataxia during the acute phase may indicate extension of stroke or severe swelling of the brain.
◆ Accompanying signs and symptoms include motor weakness, sensory loss, vertigo, nausea, vomiting, oculomotor palsy, dysphagia and, possibly, altered LOC.

Wernicke's disease

◆ Gait ataxia occurs in this thiamine deficiency disorder.
◆ With severe ataxia, the patient may not be able to stand or walk.
◆ Other signs and symptoms include nystagmus, diplopia, oculomotor palsies, confusion, tachycardia, exertional dyspnea, and orthostatic hypotension.

OTHER
Drugs

◆ Aminoglutethimide may cause ataxia that disappears 4 to 6 weeks after the drug is stopped.

◆ Toxic levels of anticonvulsants, anticholinergics, and tricyclic antidepressants may result in ataxia.

Poisoning

◆ Chronic arsenic poisoning may cause sensory ataxia along with headache, seizures, altered LOC, motor deficits, and muscle aching.
◆ Chronic mercury poisoning causes gait and limb ataxia, principally of the arms as well as dysarthria, mood changes, mental confusion, and tremors of the extremities, tongue, and lips.

NURSING CONSIDERATIONS

◆ If toxic drug levels are the cause, stop the drug.
◆ Encourage physical therapy to improve function following a stroke.
◆ If the patient has a brain tumor, prepare him for surgery, chemotherapy, or radiation therapy.
◆ Monitor neurologic status.
◆ Assist patient with activities of daily living, and assess for safety concerns.

PEDIATRIC POINTERS

◆ Acute ataxia may stem from febrile infection, brain tumors, mumps, and other disorders.
◆ Chronic ataxia may stem from Gaucher's disease, Refsum's disease, and other inborn errors of metabolism.
◆ If you suspect ataxia, refer the child for a neurologic evaluation to rule out a brain tumor.

PATIENT TEACHING

◆ Help the patient to identify rehabilitation goals.
◆ Stress safety measures.
◆ Discuss use of assistive devices.
◆ Refer the patient to counseling, as needed.

Athetosis

OVERVIEW

- Extrapyramidal sign characterized by slow, continuous, and twisting involuntary movements of the face, neck, and distal extremities
- Facial grimaces, jaw and tongue movements, and occasional phonation associated with neck movements
- Worsens during stress and voluntary activity; may subside during relaxation and disappear during sleep
- Commonly a lifelong disorder; difficult to distinguish from chorea
- Athetoid movements typically slower than choreiform movements (see *Distinguishing athetosis from chorea*)

HISTORY

- Obtain a medical history, including prenatal and postnatal complications, drug therapy, and family history.
- Determine the onset and duration of symptoms.
- Ask about the effects of rest, stress, and routine activity on symptoms.

PHYSICAL ASSESSMENT

- Test muscle strength and tone, range of motion, fine-muscle movements, and ability to perform rapidly alternating movements.
- Observe limb muscles during voluntary movements, noting the rhythm and duration of contraction and relaxation.

Distinguishing athetosis from chorea

In *athetosis*, movements are typically slow, twisting, and writhing. They're associated with spasticity and most commonly involve the face, neck, and distal extremities.

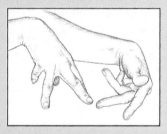

In *chorea*, movements are brief, rapid, jerky, and unpredictable. They can occur at rest or during normal movement. Typically, they involve the hands, lower arm, face, and head.

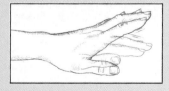

CAUSES

MEDICAL
Brain tumor
- Opposite-side choreoathetosis occurs.
- Other signs and symptoms vary with the type of tumor and degree of invasion.

Calcification of the basal ganglia
- This disorder is characterized by choreoathetosis and rigidity, it usually arises in adolescence or early adult life.

Cerebral infarction
- Opposite-side athetosis is accompanied by altered level of consciousness.
- Opposite-side paralysis of the face or limbs may also occur.

Hepatic encephalopathy
- Episodic or persistent choreoathetosis occurs in the chronic stage.
- Other signs and symptoms include cerebellar ataxia, myoclonus of the face and limbs, asterixis, dysarthria, and dementia.

Huntington's disease
- This disease is an inherited degenerative neurologic disorder.
- Athetosis and chorea progressively develop.
- Other signs and symptoms include dystonia, dysarthria, facial apraxia, rigidity, depression, and progressive mental deterioration leading to dementia.

Wilson's disease
- This is a progressive, hereditary copper metabolism disorder.
- Initially, choreoathetoid movements involve the fingers and hands and

then spread to the arms, head, trunk, and legs.
- Hepatomegaly, splenomegaly, jaundice, hematemesis, and spider angiomas may also occur.
- Other signs and symptoms include Kayser-Fleischer rings, arm and hand tremors, facial and muscular rigidity, dysarthria, dysphagia, drooling, and progressive dementia.

OTHER
Drugs
- Athetoid or choreoathetoid movements may occur with toxic levels of levodopa and phenytoin.
- Athetosis may occur with phenothiazine and other antipsychotics.

- Stop the drug that's causing the athetosis.
- Prepare the patient for diagnostic tests, such as computed tomography scanning, magnetic resonance imaging, lumbar puncture, EEG, and urine and blood studies.
- Assist with rehabilitation.
- Encourage exercise to maintain coordination, reduce the rate of deterioration, and minimize antisocial behavior.
- Encourage verbalization of feelings.
- Help the patient adapt to assistive devices to perform fine motor tasks.

PEDIATRIC POINTERS
- Athetosis may be acquired or inherited.
- Promote the patient's self-esteem and positive self-image.

GERIATRIC POINTERS
- Carefully question elderly patients about tremors; many older adults believe that tremors are a part of aging and may not report them.
- Tremors may result from vascular or neoplastic lesions, degenerative disease, drug toxicity, or hypoxia.

- Refer parents or caregivers to special education services, rehabilitation centers, and support groups.
- Give instruction in the use of assistive devices.
- Stress safety measures to prevent falls.

Aura

OVERVIEW

- A sensory or motor phenomenon, idea, or emotion that marks the initial stage of a seizure or the approach of a classic migraine headache
- May be classified as cognitive, affective, psychosensory, or psychomotor (see *Recognizing types of auras*)
- When associated with a seizure, stems from an irritable focus in the brain that spreads throughout the cortex
- Typically occurs seconds to minutes before the ictal phase
- Intensity, duration, and type dependent on the origin of the irritable focus
- Postictal phase of seizure: temporarily alters patient's level of consciousness, impairing his memory, causing him difficulty in describing event
- Aura associated with classic migraine headache: results from cranial vasoconstriction and typically involves visual disturbances; helps distinguish a classic migraine from other types of headaches; develops over 10 to 30 minutes and varies in intensity and duration

ACTION STAT! When an aura rapidly progresses to the ictal phase of a seizure, quickly evaluate the seizure and be alert for life-threatening complications, such as apnea. When an aura heralds a classic migraine, make the patient as comfortable as possible. Place him in a dark, quiet room and administer drugs to prevent the headache, if necessary.

HISTORY

- Obtain a thorough history of the patient's headaches or seizures.
- Ask the patient to describe any sensory or motor phenomena that precede each headache or seizure.
- Find out how long each headache or seizure typically lasts. Does anything make it worse, such as bright lights, noise, or caffeine? Does anything make it better?
- Ask the patient about drugs he takes for pain relief.

PHYSICAL ASSESSMENT

- Perform vision test.
- Perform complete neurologic assessment. Note sensory motor changes.

CAUSES

MEDICAL
Migraine headache, classic

- A classic migraine is preceded by a vague premonition and then, usually, a visual aura involving flashes of light.
- The aura lasts 10 to 30 minutes and may intensify until it completely obscures the patient's vision.
- When it peaks, the patient may then experience photophobia, nausea, and vomiting.
- Other signs and symptoms may include numbness or tingling of the lips, face, or hands; slight confusion; and dizziness before the characteristic unilateral, throbbing headache appears

Seizure, generalized tonic-clonic

- A generalized tonic-clonic seizure may begin with an aura.
- The patient loses consciousness and falls to the ground. His body stiffens (tonic phase); then he experiences rapid, synchronous muscle jerking and hyperventilation (clonic phase).
- The seizure usually lasts 2 to 5 minutes.

Recognizing types of auras

Determining whether an aura marks the patient's thought processes, emotions, or sensory or motor function usually requires keen observation. An aura is typically difficult to describe and is only dimly remembered when associated with seizure activity. Below you'll find the types of auras the patient may experience.

AFFECTIVE AURAS

- Fear
- Paranoia
- Other emotions

COGNITIVE AURAS

- Déjà vu (familiarity with unfamiliar events or environments)
- Flashback of past events
- *Jamais vu* (unfamiliarity with a known event)
- Time standing still

PSYCHOMOTOR AURAS

- Automatisms (inappropriate, repetitive movements): lip smacking, chewing, swallowing, grimacing, picking at clothes, climbing stairs

PSYCHOSENSORY AURAS

- Auditory: buzzing or ringing in the ears
- Gustatory: acidic, metallic, or bitter tastes
- Olfactory: foul odors
- Tactile: numbness or tingling
- Vertigo
- Visual: flashes of light (scintillations)

NURSING CONSIDERATIONS

- Advise the patient to keep a diary of factors that precipitate each headache as well as associated symptoms to help you evaluate the effectiveness of drug therapy and recommend lifestyle changes.
- Maintain safe environment to protect the seizuring patient.

PEDIATRIC POINTERS

- Watch for nonverbal clues that may be associated with an aura, such as rubbing the eyes, coughing, and spitting.
- When taking the seizure history, recognize that children—like adults—tend to forget the aura.
- Ask simple, direct questions, such as "Do you see anything funny before the seizure?" and "Do you get a bad taste in your mouth?"
- Give the child ample time to respond because he may have difficulty describing the aura.

PATIENT TEACHING

- Teach stress-reduction measures.
- Explain diagnosis and treatment options.
- Explain safety precautions to take when aura occurs.
- Teach family how to care for the patient if they witness a seizure.

Babinski's reflex

OVERVIEW

- Also known as *extensor plantar reflex* or *toe sign*
- Refers to dorsiflexion of the great toe with extension and fanning of the other toes
- Elicited by firmly stroking the side of the sole of the foot with a moderately sharp object (see *How to test for Babinski's reflex*)
- A normal response in infants; in normal adults and infants, toes curl toward the sole
- May be on one side or both
- May be temporary (occurs in the postictal stage of a seizure) or permanent (indicates corticospinal damage)

HISTORY

- Ask about recent head trauma, spinal cord injury, or animal bite.
- Find out about a personal or family history of neurologic disorders.

PHYSICAL ASSESSMENT

- Evaluate other neurologic signs.
- Evaluate muscle strength and tone in each extremity.
- Observe coordination.
- Test deep tendon reflexes (DTRs) in the elbow, antecubital area, wrist, knee, and ankle.
- Evaluate pain sensation and proprioception in the feet.

CAUSES

MEDICAL

Amyotrophic lateral sclerosis

- One-sided Babinski's reflex may occur with hyperactive DTRs and spasticity.
- Fasciculations are accompanied by muscle atrophy and weakness.
- Other signs and symptoms include incoordination; impaired speech; difficulty chewing, swallowing, and breathing; urinary frequency and urgency; and choking and excessive drooling.

Brain tumor

- Babinski's reflex may be present if the tumor involves the corticospinal tract.
- Other signs and symptoms include hyperactive DTRs, spasticity, seizures, cranial nerve dysfunction, hemiparesis or hemiplegia, decreased pain sensation, unsteady gait, incoordination, headache, emotional lability, and decreased level of consciousness (LOC).

Head trauma

- Unilateral or bilateral Babinski's may occur from primary corticospinal damage or secondary injury associated with increased intracranial pressure.
- Hyperactive DTRs, spasticity, weakness, and incoordination may occur.
- Depending on the type of head trauma, other signs and symptoms may include headache, vomiting, behavior changes, altered vital signs, and decreased LOC with abnormal pupillary size and response to light.

Meningitis

- Babinski's reflex of both feet follows fever, chills, and malaise.
- Nausea and vomiting may occur.
- As meningitis progresses, signs and symptoms include decreased LOC, nuchal rigidity, positive Brudzinski's and Kernig's signs, hyperactive DTRs, and opisthotonos.
- Other signs and symptoms include irritability, photophobia, diplopia,

TOP TECHNIQUE

How to test for Babinski's reflex

Firmly stroke the side of the sole of the patient's foot with your thumbnail or another moderately sharp object. Normally, this elicits flexion of all toes (a negative Babinski's reflex), as shown below left. With a positive Babinski's reflex, the great toe dorsiflexes, and the other toes fan out, as shown below right.

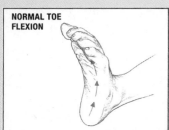

NORMAL TOE FLEXION

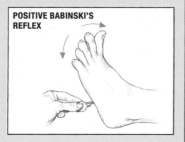

POSITIVE BABINSKI'S REFLEX

delirium, and deep stupor that may progress to coma.

Multiple sclerosis
- Progressive neurologic disease of the brain and spinal cord.
- Babinski's reflex starts in one foot but eventually occurs in both.
- Initial signs and symptoms include paresthesia, nystagmus, and blurred or double vision.
- Other signs and symptoms include scanning speech (syllables separated by pauses), dysphagia, intention tremor, weakness, incoordination, spasticity, gait ataxia, seizures, paraparesis or paraplegia, bladder incontinence, emotional lability, and loss of pain and temperature sensation and proprioception.

Pernicious anemia
- Babinski's reflex occurs in both feet late in the progression of the disorder.
- Weakness; sore, burning tongue; and numbness and tingling in the extremities are the classic triad of symptoms in this disorder.
- Other signs and symptoms include constipation, diarrhea, abdominal pain, nausea and vomiting, bleeding gums, ataxia, anorexia, diplopia and blurred vision, positive Romberg's sign, tachycardia, irritability, headache, malaise, and fatigue.

Rabies
- Babinski's reflex occurs in both feet during the excitation phase—2 to 10 days after the onset of symptoms.
- Such prodromal findings as fever, malaise, and irritability occur 30 to 40 days after a bite from an infected animal.
- Restlessness and extremely painful pharyngeal muscle spasms may occur.
- Other signs and symptoms may include difficulty swallowing, excessive drooling, hydrophobia, seizures, and hyperactive DTRs.

Spinal cord injury
- Babinski's reflex can be elicited as spinal shock resolves.

- Babinski's reflex occurs on one side if injury affects only one side of the spinal cord (Brown-Séquard's syndrome) and both sides if injury affects both sides.
- Horner's syndrome—marked by one-sided ptosis, pupillary constriction, and facial anhidrosis—may occur with lower cervical cord injury.
- Other signs and symptoms include hyperactive DTRs, spasticity, and variable or total loss of pain and temperature sensation, proprioception, and motor function.

Spinal cord tumor
- Babinski's reflex occurs in both feet with paresis and paralysis below the level of the tumor.
- Other signs and symptoms include spasticity, hyperactive DTRs, absent abdominal reflexes, incontinence, and diffuse pain at the level of the tumor.

Stroke
- Cerebral involvement produces Babinski's reflex in one foot with hemiplegia or hemiparesis, one-sided hyperactive DTRs, hemianopsia, and aphasia.
- Brain stem involvement produces Babinski's reflex in both feet with weakness or paralysis, bilateral hyperactive DTRs, cranial nerve dysfunction, incoordination, and unsteady gait.
- Generalized signs and symptoms include headache, vomiting, fever, disorientation, nuchal rigidity, seizures, and coma.

NURSING CONSIDERATIONS
- Assist the patient with activity.
- Keep his environment free from obstructions.

PEDIATRIC POINTERS
- Babinski's reflex occurs normally in infants up to age 2, reflecting immaturity of the corticospinal tract.
- After age 2, Babinski's reflex is pathologic and may result from hydrocephalus or any of the causes more commonly seen in adults.

PATIENT TEACHING
- Instruct the patient about the need to call for assistance when getting out of bed.
- Discuss ways to maintain a safe environment.
- Instruct the patient in the use of adaptive devices.
- Discuss underlying condition, diagnostic tests, and treatment options.

Back pain

OVERVIEW

- Affects about 80% of the U.S. population
- May be acute or chronic and constant or intermittent
- May be localized or radiate along the spine or legs
- May be referred from abdomen or flank, possibly signaling a life-threatening disorder (see *Managing acute, severe back pain*)

HISTORY

- Obtain a medical, family, and drug history.
- Ask about unusual sensations in the legs.
- Ask about diet and alcohol use.

PHYSICAL ASSESSMENT

- Observe skin color, especially in the legs.
- Observe posture and body alignment.
- Palpate skin temperature and femoral, popliteal, posterior tibial, and pedal pulses.
- Ask the patient to bend forward, backward, and side to side while you palpate for paravertebral muscle spasms.
- Palpate the dorsolumbar spine for point tenderness.
- Ask the patient to walk—first on heels, then on toes.
- Evaluate patellar tendon (knee), Achilles tendon, and Babinski's reflexes.
- Evaluate the strength of the extensor hallucis longus by asking the patient to hold up his big toe against resistance.
- Measure leg length and hamstring and quadriceps muscles.
- Help the patient into the supine position. Then, grasp his heel and slowly lift his leg. Note the pain's exact location and the angle between the table and his leg when it occurs.

Repeat this maneuver with the opposite leg.
- Note range of motion of the hip and knee.
- Palpate and percuss the flanks to elicit costovertebral angle tenderness.

CAUSES

MEDICAL

Abdominal aortic aneurysm, dissecting
- In this life-threatening disorder, initially lower back pain or dull abdominal pain may occur; however, upper abdominal pain is more common.
- A pulsating epigastrium mass may be palpated; pulsating stops after rupture.
- Other signs and symptoms include mottled skin below the waist, absent femoral and pedal pulses, lower blood pressure in the legs than in the arms, abdominal rigidity, mild to moderate tenderness with guarding, and shock (if blood loss is significant).

Ankylosing spondylitis
- Sacroiliac pain radiates up the spine and is aggravated by pressure on the side of the pelvis.
- Pain is usually most severe in the morning or after a period of inactivity and isn't relieved by rest.
- Abnormal rigidity of the lumbar spine with forward flexion is common.
- Other signs and symptoms include local tenderness, fatigue, fever, anorexia, weight loss, and occasional iritis.

Intervertebral disk rupture
- Gradual or sudden lower back pain occurs with or without sciatica.
- Pain begins in the back and radiates to the buttocks and legs.
- Pain is exacerbated by activity, coughing, and sneezing and is eased by rest.
- The patient walks slowly and rises from sitting to standing with extreme difficulty.

 ACTION STAT!

Managing acute, severe back pain

If the patient reports acute, severe back pain, quickly take his vital signs; then perform a rapid assessment to rule out life-threatening causes:

- Ask him when the pain began. Can he relate it to any causes? For example, did the pain occur after eating? After falling on ice?
- Ask the patient to describe the pain. Is it burning, stabbing, throbbing, or aching? Is it constant or intermittent? Does it radiate to the buttocks or legs? Does he have leg weakness? Does the pain seem to originate in the abdomen and radiate to the back? Has he had a pain like this before? What makes it better or worse? Is it affected by activity or rest? Is it worse in the morning or evening? Does it wake him up? Typically, visceral-referred back pain is unaffected by activity and rest. In contrast, spondylogenic-referred back pain worsens with activity and improves with rest. Pain of

neoplastic origin is usually relieved by walking and worsens at night.

If the patient describes deep lumbar pain unaffected by activity, palpate for a pulsating epigastric mass. If this sign is present, suspect dissecting abdominal aortic aneurysm. Withhold food and fluid in anticipation of emergency surgery. Prepare for I.V. fluid replacement and for oxygen administration.

If the patient describes severe epigastric pain that radiates through the abdomen to the back, assess him for absent bowel sounds and for abdominal rigidity and tenderness. If these are present, suspect perforated ulcer or acute pancreatitis. Start an I.V. line for fluids and drugs, administer oxygen, and insert a nasogastric tube while withholding food.

◆ Other signs and symptoms include paresthesia, paravertebral muscle spasm, and decreased reflexes on the affected side.

Lumbosacral sprain

◆ Aching, localized pain and tenderness is associated with muscle spasm upon sideways motion.
◆ Flexion of the spine and movement intensify the pain; rest and lying recumbent with knees and hips flexed relieves it.

Pancreatitis, acute

◆ In this life-threatening disorder, upper abdominal pain may radiate to the flanks and back.
◆ Bending forward, drawing the knees to the chest, or moving around may relieve pain.
◆ Early signs and symptoms include abdominal tenderness, nausea, vomiting, fever, pallor, tachycardia, hypoactive bowel sounds, rebound tenderness, and abdominal guarding and rigidity.
◆ Turner's sign (ecchymosis of the abdomen or flank) or Cullen's sign (bluish discoloration of skin around the umbilicus and in both flanks) signals hemorrhagic pancreatitis.

Perforated ulcer

◆ In this life-threatening disorder, sudden, prostrating epigastric pain may radiate throughout the abdomen and to the back.
◆ Other signs and symptoms include boardlike abdominal rigidity, tenderness with guarding, generalized rebound tenderness, absent bowel sounds, fever, tachycardia, hypotension, and grunting, shallow respirations.

Prostate cancer

◆ Chronic, aching back pain may be the only symptom, appearing in the advanced stages.
◆ Other late signs and symptoms include hematuria, difficulty initiating a urine stream, dribbling, urine retention, unexplained cystitis, and a decrease in the urine stream.

Pyelonephritis, acute

◆ Progressive flank and lower abdominal pain accompanies back pain or tenderness (especially over the costovertebral angle).
◆ Other signs and symptoms include high fever and chills, nausea, vomiting, flank and abdominal tenderness, and urinary frequency and urgency.

Renal calculi

◆ Colicky pain travels from the costovertebral angle to the flank, suprapubic region, and external genitalia.
◆ If calculi travel down a ureter, the patient may feel excruciating pain.
◆ If calculi are in the renal pelvis and calyces, the patient may feel dull and constant flank pain.
◆ Other signs and symptoms include nausea, vomiting, urinary urgency, hematuria, and agitation.

Sacroiliac strain

◆ Sacroiliac pain may radiate to the buttock, hip, and lateral aspect of the thigh.
◆ Weight bearing on the affected side and abduction with resistance of the leg aggravates the pain.

Spinal stenosis

◆ Back pain occurs with or without sciatica.
◆ Pain may radiate to the toes and, if the patient doesn't rest, may progress to numbness or weakness.

Transverse process fractures and vertebral compression fractures

◆ Severe, localized back pain occurs with muscle spasm and hematoma in a transverse process fracture.
◆ Pain may not occur for several weeks in a vertebral compression fracture; then, back pain aggravated by weight bearing and local tenderness occurs.

Vertebral osteoporosis

◆ Chronic, aching back pain is aggravated by activity and relieved (somewhat) by rest.
◆ Vertebral collapse, causing a backache with pain that radiates around the trunk, is the most common characteristic.

NURSING CONSIDERATIONS

◆ If the cause is life-threatening, monitor the patient closely.
◆ Look for increasing pain, altered neurovascular condition of the legs, loss of bowel or bladder control, altered vital signs, sweating, and cyanosis.
◆ Withhold food and fluids in case surgery is needed.
◆ Elevate the head of the bed and place a pillow under the knees.
◆ Fit the patient for a corset or lumbosacral support, as needed.
◆ Apply heat or cold therapy, backboard, foam mattress, or pelvic traction.

PEDIATRIC POINTERS

◆ Back pain may stem from diskitis, neoplasms, idiopathic juvenile osteoporosis, and spondylolisthesis.

PATIENT TEACHING

◆ Provide information about the use of anti-inflammatory drugs and analgesics.
◆ Discuss lifestyle changes, such as losing weight or correcting posture.
◆ Teach relaxation techniques, such as deep breathing.
◆ Instruct the patient on correct use of corset or lumbosacral support.
◆ Provide information about alternatives to drug therapy, such as biofeedback and transcutaneous electrical nerve stimulation.

Barrel chest

OVERVIEW

- A rounded chest in which the antero-posterior diameter enlarges to approximate the transverse diameter
- A late sign of chronic obstructive pulmonary disease (COPD), which results from increased lung volumes from chronic airflow obstruction (see *Recognizing barrel chest*)

HISTORY

- Ask about a history of pulmonary disease.
- Note chronic exposure to environmental irritants, such as asbestos.
- Ask about smoking habits.
- Inquire about a cough and, if it's productive, about the color and consistency of the sputum.
- Ask if dyspnea or shortness of breath is present at rest or with activity.

PHYSICAL ASSESSMENT

- Auscultate for abnormal breath sounds.
- Percuss the chest for hyperresonant sounds (indicating trapped air) and dull or flat sounds (indicating consolidation).
- Observe for accessory muscle use, intercostal retractions, and tachypnea.
- Note if central cyanosis of the cheeks, nose, and oral mucosa is present.
- Check for peripheral cyanosis of the nail beds.
- Observe for finger clubbing, a late sign of COPD.

Recognizing barrel chest

In the normal adult chest, the ratio of anteroposterior to transverse (or lateral) diameter is 1:2. In patients with barrel chest, this ratio approaches 1:1 as the anteroposterior diameter enlarges.

NORMAL CHEST

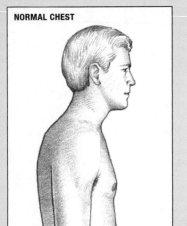

BARREL CHEST

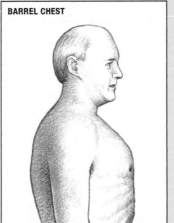

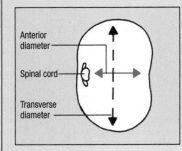

Anterior diameter

Spinal cord

Transverse diameter

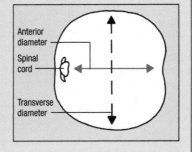

Anterior diameter

Spinal cord

Transverse diameter

CAUSES

MEDICAL
Asthma
- Barrel chest develops with chronic asthma.
- Severe dyspnea, wheezing, and a productive cough occur with an acute asthma attack.
- Other signs and symptoms include prolonged expiratory time, accessory muscle use, tachycardia, perspiration, and flushing.

Chronic bronchitis
- Barrel chest, a late sign, is preceded by dyspnea and a productive cough.
- Other signs and symptoms include cyanosis, tachypnea, wheezing, prolonged expiratory time, and accessory muscle use.

Emphysema
- Barrel chest is a late sign.
- Dyspnea is the initial symptom.
- Eventually, other signs and symptoms include anorexia, weight loss, malaise, accessory muscle use, pursed-lip breathing, tachypnea, peripheral cyanosis, clubbing of fingers, and a chronic cough.

NURSING CONSIDERATIONS

- Have the patient sit forward with his hands on his knees to support the upper torso and ease breathing.
- Closely monitor respiratory status.

PEDIATRIC POINTERS
- In infants, the ratio of anteroposterior to transverse diameter is normally 1:1.
- By age 5 or 6, this ratio gradually changes to 1:2.
- Cystic fibrosis and chronic asthma may cause barrel chest in a child.

GERIATRIC POINTERS
- Senile kyphosis of the thoracic spine may be mistaken for barrel chest in an elderly patient, but signs of pulmonary disease are absent.

PATIENT TEACHING

- Explain how to avoid bronchial irritants that may exacerbate COPD.
- Emphasize the importance of quitting smoking, and provide information about resources to assist with this goal.
- Tell the patient the signs and symptoms of upper respiratory infection he should report.
- Discuss the pacing of activities to minimize exertional dyspnea.
- Discuss proper nutrition and eating more frequent, smaller meals.

Battle's sign

OVERVIEW

- Ecchymosis over the temporal bone's mastoid process
- Develops 24 to 36 hours after a basilar skull fracture and is commonly the only outward sign of basilar skull fracture

 ACTION STAT! *Basilar skull fracture, if untreated, can be fatal. Place the patient flat on his back in bed and monitor his neurologic status. If the patient has a large dural tear, prepare him for a craniotomy.*

HISTORY

- Ask about recent trauma, such as a severe blow to the head or a motor vehicle accident.

PHYSICAL ASSESSMENT

- Perform a complete neurologic examination, including mental status and speech, cranial nerve function, sensory and motor function, and reflexes. (See *Reviewing cranial nerves.*)
- Assess level of consciousness (LOC).
- Check vital signs, and look for signs of increased intracranial pressure (ICP). (See *Signs of increased ICP.*)
- Evaluate pupillary size, response to light, and motor and verbal responses; relate data to the Glasgow Coma Scale.
- Note cerebrospinal fluid (CSF) leakage from the nose or ears.
- Test leakage with a glucose reagent strip to confirm that it's CSF. (If it's CSF, the strip will indicate presence of glucose.)
- Look for the "halo" sign on bed linens or dressings.
- Perform a complete physical examination of all body systems.

Reviewing cranial nerves

The cranial nerves have either sensory or motor function or both. The function of each cranial nerve is listed below.

- CN I: Olfactory
Smell
- CN II: Optic
Vision
- CN III: Oculomotor
Most eye movement, pupillary constriction, upper eyelid elevation
- CN IV: Trochlear
Downward and inward eye movement
- CN V: Trigeminal
Chewing, corneal reflex, face and scalp sensations
- CN VI: Abducens
Lateral eye movement
- CN VII: Facial
Expressions in forehead, eye, and mouth; taste
- CN VIII: Acoustic
Hearing and balance
- CN IX: Glossopharyngeal
Swallowing, salivating, and tasting
- CN X: Vagus
Swallowing, gag reflex, talking; sensations of throat, larynx, and abdominal viscera; activities of thoracic and abdominal viscera, such as heart rate and peristalsis
- CN XI: Spinal accessory
Shoulder movement and head rotation
- CN XII: Hypoglossal
Tongue movement

Signs of increased ICP

The earlier you can spot signs of increased intracranial pressure (ICP), the quicker you can intervene and the better your patient's chance of recovery. By the time late signs appear, interventions may be futile.

ASSESSMENT AREA	EARLY SIGNS	LATE SIGNS
Level of consciousness	• Need for increased stimulation • Subtle orientation loss • Restlessness and anxiety • Sudden quietness	• Unable to be roused
Pupils	• Changes in pupil on side of lesion • Abnormal and exaggerated rhythmic contraction and dilation of one pupil (unilateral hippus) • Sluggish reaction of both pupils • Unequal pupils	• Pupils fixed and dilated
Motor response	• Sudden weakness • Motor changes on side opposite the lesion • Positive pronator drift: with palms up, one hand pronates	• Profound weakness
Vital signs	• Intermittent increases in blood pressure	• Increased systolic pressure with widening pulse pressure, bradycardia, and abnormal respirations (Cushing's triad)

CAUSES

MEDICAL
Basilar skull fracture
◆ Battle's sign may be the only outward sign.
◆ Other signs and symptoms include periorbital ecchymosis ("raccoon" eyes), conjunctival hemorrhage, nystagmus, ocular deviation, epistaxis, anosmia, visible fracture lines on the external auditory canal, tinnitus, difficulty hearing, facial paralysis, vertigo, and a bulging tympanic membrane (from accumulation of CSF or blood).

NURSING CONSIDERATIONS

◆ Keep the patient flat to decrease pressure on dural tears and to minimize CSF leakage.
◆ Monitor neurologic status.
◆ Avoid nasogastric intubation and nasopharyngeal suction, either of which may cause cerebral infection.
◆ Caution the patient against blowing his nose, which may worsen a dural tear.
◆ Prepare the patient for diagnostic tests, such as skull X-rays and computed tomography scan.
◆ Explain to the patient that basilar skull fracture and associated dural tears typically heal spontaneously within several days to weeks.
◆ Because a large dural tear may require a craniotomy to repair the tear with a graft patch, prepare the patient for surgery, as indicated.

PEDIATRIC POINTERS
◆ Victims of abuse frequently sustain basilar skull fractures.
◆ If you suspect abuse, follow protocol for reporting the incident.

PATIENT TEACHING

◆ Explain what activities the patient should avoid, and emphasize the importance of bed rest.
◆ Explain to the patient (or caregiver) the signs and symptoms to look for and report, such as changes in mental status, LOC, or breathing.
◆ Tell the patient to take acetaminophen for headaches.
◆ Explain what diagnostic tests the patient may need.
◆ Discuss the prospect of surgery with the patient, and answer his questions and concerns.

Biot's respirations

OVERVIEW

- A late and ominous sign of neurologic deterioration
- Characterized by an irregular and unpredictable rate, rhythm, and depth
- May appear abruptly and may reflect increased pressure on the medulla coinciding with brain stem compression

ACTION STAT! Observe the patient's breathing pattern for several minutes to avoid confusing Biot's respirations with other respiratory patterns. (See Identifying Biot's respirations.) Assess the patient's respiratory status and prepare to intubate him and provide mechanical ventilation. Next, take his vital signs, noting especially increased systolic pressure.

HISTORY

- Ask about onset and duration of altered breathing pattern and neurologic changes.
- If the patient isn't capable of communicating, question family members.
- Obtain a medical history.

PHYSICAL ASSESSMENT

- Assess respiratory rate, rhythm, and depth.
- Take vital signs.
- Assess neurologic status and level of consciousness.

Identifying Biot's respirations

Biot's respirations, also known as *ataxic respirations,* have a completely irregular pattern. Shallow and deep breaths occur randomly, with haphazard, irregular pauses. The respiratory rate tends to be slow and may progressively decelerate to apnea.

├─── 1 minute ───┤

CAUSES

MEDICAL
Brain stem compression
◆ Biot's respirations are characteristic in brain stem compression, a neurologic emergency.
◆ Rapidly enlarging lesions may cause ataxic respirations and lead to complete respiratory arrest.

NURSING CONSIDERATIONS

◆ Monitor the patient's vital signs frequently, including oxygen saturation.
◆ Elevate the head of the patient's bed 30 degrees to help reduce intracranial pressure.
◆ Prepare the patient for emergency surgery to relieve pressure on the brain stem.
◆ Computed tomography scans or magnetic resonance imaging may confirm the cause of brain stem compression.
◆ Because Biot's respirations typically reflect a grave prognosis, give the patient's family information and emotional support.

PEDIATRIC POINTERS
◆ Biot's respirations are rarely seen in children.

PATIENT TEACHING

◆ Explain all tests and procedures to the patient and family members.
◆ Teach the patient and family about the diagnosis, treatments, and prognosis.

Bladder distention

OVERVIEW

- Abnormal enlargement of the bladder
- Results from an inability to urinate
- Caused by a mechanical or anatomic obstruction, neuromuscular disorder, or the use of certain drugs
- If severe distention isn't corrected promptly, renal impairment can occur.
- Gradual distention: no symptoms until the stretched bladder produces discomfort
- Acute distention: suprapubic fullness, pressure, and pain

ACTION STAT! With severe distention, insert an indwelling urinary catheter to relieve discomfort and prevent bladder rupture. If more than 700 ml is emptied when the catheter is inserted, compressed blood vessels dilate and may make the patient feel faint. Clamp the indwelling urinary catheter for 30 to 60 minutes, then resume draining.

HISTORY

- Ask about voiding patterns and characteristics.
- Find out the time and amount of last voiding.
- Determine the amount of fluid consumed since last voiding.
- Obtain a medical history, including urinary tract obstruction or infections; sexually transmitted disease; neurologic, intestinal, or pelvic surgery; lower abdominal or urinary tract trauma; and systemic or neurologic disorders.
- Note drug history, including use of over-the-counter drugs.

PHYSICAL ASSESSMENT

- Take vital signs.
- Percuss and palpate the bladder.
- Inspect the urethral meatus and measure its diameter.
- Note the appearance and amount of discharge.
- Test for perineal sensation and anal sphincter tone.
- Digitally examine the prostate gland (in men).

MEDICAL

Benign prostatic hyperplasia

◆ Bladder distention develops gradually as the prostate enlarges.

◆ Initial signs and symptoms include urinary hesitancy, straining, and frequency; reduced force of the urine stream and the inability to stop the stream; nocturia; and postvoiding dribbling.

◆ Later signs and symptoms include prostate enlargement, perineal pain, constipation, hematuria, and sensations of suprapubic fullness and incomplete bladder emptying.

Bladder cancer

◆ Neoplasms can cause bladder distention by blocking the urethra.

◆ A mass may be palpable on manual examination.

◆ Other signs and symptoms include hematuria (the most common sign); urinary frequency and urgency; nocturia; dysuria; pyuria; pain in the bladder, rectum, pelvis, flank, back, or legs; vomiting; diarrhea; and sleeplessness.

Multiple sclerosis

◆ Urine retention and bladder distention result from interrupted upper-motor-neuron control of the bladder.

◆ Other signs and symptoms include optic neuritis, paresthesia, impaired senses of position and vibration, diplopia, nystagmus, dizziness, abnormal reflexes, dysarthria, muscle weakness, emotional lability, Lhermitte's sign (transient, electric-like shocks that spread down the body when the head is dropped forward), Babinski's sign, and ataxia.

Prostatitis

◆ Bladder distention occurs rapidly along with perineal discomfort and suprapubic fullness.

◆ Other signs and symptoms include perineal pain; tense, boggy, tender, and warm enlarged prostate; decreased libido; impotence; decreased force of the urine stream; dysuria; hematuria; urinary frequency and urgency; fatigue; malaise; myalgia; fever; chills; nausea; and vomiting.

Spinal neoplasms

◆ Upper-neuron control of the bladder is disrupted, causing neurogenic bladder and distention.

◆ Other signs and symptoms include a sense of pelvic fullness, continuous overflow dribbling, back pain that typically mimics sciatic pain, constipation, tender vertebral processes, sensory deficits, and muscle weakness, flaccidity, and atrophy.

Urethral calculi

◆ Urethral obstruction causes bladder distention and interrupted urine flow.

◆ Pain from the obstruction radiates to the penis or vulva and then to the perineum or rectum.

◆ A palpable calculus and urethral discharge may also be present.

Urethral stricture

◆ Urine retention and bladder distention result.

◆ Urethral discharge and urinary frequency are common signs.

OTHER

Catheterization

◆ Urine retention and bladder distention may occur from a kinked tube or an occluded lumen.

Drugs

◆ Anesthetics, anticholinergics, ganglionic blockers, opiates, parasympatholytics, and sedatives may cause urine retention and bladder distention.

◆ Monitor vital signs, intake and output, and the extent of bladder distention.

◆ Encourage the patient to change positions to alleviate discomfort.

◆ Give analgesics, if needed.

◆ Prepare the patient for surgery, as needed.

◆ Provide privacy for voiding and encourage a normal voiding position.

PEDIATRIC POINTERS

◆ Look for urine retention and bladder distention in any infant who fails to void normal amounts of urine.

◆ In boys, posterior urethral valves, meatal stenosis, phimosis, spinal cord anomalies, bladder diverticula, and other congenital defects may cause urinary obstruction and resultant bladder distention.

GERIATRIC POINTERS

◆ Bladder distention is most common in elderly men with prostate disorders that cause urine retention.

◆ Teach the patient to use Valsalva's maneuver or Credé's method to empty the bladder.

◆ Explain how to stimulate voiding.

◆ Discuss underlying condition, diagnostic tests, and treatment options.

Blood pressure decrease

OVERVIEW

- Inadequate intravascular pressure to maintain oxygen requirements
- Also called *hypotension*
- Typically defined as a reading below 90/60 mm Hg or a drop of 30 mm Hg from the baseline
- May affect the kidneys, brain, and heart, and may lead to a change in level of consciousness (LOC) or to myocardial ischemia
- May reflect an expanded intravascular space or reduced intravascular volume and cardiac output

 ACTION STAT! *If the patient's systolic blood pressure is less than 80 mm Hg, or 30 mm Hg below baseline, suspect shock. Quickly evaluate the patient for decreased LOC. Check the apical pulse for tachycardia; check respirations for tachypnea. Inspect for cool, clammy skin. Elevate the patient's legs above the level of his heart, or place him in Trendelenburg's position. Start an I.V. line using a large-bore needle to replace fluids and blood or to give drugs. Administer oxygen. Mechanical ventilation may be necessary. Monitor intake of fluids and output of urine. Prepare for cardiac or hemodynamic monitoring. Insert a nasogastric tube to prevent aspiration in the comatose patient. Insert an indwelling urinary catheter to measure hourly urine output.*

HISTORY

- Ask about such symptoms as weakness, nausea, dizziness, and chest pain.
- Ask about recent illnesses.

PHYSICAL ASSESSMENT

- Obtain vital signs and weight.
- Inspect skin for pallor, sweating, and clamminess.
- Palpate peripheral pulses.
- Auscultate for abnormal heart, breath, and bowel sounds and abnormal heart and breath rates, and rhythms.
- Look for signs of hemorrhage.

TOP TECHNIQUE

Ensuring accurate blood pressure measurement

When taking the patient's blood pressure, begin by applying the cuff properly, as shown here.

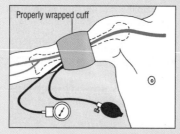

Properly wrapped cuff

Then be alert for these common pitfalls to avoid recording an inaccurate blood pressure measurement.

- *Wrong-sized cuff.* Select the appropriate-sized cuff for the patient. This ensures that adequate pressure is applied to compress the brachial artery during cuff inflation. If the cuff bladder is too narrow, a false-high reading will be obtained; too wide, a false-low reading. The cuff bladder width should be about 40% of the circumference of the midpoint of the limb; bladder length should be twice the width. If the arm circumference is less than 13″ (33 cm), select a regular-sized cuff; if it's between 13″ and 16″ (33 to 40.5 cm), a large-sized cuff; if it's more than 16″, a thigh cuff. Pediatric cuffs are also available.
- *Slow cuff deflation, causing venous congestion in the extremity.* Don't deflate the cuff more slowly than 2 mm Hg/heartbeat because you'll get a false-high reading.
- *Cuff wrapped too loosely, reducing its effective width.* Tighten the cuff to avoid a false-high reading.
- *Mercury column not read at eye level.* Read the mercury column at eye level. If the column is below eye level, you may record a false-low reading; if it's above eye level, a false-high reading.
- *Tilted mercury column.* Keep the mercury column vertical to avoid a false-high reading.
- *Poorly timed measurement.* Don't take the patient's blood pressure if he appears anxious or has just eaten or ambulated; you'll get a false-high reading.
- *Incorrect position of the arm.* Keep the patient's arm level with his heart to avoid a false-low reading.
- *Cuff overinflation, causing venospasm or pain.* Don't overinflate the cuff because you'll get a false-high reading.
- *Failure to notice an auscultatory gap* (sound fades out for 10 to 15 mm Hg, then returns). To avoid missing the top Korotkoff's sound, estimate systolic pressure by palpation first. Then inflate the cuff rapidly—at a rate of 2 to 3 mm Hg/second—to about 30 mm Hg above the palpable systolic pressure.
- *Inaudibility of feeble sounds.* Before reinflating the cuff, have the patient raise his arm to reduce venous pressure and amplify low-volume sounds. After inflating the cuff, lower the patient's arm; then deflate the cuff and listen. Alternatively, with the patient's arm positioned at heart level, inflate the cuff and have the patient make a fist. Have him rapidly open and close his hand 10 times before you begin to deflate the cuff, and then listen. Make sure to document that the blood pressure reading was augmented.

- Assess for abdominal rigidity and rebound tenderness and possible sources of infection.
- If patient has episodes of dizziness when standing up suddenly, take blood pressure while he's lying down, sitting, and then standing. Compare readings. (See *Ensuring accurate blood pressure measurement*.)
- Obtain an electrocardiogram and, urine and serum samples as needed.

CAUSES

MEDICAL
Acute adrenal insufficiency
- Orthostatic hypotension is a characteristic sign.
- Other signs and symptoms include fatigue; weakness; nausea; vomiting; abdominal discomfort; weight loss; fever; tachycardia; pale, cool, clammy skin; restlessness; decreased urine output; tachypnea; hyperpigmentation of fingers, nails, scars, nipples, and body folds; and coma.

Anaphylactic shock
- Blood pressure falls dramatically and pulse pressure narrows, due to vasodilitation.
- Initially, anxiety, restlessness, intense itching, pounding headache, and a feeling of doom occur.
- Other later signs and symptoms include weakness, sweating, nasal congestion, coughing, difficulty breathing, nausea, abdominal cramps, involuntary defecation, seizures, flushing, change or loss of voice, urinary incontinence, and tachycardia.

Anthrax, inhalation
- Initial signs and symptoms are flulike and include fever, chills, weakness, cough, and chest pain.
- The second stage develops abruptly with rapid deterioration marked by fever, dyspnea, stridor, and hypotension.

Cardiac arrhythmia
- Blood pressure fluctuates between normal and low.
- Dizziness, chest pain, difficulty breathing, light-headedness, weakness, fatigue, and palpitations occur.
- Pulse rhythm is irregular, and heart rate is greater than 100 beats/minute or less than 60 beats/minute, causing inefficient heart contraction.

Cardiac tamponade
- Compression of the heart due to critical increase in fluid volume in the pericardium.
- Systolic pressure falls more than 10 mm Hg during inspiration (paradoxical pulse).
- Other signs and symptoms include restlessness, cyanosis, tachycardia, jugular vein distention, muffled heart sounds, dyspnea, and Kussmaul's sign.

Cardiogenic shock
- Systolic pressure falls to less than 80 mm Hg or to 30 mm Hg less than baseline, secondary to serious heart disease.
- Tachycardia; narrowed pulse pressure; diminished Korotkoff sounds; peripheral cyanosis; restlessness and anxiety, which may progress to disorientation and confusion; and pale, cool, clammy skin occur.
- Other signs and symptoms include angina, dyspnea, jugular vein distention, oliguria, ventricular gallop, tachypnea, and weak, rapid pulse.

Cholera
- This life-threatening disorder causes watery diarrhea and vomiting.
- Water and electrolyte losses cause thirst, weakness, muscle cramps, decreased skin turgor, oliguria, tachycardia, and hypotension.
- Without treatment, death occurs within hours.

Dehydration
- Decreased intravascular fluid volume due to loss of body fluid causes drop in blood pressure.
- May be insidious loss due to diaphoresis, fever, overdiuresis, poor intake due to mentation changes.
- Signs and symptoms include dizziness, weakness, extreme thirst, fever, dry skin, dry mucous membranes, and poor skin turgor.
- If untreated, may progress to hypovolemic shock.

Diabetic ketoacidosis
- Hypovolemia—triggered by osmotic diuresis in hyperglycemia—causes low blood pressure.
- Other signs and symptoms include polydipsia, polyuria, polyphagia, dehydration, weight loss, abdominal pain, nausea, vomiting, breath with fruity odor, Kussmaul's respirations, tachycardia, seizures, confusion, and stupor that may progress to coma.

Heart failure
- Blood pressure fluctuates between normal and low.
- Auscultation reveals ventricular gallop, tachycardia, crackles, and tachypnea.
- Dependent edema, jugular vein distention, and hepatomegaly may also occur.
- Other signs and symptoms include dyspnea of abrupt or gradual onset, exertional dyspnea, orthopnea, paroxysmal nocturnal dyspnea, fatigue, weight gain, pallor or cyanosis, sweating, and anxiety.

Hypovolemic shock
- Systolic pressure falls to less than 80 mm Hg, or 30 mm Hg less than the patient's baseline, because of acute blood loss or dehydration.
- Other signs and symptoms include diminished Korotkoff sounds; narrowed pulse pressure; cyanosis of the extremities; pale, cool, clammy skin; rapid, weak, and irregular pulse; olig-

(continued)

uria; confusion; disorientation; restlessness; and anxiety.

Hypoxemia
◆ Initially, blood pressure may be normal or slightly elevated.
◆ Blood pressure drops as hypoxemia becomes pronounced.
◆ Other signs and symptoms include tachycardia, tachypnea, dyspnea, confusion, and stupor that may progress to coma.

Myocardial infarction
◆ In this life-threatening disorder, blood pressure may be low or high.
◆ A precipitous drop in blood pressure may signal cardiogenic shock.
◆ Other signs and symptoms include chest pain that may radiate to the jaw, shoulder, arm, or epigastrium; dyspnea; anxiety; nausea or vomiting; sweating; and cool, pale, or cyanotic skin.

Neurogenic shock
◆ Low blood pressure and bradycardia occur.
◆ Other signs and symptoms include warm, dry skin and, possibly, motor weakness of the limbs or diaphragm, depending on the cause of shock.

Pulmonary embolism
◆ Low blood pressure with narrowed pulse pressure and diminished Korotkoff sounds occur.
◆ Early signs and symptoms include sharp chest pain, dyspnea, and cough.
◆ Other signs and symptoms include tachycardia, tachypnea, paradoxical pulse, jugular vein distention, and hemoptysis.

Septic shock
◆ Initially, fever and chills occur.
◆ Low blood pressure, tachycardia, and tachypnea may also develop early, but the skin remains warm.
◆ Blood pressure continues to decrease, accompanied by a narrowed pulse pressure.
◆ Other late signs and symptoms include pale skin, cyanotic extremities, apprehension, thirst, oliguria, and coma.

Vasovagal syncope
◆ Low blood pressure, pallor, cold sweats, nausea, palpitations or slowed heart rate, and weakness follow stressful, painful, or claustrophobic experiences.

OTHER
Diagnostic tests
◆ A gastric acid stimulation test, using histamine, and X-ray studies, using contrast media, may cause low blood pressure.

Drugs
◆ Alpha and beta blockers, anxiolytics, calcium channel blockers, diuretics, general anesthetics, most I.V. antiarrhythmics, monoamine oxidase inhibitors, opioid analgesics, tranquilizers, and vasodilators can cause low blood pressure.

Normal pediatric blood pressure

AGE	NORMAL SYSTOLIC PRESSURE	NORMAL DIASTOLIC PRESSURE
Birth to 3 months	40 to 80 mm Hg	Not detectable
3 months to 1 year	80 to 100 mm Hg	Not detectable
1 to 4 years	100 to 108 mm Hg	60 mm Hg
4 to 12 years	108 to 120 mm Hg	60 to 70 mm Hg

NURSING CONSIDERATIONS

♦ Check vital signs frequently to determine if low blood pressure is constant or intermittent.
♦ If blood pressure remains extremely low, an arterial catheter to allow close monitoring may be inserted.
♦ Maintain bed rest, if indicated.
♦ Assist ambulatory patients, as needed.
♦ Don't leave a dizzy patient unattended when he's sitting or walking.
♦ Monitor intake and output, and daily weight.
♦ Administer I.V. fluids, as prescribed.
♦ If blood pressure remains low after fluid resusitation, administer vasopressors, as prescribed.

PEDIATRIC POINTERS

♦ Normal blood pressure is lower than that in adults. (See *Normal pediatric blood pressure.*)
♦ Suspect trauma or shock as a possible cause of low blood pressure.
♦ Dehydration may also cause low blood pressure.

GERIATRIC POINTERS

♦ Low blood pressure may occur as a result of taking several drugs that have such an adverse effect.
♦ Orthostatic hypotension may occur because of autonomic dysfunction.
♦ May have reduced sense of thirst.

PATIENT TEACHING

♦ Advise the patient with orthostatic hypotension to stand up slowly from a sitting position and to dangle his feet and rise slowly when getting out of bed.
♦ For patients with vasovagal syncope, discuss how to avoid triggers.
♦ Discuss the need for a cane or walker.
♦ Discuss maintaining adequate hydration.
♦ Instruct in home monitoring of the patient's blood pressure as appropriate.
♦ Discuss underlying condtion, diagnostic tests, and treatment options.

Blood pressure increase

- Intermittent or sustained increase in blood pressure exceeding 140/90 mm Hg
- Affects men more than women
- May develop gradually or suddenly (see *Pathophysiology of elevated blood pressure*)
- May indicate life-threatening condition if rise in blood pressure is sudden and severe (see *Managing elevated blood pressure*)

ACTION STAT! *If blood pressure rises above 180/110 mm Hg, suspect hypertensive crisis and treat immediately. Maintain a patent airway in case the patient vomits, and use seizure precautions. Give an I.V. antihypertensive and a diuretic, as ordered. Insert an indwelling urinary catheter to monitor urine output.*

Pathophysiology of elevated blood pressure

Blood pressure—the force blood exerts on vessels as it flows through them—depends on cardiac output, peripheral resistance, and blood volume. A brief review of its regulating mechanisms—nervous system control, capillary fluid shifts, kidney excretion, and hormonal changes—will help you understand how elevated blood pressure develops.

- *Nervous system control* involves the sympathetic system, chiefly baroreceptors and chemoreceptors, which promotes moderate vasoconstriction to maintain normal blood pressure. When this system responds inappropriately, increased vasoconstriction enhances peripheral resistance, resulting in elevated blood pressure.
- *Capillary fluid shifts* regulate blood volume by responding to arterial pressure. Increased pressure forces fluid into the interstitial space; decreased pressure allows it to be drawn back into the arteries by osmosis. However, this fluid shift may take several hours to adjust blood pressure.
- *Kidney excretion* also helps regulate blood volume by increasing or decreasing urine formation. Normally, an arterial pressure of about 60 mm Hg maintains urine output. When

pressure drops below this reading, urine formation ceases, thereby increasing blood volume. Conversely, when arterial pressure exceeds this reading, urine formation increases, thereby reducing blood volume. Like capillary fluid shifts, this mechanism may take several hours to adjust blood pressure.
- *Hormonal changes* reflect stimulation of the kidney's renin-angiotensin-aldosterone system in response to low arterial pressure. This system affects vasoconstriction, which increases arterial pressure, and stimulates aldosterone release, which regulates sodium retention—a key determinant of blood volume.

Elevated blood pressure signals the breakdown or inappropriate response of these pressure-regulating mechanisms. Its associated signs and symptoms concentrate in the target organs and tissues illustrated below.

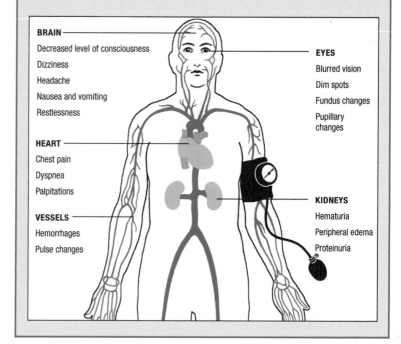

BRAIN
Decreased level of consciousness
Dizziness
Headache
Nausea and vomiting
Restlessness

HEART
Chest pain
Dyspnea
Palpitations

VESSELS
Hemorrhages
Pulse changes

EYES
Blurred vision
Dim spots
Fundus changes
Pupillary changes

KIDNEYS
Hematuria
Peripheral edema
Proteinuria

- Obtain a medical history, noting incidence of diabetes or cardiovascular, cerebrovascular, or renal disease or a family history of high blood pressure.
- Ask the patient about the onset of high blood pressure.
- Note associated signs and symptoms, including headache, palpitations, blurred vision, sweating, wine-colored urine, and decreased urine output.
- Take a drug history, including past and present prescriptions, herbal preparations, and over-the-counter (OTC) drugs.

- If the patient is taking antihypertensives, determine compliance to the drug regimen.
- Explore psychosocial or environmental factors that affect blood pressure control.

PHYSICAL ASSESSMENT

- Perform a funduscopic (ophthalmoscopic) examination.
- Perform a cardiovascular assessment; check for carotid bruits, peripheral edema, and jugular vein distention.
- Assess skin color, temperature, and turgor.
- Palpate peripheral pulses.
- Auscultate for abnormal heart sounds, rate, or rhythm.
- Auscultate for abnormal breath sounds, rate, or rhythm.
- Auscultate for abdominal bruits.
- Palpate the abdomen for tenderness, masses, and liver or kidney enlargement.

 ACTION STAT!

Managing elevated blood pressure

Elevated blood pressure can signal various life-threatening disorders. However, if pressure exceeds 180/110 mm Hg, the patient may be experiencing hypertensive crisis and may require prompt treatment. Maintain a patent airway in case the patient vomits, and institute seizure precautions. Prepare to administer an I.V. antihypertensive and diuretic. You'll also need to insert an indwelling urinary catheter to accurately monitor urine output.

If blood pressure is less severely elevated, continue to rule out other life-threatening causes. If the patient is pregnant, suspect preeclampsia or eclampsia. Place her on bed rest, and insert an I.V. line. Administer magnesium sulfate (to decrease neuromuscular irritability) and an antihypertensive. Monitor her vital signs closely for the next 24 hours. If diastolic blood pressure continues to exceed 100 mm Hg despite drug therapy, you may need to prepare the patient for induced labor and delivery or for cesarean birth. Offer emotional support if she must face delivery of a premature neonate.

If the patient isn't pregnant, quickly observe for equally obvious clues. Assess the patient for exophthalmos and an enlarged thyroid gland. If these signs are present, ask about a history of hyperthyroidism. Then look for other associated signs and symptoms, including

tachycardia, widened pulse pressure, palpitations, severe weakness, diarrhea, fever exceeding 100° F (37.8° C), and nervousness. Prepare to administer an antithyroid drug orally or by nasogastric tube, if necessary. Also, evaluate fluid status; look for signs of dehydration, such as poor skin turgor. Prepare the patient for I.V. fluid replacement and temperature control using a cooling blanket, if necessary.

If the patient shows signs of increased intracranial pressure (such as a decreased level of consciousness and fixed or dilated pupils), ask him or a family member if he has recently experienced head trauma. Then check for an increased respiratory rate and bradycardia. You'll need to maintain a patent airway in case the patient vomits. In addition, institute seizure precautions, and prepare to give an I.V. diuretic. Insert an indwelling urinary catheter, and monitor intake and output. Check his vital signs every 15 minutes until he's stable.

If the patient has absent or weak peripheral pulses, ask about chest pressure or pain, which suggests a dissecting aortic aneurysm. Enforce bed rest until a diagnosis has been established. As appropriate, give the patient an I.V. antihypertensive or prepare him for surgery.

(continued)

MEDICAL
Anemia
◆ Elevated systolic pressure may occur.
◆ Other signs and symptoms include pulsations in the capillary beds, bounding pulse, tachycardia, systolic ejection murmur, and pale mucous membranes.

Aortic aneurysm, dissecting
◆ Initially, a sudden rise in systolic pressure occurs, but diastolic pressure remains stable.
◆ Hypotension occurs as the body's ability to compensate fails.
◆ With an abdominal aneursym, associated signs and symptoms include abdominal and back pain, weakness, sweating, tachycardia, dyspnea, a pulsating abdominal mass, restlessness, confusion, and cool, clammy skin may occur.
◆ With a thoracic aneurysm, associated signs and symptoms include a ripping or tearing sensation in the chest, which may radiate to the neck, shoulders, lower back, or abdomen; pallor; syncope; blindness; loss of consciousness; sweating; dyspnea; tachycardia; cyanosis; leg weakness; murmur; and absent radial and femoral pulses.

Atherosclerosis
◆ Systolic pressure rises, but diastolic pressure remains normal or slightly elevated.
◆ The patient may be asymptomatic.
◆ Other signs and symptoms may include a weak pulse, flushed skin, tachycardia, angina, and claudication.

Cushing's syndrome
◆ Blood pressure elevates and pulse pressure widens due to abnormal hormone levels.
◆ Other findings include truncal obesity, "moon" face, and other cushingoid signs.

Hypertension
◆ Essential hypertension develops insidiously; blood pressure increases gradually.
◆ The patient may be asymptomatic.
◆ Malignant hypertension results when diastolic pressure abruptly rises above 120 mm Hg; systolic pressure may exceed 200 mm Hg.
◆ Pulmonary edema is a common sign.
◆ Other signs and symptoms include severe headache, confusion, blurred vision, tinnitus, epistaxis, muscle twitching, chest pain, nausea, and vomiting.

Increased intracranial pressure
◆ Respiratory rate increases initially, followed by increased systolic pressure and widened pulse pressure.
◆ Bradycardia is a late sign.
◆ Other signs and symptoms include headache, projectile vomiting, decreased level of consciousness, and fixed or dilated pupils.

Myocardial infarction
◆ Blood pressure may be high or low.
◆ Crushing chest pain may radiate to the jaw, shoulder, arm, or epigastrium.
◆ Other signs and symptoms include dyspnea, anxiety, nausea, vomiting, weakness, diaphoresis, atrial gallop, and murmurs.

Pheochromocytoma
◆ Paroxysmal or sustained elevated blood pressure occurs with possible orthostatic hypotension.
◆ Other findings include anxiety, diaphoresis, palpitations, tremors, pallor, nausea, weight loss, and headache.
◆ Hematuria, life-threatening retroperitoneal bleeding, proteinuria, and colicky abdominal pain may occur in advanced stages.

Preeclampsia and eclampsia
◆ Blood pressure increases to 140/90 mm Hg or more in the first trimester of pregnancy; to 130/80 mm Hg or more in the second or third trimester; to 30 mm Hg above baseline systolic pressure; or to 15 mm Hg above baseline diastolic pressure.
◆ Other signs and symptoms include generalized edema, sudden weight gain of 3 lb (1.4 kg) or more per week during the second or third trimester, severe frontal headache, blurred or double vision, decreased urine output, proteinuria, midabdominal pain, neuromuscular irritability, nausea, and seizures.

Renovascular stenosis
◆ Systolic and diastolic pressure rise abruptly.
◆ Other characteristic signs and symptoms include bruits over the upper abdomen or in the costovertebral angles, hematuria, and acute flank pain.

Thyrotoxicosis
◆ In this life-threatening disorder, elevated systolic pressure occurs.
◆ Other signs and symptoms include widened pulse pressure, tachycardia, bounding pulse, pulsations in the capillary nail beds, palpitations, weight loss, exophthalmos, enlarged thyroid gland, weakness, diarrhea, fever, nervousness, emotional instability, heat intolerance, exertional dyspnea, decreased or absent menses, and warm, moist skin.

OTHER
Drugs
◆ Central nervous system stimulants, corticosteroids, hormonal contraceptives, monoamine oxidase inhibitors, nonsteroidal anti-inflammatory drugs, sympathomimetics, and OTC cold remedies can increase blood pressure.
◆ Cocaine use may increase blood pressure.

Treatments
◆ Kidney dialysis or transplant may cause temporary elevation of blood pressure.

NURSING CONSIDERATIONS

◆ Stress the need for follow-up diagnostic tests.
◆ Monitor cardiovascular status closely.

PEDIATRIC POINTERS

◆ Elevated blood pressure may result from such conditions as lead or mercury poisoning, chronic pyelonephritis, coarctation of the aorta, patent ductus arteriosus, glomerulonephritis, adrenogenital syndrome, or neuroblastoma.

GERIATRIC POINTERS

◆ Atherosclerosis produces isolated systolic hypertension.

PATIENT TEACHING

◆ Emphasize the importance of weight loss and exercise.
◆ Explain the need for sodium restriction.
◆ Discuss stress management.
◆ Discuss ways of reducing other risk factors for coronary artery disease.
◆ Discuss the importance of regular blood pressure monitoring.
◆ Explain how to take prescribed antihypertensives correctly.
◆ Explain what adverse drug reactions the patient should report.
◆ Emphasize the importance of long-term follow-up care.

Bowel sounds, absent (silent)

OVERVIEW

- Characterized by an inability to hear bowel sounds in any quadrant with a stethoscope after listening for at least 5 minutes (see *Are bowel sounds really absent?*)
- When mechanical or vascular obstruction or neurogenic inhibition halts peristalsis, bowel sounds absent
- Life-threatening complications: bowel perforation, peritonitis, sepsis, and hypovolemic shock
- Life-threatening crisis: abrupt stopping of bowel sounds with abdominal pain, rigidity, and distention
- Absent bowel sounds following a period of hyperactive sounds: bowel strangulation or a mechanically obstructed bowel

 ACTION STAT! *If accompanied by sudden, severe abdominal pain and cramping or severe abdominal distention, insert a nasogastric (NG) or intestinal tube to suction lumen contents and decompress the bowel. Give I.V. fluids and electrolytes. Withhold oral intake in the event that surgery is warranted. Take the patient's vital signs, and watch for signs of shock, such as hypotension, tachycardia, and cool, clammy skin. Measure abdominal girth to establish a baseline.*

HISTORY

- Ask about the onset and description of abdominal pain.
- Obtain a description of bowel movements and ask the patient if he has had diarrhea or has passed pencil-thin stools (a possible sign of a developing luminal obstruction).
- Obtain a medical and surgical history, including recent accidents, abdominal tumors, hernias, adhesions from past surgery, acute pancreatitis, diverticulitis, gynecologic infection, uremia, or spinal cord injury.

 TOP TECHNIQUE

Are bowel sounds really absent?

Before concluding that your patient has absent bowel sounds, ask yourself these three questions:
- Did I use the diaphragm of my stethoscope to auscultate for the bowel sounds? The diaphragm detects high-frequency sounds, such as bowel sounds, whereas the bell detects low-frequency sounds, such as a vascular bruit or a venous hum.
- Did I listen for at least 5 minutes for the presence of bowel sounds? Normally, bowel sounds occur every 5 to 15 seconds, but the duration of a single sound may be less than 1 second.
- Did I listen for bowel sounds in all quadrants? Bowel sounds may be absent in one quadrant but present in another.

PHYSICAL ASSESSMENT

- Inspect abdominal contour.
- Observe for distention.
- Gently percuss and palpate the abdomen.
- Listen for dullness over fluid-filled areas and for tympany over pockets of gas.
- Palpate for abdominal rigidity and guarding.
- Obtain vital signs.

MEDICAL
Abdominal surgery
◆ Bowel sounds are normally temporarily absent after abdominal surgery.

Complete mechanical intestinal obstruction
◆ In this potentially life-threatening condition, absent bowel sounds follow hyperactive sounds.
◆ Colicky abdominal pain, which may radiate, arises in the quadrant with the obstruction.
◆ Signs of shock, fever, rebound tenderness, and abdominal rigidity may occur in later stages.
◆ Other signs and symptoms include abdominal distention, bloating, constipation, nausea, and vomiting.

Mesenteric artery occlusion
◆ Bowel sounds disappear after a brief period of hyperactive sounds.
◆ Midepigastric or periumbilical pain occurs next, followed by abdominal distention, bruits, vomiting, constipation, and signs of shock.
◆ Abdominal rigidity may appear later.

Paralytic ileus
◆ Absent bowel sounds are a hallmark sign.
◆ If paralytic ileus follows acute abdominal infection, fever and abdominal pain may occur.
◆ Other signs and symptoms include abdominal distention, generalized discomfort, and constipation or passage of small, liquid stools.

◆ After NG or intestinal tube insertion, elevate the head of the bed at least 30 degrees.
◆ Turn the patient to facilitate passage of the tube through the GI tract.
◆ Ensure tube patency.
◆ Continue to give I.V. fluids and electrolytes, as prescribed.
◆ Once mechanical obstruction and intra-abdominal sepsis have been ruled out, give drugs to control pain and stimulate peristalsis.

PEDIATRIC POINTERS
◆ Absent bowel sounds in children may result from Hirschsprung's disease or intussusception; these conditions may lead to life-threatening obstruction.

GERIATRIC POINTERS
◆ If a bowel obstruction doesn't respond to decompression, early surgical intervention should be considered to avoid the risk of bowel infarct

◆ Explain diagnostic tests and therapeutic procedures that are needed.
◆ Explain which foods and fluids the patient should avoid.
◆ Explain the need for postoperative ambulation.

Bowel sounds, hyperactive

- Reflect increased intestinal motility
- Characterized as rapid, rushing, gurgling waves of sounds (see *Characterizing bowel sounds*)
- May be caused by life-threatening disorder or a chronic disease

ACTION STAT! *Take the patient's vital signs, and ask him about other symptoms, such as abdominal pain, vomiting, and diarrhea. If he has cramping abdominal pain or is vomiting, continue to auscultate for bowel sounds. If bowel sounds stop abruptly, suspect complete bowel obstruction. Assist with GI suction and decompression, give I.V. fluids and electrolytes, and prepare the patient for surgery.*

If the patient has diarrhea, record its frequency, amount, color, and consistency. If you detect excessive watery diarrhea or bleeding, give an antidiarrheal, I.V. fluids and electrolytes and, possibly, blood transfusions.

HISTORY

- Obtain a medical and surgical history, including abdominal surgeries or previous inflammatory bowel disease.
- Ask the patient about recent exposure to gastroenteritis.
- Determine whether the patient has traveled recently.
- Inquire about possible stress factors.
- Ask about allergies and recent food and fluid consumption.

PHYSICAL ASSESSMENT

- Take vital signs.
- Check for fever.
- After auscultation, gently inspect, percuss, and palpate the abdomen.

CAUSES

MEDICAL
Crohn's disease
- Hyperactive bowel sounds arise insidiously, due to this inflammatory disorder.
- Muscle wasting, weight loss, and signs of dehydration may occur as the disease progresses.
- Other signs and symptoms include diarrhea, anorexia, low-grade fever, abdominal distention and tenderness, cramping abdominal pain that may be relieved by defecation, and a fixed mass in the right lower quadrant of the abdomen.

Gastroenteritis
- Hyperactive bowel sounds follow sudden nausea and vomiting.
- The patient has explosive diarrhea.
- Abdominal cramping or pain is common.
- Fever may occur, depending on the causative organism.

GI hemorrhage
- Hyperactive bowel sounds indicate upper GI bleeding.
- Decreased urine output, tachycardia, and hypotension accompany blood loss.
- Other signs and symptoms include hematemesis, coffee-ground vomitus, abdominal distention, bloody diarrhea, rectal passage of bright red clots and jellylike material or melena, and pain.

Malabsorption
- Lactose intolerance typically results in hyperactive bowel sounds.
- Other signs and symptoms include diarrhea and, possibly, nausea and vomiting, angioedema, and urticaria.

Mechanical intestinal obstruction
- A potentially life-threatening disorder, hyperactive bowel sounds occur with cramping abdominal pain every few minutes.
- Bowel sounds may later become hypoactive and then disappear.

TOP TECHNIQUE

Characterizing bowel sounds

The sounds of swallowed air and fluid moving through the GI tract are known as bowel sounds. These sounds usually occur every 5 to 15 seconds, but their frequency may be irregular. For example, bowel sounds are normally more active just before and after a meal. Bowel sounds may last less than 1 second or up to several seconds.

To accurately assess bowel sounds, you need to be aware of the various types:

- *Normal bowel sounds* can be characterized as murmuring, gurgling, or tinkling.
- *Hyperactive bowel sounds* can be characterized as loud, gurgling, splashing, and rushing; they're higher pitched and occur more frequently than normal sounds.
- *Hypoactive bowel sounds* can be characterized as softer or lower in tone and less frequent than normal sounds.

- Nausea and vomiting occur earlier and with greater severity in small-bowel obstruction than in large-bowel obstruction.
- Abdominal distention and constipation accompany hyperactive bowel sounds in complete obstruction, although the bowel furthest from the obstruction may continue to empty for up to 3 days.

Ulcerative colitis, acute
- Hyperactive bowel sounds arise abruptly.
- Bloody diarrhea occurs, with accompanying anorexia, abdominal pain, nausea and vomiting, fever, and tenesmus.
- Weight loss, arthralgia, and arthritis may also occur.

NURSING CONSIDERATIONS

If the patient has GI bleeding:
- Insert an I.V. line for giving fluids and blood.
- Restrict food and oral fluids.
- Give drugs, such as vasopressin to manage bleeding.
- Insert a nasogastric tube to suction and monitor drainage.

PEDIATRIC POINTERS
- Hyperactive bowel sounds in children usually result from gastroenteritis, erratic eating habits, excessive ingestion of certain foods, or food allergy.

PATIENT TEACHING

- Explain dietary changes that are necessary or beneficial.
- Explain what physical activity the patient should avoid.
- Discuss stress reduction techniques.
- Discuss underlying condition, diagnostic tests, and treatment options.

Bowel sounds, hypoactive

OVERVIEW

- Bowel sounds diminished in regularity, tone, and loudness
- Result if peristalsis is decreased, a situation that may occur as a result of bowel obstruction
- May precede absent bowel sounds, a possible sign of a life-threatening condition

HISTORY

- Ask about the location, onset, frequency, and severity of pain—cramping or colicky abdominal pain usually indicates mechanical bowel obstruction; whereas diffuse abdominal pain usually indicates intestinal distention from paralytic ileus.
- Obtain a description of any recent vomiting or constipation.
- Obtain a medical and surgical history, including conditions that may cause mechanical bowel obstruction.
- Note the patient's treatment history, including radiation and drug therapy.

PHYSICAL ASSESSMENT

- Inspect the abdomen for distention, noting surgical incisions and obvious masses.
- Gently percuss and palpate the abdomen for masses, gas, fluid, tenderness, and rigidity.
- Measure abdominal girth.
- Check for signs of dehydration and electrolyte imbalance.

CAUSES

MEDICAL

Mechanical intestinal obstruction

◆ Bowel sounds may become hypoactive after a period of hyperactive bowel sounds.
◆ If obstruction becomes complete, signs of shock may occur.
◆ Other signs and symptoms include acute colicky abdominal pain in the quadrant with obstruction, possibly radiating to the flank or lumbar region; nausea and vomiting; and abdominal distention and bloating.

Mesenteric artery occlusion

◆ Bowel sounds become hypoactive after a brief period of hyperactivity and then quickly disappear, signifying a life-threatening crisis.
◆ Abdominal rigidity is a late sign.
◆ Other signs and symptoms include fever; a history of colicky abdominal pain leading to sudden and severe midepigastric or periumbilical pain, followed by abdominal distention and possible bruits; vomiting; constipation; and signs of shock.

Paralytic ileus

◆ Bowel sounds are hypoactive and may become absent.
◆ If the disorder follows acute abdominal infection, fever and abdominal pain may occur.
◆ Other signs and symptoms include abdominal distention and constipation or passage of small, liquid stools and flatus.

OTHER

Drugs

◆ Anticholinergics, general or spinal anesthetics, opiates, phenothiazine, and vinca alkaloids may cause hypoactive bowel sounds.

Surgery

◆ Surgery involving the bowel may produce hypoactive bowel sounds from manipulation of the bowel. Motility and bowel sounds in the small intestine usually resume within 24 hours; colonic bowel sounds, in 3 to 5 days.

NURSING CONSIDERATIONS

◆ Frequently evaluate for signs and symptoms of shock.
◆ Be alert for sudden absence of bowel sounds; monitor vital signs, and auscultate for bowel sounds every 2 to 4 hours.
◆ If GI suction and decompression are needed, maintain tube patency and provide oral and nasal hygiene.
◆ Withhold food and oral fluids.
◆ If severe pain, abdominal rigidity, guarding, and fever accompany hypoactive bowel sounds, perform emergency interventions to treat paralytic ileus from peritonitis.
◆ Give I.V. fluids and electrolytes.
◆ Prepare the patient for diagnostic studies, such as X-rays and endoscopic procedures.

PEDIATRIC POINTERS

◆ Hypoactive bowel sounds in a child may be caused by bowel distention from excessive swallowing of air while eating or crying.
◆ Observe the child for further signs of illness.

PATIENT TEACHING

◆ Tell the caregiver that ambulation or frequent turning are important.
◆ Teach the patient or caregiver about the need for diagnostic tests and procedures.
◆ Tell the patient or caregiver to maintain food and fluid restrictions.

Bradycardia

OVERVIEW

- Refers to a heart rate of fewer than 60 beats/minute
- Occurs normally but can also result from pathologic causes (see *Managing life-threatening bradycardia*)

HISTORY

- Ask about a family history of slow pulse rate.
- Obtain a medical history, including underlying metabolic disorders.
- Ask about current drugs and the patient's compliance.
- Find out if the patient is an athlete and his degree of physical activity.

PHYSICAL ASSESSMENT

- Monitor vital signs and oxygen saturation.
- Perform a complete cardiac assessment.
- After detecting bradycardia, look for related signs and symptoms to identify the cause.

ACTION STAT!

Managing life-threatening bradycardia

Bradycardia can signal a life-threatening disorder when accompanied by pain, shortness of breath, dizziness, syncope, or other symptoms; prolonged exposure to cold; or head or neck trauma. In such patients, quickly take vital signs. Connect the patient to a cardiac monitor, and insert an I.V. line. Depending on the cause of bradycardia, you'll need to administer fluids, atropine, steroids, or thyroid medication. If indicated, insert an indwelling urinary catheter. Intubation and mechanical ventilation may be necessary if the patient's respiratory rate falls. Assist with the placement of a pacemaker if medications don't increase the heart rate.

Perform a focused assessment to help locate the cause of bradycardia. For example, ask about pain. Viselike pressure or crushing or burning chest pain that radiates to the arms, back, or jaw may indicate an acute myocardial infarction (MI); a severe headache may indicate increased intracranial pressure. Also, ask about nausea, vomiting, or shortness of breath—signs and symptoms associated with an acute MI and cardiomyopathy. Observe the patient for peripheral cyanosis, edema, or jugular vein distention, any of which may indicate cardiomyopathy. Look for a thyroidectomy scar because severe bradycardia may result from hypothyroidism caused by failure to take thyroid hormone replacements.

If the cause of bradycardia is evident, provide supportive care. For example, keep the hypothermic patient warm by applying blankets, and monitor his core temperature until it reaches 99° F (37.2° C); stabilize the head and neck of a trauma patient until cervical spinal injury is ruled out.

MEDICAL

Cardiac arrhythmia

◆ Bradycardia may be transient or sustained, benign, or life-threatening.
◆ Other signs and symptoms include hypotension, palpitations, dizziness, weakness, dyspnea, chest pain, decreased urine output, altered level of consciousness (LOC), syncope, and fatigue.

Cardiomyopathy

◆ A life-threatening disorder, transient or sustained bradycardia may occur.
◆ Other signs and symptoms include dizziness, syncope, edema, fatigue, jugular vein distention, orthopnea, dyspnea, and peripheral cyanosis.

Cervical spinal injury

◆ Bradycardia may be transient or sustained, depending on the severity of the injury.
◆ Other signs and symptoms include hypotension, decreased body temperature, slowed peristalsis, leg paralysis, and partial arm and respiratory muscle paralysis.

Hypothermia

◆ If the patient's core temperature drops below 86° F (30° C), he may not have a palpable pulse or audible heart sounds.
◆ Other signs and symptoms include shivering, peripheral cyanosis, muscle rigidity, bradypnea, and confusion leading to stupor.

Hypothyroidism

◆ Severe bradycardia is accompanied by fatigue, constipation, unexplained weight gain, and sensitivity to cold.
◆ Related signs and symptoms include cool, dry, thick skin; sparse, dry hair; facial swelling; periorbital edema; thick, brittle nails; and confusion leading to stupor.

Myocardial infarction

◆ Sinus bradycardia is common.
◆ Abnormal heart sounds may be heard on auscultation.

◆ Other signs and symptoms include an aching, burning, or viselike pressure in the chest, which may radiate to the jaw, shoulder, arm, back, or epigastric area; nausea and vomiting; cool, clammy, and pale or cyanotic skin; anxiety; and dyspnea.

OTHER

Diagnostic tests

◆ Cardiac catheterization and electrophysiologic studies can induce temporary bradycardia.

Drugs

◆ Protamine and some antiarrhythmics, beta blockers, cardiac glycosides, calcium channel blockers, sympatholytics, and topical miotics may cause transient bradycardia.
◆ Not taking a thyroid replacement may cause bradycardia.

Invasive treatments

◆ Cardiac surgery can result in edema or damage to the conduction tissue, causing bradycardia.
◆ Suctioning can induce hypoxia and vagal stimulation, causing bradycardia.

◆ Look for changes in cardiac rhythm, respiratory rate, and LOC.
◆ Prepare the patient for 24-hour Holter monitoring.

PEDIATRIC POINTERS

◆ Fetal bradycardia, characterized by heart rate less than 120 beats/minute, may occur during prolonged labor or complications of delivery.
◆ Intermittent bradycardia commonly occurs in premature infants.
◆ Congenital heart defects, acute glomerulonephritis, and transient or complete heart block associated with cardiac catheterization or cardiac surgery can cause bradycardia in full-term infants and in children.

GERIATRIC POINTERS

◆ Sinus node dysfunction is the most common bradyarrhythmia in elderly patients.
◆ Carefully scrutinize the patient's drug regimen.

◆ Inform the patient about signs and symptoms he should report.
◆ Give instructions for pulse measurement, and explain the parameters for calling the physician and seeking emergency care.
◆ If a patient is getting a pacemaker, explain its use, postoperative care, and required follow-up assessments.

Bradypnea

- Involves a pattern of regular respirations with a rate of less than 10 breaths/minute
- May precede life-threatening apnea or respiratory arrest
- Results from neurologic and metabolic disorders and drug overdose, which depress the brain's respiratory control centers (see *Understanding how the nervous system controls breathing*)

 ACTION STAT! *If the patient requires constant stimulation to breathe, try to rouse him by shaking him and telling him to breathe. Quickly assess his vital signs and neurologic status. Place the patient on a pulse oximeter or apnea monitor, keep emergency airway equipment readily available, and assist with intubation and mechanical ventilation. To prevent aspiration, position the patient on his side or keep his head elevated 30 degrees. Suction the airway, if needed.*

HISTORY

- Ask about whether a drug overdose is possible; find out the names, doses, time frames, and routes of the drugs taken.
- Obtain a medical history.

PHYSICAL ASSESSMENT

- Assess vital signs.
- Perform a complete physical assessment, paying particular attention to the cardiopulmonary portion.

Understanding how the nervous system controls breathing

Stimulation from the external sources and from higher brain centers acts on respiratory centers in the pons and medulla. These centers, in turn, send impulses to the various parts of the respiratory system to alter respiration patterns.

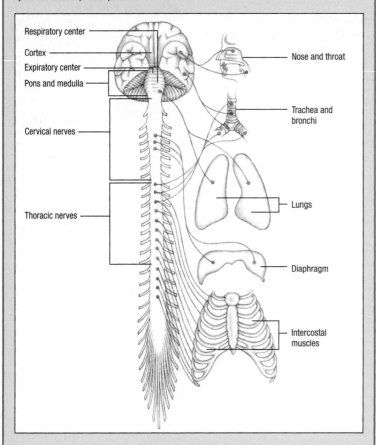

Respiratory center
Cortex
Expiratory center
Pons and medulla
Cervical nerves
Thoracic nerves

Nose and throat
Trachea and bronchi
Lungs
Diaphragm
Intercostal muscles

CAUSES

MEDICAL
Diabetic ketoacidosis
- In patients with severe, uncontrolled diabetes, bradypnea occurs late.
- Other signs and symptoms include decreased LOC, fatigue, weakness, fruity breath odor, and oliguria.

Increased intracranial pressure
- Bradypnea is a late sign.
- Bradypnea is preceded by decreased LOC, deteriorating motor function, and fixed, dilated pupils.
- The triad of bradypnea, bradycardia, and hypertension is a classic sign of late medullary strangulation.

Respiratory failure
- Bradypnea occurs during end-stage respiratory failure.
- Restlessness, confusion, irritability, and a decreased LOC may also occur.
- Other signs and symptoms include cyanosis, diminished breath sounds, tachycardia, and mildly increased blood pressure.

OTHER
Drugs
- Overdose with an opioid analgesic, sedative, barbiturate, phenothiazine, or another central nervous system (CNS) depressant can cause bradypnea.
- Use of alcohol with these drugs can also cause bradypnea.

NURSING CONSIDERATIONS

- Check respiratory status frequently, and give ventilatory support, if needed.
- Monitor arterial blood gas analysis, electrolyte studies, and drug screening.
- Give oxygen and prescribed drugs, avoiding CNS depressants, which can exacerbate bradypnea.
- Review all drugs and dosages taken during the last 24 hours.

PEDIATRIC POINTERS
- Because respiratory rates are higher in children than in adults, bradypnea in children is defined according to age. (See *Respiratory rates in children.*)

GERIATRIC POINTERS
- Older patients have a higher risk of developing bradypnea from drug toxicity.

PATIENT TEACHING

- Explain the complications of opioid therapy—such as bradypnea.
- Discuss the signs and symptoms of opioid toxicity.
- Discuss underlying disorder, diagnostic tests, and treatment options.

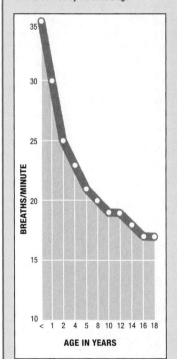

Respiratory rates in children

This graph shows normal respiratory rates in children, which are higher than normal rates in adults. Accordingly, bradypnea in a child is defined by the child's age.

Breast dimpling

- Puckering or retraction of skin on the breast
- Results from abnormal attachment of the skin to underlying tissue
- Suggests an inflammatory or malignant mass beneath the skin surface and usually represents a late sign of breast cancer
- Usually affects women older than age 40, but it also occasionally affects men

HISTORY

- Obtain a medical, reproductive, and family history, noting factors that increase the patient's risk of breast cancer.
- Obtain a pregnancy history because women who haven't had a full-term pregnancy before age 30 have a higher risk of developing breast cancer.
- Ask about the patient's dietary habits because a high-fat diet predisposes women to breast cancer.
- Ask the patient if she has noticed any changes in the shape of her breast or if there are any painful or tender areas.
- If she's breast-feeding, ask if she recently experienced high fever, chills, malaise, muscle aches, fatigue, or other flulike signs or symptoms.

PHYSICAL ASSESSMENT

- Inspect the dimpled area for redness, swelling, warmth, bruises or contusions.
- Ask the patient to tense her pectoral muscles by pressing her hips with both hands or by raising her hands over her head and see if the puckering increases. Gently pull the skin upward toward the clavicle and observe for exaggerated dimpling.
- Observe the breast for nipple retraction, nipple discharge, and breast symmetry.
- Examine both breasts with the patient supine, sitting, and then leaning forward. If you can palpate a lump, describe its size, location, consistency, mobility, and delineation.
- Examine breast and axillary lymph nodes, noting any enlargement.

CAUSES

MEDICAL
Breast abscess
- Breast dimpling sometimes accompanies a chronic breast abscess.
- Axillary lymph nodes may be enlarged.
- Other findings include a firm, irregular, nontender lump and signs of nipple retraction, such as deviation, inversion, or flattening.

Breast cancer
- Breast dimpling is an important but somewhat late sign of breast cancer.
- A neoplasm that causes dimpling is usually close to the skin and at least 1 cm in diameter. It feels irregularly shaped and fixed to underlying tissue, and it's usually painless.
- Axillary lymph nodes may be enlarged.
- Pain may be present but isn't a reliable symptom of breast cancer.
- A breast ulcer may appear as a late sign.
- Other signs and symptoms include peau d'orange, changes in breast symmetry or size, nipple retraction, and a unilateral, spontaneous, nonmilky nipple discharge that's serous or bloody. (A bloody nipple discharge in the presence of a lump is a classic sign of breast cancer.)

Fat necrosis
- Breast dimpling due to fat necrosis follows inflammation and trauma to the fatty tissue of the breast (although the patient usually can't remember such trauma).
- Tenderness, erythema, bruising, and contusions may occur.
- Other signs and symptoms include a firm, irregular, fixed mass and skin retraction signs, such as skin dimpling and nipple retraction. (Fat necrosis is difficult to differentiate from breast cancer.)

Mastitis

- Breast dimpling may signal bacterial mastitis, which usually results from duct obstruction and milk stasis during lactation.
- Signs and symptoms include heat, erythema, swelling, induration, pain, and tenderness.
- Dimpling is more likely to occur with diffuse induration than with a single hard mass. The skin on the breast may feel fixed to underlying tissue.
- Other possible signs and symptoms include nipple retraction, nipple cracks, a purulent discharge, and enlarged axillary lymph nodes. Flulike signs and symptoms (such as fever, malaise, fatigue, and aching) are common.

NURSING CONSIDERATIONS

- Remember that any breast problem can arouse fears of mutilation, loss of sexuality, and death. Allow the patient to express her feelings.

PEDIATRIC POINTERS

- Because breast cancer, the most likely cause of dimpling, is extremely rare in children, consider trauma as a likely cause.
- As in adults, breast dimpling may occur in adolescents from fatty tissue necrosis due to trauma.

PATIENT TEACHING

- Provide a clear explanation of diagnostic tests that may be ordered, such as mammography, thermography, ultrasonography, cytology of nipple discharge, and biopsy.
- Discuss breast self-examination, and provide follow-up teaching when the patient expresses a readiness to learn.

Breast nodule

OVERVIEW

- Also known as *breast lumps*
- Two chief causes: benign breast disease and cancer
- Less than 20% malignant

HISTORY

- Ask the patient for a description of the lump and how long she's had it.
- Ask the patient about other signs and symptoms.
- Determine whether the patient has ever breast-fed.
- Obtain a medical and family history.
- Determine the patient's risk factors for breast cancer risk.

PHYSICAL ASSESSMENT

- Perform a thorough breast examination.
- Carefully palpate a suspected breast nodule, noting its location, shape, size, consistency, mobility, and delineation.
- Inspect and palpate the skin over the nodule for warmth, redness, and edema.
- Palpate the lymph nodes of the breast and axilla for enlargement.
- Observe the contour of the breasts, looking for asymmetry and irregularities.
- Look for signs of retraction, such as skin dimpling and nipple deviation or flattening.
- Note any nipple discharge that occurs spontaneously, comes from only one breast, and isn't milky.

MEDICAL

Adenofibroma

◆ The nodule usually occurs singly and feels firm, slippery, elastic, and round or lobular, with well-defined margins.
◆ The nodule is painless, grows rapidly, and usually lies around the nipple or upper outer quadrant.

Areolar gland abscess

◆ A tender, palpable abscess on the border of the areola develops following an inflammation of Montgomery's glands.
◆ Fever, local swelling, drainage, and malaise may also occur.

Breast abscess

◆ The nodule is localized, hot, tender, and fluctuant, with erythema and peau d'orange.
◆ With a chronic abscess, the nodule is nontender, irregular, firm, and may feel like a thick wall of fibrous tissue; other findings include skin dimpling, peau d'orange, nipple retraction, and axillary lymphadenopathy.
◆ Associated signs and symptoms include fever, chills, malaise, and generalized discomfort.

Breast cancer

◆ The nodule is hard, poorly delineated, and fixed to the skin or underlying tissue.
◆ Nodules usually occur singly, developing in the upper outer quadrant 40% to 50% of the time.
◆ Satellite nodules may surround the main one.
◆ Breast ulcer is a late sign.
◆ Other signs and symptoms include serous or bloody nipple discharge (common); breast dimpling; nipple deviation or retraction; flattening of the nipple or breast contour; peau d'orange; erythema; tenderness; and axillary lymphadenopathy.

Fibrocystic breast disease

◆ Smooth, round, slightly elastic nodules, increase in size and tenderness just before menstruation.
◆ Nodules are mobile, which differentiates them from malignant nodules.
◆ They may occur in fine, granular clusters in both breasts or as widespread, well-defined lumps in varying sizes.
◆ Other findings include thickening of adjacent tissue and premenstrual syndrome.

Intraductal papilloma

◆ Nodules are tiny, benign, soft, poorly delineated, and usually resist palpation.
◆ Serous or bloody nipple discharge is the primary sign.
◆ Breast pain and tenderness may occur.

Mammary duct ectasia

◆ A rubbery breast nodule lies under the areola.
◆ Other signs and symptoms include transient pain, itching, tenderness, and erythema of the areola; thick, sticky, multicolored nipple discharge from multiple ducts; nipple retraction; bluish green or peau d'orange skin over the mass; and lymphadenopathy.

Mastitis

◆ Nodules feel firm and hard or tender, flocculent, and discrete.
◆ Skin dimpling; nipple deviation, retraction, or flattening; and nipple crack or abrasion may occur.
◆ Other signs and symptoms include breast warmth, erythema, tenderness, peau d'orange, high fever, chills, malaise, and fatigue.

Paget's disease

◆ Paget's disease is characterized by a scaling, eczematoid, single nipple lesion that progresses to a deep mass.
◆ Later, the nipple becomes reddened and excoriated and may eventually be completely destroyed.

◆ Provide a simple explanation of your examination.
◆ Encourage the patient to express feelings about nodules.
◆ Although most nodules in breast-feeding women are from mastitis, the possibility of cancer demands careful evaluation.

PEDIATRIC POINTERS

◆ Most nodules in children and adolescents reflect the normal response of breast tissue to hormonal fluctuations.

GERIATRIC POINTERS

◆ In women age 70 and older, 75% of all breast lumps are malignant.

◆ Teach the patient the techniques of breast self-examination.
◆ Explain how to treat mastitis.
◆ Discuss underlying condition, diagnostic tests, and treatment options.

Breast pain

OVERVIEW

- Also called *mastalgia*
- Commonly results from benign breast disease
- May occur during rest or movement
- May be aggravated by manipulation or palpation
- May be in one or both breasts
- May be cyclic; intermittent or constant; dull or sharp
- May occur normally before menstruation as a result of increased mammary blood flow caused by hormonal changes
- May occur normally during pregnancy as a result of hormonal changes

HISTORY

- Ask the patient when the pain started and to describe it.
- Ask about duration of pain (constant or intermittent).
- Find out if the patient is nursing, pregnant, menopausal, or post-menopausal.
- Question the patient about injury or changes to breast.

PHYSICAL ASSESSMENT

- With the patient standing or sitting with arms at the sides, note breast size, symmetry, and contour, and the appearance of the skin.
- Note the size, shape, and symmetry of the nipples and areolae.
- Repeat your inspection with the patient's arms raised over the head and then with the hands pressed against the hips.
- Palpate the breasts with the patient seated and then lying down with a pillow placed under the shoulder on the side being examined.
- Palpate the nipple, noting tenderness and nodules; check for discharge.
- Palpate axillary lymph nodes, noting any enlargement.

MEDICAL
Areolar gland abscess
◆ Montgomery's glands become inflamed.
◆ Abscess is tender and palpable and is located on the periphery of the areola.
◆ Other signs and symptoms include fever, local swelling, drainage, and malaise.

Breast abscess, acute
◆ Local pain, tenderness, erythema, peau d'orange, and warmth are associated with a nodule.
◆ Other signs and symptoms include malaise, fever, chills, and enlarged axillary nodes.

Fat necrosis
◆ Local pain and tenderness may develop.
◆ Other signs and symptoms include ecchymosis; erythema; a firm, irregular, fixed mass; skin dimpling; and nipple retraction.

Fibrocystic breast disease
◆ Cysts may cause pain before menstruation and produce no symptoms afterward.
◆ Later, pain may persist throughout the cycle.
◆ Cysts feel firm, mobile, and well-defined.
◆ A clear, serous nipple discharge may come from one or both breasts.
◆ The patient may experience signs and symptoms of premenstrual syndrome.

Intraductal papilloma
◆ Breast pain or tenderness may occur in one breast.
◆ Serous or bloody nipple discharge is the primary sign.
◆ Other findings include a small, soft, poorly delineated mass in the ducts beneath the areola.

Mammary duct ectasia
◆ Burning pain and itching around the areola may occur.
◆ Inflammation with pain, tenderness, erythema, and acute fever, or with pain and tenderness alone, may develop and subside in 7 to 10 days.
◆ Other signs and symptoms include a rubbery, subareolar breast nodule; swelling and erythema around the nipple; nipple retraction; a bluish green discoloration or peau d'orange of the skin overlying the nodule; a thick, sticky, multicolored nipple discharge from multiple ducts; axillary lymphadenopathy; and breast ulcer (late sign).

Mastitis
◆ Pain in one breast may be severe.
◆ Skin is typically red and warm at the inflammation site.
◆ High fever, chills, malaise, and fatigue are systemic findings.
◆ Other signs and symptoms include peau d'orange, breast dimpling, a firm area of induration, and nipple deviation, inversion, or flattening.

Sebaceous cyst, infected
◆ Pain may be reported with this cutaneous cyst.
◆ Other signs and symptoms include a small, well-delineated nodule, localized erythema, and induration.

◆ Provide emotional support for the patient.
◆ Emphasize the importance of monthly breast self-examinations.

PEDIATRIC POINTERS
◆ Transient gynecomastia can cause breast pain in boys during puberty.

GERIATRIC POINTERS
◆ Breast pain from benign breast disease is rare in postmenopausal women.
◆ Breast pain can be due to trauma from falls or physical abuse.
◆ Because of decreased pain perception and decreased cognitive function, elderly patients may not report breast pain.

◆ Instruct the patient on correct type of brassiere.
◆ Explain the use of warm or cold compresses.
◆ Teach the techniques of breast self-examination, and stress the importance of monthly self-examinations.
◆ Explain underlying disorder, diagnostic tests, and treatment options.

Breast ulcer

OVERVIEW

- Appears on the nipple, areola, or the breast itself
- Indicates destruction of the skin and subcutaneous tissue
- Usually a late sign of cancer, appearing well after the confirming diagnosis
- Can also result from trauma, infection, or radiation

HISTORY

- Obtain a patient history including when the patient first noticed the ulcer. Ask if it's improving or getting worse, is it painful or draining, and is it accompanied by nodules, edema, or nipple discharge, deviation, or retraction.
- Review the patient's personal and family history for factors that increase the risk of breast cancer.
- Ask about breast-feeding, weaning, diabetes and if she's currently taking an oral antibiotic as these factors predispose the patient to Candida infections.

PHYSICAL ASSESSMENT

- Inspect the patient's breast, noting any asymmetry or flattening.
- Look for a rash, scaling, cracking, or red excoriation on the nipples, areola, and inframammary fold.
- Check especially for skin changes, such as warmth, erythema, or peau d'orange.
- Palpate the breast for masses, noting any induration beneath the ulcer. Then carefully palpate for tenderness or nodules around the areola and the axillary lymph nodes.

MEDICAL
Breast cancer

◆ A breast ulcer that doesn't heal within a month usually indicates cancer. Ulceration along a mastectomy scar may indicate metastatic cancer; a nodule beneath the ulcer may be a late sign of a fulminating tumor.
◆ A breast ulcer may be the presenting sign of breast cancer in men, who are more apt to miss or dismiss earlier breast changes.
◆ Other signs and symptoms include a palpable breast nodule, skin dimpling, nipple retraction, bloody or serous nipple discharge, erythema, peau d'orange, and enlarged axillary lymph nodes.

Breast trauma

◆ Tissue destruction with inadequate healing may produce breast ulcers.
◆ Associated signs depend on the type of trauma, but may include ecchymosis, lacerations, abrasions, swelling, and hematoma.

Candida albicans *infection*

◆ Severe *Candida* infection can cause maceration of breast tissue followed by ulceration.
◆ Well-defined, bright-red papular patches—usually with scaly borders—characterize the infection, which can develop in the breast folds.
◆ In breast-feeding women, cracked nipples predispose them to infection.Women describe the pain, felt when the infant sucks, as a burning pain that penetrates into the chest wall.

Paget's disease

◆ Bright-red nipple excoriation can extend to the areola and ulcerate.
◆ Serous or bloody nipple discharge and extreme nipple itching may accompany ulceration.
◆ Symptoms are usually unilateral.

OTHER
Radiation therapy

◆ After treatment, the breasts appear "sunburned." Subsequently, the skin ulcerates and the surrounding area becomes red and tender.

NURSING CONSIDERATIONS

◆ If breast cancer is suspected, provide emotional support and encourage the patient to express her feelings.
◆ Prepare her for diagnostic tests, such as ultrasonography, thermography, mammography, nipple discharge cytology, and breast biopsy.
◆ If a Candida infection is suspected, prepare her for skin or blood cultures.

GERIATRIC POINTERS

◆ Because of the increased breast cancer risk in this population, breast ulcers should be considered cancerous until proven otherwise.
◆ Ulcers can also result from normal skin changes in the elderly, such as thinning, decreased vascularity, and loss of elasticity as well as from poor skin hygiene.
◆ Pressure ulcers may result from restraints and tight brassieres; traumatic ulcers, from falls or abuse.

PATIENT TEACHING

◆ Because breast ulcers become infected easily, teach the patient how to apply a topical antifungal or antibacterial ointment or cream.
◆ Instruct her to keep the ulcer dry to reduce chafing and to wear loose-fitting undergarments.
◆ Discuss underlying condition, diagnostic tests, and treatment options.

Breath with ammonia odor

OVERVIEW

- Described as urinous or "fishy" breath and occurs in end-stage chronic renal failure
- Improves slightly after hemodialysis, but persists throughout the course of the disorder
- Reflects long-term metabolic disturbances and biochemical abnormalities associated with uremia and end-stage chronic renal failure
- Produced by metabolic end products blown off by the lungs and the breakdown of urea (to ammonia) in the saliva; however, specific uremic toxin not yet identified
- Breath odor analysis in animals: reveals toxic metabolites, such as dimethylamine and trimethylamine, that contribute to "fishy" odor; source of amines may be intestinal bacteria acting on dietary chlorine

HISTORY

- Obtain a medical history, noting a diagnosis of chronic renal failure.
- Ask the patient if he has experienced a metallic taste, loss of smell, increased thirst, heartburn, difficulty swallowing, loss of appetite at the sight of food, or early morning vomiting.
- Because GI bleeding is common in patients with chronic renal failure, ask about bowel habits, noting especially melena or constipation.
- Ask about associated GI symptoms so that palliative care and support can be individualized.

PHYSICAL ASSESSMENT

- Inspect the patient's oral cavity for bleeding, swollen gums or tongue, and ulceration with drainage.
- Take the patient's vital signs. Watch for any indications of hypertension (the patient with end-stage chronic renal failure is usually somewhat hypertensive) or hypotension.
- Be alert for other signs of shock (such as tachycardia, tachypnea, and cool, clammy skin) and altered mental status. Any significant changes can indicate complications, such as massive GI bleeding or pericarditis with tamponade.

MEDICAL
End-stage chronic renal failure

◆ Ammonia breath odor is a late finding in end-stage chronic renal failure.
◆ Accompanying signs and symptoms include anuria, skin pigmentation changes and excoriation, brown arcs under the nail margins, tissue wasting, Kussmaul's respirations, neuropathy, lethargy, somnolence, confusion, disorientation, behavior changes, irritability, and emotional lability.
◆ Later neurologic signs and symptoms that signal impending uremic coma include muscle twitching and fasciculations, asterixis, paresthesia, and footdrop.
◆ Cardiovascular findings include hypertension, myocardial infarction, signs of heart failure, pericarditis, and even sudden death and stroke.
◆ GI findings include anorexia, weight loss, nausea, heartburn, vomiting, constipation, hiccups, and a metallic taste; the patient is also at increased risk for peptic ulceration and acute pancreatitis.
◆ Oral signs and symptoms may include stomatitis, gum ulceration and bleeding, and a coated tongue.
◆ Uremic frost, pruritus, and signs of hormonal changes, such as impotence or amenorrhea, may also appear.

◆ Ammonia breath odor is offensive to others, but the patient may become accustomed to it. As a result, remind him to perform frequent mouth care, particularly before meals because reducing the foul taste and odor may stimulate his appetite.
◆ A half-strength hydrogen peroxide mixture or lemon juice gargle helps neutralize the ammonia; the patient may also want to use commercial lozenges or breath sprays or to suck on hard candy.
◆ Advise him to use a soft-bristled toothbrush or sponge to prevent trauma.
◆ Maximize dietary intake by offering the patient frequent small meals of his favorite foods, within dietary limitations.

PEDIATRIC POINTERS
◆ Ammonia breath odor also occurs in children with end-stage chronic renal failure.
◆ Provide hard candy to relieve bad taste and odor.
◆ If the child can gargle, try mixing hydrogen peroxide with flavored mouthwashes.

◆ If the patient can't perform mouth care, teach his family members how to assist him.
◆ Involve the patient at an early stage in the various aspects of treatment to help prepare him for any complicated training that may be needed later—for example, if he needs dialysis or transplantation.
◆ Explain dietary and drug therapies.

Breath with fecal odor

- Typically occurs with fecal vomiting associated with a long-standing intestinal obstruction or gastrojejuno-colic fistula
- May indicate a late diagnostic clue to a life-threatening GI disorder (see *Managing fecal breath odor*)

- Ask about previous abdominal surgeries.
- Note the onset, duration, and location of abdominal pain.
- Find out about bowel habits, including time and description of last bowel movement.
- Ask about any loss of appetite.

- Auscultate for bowel sounds.
- Inspect the abdomen, noting its contour and surgical scars.
- Measure abdominal girth to provide a baseline.
- Percuss for tympany or dullness.
- Palpate for tenderness, distention, and rigidity.
- Rectal and pelvic examinations should also be performed.

ACTION STAT!

Managing fecal breath odor

Because fecal breath odor can signal a life-threatening intestinal obstruction, you'll need to quickly assess your patient's condition. Monitor his vital signs, and look for signs of shock, such as hypotension, tachycardia, narrowed pulse pressure, and cool, clammy skin. Ask the patient if he's nauseated or has vomited. Find out the frequency of vomiting as well as the color, odor, amount, and consistency of the vomitus. Have an emesis basin nearby to collect and accurately measure the vomitus.

Withhold all food and fluids because surgery may be necessary to relieve an obstruction or repair a fistula. Insert a nasogastric or intestinal tube for GI tract decompression. Insert a peripheral I.V. line for vascular access, or assist with central line insertion for large-bore access and central venous pressure monitoring. Obtain a blood sample and send it to the laboratory for complete blood count and electrolyte analysis. Maintain adequate hydration and support circulatory status with additional fluids. Give a physiologic solution—such as lactated Ringer's solution, normal saline solution, or human plasma protein fraction (Plasmanate)—to prevent metabolic acidosis from gastric losses and metabolic alkalosis from intestinal fluid losses.

MEDICAL
Distal small-bowel obstruction
- Fecal breath odor results from vomiting of fecal contents after vomiting of gastric contents and bilious contents.
- Other symptoms include achiness, malaise, drowsiness, and polydipsia.
- Bowel changes (ranging from diarrhea to constipation) are accompanied by abdominal distention, persistent epigastric or periumbilical colicky pain, and hyperactive bowel sounds and borborygmi.
- Bowel sounds become hypoactive or absent as obstruction becomes complete.
- Fever, hypotension, tachycardia, and rebound tenderness may indicate strangulation or perforation.

Gastrojejunocolic fistula
- Fecal vomiting with resulting fecal breath odor may occur.
- Diarrhea with abdominal pain is the most common complaint.
- Other signs and symptoms include anorexia, weight loss, abdominal distention, and marked malabsorption.

Large-bowel obstruction
- Fecal vomiting with fecal breath odor occurs as a late sign.
- Colicky abdominal pain appears suddenly, followed by continuous hypogastric pain.
- Marked abdominal distention and tenderness occur.
- Constipation develops, but defecation of stool below obstruction may continue for up to 3 days.
- Leakage of stool is common with partial obstruction.

After a nasogastric or intestinal tube has been inserted:
- Keep the head of the bed elevated at least 30 degrees.
- Turn the patient to facilitate passage of the intestinal tube through the GI tract.
- Don't tape the intestinal tube to the patient's face, so that it can continue to advance.
- Ensure tube patency by monitoring drainage and checking that suction devices function properly.
- Irrigate tube as needed.
- Monitor GI drainage.
- At least once per day, send serum specimens to the laboratory for electrolyte analysis.

PEDIATRIC POINTERS
- Carefully monitor the child's fluid and electrolyte status, because dehydration can develop rapidly from persistent vomiting.
- Signs of dehydration include the absence of tears and dry or parched mucous membranes.

GERIATRIC POINTERS
- Early surgical intervention may be necessary for a bowel obstruction that doesn't respond to decompression because of the high risk of bowel infarct.

- Explain to the patient the procedures and treatments he needs.
- Teach the patient the techniques of good oral hygiene.
- Explain to the patient the food and fluid restrictions that are needed.

Breath with fruity odor

OVERVIEW

- Results from respiratory elimination of excess acetone
- Characteristically occurs with ketoacidosis, a potentially life-threatening condition (see *Managing fruity breath odor*)

HISTORY

- Ask about the onset and duration of odor.
- Find out about changes in breathing patterns.
- Review other signs and symptoms, including increased thirst, frequent urination, weight loss, fatigue, and abdominal pain.
- Ask the female patient if she has had candidal vaginitis or vaginal secretions with itching.
- If the patient has a history of diabetes mellitus, ask about stress, infections, and noncompliance to the treatment regimen.
- If anorexia nervosa is suspected, obtain a dietary and weight history.

PHYSICAL ASSESSMENT

- Take vital signs.
- Perform a physical examination.

 ACTION STAT!

Managing fruity breath odor

Check for Kussmaul's respirations, and examine the patient's level of consciousness. Take vital signs and check skin turgor. Check for rapid, deep respirations; stupor; and poor skin turgor. Obtain a brief history, noting especially diabetes mellitus, nutritional problems such as anorexia nervosa, and fad diets with scant or no carbohydrates. Obtain venous and arterial blood samples for complete blood count and glucose, electrolyte, acetone, and arterial blood gas (ABG) levels. Also obtain a urine specimen to test for glucose and acetone. Administer I.V. fluids and electrolytes to maintain hydration and electrolyte balance and, in patients with diabetic ketoacidosis, give regular insulin to reduce glucose levels.

If the patient is obtunded, insert endotracheal and nasogastric tubes. Suction as needed. Insert an indwelling urinary catheter, and monitor fluid intake and urine output. Insert central venous pressure and arterial lines to monitor the patient's fluid status and blood pressure. Place the patient on a cardiac monitor, monitor vital signs and neurologic status, and draw blood hourly to check glucose, electrolyte, acetone, and ABG levels.

CAUSES

MEDICAL

Anorexia nervosa

◆ Severe weight loss may produce fruity breath odor.
◆ Nausea, constipation, and cold intolerance may be present.
◆ Dental enamel erosion and scars or calluses in the dorsum of the hand may indicate induced vomiting.

Ketoacidosis

◆ With alcoholic ketoacidosis, fruity breath odor occurs with vomiting, abdominal pain, abrupt onset of Kussmaul's respirations, signs of dehydration, minimal food intake over several days, and normal or slightly decreased blood glucose levels.
◆ With starvation ketoacidosis, fruity breath odor occurs with signs of cachexia and dehydration, decreased level of consciousness, bradycardia, and a history of severely limited food intake.
◆ With diabetic ketoacidosis (DKA), fruity breath odor occurs as DKA develops over 1 or 2 days.
◆ Other signs and symptoms of DKA include polydipsia, polyuria, nocturia, weak and rapid pulse, hunger, weight loss, weakness, fatigue, nausea, vomiting, abdominal pain, and, eventually, Kussmaul's respirations, orthostatic hypotension, dehydration, tachycardia, confusion, stupor, and coma.

OTHER

Drugs

◆ Drugs that cause metabolic acidosis, such as nitroprusside and salicylates, can result in fruity breath odor.
◆ Low-carbohydrate diets may cause ketoacidosis and a fruity breath odor.

NURSING CONSIDERATIONS

◆ When the patient is more alert and his condition stabilizes, remove the nasogastric tube and start him on an appropriate diet.
◆ Switch his insulin from I.V. to subcutaneous.

PEDIATRIC POINTERS

◆ Fruity breath odor in an infant or a child usually stems from uncontrolled diabetes mellitus.
◆ Ketoacidosis develops rapidly because of low glycogen stores in this age-group.

GERIATRIC POINTERS

◆ Consider such factors as poor oral hygiene, increased dental caries, decreased salivary function, poor dietary intake, and use of multiple drugs when evaluating the condition of an elderly patient with mouth odor.

PATIENT TEACHING

◆ Explain the signs of hyperglycemia.
◆ Emphasize the importance of wearing medical identification.
◆ Refer the patient to psychologist or support group, as needed.
◆ Provide dietary instruction and referral to nutritionist as appropriate.

Brudzinski's sign

OVERVIEW

- Causes hips and knees to go into flexion in response to passive flexion of the neck
- Signals meningeal irritation
- Early indicator of life-threatening meningitis and subarachnoid hemorrhage (see *Testing for Brudzinski's sign*)

 ACTION STAT! *Ask the patient about signs of increased intracranial pressure (ICP), such as headache, neck pain, nausea, and vision disturbances. Observe for altered level of consciousness (LOC), pupillary changes, bradycardia, widened pulse pressure, Cheyne-Stokes or Kussmaul's respirations, vomiting, and moderate fever.*

Keep artificial airways, intubation equipment, a handheld resuscitation bag, and suction equipment on hand. Elevate the head of the patient's bed 30 to 60 degrees to promote venous return. Give an osmotic diuretic to reduce cerebral edema. Monitor and look for ICP that continues to rise. You may have to provide mechanical ventilation and give a barbiturate and additional doses of a diuretic. You may also need to prepare patient for procedure to drain cerebrospinal fluid.

 TOP TECHNIQUE

Testing for Brudzinski's sign

Here's how to test for Brudzinski's sign when you suspect meningeal irritation:

With the patient in a supine position, place your hands behind her neck and lift her head toward her chest.

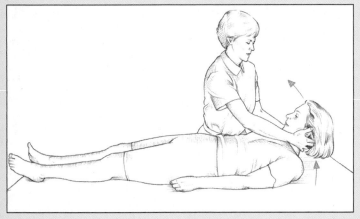

If your patient has meningeal irritation, she'll flex her hips and knees in response to the passive neck flexion.

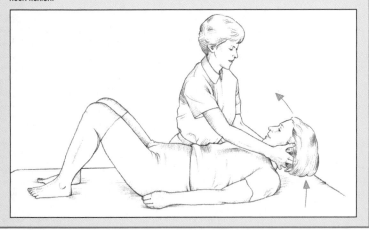

HISTORY

- Ask about a history of hypertension, spinal arthritis, recent head trauma, open-head injury, dental work or abscessed teeth, endocarditis, or I.V. drug abuse.
- Ask about the sudden onset of headaches.

PHYSICAL ASSESSMENT

- Evaluate cranial nerve function, noting any motor or sensory deficits.
- Look for Kernig's sign (resistance to knee extension after flexion of the hip), which is a further indication of meningeal irritation.
- Look for signs of central nervous system infection, such as fever and nuchal rigidity.
- Obtain vital signs.

CAUSES

MEDICAL
Meningitis

◆ A life-threatening disorder, a positive Brudzinski's sign can usually be elicited 24 hours after onset.
◆ As ICP rises, arterial hypertension, bradycardia, widened pulse pressure, Cheyne-Stokes or Kussmaul's respirations, and coma may develop.
◆ Other signs and symptoms include headache, a positive Kernig's sign, nuchal rigidity, irritability or restlessness, deep stupor or coma, vertigo, fever, chills, malaise, hyperalgesia, muscular hypotonia, opisthotonos, symmetrical deep tendon reflexes, papilledema, ocular and facial palsies, nausea, vomiting, photophobia, diplopia, and unequal, sluggish pupils.

Subarachnoid hemorrhage

◆ A life-threatening disorder, Brudzinski's sign may be elicited within minutes after initial bleeding.
◆ Focal signs, such as hemiparesis, vision disturbances, or aphasia, may occur.
◆ As ICP rises, arterial hypertension, bradycardia, widened pulse pressure, Cheyne-Stokes or Kussmaul's respirations, and coma may develop.
◆ Other signs and symptoms include sudden onset of severe headache, nuchal rigidity, altered LOC, dizziness, photophobia, cranial nerve palsies, nausea, vomiting, fever, and a positive Kernig's sign.

NURSING CONSIDERATIONS

◆ Provide constant ICP monitoring and perform frequent neurologic checks.
◆ Monitor vital signs, fluid intake and urine output, and cardiorespiratory status.
◆ Maintain low lights and minimal noise and elevate the head of the bed to make the patient more comfortable.

PEDIATRIC POINTERS

◆ Bulging fontanels, a weak cry, fretfulness, vomiting, and poor feeding appear earlier in infants with meningeal irritation than does Brudzinski's sign.

PATIENT TEACHING

◆ Discuss the signs and symptoms of meningitis and subdural hematoma.
◆ Tell the patient when to seek immediate medical attention.
◆ Discuss diagnostic tests needed and treatment options.

Bruit

OVERVIEW

- Swishing sound caused by turbulent blood flow
- Characterized by location, duration, intensity, pitch, and time of onset in the cardiac cycle
- May indicate life- or limb-threatening vascular disease
- Loud bruits: produce a strong thrill
- Diagnostically significant when heard over the abdominal aorta; the thyroid gland; the renal, carotid, femoral, popliteal, or subclavian artery; or, when heard consistently despite changes in patient's position and during diastole (see *Preventing false bruits*)

HISTORY

- Obtain a medical history, noting past injuries, illnesses, surgeries, and family medical history.
- Ask about alcohol use and diet.
- Take a drug and social history.

PHYSICAL ASSESSMENT

- Perform cardiac and vascular assessment.
- Obtain vital signs.

FOR BRUITS OVER ABDOMINAL AORTA

- Check for a pulsating mass, Cullen's sign, or severe, tearing pain in the abdomen, flank, or lower back.
- Check peripheral pulses, comparing intensity in the upper versus lower extremities.
- Look for signs and symptoms of hypovolemic shock and dissection.

FOR BRUITS OVER THYROID GLAND

- Ask the patient about history of hyperthyroidism.
- Watch for signs and symptoms of life-threatening thyroid storm.

FOR CAROTID ARTERY BRUITS

- Be alert for signs and symptoms of a transient ischemic attack (TIA).
- Evaluate frequently for changes in level of consciousness and muscle function.

FOR BRUITS OVER FEMORAL, POPLITEAL, OR SUBCLAVIAN ARTERY

- Watch for signs and symptoms of decreased or absent peripheral circulation.
- Ask the patient about a history of intermittent claudication.
- Frequently check distal pulses and skin color and temperature.
- Watch for pallor, coolness, or the sudden absence of pulse.

 TOP TECHNIQUE

Preventing false bruits

Auscultating bruits accurately requires practice and skill. These sounds typically stem from arterial luminal narrowing or arterial dilation, but they can also result from excessive pressure applied to the stethoscope's bell during auscultation. This pressure compresses the artery, creating turbulent blood flow and a false bruit.

To prevent false bruits, place the bell lightly on the patient's skin. Also, if you're auscultating for a popliteal bruit, help the patient to a supine position, place your hand behind his ankle, and lift his leg slightly before placing the bell behind the knee.

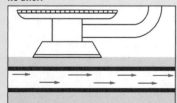

NORMAL BLOOD FLOW, NO BRUIT

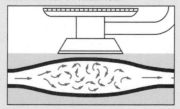

TURBULENT BLOOD FLOW AND RESULTANT BRUIT CAUSED BY ANEURYSM

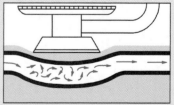

TURBULENT BLOOD FLOW AND FALSE BRUIT CAUSED BY COMPRESSION OF ARTERY

MEDICAL

Abdominal aortic aneurysm

◆ A systolic bruit over the aorta accompanies a pulsating periumbilical mass.
◆ Sharp, tearing pain in the abdomen, flank, or lower back signals imminent dissection.
◆ Other signs and symptoms include a rigid, tender abdomen; mottled skin; diminished peripheral pulses; and claudication.

Abdominal aortic atherosclerosis

◆ Loud systolic bruits in the epigastric and midabdominal areas are common findings.
◆ Other signs and symptoms may include leg weakness, numbness, paresthesia, or paralysis; leg pain; or decreased or absent femoral, popliteal, or pedal pulses.

Carotid artery stenosis

◆ Systolic bruits heard over one or both carotid arteries may be the only sign of this disorder.
◆ Dizziness, vertigo, headache, syncope, aphasia, dysarthria, sudden vision loss, hemiparesis, or hemiparalysis signals TIA and may signal an impending stroke.

Peripheral arteriovenous fistula

◆ A rough, continuous bruit with systolic accentuation may be heard over the fistula.
◆ A palpable thrill is also common.
◆ Other signs and symptoms depend on the location of the fistula, but may include claudication, absent pulses, and cool skin.

Peripheral vascular disease

◆ Bruits may be heard over the femoral artery and other arteries in the legs.
◆ Lower-leg ulcers that are difficult to heal may also occur.
◆ Other signs and symptoms include diminished or absent femoral, popliteal, or pedal pulses; intermittent claudication; numbness, weakness, pain, and cramping in the legs, feet, and hips; and cool, shiny skin and hair loss on the affected extremity.

Renal artery stenosis

◆ Systolic bruits are heard over abdominal midline and flank on affected side.
◆ Hypertension commonly accompanies stenosis.
◆ Other signs and symptoms include headache, palpitations, tachycardia, anxiety, dizziness, retinopathy, hematuria, and mental sluggishness.

Subclavian steal syndrome

◆ Systolic bruit may be heard over the subclavian artery due to narrowing of the subclavian artery and retrograde blood flow from the vertebral artery.
◆ Other signs and symptoms include decreased blood pressure and claudication in the affected arm, hemiparesis, vision disturbances, vertigo, and dysarthria.

Thyrotoxicosis

◆ Systolic bruit is heard over the thyroid gland.
◆ Characteristic signs and symptoms include thyroid enlargement, fatigue, nervousness, tachycardia, heat intolerance, sweating, tremor, diarrhea, exophthalmos, and weight loss despite increased appetite.

◆ Frequently check vital signs, and auscultate over affected arteries.
◆ Check for bruits that become louder or develop a diastolic component.
◆ Administer drugs, such as a vasodilator, anticoagulant, antihypertensive, or antiplatelet.

PEDIATRIC POINTERS

◆ Bruits are common in young children and usually of little significance.
◆ Auscultate for bruits in a child with port-wine spots or cavernous or diffuse hemangiomas.

GERIATRIC POINTERS

◆ Elderly patients with atherosclerosis may experience bruits over several arteries.
◆ Bruits from carotid artery stenosis are associated with stroke; therefore, close follow-up and prompt surgical referral are essential.

◆ Tell the patient the signs and symptoms of stroke to report immediately.
◆ Discuss lifestyle changes, such as quitting smoking, exercising regularly, and eating a balanced, healthy diet.

Buffalo hump

OVERVIEW

- Characterized by an accumulation of cervicodorsal fat
- May indicate hypercortisolism (Cushing's syndrome), which may result from long-term glucocorticoid therapy, adrenal carcinoma, adrenal adenoma, ectopic corticotropin production, or excessive pituitary secretion of corticotropin (Cushing's disease)
- Doesn't help distinguish between underlying causes of hypercortisolism, but may help direct diagnostic testing

HISTORY

- Obtain a patient history, asking about recent weight gain, changes in diet, and when he first noticed the buffalo hump.
- Typically, a history of moderate to extreme obesity, with accumulation of adipose tissue in the nape of the neck, face, and trunk and thinning of the arms and legs, indicates hypercortisolism. (See *Recognizing hypercortisolism.*)
- If the patient has an old photograph, use it to compare his current and former weight and distribution of adipose tissue.
- Ask if the patient or any family member has a history of endocrine disorders, cancer, or obesity.
- If the patient is a female of childbearing age, ask the date of her last menses and about any changes in her normal menstrual pattern.
- If the patient is receiving glucocorticoid therapy, ask about the dosage, schedule, administration route, and any recent changes in therapy.

PHYSICAL ASSESSMENT

- Take the patient's vital signs, height, and weight.
- Note obvious signs of hypercortisolism, such as hirsutism, diaphoresis, and moon (roundish) face.
- Inspect the arms, legs, and trunk for striae, and note skin turgor for thin skin.
- Assess muscle function by asking the patient to rise from a squatting position; note any difficulty because this may indicate quadriceps muscle weakness. These patients will typically have proximal muscle weakness (for example, limb or girdle weakness).
- Observe the patient's behavior; extreme emotional lability along with depression, irritability, or confusion may signal hypercortisolism.

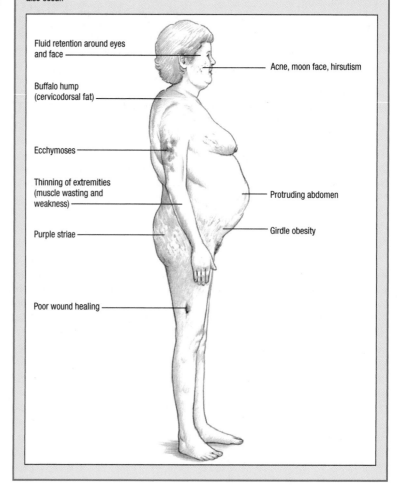

Recognizing hypercortisolism

Buffalo hump, moon face, and truncal obesity are the cardinal signs of hypercortisolism. In addition to these and the other signs shown here, hypertension, osteoporosis, and emotional lability may also occur.

Fluid retention around eyes and face

Buffalo hump (cervicodorsal fat)

Ecchymoses

Thinning of extremities (muscle wasting and weakness)

Purple striae

Poor wound healing

Acne, moon face, hirsutism

Protruding abdomen

Girdle obesity

MEDICAL

Hypercortisolism

◆ Buffalo hump varies in size, depending on the severity of hypercortisolism and the amount of weight gain.
◆ It's commonly accompanied by hirsutism, moon face, and truncal obesity with slender arms and legs.
◆ The skin may appear transparent, with purple striae and ecchymoses.
◆ Other signs and symptoms include acne, muscle weakness and wasting, fatigue, poor wound healing, elevated blood pressure, personality changes, and amenorrhea or oligomenorrhea in women or impotence in men.

Morbid obesity

◆ The size of the buffalo hump depends on the amount of weight gain and the distribution of adipose tissue.
◆ Associated signs and symptoms include generalized adiposity, silver striae, elevated blood pressure, and hypogonadism.

OTHER

Drugs

◆ Buffalo hump may result from excessive doses of a glucocorticoid, such as cortisone, hydrocortisone, prednisone, or dexamethasone. Long-term glucocorticoid therapy is the most common cause of buffalo hump in the United States.

◆ Prepare the patient for diagnostic tests.
◆ Blood and urine tests can confirm hypercortisolism; ultrasonography, computed tomography (CT) scan, or arteriography can localize adrenal tumors.
◆ Chest X-rays, bronchography, and an abdominal CT scan can determine ectopic involvement.
◆ Visual field testing and a skull CT scan can identify pituitary tumors.

PEDIATRIC POINTERS

◆ In children older than age 7, this sign usually results from pituitary over-secretion of corticotropin in bilateral adrenal hyperplasia.
◆ In younger children, it commonly results from glucocorticoid therapy— for example, overuse of glucocorticoid eyedrops.

◆ Advise the patient about proper diet, drug therapy, and exercise.
◆ Provide education and intervention for emotional lability.

Butterfly rash

- Signals systemic lupus erythematosus (SLE) or dermatologic disorders
- Appears in a malar distribution across the nose and cheeks (see *Recognizing butterfly rash*)

HISTORY

- Ask about the onset and extent of rash.
- Ask the patient about recent exposure to the sun.
- Determine whether the patient has had recent weight or hair loss.
- Ask about a family history of SLE.
- Note whether the patient is taking hydralazine or procainamide.

PHYSICAL ASSESSMENT

- Inspect the rash, noting macules, papules, pustules, scaling, hypopigmentation, or hyperpigmentation.
- Look for blisters or ulcers in the mouth.
- Note inflamed lesions.
- Check for rashes elsewhere on the body.

Recognizing butterfly rash

With classic butterfly rash, lesions appear on the cheeks and the bridge of the nose, creating a characteristic butterfly pattern. The rash may vary in severity from malar erythema to discoid lesions (plaques).

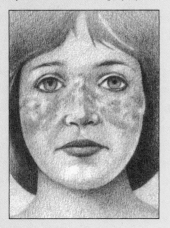

MEDICAL

Discoid lupus erythematosus

◆ A localized form of lupus erythematosus characterized by one-sided rash or butterfly rash with erythematous, raised, sharply demarcated plaques, follicular plugging, and central atrophy of the plaque.
◆ Affected areas include the scalp, ears, chest, or other areas exposed to the sun.
◆ Later signs and symptoms include telangiectasia, scarring, alopecia, and hypopigmentation or hyperpigmentation.
◆ Other signs and symptoms include conjunctival redness, dilated capillaries of the nail fold, parotid gland enlargement, oral lesions, and mottled, reddish-blue skin on the legs.

Erysipelas

◆ Rosy or crimson swollen lesions develop on the neck and head and along the nasolabial fold.
◆ The condition occurs primarily in infants and in adults older than age 30 and usually follows a streptococcal infection.
◆ Other signs and symptoms include fever, chills, cervical lymphadenopathy, and malaise.

Rosacea

◆ Initially, the rash may appear as a prominent, nonscaling, intermittent erythema limited to the lower half of the nose or including the chin, cheeks, and central forehead.
◆ As the rash develops, it remains longer, and, instead of disappearing after each episode, it merely subsides then rises again; it's often seen with telangiectasia.
◆ In advanced stages, the skin is oily, with papules, pustules, nodules, and telangiectasis only on the central oval of the face.

Seborrheic dermatitis

◆ The rash appears as greasy, scaling, slightly yellow macules and papules of varying size on the cheeks and the bridge of the nose.
◆ The scalp, beard, eyebrows, portions of the forehead above the bridge of the nose, the nasolabial fold, or the trunk may be involved.
◆ Other signs and symptoms include crusts and fissures, pruritus, redness, blepharitis, styes, severe acne, and oily skin.

Systemic lupus erythematosus

◆ This is a chronic inflammatory connective tissue disease.
◆ The rash appears as a red, scaly, sharply demarcated macular eruption.
◆ The rash may progress slowly to include the forehead, chin, the area around the ears, and other exposed areas.
◆ Joint pain, stiffness, and deformities, particularly an ulnar deviation of the fingers and subluxation of the proximal interphalangeal joints, may accompany the rash.
◆ Related signs and symptoms include scaling, patchy alopecia, mucous membrane lesions, mottled erythema of the palms and fingers, periungual erythema with edema, reddish purple macular lesions on the palm side of the fingers, telangiectasis of the base of the nails or of the eyelids, purpura, petechiae, and ecchymoses.
◆ Generalized signs and symptoms include periorbital and facial edema, dyspnea, low-grade fever, malaise, weakness, fatigue, weight loss, anorexia, nausea, vomiting, lymphadenopathy, photosensitivity, and hepatosplenomegaly.

OTHER

Drugs

◆ Hydralazine and procainamide can cause a lupuslike syndrome.

◆ Withhold photosensitizing drugs.
◆ Prepare patient for immunologic and other studies.

PEDIATRIC POINTERS

◆ Rarely, butterfly rash may occur as part of an infectious disease such as erythema infectiosum.

◆ Urge the use of sunscreen.
◆ Stress the need to avoid sun exposure.
◆ Encourage the use of hypoallergenic makeup to conceal facial lesions.
◆ Inform the patient about sources of support such as Lupus Foundation of America.

Café-au-lait spots

OVERVIEW

- Important indicator of neurofibromatosis and other congenital melanotic disorders
- Appear as flat, light brown, uniformly hyperpigmented macules or patches on the skin surface, usually appearing during the first 3 years of life but possibly developing at any age
- Differentiated from freckles and other benign birthmarks by their larger size (0.5 mm or larger in diameter) and irregular shape
- Usually have no significance; however, six or more spots possibly associated with underlying neurologic disorder

HISTORY

- Ask when the café-au-lait spots first appeared.
- Ask about a family history of these spots and of neurofibromatosis.
- Obtain history for seizures, frequent fractures, or mental retardation.

PHYSICAL ASSESSMENT

- Inspect the skin, noting the location and pattern of the spots.
- Look for distinctive skin lesions, such as axillary freckling, mottling, small spherical patches, and areas of depigmentation; large lesions should be measured along the longest axis.
- Perform a Wood's light examination to help visualize lesions in pale-skinned individuals.
- Check for subcutaneous neurofibromas along major nerve branches, especially on the trunk.
- Check for bony abnormalities, such as scoliosis or kyphosis.

| CAUSES | NURSING CONSIDERATIONS | PATIENT TEACHING |

CAUSES

MEDICAL

Albright's syndrome

◆ Spots are smaller (about ⅜″ [1 cm] in diameter) and more irregularly shaped than those in neurofibromatosis.
◆ Spots may stop abruptly at the midline and seem to follow a dermatomal distribution.
◆ Usually, fewer than six spots appear, unilaterally on the forehead, neck, and lower back.
◆ When they occur on the scalp, the hair overlying them may be more deeply pigmented.
◆ Other signs and symptoms include skeletal deformities, frequent fractures, and sexual precocity (more common in girls than boys).

Neurofibromatosis

◆ This disorder (also called *von Recklinghausen's disease*), which develops during childhood, is characterized by six or more large, smooth-bordered spots more than 0.5 mm in diameter in prepubertal children and more than ⅝″ (1.5 mm) in diameter in postpubertal children.
◆ The nodules proliferate throughout life, affecting all body tissues and causing marked deformity; the spots may grow to ⅝″ or larger in adults.
◆ Mental impairment, seizures, hearing loss, exophthalmos, decreased visual acuity, and GI bleeding can eventually occur.
◆ Other signs and symptoms include axillary and inguinal freckling; irregular, hyperpigmented, and mottled skin; and multiple skin-colored pedunculated nodules clustered along nerve sheaths.

Tuberous sclerosis

◆ Mental retardation and seizures characteristically appear first, followed several years later by cutaneous facial lesions—multiple café-au-lait spots, spherical areas of rough skin, and areas of yellow-red or depigmented nevi.

NURSING CONSIDERATIONS

◆ Although café-au-lait spots require no treatment, you'll need to provide emotional support for the patient and his family.
◆ Refer patient and family for genetic counseling.

PATIENT TEACHING

◆ Teach the patient about diagnostic tests, such as tissue biopsy and radiographic studies.
◆ Teach the patient and family about underlying diagnosis.
◆ Teach the patient about genetic counseling.

Capillary refill time, increased

OVERVIEW

- Increased time required for color to return to the nail bed after application of slight pressure
- Reflects the quality of peripheral vasomotor function
- Signals obstructive peripheral arterial disease or decreased cardiac output
- Normal capillary refill time is less than 3 seconds

HISTORY

- Take a medical history, including previous peripheral vascular disease.
- Obtain a drug history, including tobacco use.
- Ask about pain or other sensations in fingers or toes.

PHYSICAL ASSESSMENT

- Perform a complete cardiovascular examination. (See *Assessing capillary refill*.)
- Observe skin color and check for edema.
- Check pulses in the affected limb.

CAUSES

MEDICAL
Aortic aneurysm, dissecting
- If aneurysm is in the thoracic aorta, capillary refill time is increased in the fingers and toes.
- If aneurysm is in the abdominal aorta, capillary refill time is increased in the toes.
- Other signs and symptoms include a pulsating abdominal mass, systolic bruit, and substernal, back, or abdominal pain.

Aortic arch syndrome
- Increased capillary refill time n the fingers occurs early.
- Carotid pulses are absent, and radial pulses may be uneven.
- Other signs and symptoms usually precede loss of pulses and include fever, night sweats, arthralgia, weight loss, anorexia, nausea, malaise, skin rash, splenomegaly, and pallor.

Arterial occlusion, acute
- Capillary refill time is increased (early) in the affected limb.
- Arterial pulses are usually absent distal to the obstruction.
- The affected limb appears cool and pale or cyanotic.
- Other signs and symptoms may include intermittent claudication, moderate to severe pain, numbness, and paresthesia or paralysis of the affected limb.

Buerger's disease
- Capillary refill time is increased in the toes.
- With exposure to low temperatures, feet turn cold, cyanotic, and numb; later, feet redden, become hot, and tingle.
- Ulceration, muscle atrophy, and gangrene may occur in later stages.
- Other signs and symptoms include intermittent claudication of the instep, weak peripheral pulses, and painful fingertip ulceration (if hands are affected).

TOP TECHNIQUE

Assessing capillary refill

Fingernails normally appear pinkish with no markings. To estimate the rate of peripheral blood flow, assess capillary refill in the fingernails (or toenails) by applying pressure to the nail for about 5 seconds, then assess the time it takes for color to return. In a patient with good arterial blood supply, the color should return in less than 3 seconds.

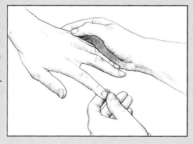

Cardiac tamponade
◆ Increased capillary refill time represents a late sign of decreased cardiac output.
◆ Other signs and symptoms include paradoxical pulse, tachycardia, cyanosis, dyspnea, jugular vein distention, and hypotension.

Hypothermia
◆ Increased capillary refill time may appear as an early response.
◆ Other signs and symptoms include shivering, fatigue, weakness, decreased level of consciousness (LOC), slurred speech, ataxia, muscle stiffness or rigidity, tachycardia or bradycardia, hyporeflexia or areflexia, diuresis, oliguria, bradypnea, decreased blood pressure, and cold, pale skin.

Peripheral arterial trauma
◆ Trauma to a peripheral artery that reduces blood flow increases capillary refill time in the affected extremity.
◆ Other signs and symptoms in the affected extremity include bruising, pulsating bleeding, weakened pulse, cyanosis, sensory loss, and cool, pale skin.

Raynaud's phenomenon
◆ Capillary refill time is increased in the fingers.
◆ Exposure to cold or stress initially produces blanching in the fingers, then cyanosis and, finally, erythema, before the fingers return to normal temperature.
◆ Skin and other changes from poor circulation may occur with chronic disease.

Shock
◆ Increased capillary refill time appears late in almost all types of shock.
◆ Other signs and symptoms include hypotension, tachycardia, tachypnea, and cool, clammy skin.

OTHER
Diagnostic tests
◆ Cardiac catheterization can cause arterial hematoma or clot formation and increased capillary refill time.

Drugs
◆ Drugs that cause vasoconstriction (particularly alpha blockers) increase capillary refill.

Treatments
◆ Arterial or umbilical lines can cause arterial hematoma and obstructed blood flow, leading to increased capillary refill time.
◆ Improperly fitting casts can constrict circulation.

NURSING CONSIDERATIONS

◆ Frequently assess vital signs, LOC, and the affected extremity; report any changes.
◆ Prepare the patient for tests, which may include arteriography or Doppler ultrasonography.

PEDIATRIC POINTERS
◆ Increased capillary refill time is normal in neonates with acrocyanosis.
◆ Cardiac surgery is also a common cause.

PATIENT TEACHING

◆ Explain the signs and symptoms the patient needs to report.
◆ Discuss with the patient ways to reduce the risk of aggravating or reintroducing the underlying disorder.
◆ Instruct the patient in ways to promote circulation.
◆ Stress to the patient the importance of quitting smoking.

Carpopedal spasm

OVERVIEW

- Violent, painful contraction of muscles in the hands and feet (see *Recognizing carpopedal spasm*)
- Commonly associated with hypocalcemia
- Indicates tetany, a potentially life-threatening disorder
- If left untreated, resulting laryngospasm, seizures, cardiac arrhythmias, and cardiac and respiratory arrest

ACTION STAT! *Look for signs of respiratory distress or cardiac arrhythmias. Obtain blood samples for electrolyte analysis, especially for calcium, and obtain an electrocardiogram. Connect the patient to a monitor to watch for arrhythmias. Infuse I.V. calcium and provide emergency respiratory and cardiac support. If the calcium infusion doesn't control seizures, give a sedative.*

HISTORY

- Ask about the onset and duration of spasms.
- Explore the extent of pain.
- Note related signs and symptoms of hypocalcemia.
- Obtain the patient's immunization history, especially tetanus vaccine.
- Ask about previous neck surgery, calcium or magnesium deficiency, tetanus exposure, hypoparathyroidism, or recent puncture wounds.

PHYSICAL ASSESSMENT

- Perform a complete physical examination, including taking vital signs.
- Check for Chvostek's and Trousseau's signs.
- Inspect the patient's skin and fingernails, noting any dryness or scaling or ridged, brittle nails caused by hypocalcemia.
- Assess his mental status and behavior.

Recognizing carpopedal spasm

In the hand, carpopedal spasm involves adduction of the thumb over the palm, followed by flexion of the metacarpophalangeal joints, extension of the interphalangeal joints (fingers together), adduction of the hyperextended fingers, and flexion of the wrist and elbow joints. Similar effects occur in the joints of the feet.

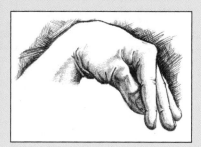

MEDICAL
Hypocalcemia
◆ Carpopedal spasm is an early sign.
◆ Paresthesia of the fingers, toes, and perioral area; muscle weakness, twitching, and cramping; hyper-reflexia; chorea; fatigue; and palpitations occur.
◆ Positive signs can be elicited.
◆ In chronic hypocalcemia, mental status changes; cramps; dry, scaly skin; brittle nails; and thin, patchy hair and eyebrows may occur.
◆ In severe hypocalcemia, laryngospasm, stridor, and seizures may appear.

Tetanus
◆ Muscle spasms and seizures develop.
◆ Other signs and symptoms include difficulty swallowing and a low-grade fever.

OTHER
Surgery
◆ Surgery that impairs calcium absorption may cause hypocalcemia.

Treatments
◆ Multiple blood transfusions and parathyroidectomy may cause hypocalcemia.

◆ If hyperventilation occurs, help the patient slow his breathing.
◆ To reduce the patient's anxiety, provide a quiet, dark environment.
◆ Administer calcium replacement, as prescribed.

PEDIATRIC POINTERS
◆ Monitor children with hypocalcemia caused by idiopathic hypoparathyroidism; carpopedal spasm may precede the onset of epileptiform seizures or generalized tetany.

GERIATRIC POINTERS
◆ Suspect tetanus in anyone with carpopedal spasm, difficulty swallowing, and seizures.
◆ Ask the elderly patient about his immunization record and recent wounds.

◆ Explain the importance of tetanus immunization and keeping an up-to-date immunization record and schedule.
◆ Discuss dietary sources of calcium and daily requirements, as appropriate.

Cat's cry

OVERVIEW

- Occurs during infancy; syndrome indicated by mewing, kittenlike sound (also known as *cri du chat*)
- Affects about 1 in 50,000 neonates and affects females more commonly than males
- May result from abnormal laryngeal development
- Commonly seen with profound mental retardation and failure to thrive
- Of those affected, normal life span in some; serious organ defects and other life-threatening medical conditions in others
- Chromosomal defect responsible (deletion of short arm of chromosome 5) usually appearing spontaneously, but may be inherited from carrier parent

ACTION STAT! *Be alert for signs of respiratory distress, such as nasal flaring; irregular, shallow respirations; cyanosis; and a respiratory rate over 60 breaths/minute. Be prepared to suction the neonate and to administer warmed oxygen. Keep emergency resuscitation equipment nearby because bradycardia may develop.*

HISTORY

- If you detect cat's cry in an older infant, ask the parents when it developed. The sudden onset of an abnormal cry in an infant with a previously normal, vigorous cry suggests other disorders.

PHYSICAL ASSESSMENT

- Perform a complete physical examination, and note abnormalities.

CAUSES

MEDICAL
Cat's cry syndrome
- A kittenlike cry begins at birth or shortly thereafter.
- Typically, the neonate has a round face with wide-set eyes; strabismus; a broad-based nose with oblique or down-sloping epicanthal folds; abnormally shaped, low-set ears; and an unusually small jaw; other abnormalities include a short neck, webbed fingers, a simian crease, heart defects, and GI problems.
- Associated signs and symptoms include profound mental retardation, microcephaly, low birth weight, hypotonia, failure to thrive, and feeding difficulties.

NURSING CONSIDERATIONS

- Connect the neonate to an apnea monitor, and check for signs of respiratory distress.
- Keep suction equipment and warmed oxygen available.
- Obtain a blood sample for chromosomal analysis.
- Prepare the neonate for a computed tomography scan to rule out other causes of microcephaly and for an ear, nose, and throat examination to evaluate vocal cords.
- Because the neonate with cat's cry syndrome is usually a poor eater, monitor intake, output, and weight. Instruct the parents to offer small, frequent feedings.

PATIENT TEACHING

- Teach the parents and family members about the disease, its long-term effects, and the prognosis.
- Prepare the parents to work with a team of specialists in such various fields as genetics, neurology, cardiology, and speech and language. Instruct them on the purpose of the team members.
- Inform the parents and family about available support groups and counselors.

Chest expansion, asymmetrical

OVERVIEW

- Uneven extension of portions of the chest wall during inspiration
- May develop suddenly or gradually and may affect one or both sides of the chest wall
- May be a sign of a potentially life-threatening disorder (see *Recognizing life-threatening causes of asymmetrical chest expansion*)

◆ **ACTION STAT!** *Always suspect flail chest and treat as a life-threatening emergency. Take the patient's vital signs, and look for signs of acute respiratory distress. Use tape or sandbags to temporarily splint the unstable flail segment. Administer oxygen by nasal cannula, mask, or mechanical ventilation, depending on the severity of respiratory distress. Insert an I.V. catheter to allow fluid replacement and administration of drugs for pain. Draw a blood sample for arterial blood gas analysis, and connect the patient to a cardiac monitor. Continue to watch for signs of respiratory distress.*

HISTORY

- Ask about the onset, duration, aggravating and alleviating factors, and extent of dyspnea or pain during breathing.
- Obtain a history of pulmonary or systemic illness, thoracic surgery, or blunt or penetrating chest trauma.
- Obtain an occcupational history, asking about exposure to potentially hazardous chemicals and biohazards.

PHYSICAL ASSESSMENT

- Palpate the trachea for midline positioning.
- Examine the anterior and posterior chest wall for tenderness or deformity.
- Evaluate the extent of asymmetrical chest expansion.
- Palpate for vocal or tactile fremitus on both sides of the chest. Note asymmetrical vibrations and areas of enhanced, diminished, or absent fremitus.
- Percuss and auscultate to detect air and fluid in the lungs and pleural spaces.
- Auscultate all lung fields for abnormal breath sounds.

Recognizing life-threatening causes of asymmetrical chest expansion

Asymmetrical chest expansion can result from several life-threatening disorders. Two common causes—bronchial obstruction and flail chest—produce distinctive chest wall movements that provide important clues about the underlying disorder.

With *bronchial obstruction*, only the unaffected portion of the chest wall expands during inspiration. Intercostal bulging during expiration may indicate that the air is trapped in the chest.

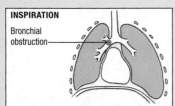

INSPIRATION
Bronchial obstruction

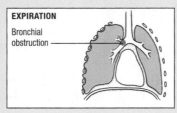

EXPIRATION
Bronchial obstruction

With *flail chest*—a disruption of the thorax due to multiple rib fractures—the unstable portion of the chest wall collapses inward at inspiration and balloons outward at expiration.

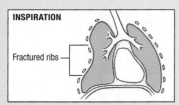

INSPIRATION

Fractured ribs

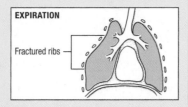

EXPIRATION

Fractured ribs

CAUSES

MEDICAL
Bronchial obstruction
◆ A life-threatening disorder, lack of chest movement indicates complete obstruction; lagging chest signals partial obstruction.
◆ Intercostal bulging during expiration and hyperresonance on percussion suggests air trapped in the chest.
◆ Other signs and symptoms may include dyspnea, accessory muscle use, decreased or absent breath sounds, and suprasternal, substernal, or intercostal retractions.

Flail chest
◆ A life-threatening disorder, the unstable portion of the chest wall collapses inward during inspiration and balloons outward during expiration.
◆ Ecchymoses and severe localized pain occur with traumatic injury to the chest wall.
◆ Rapid and shallow respirations, tachycardia, and cyanosis may also occur.

Hemothorax
◆ A life-threatening disorder, bleeding into the pleural space causes the chest to lag during inspiration.
◆ Other signs and symptoms include signs of traumatic chest injury, stabbing pain at the injury site, anxiety, dullness on percussion, tachypnea, tachycardia, hypoxemia, and signs of shock.

Kyphoscoliosis
◆ Lateral and posterior curvature of the spine causes compression of the lung.
◆ Chest wall movement is decreased on the compressed-lung side, and intercostal muscles expand during inspiration on the opposite side.

Myasthenia gravis
◆ Progressive loss of ventilatory muscle function produces asynchrony of the chest and abdomen during inspiration.

◆ Shallow respirations and increased muscle weakness cause severe dyspnea, tachypnea, and possible apnea.

Phrenic nerve dysfunction
◆ The paralyzed hemidiaphragm fails to contract downward; onset may be gradual or sudden.
◆ Asynchrony of thorax and upper abdomen during inspiration develops on the affected side.

Pneumonia
◆ Inspiratory lagging chest or chest-abdomen asynchrony occurs.
◆ Other signs and symptoms include fever, chills, tachycardia, fatigue, productive cough with rust-colored sputum, tachypnea, dyspnea, crackles, rhonchi, and chest pain that worsens with deep breathing.

Pneumothorax
◆ This life-threatening disorder can occur, in which free air enters the pleural cavity, collapsing the lung and lagging the chest at end-inspiration.
◆ Sudden, stabbing chest pain that may radiate to the arms, face, back, or abdomen occurs.
◆ Other signs and symptoms include tachypnea, decreased tactile fremitus, tympany on percussion, decreased or absent breath sounds over the trapped air, tachycardia, restlessness, and anxiety.
◆ In tension pneumothorax, the same findings occur as in pneumothorax but are more severe.
◆ Other signs and symptoms of tension pneumothorax include cyanosis; hypotension; subcutaneous crepitation of the upper trunk, neck, and face; mediastinal and tracheal deviation from the affected side; and a crunching sound on auscultation over the precordium with each heartbeat.

OTHER
Treatments
◆ Pneumonectomy and surgical removal of several ribs can cause asymmetrical chest expansion.

◆ Mainstem bronchial intubation may also cause chest lag or the absence of chest movement.

NURSING CONSIDERATIONS

◆ Prepare the patient for pulmonary studies.
◆ Auscultate all lung fields.
◆ Give supplemental oxygen during acute events.
  If the patient has a chest tube:
◆ Maintain the water seal.
◆ Check the system for air leaks.
◆ Monitor drainage.

PEDIATRIC POINTERS
◆ Asymmetrical chest expansion may develop with acute respiratory illnesses, congenital abnormalities, cerebral palsy, and life-threatening diaphragmatic hernia.

GERIATRIC POINTERS
◆ Asymmetrical chest expansion may be more difficult to determine because of the structural deformities associated with aging.

PATIENT TEACHING

◆ Explain to the patient or caregiver how to recognize early signs and symptoms of respiratory distress and what to do if they occur.
◆ Teach the patient coughing and deep-breathing exercises.
◆ Teach the patient techniques that can help reduce his anxiety.
◆ Teach the patient about all hospital procedures, tests, and interventions, such as chest tube insertion and oxygen administration.

Chest pain

- Results from disorders that affect thoracic or abdominal organs
- May be sudden or gradual in onset
- May radiate to the arms, neck, jaw, or back
- Can be steady or intermittent, mild or acute
- May be an indicator of acute and life-threatening disorders (see *Managing severe chest pain*)

HISTORY

- Ask about the onset and radiation of pain and its duration, quality, quantity, and what aggravates or alleviates it. (See *Atypical chest pain in women* and *Understanding chest pain.*)
- Obtain a history of cardiac or pulmonary disease, chest trauma, GI disease, or sickle cell anemia or anxiety disorders.
- Obtain a drug history, including tobacco use.

PHYSICAL ASSESSMENT

- Take vital signs; note tachypnea, fever, tachycardia, oxygen saturation, paradoxical pulse, and hypertension or hypotension.
- Look for jugular vein distention and peripheral edema.
- Observe breathing pattern; inspect the chest for asymmetrical expansion.
- Auscultate for pleural rub, crackles, rhonchi, wheezing, and diminished or absent breath sounds.
- Auscultate for murmurs, clicks, gallops, and pericardial rub.
- Palpate for lifts, heaves, thrills, gallops, tactile fremitus, and abdominal masses or tenderness.

CAUSES

MEDICAL
Angina pectoris
- Chest discomfort may be described as pain or a sensation of indigestion or expansion.

- Pain usually occurs in the retrosternal region behind the sternum and typically lasts 2 to 10 minutes.
- Pain may radiate to the neck, jaw, and arms.
- Emotional stress, exertion, or a heavy meal may provoke anginal pain.
- Other signs and symptoms include dyspnea, nausea, vomiting, tachycardia, dizziness, diaphoresis, belching, and palpitations.
- With Prinzmetal's angina, pain occurs at rest and with shortness of breath, nausea, vomiting, dizziness, and palpitations.

Anthrax, inhalation
- Early signs and symptoms include low-grade fever, chills, cough, and chest pain.
- Later signs and symptoms are characterized by abrupt development and rapid deterioration, including high fever, dyspnea, stridor, and hypotension, generally leading to death within 24 hours.

Anxiety
- Intermittent, sharp, stabbing pain that often occurs behind the left breast.
- Other signs and symptoms include precordial tenderness, palpitations, fatigue, headache, insomnia, breathlessness, nausea, vomiting, diarrhea, and tremors.

ACTION STAT!

Managing severe chest pain

If the patient reports a sudden onset of pleuritic chest pain, described as crushing, shooting, and deep, assess him for diaphoresis, dyspnea, hemoptysis, and tachycardia. If you detect these signs and symptoms, suspect *pulmonary embolism*.

If the patient tells you his chest pain started suddenly and describes it as tearing, ripping, or stabbing, question him about syncope and hemiplegia. Check for differences in blood pressure between legs and arms as well as weak or absent femoral or pedal pulses. Begin interventions for *aortic aneurysm* if you assess these signs.

If the patient reports the sudden onset of severe substernal pain that radiates to his left arm, jaw, neck, or shoulder blades that he describes as squeezing, viselike, or burning, have him lie down. Assess for pallor, diaphoresis, nausea, vomiting, apprehension, weakness, fatigue, and dyspnea. If you detect these signs and symptoms, suspect *myocardial infarction*.

If you suspect any of these life-threatening disorders, quickly take the patient's vital signs. Obtain a 12-lead electrocardiogram. Insert an I.V. catheter to administer fluids and drugs, and give oxygen. Check the patient's vital signs frequently to detect changes from baseline. Begin cardiac monitoring to detect arrhythmias. As appropriate, prepare the patient for emergency surgery.

If the patient reports a sudden onset of diffuse chest tightness, assess for wheezing, dry cough, dyspnea, tachycardia, and hyperventilation. The presence of these signs and symptoms suggests an acute *asthmatic attack*. Try to calm the patient to slow his respiratory rate. Ask him if he has ever had this pain before and, if so, what eased it. Give oxygen and insert an I.V. catheter to administer fluids and drugs. Expect to give epinephrine and a bronchodilator and to begin respiratory therapy.

Atypical chest pain in women

Women with coronary artery disease may experience typical chest pain (crushing chest pain that radiates down the arm or to the jaw), but commonly experience atypical chest pain, vague chest pain, or a lack of chest pain.

Atypical symptoms may include upper back discomfort between the shoulder blades, palpitations, feeling of fullness in the neck, nausea, dizziness, unexplained fatigue, and exhaustion or shortness of breath.

Aortic aneurysm, dissecting

◆ A life-threatening disorder, excruciating tearing, ripping, stabbing chest and neck pain begins suddenly and radiates to the upper and lower back and abdomen.
◆ Other signs and symptoms include abdominal tenderness; tachycardia; murmurs; syncope; blindness; loss of consciousness; weakness or transient paralysis of the arms or legs; hypotension; asymmetrical brachial pulses; lower blood pressure in the legs than in the arms; pale, cool, diaphoretic, and mottled skin below the waist; weak or absent femoral or pedal pulses; a palpable abdominal mass; and systolic bruit.

Asthma

◆ Diffuse and painful chest tightness, dry cough, and mild wheezing arise suddenly.
◆ Signs may progress to a productive cough, audible wheezing, and severe dyspnea.
◆ Associated respiratory signs and symptoms include rhonchi, crackles, prolonged expirations, intercostal and supraclavicular retractions on inspiration, accessory muscle use, flaring nostrils, and tachypnea.
◆ Other signs and symptoms include anxiety, tachycardia, diaphoresis, flushing, and cyanosis.
◆ Asthma may be associated with exercise, cold air, or environmental triggers.

Bronchitis

◆ The acute form produces a burning chest pain or a sensation of substernal tightness.
◆ Cough is initially dry but later productive.
◆ Other signs and symptoms include a low-grade fever, chills, sore throat, tachycardia, muscle and back pain, rhonchi, crackles, and wheezing.

Cardiomyopathy

◆ Hypertrophic cardiomyopathy may cause angina-like chest pain, dyspnea, cough, dizziness, syncope, gallops, murmurs, and bradycardia associated with tachycardia.
◆ A medium-pitched systolic ejection murmur may be heard along the left sternal border and top of the heart.
◆ Palpation of peripheral pulses reveals a characteristic double impulse (*pulsus biferiens*).
◆ The patient has a laterally displaced point of maximal impulse.

Cholecystitis

◆ Epigastric or right-upper-quadrant pain occurs abruptly because of gallbladder inflammation.
◆ Pain may be sharp or intensely aching, steady or intermittent.
◆ Pain may radiate to the back or right shoulder.
◆ An abdominal mass, rigidity, distention, or tenderness may be palpable in the right upper abdomen.
◆ Other signs and symptoms include Murphy's sign, nausea, vomiting, fever, diaphoresis, and chills.

(continued)

Understanding chest pain

DESCRIPTION	LOCATION	CAUSES
Aching, squeezing, pressure, heaviness, and burning pain; usually subsides within 10 minutes	Substernal; may radiate to jaw, neck, arms, and back	Angina pectoris
Tightness or pressure; burning, aching pain, possibly accompanied by shortness of breath, diaphoresis, weakness, anxiety, or nausea; sudden onset; lasts 30 minutes to 2 hours	Typically across chest but may radiate to jaw, neck, arms, or back	Acute myocardial infarction
Sharp and continuous; may be accompanied by friction rub; sudden onset, may be positional	Substernal; may radiate to neck or left arm	Pericarditis
Excruciating, tearing pain; may be accompanied by blood pressure difference between right and left arm; sudden onset	Retrosternal, upper abdominal, or epigastric; may radiate to back, neck, or shoulders	Dissecting aortic aneurysm
Sudden, stabbing pain; may be accompanied by cyanosis, dyspnea, or cough with hemoptysis	Over lung area	Pulmonary embolus
Sudden and severe pain, sometimes accompanied by dyspnea, increased pulse rate, decreased breath sounds (especially on one side), or deviated trachea	Lateral thorax	Pneumothorax
Dull, squeezing pain or pressure	Substernal, epigastric areas	Esophageal spasm
Sharp, severe pain	Lower chest or upper abdomen	Hiatal hernia
Burning feeling after eating that's sometimes accompanied by hematemesis or tarry stools; sudden onset; generally subsides within 15 to 20 minutes	Epigastric	Peptic ulcer
Gripping, sharp pain, possibly accompanied by nausea and vomiting. especially following meals	Right epigastric or abdominal areas; may radiate to shoulders	Cholecystitis
Continuous or intermittent sharp pain; possibly tender to touch; gradual or sudden onset	Anywhere in chest	Chest-wall syndrome
Dull or stabbing pain usually accompanied by hyperventilation or breathlessness; sudden onset; lasting less than 1 minute or as long as several days	Anywhere in chest	Acute anxiety

Costochondritis

◆ Pain and tenderness due to inflammation occur at the costochondral junctions, especially at the second costicartilage.
◆ Pain is elicited by palpating the inflamed joint and worsens with movement.

Esophageal spasm

◆ Substernal chest pain mimics angina.
◆ Pain may last up to an hour and can radiate to the neck, jaw, arms, or back.
◆ Other findings include dysphagia for solid foods, bradycardia, and nodal rhythm.

Herpes zoster, shingles

◆ This infection caused by a herpes virus leads to inflammation of ganglia and nerve roots.
◆ Initially, pain is sharp, shooting, and one-sided; it may mimic myocardial infarction.
◆ About 4 to 5 days after onset, chest pain becomes burning, and small, red, nodular lesions erupt on the painful areas.
◆ Other signs and symptoms include fever, malaise, pruritus, and paresthesia or hyperesthesia of the affected areas.

Hiatal hernia

◆ Heartburn and sternal ache or pressure occur and may radiate to left shoulder and arm.
◆ Pain occurs after a meal and with bending or lying down.
◆ Other findings include a bitter taste and pain while eating or drinking.

Interstitial lung disease

◆ Pleuritic chest pain, progressive dyspnea, "cellophane" crackles, nonproductive cough, fatigue, weight loss, decreased exercise tolerance, clubbing, and cyanosis occur.

Legionnaires' disease

◆ Pleuritic chest pain, malaise, headache, and general weakness develop early in this bacterial infection.

◆ Within 2 to 10 days of exposure, a sudden high fever; chills; a nonproductive cough that eventually yields mucoid and then mucopurulent sputum; and, possibly hemoptysis, occur.
◆ Other signs and symptoms include diarrhea, flushed skin, diaphoresis, prostration, anorexia, nausea, vomiting, diffuse myalgia, mild temporary amnesia, confusion, dyspnea, crackles, tachypnea, and tachycardia.

Mediastinitis

◆ Severe retrosternal chest pain radiates to the epigastrium, back, or shoulder.
◆ Pain may worsen with breathing, coughing, or sneezing.
◆ Chills, fever, and dysphagia may also occur.

Mitral valve prolapse

◆ Sharp, stabbing precordial chest pain or precordial ache may occur.
◆ A midsystolic click is followed by a systolic murmur at the apex.
◆ Other signs and symptoms include cardiac awareness, migraine headache, dizziness, weakness, episodic severe fatigue, dyspnea, tachycardia, anxiety, mood swings, and palpitations.

Muscle strain

◆ A superficial and continuous ache or pulling sensation in the chest may result from strain.
◆ Lifting, pulling, or pushing heavy objects may aggravate this discomfort.
◆ Fatigue, weakness, and rapid swelling of the affected area occur with acute strain.

Myocardial infarction

◆ Crushing substernal pain occurs that isn't relieved by nitroglycerin.
◆ Pain lasts 15 minutes to hours and may radiate to the left arm, jaw, neck, or shoulder blades.
◆ Other signs and symptoms include pallor, clammy skin, dyspnea, diaphoresis, nausea, vomiting, anxiety, restlessness, murmurs, crackles, hypotension or hypertension, a feeling

of impending doom, and an atrial gallop.

Pancreatitis

◆ Acute form causes intense pain in the epigastric area.
◆ Pain radiates to the back and worsens in a supine position.
◆ Extreme restlessness, mottled skin, tachycardia, and cold, sweaty extremities may occur with severe pancreatitis.
◆ Massive hemorrhage, with resultant shock and coma, occurs with sudden, severe pancreatitis.
◆ Other signs and symptoms include nausea, vomiting, fever, abdominal tenderness and rigidity, diminished bowel sounds, and crackles at the lung bases.

Peptic ulcer

◆ Sharp and burning pain arises in the epigastric region hours after food intake, commonly during the night.
◆ Pain is relieved by food or antacids.
◆ Other signs and symptoms include nausea, vomiting, melena, and epigastric tenderness.

Pericarditis

◆ Sharp or cutting precordial or retrosternal pain is aggravated by deep breathing, coughing, and position changes.
◆ Pain radiates to the shoulder and neck.
◆ Other signs and symptoms include pericardial rub, fever, tachycardia, and dyspnea.

Pleurisy

◆ Sharp, usually one-sided, pain in the lower aspects of the chest arises abruptly, reaching maximum intensity within a few hours.
◆ Deep breathing, coughing, or thoracic movement aggravates pain.
◆ Decreased breath sounds, inspiratory crackles, and a pleural rub may be heard on auscultation.
◆ Other signs and symptoms include dyspnea, shallow breathing, cyanosis, fever, and fatigue.

Pneumonia

◆ Pleuritic chest pain increases with deep inspiration.
◆ Shaking chills, fever, and a dry, hacking cough that later becomes productive occur.
◆ Other signs and symptoms include crackles, rhonchi, tachycardia, tachypnea, myalgia, fatigue, headache, dyspnea, abdominal pain, anorexia, cyanosis, decreased breath sounds, and diaphoresis.

Pneumonic plague

◆ Signs and symptoms include productive cough, chest pain, tachypnea, dyspnea, hemoptysis, increasing respiratory distress, and cardiopulmonary insufficiency.

Pneumothorax

◆ A life-threatening disorder, sudden, severe, sharp chest pain typically presents on one side and increases with chest movement.
◆ Dyspnea and cyanosis progressively worsen.
◆ Breath sounds are decreased or absent on the affected side, with hyperresonance or tympany, subcutaneous crepitation, and decreased vocal fremitus.
◆ Other signs and symptoms include asymmetrical chest expansion, accessory muscle use, a nonproductive cough, tachypnea, tachycardia, anxiety, and restlessness.

Pulmonary embolism

◆ Sudden dyspnea occurs with intense angina-like or pleuritic pain that's aggravated by deep breathing and thoracic movement.
◆ Cyanosis and distended neck veins occur with a large embolus.
◆ Other signs and symptoms include a choking sensation, tachycardia, tachypnea, cough, low-grade fever, restlessness, diaphoresis, crackles, pleural rub, diffuse wheezing, dullness on percussion, signs of respiratory collapse, paradoxical pulse, signs of cerebral ischemia, and signs of hypoxia.

Pulmonary hypertension, primary

◆ Angina-like pain develops late and typically occurs on exertion.
◆ Pain may radiate to the neck.
◆ Other signs and symptoms include exertional dyspnea, fatigue, syncope, weakness, cough, and hemoptysis.

Q fever

◆ This acute systemic disease is caused by *Coxiella burnetii* infection.
◆ Fever, chills, severe headache, myalgia, malaise, chest pain, nausea, vomiting, and diarrhea occur.
◆ Hepatitis or pneumonia may develop in severe cases.

Rib fracture

◆ Chest pain is usually sharp, severe, and aggravated by inspiration, coughing, or pressure on the affected area.
◆ Other signs and symptoms include dyspnea, cough, tenderness and slight edema at the fracture site, and shallow, splinted breathing.

Sickle cell crisis

◆ Pain may be vague at first and located in the back, hands, or feet.
◆ As pain worsens, it becomes generalized or localized to the abdomen or chest, causing severe pleuritic pain.
◆ Other signs and symptoms may include abdominal distention and rigidity, dyspnea, fever, and jaundice.

Tuberculosis

◆ Pleuritic chest pain and fine crackles occur after coughing.
◆ Other signs and symptoms include night sweats, anorexia, weight loss, fever, malaise, dyspnea, fatigue, mild to severe productive cough, hemoptysis, dullness on percussion, increased tactile fremitus, and amphoric breath sounds.

OTHER
Drugs

◆ Abrupt withdrawal from a beta-adrenergic blocker can cause rebound angina in the patient with coronary heart disease.

NURSING CONSIDERATIONS

◆ Prepare the patient for cardiopulmonary studies.
◆ Perform a venipuncture to collect a serum specimen for cardiac enzyme and other studies.
◆ Maintain cardiac monitoring and I.V.; assess as appropriate.

PEDIATRIC POINTERS

◆ A child may complain of chest pain in an attempt to get attention or to avoid attending school.

GERIATRIC POINTERS

◆ Because older patients have a higher risk of developing life-threatening conditions, carefully evaluate reports of chest pain.

PATIENT TEACHING

◆ Alert the patient or caregiver to signs and symptoms that require immediate medical attention.
◆ Explain the diagnostic tests the patient needs.
◆ Provide details to the patient about his prescribed drugs and how to take them.
◆ Teach the patient about the underlying diagnosis and ways to prevent chest pain in the future.

Cheyne-Stokes respirations

OVERVIEW

◆ A waxing and waning period of hyperpnea that alternates with a shorter period of apnea (see *Respiratory pattern of Cheyne-Stokes*)
◆ May occur normally in patients with heart or lung disease or those who live at high altitudes
◆ Usually indicate increased intracranial pressure (ICP) from a deep cerebral or brain stem lesion or a metabolic disturbance in the brain

■■ **ACTION STAT!** *In a patient with a history of head trauma, recent brain surgery, or another brain insult, quickly take his vital signs. Elevate the head of the bed 30 degrees, and perform a rapid neurological examination. Watch for signs of rising ICP, and anticipate ICP monitoring.*

Time the periods of hyperpnea and apnea, being alert for prolonged periods of apnea. Assess vital signs and neurological status frequently to detect changes. Maintain airway patency, and administer oxygen, as needed. Mechanical ventilation may be necessary if the patient's condition worsens.

HISTORY

◆ Obtain a medical and surgical history.
◆ Ask about drug use.

PHYSICAL ASSESSMENT

◆ Perform a complete physical examination, focusing on the neurologic and cardiorespiratory systems.

Respiratory pattern of Cheyne-Stokes

When assessing a patient's respirations, you should determine the rate, rhythm, and depth. This schematic diagram shows respiratory pattern of Cheyne-Stokes—respirations that gradually become faster and deeper than normal, then slow to brief periods of apnea.

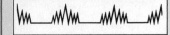

MEDICAL
Adams-Stokes syndrome
◆ Adams-Stokes attacks may precede Cheyne-Stokes respirations.
◆ A syncopal episode associated with atrioventricular block occurs.
◆ Other signs and symptoms include hypotension, a heart rate between 20 and 50 beats/minute, confusion, shaking, and paleness.

Heart failure
◆ Cheyne-Stokes respirations may occur with exertional dyspnea and orthopnea in left-sided heart failure.
◆ Other signs and symptoms include fatigue, weakness, tachycardia, tachypnea, and crackles.

Hypertensive encephalopathy
◆ A life-threatening disorder, severe hypertension precedes Cheyne-Stokes respirations.
◆ Other signs and symptoms include decreased level of consciousness (LOC), vomiting, seizures, severe headaches, vision disturbances, and transient paralysis.

Increased ICP
◆ Cheyne-Stokes respirations are the first irregular respiratory pattern to occur as ICP rises.
◆ Bradycardia and widened pulse pressure are late signs of increased ICP.
◆ Accompanying signs and symptoms include decreased LOC, hypertension, headache, vomiting, impaired motor movement, and vision disturbances.

Renal failure
◆ Cheyne-Stokes respirations occur with end-stage chronic renal failure.
◆ Other signs and symptoms include bleeding gums, oral lesions, ammonia breath odor, and marked changes in every body system.

OTHER
Drugs
◆ Large doses of an opioid, hypnotic, or barbiturate can precipitate Cheyne-Stokes respiratory pattern.

NURSING CONSIDERATIONS

◆ Don't mistake periods of hypoventilation or decreased tidal volume for complete apnea.

PEDIATRIC POINTERS
◆ Cheyne-Stokes respirations rarely occur in children except during late heart failure.

GERIATRIC POINTERS
◆ Cheyne-Stokes respirations may occur normally in elderly people during sleep.

PATIENT TEACHING

◆ Teach the patient and a responsible person to recognize the difference between sleep apnea and Cheyne-Stokes respirations.
◆ Explain the causes and treatments of conditions leading to Cheyne-Stokes respirations.

Chills

OVERVIEW

- Extreme, involuntary muscle contractions with paroxysms of violent shivering and teeth chattering
- Signal onset of infection
- Commonly accompanied by fever (see *Why chills accompany fever*)

HISTORY

- Ask about the onset and duration of chills (continuous or intermittent).
- Inquire about related signs and symptoms.
- Obtain a history of allergies or infectious disorders.

- Take a drug history.
- Ask about recent treatments (such as chemotherapy), travel, and exposure to animals or infection. (See *Rare causes of chills*.)

PHYSICAL ASSESSMENT

- Take vital signs.
- Note the pattern of temperature changes.
- Assess the skin, mucous membranes, liver, spleen, and lymph nodes.
- Check for drainage from skin lesions.
- Note skin color, temperature, and turgor.
- Percuss for costovertebral angle tenderness to determine if cystitis is present.
- Assess level of consciousness (LOC).

CAUSES

MEDICAL

Acquired immunodeficiency syndrome
- Signs and symptoms include fatigue, fever, chills, anorexia, weight loss, diarrhea, diaphoresis, skin disorders, lymphadenopathy, and upper respiratory tract infection.

Why chills accompany fever

Fever usually occurs when exogenous pyrogens activate endogenous pyrogens to reset the body's thermostat to a higher level. At this higher thermostatic setpoint, the body feels cold and responds through several compensatory mechanisms, including rhythmic muscle contractions, or chills. These muscle contractions in turn generate body heat and help produce fever. This flowchart outlines the events that link chills to fever.

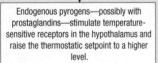

| Exogenous pyrogens (infectious organisms, immune complexes, toxins) enter the body. |

↓

| Phagocytic leukocytes release endogenous pyrogens. |

↓

| Endogenous pyrogens—possibly with prostaglandins—stimulate temperature-sensitive receptors in the hypothalamus and raise the thermostatic setpoint to a higher level. |

↓

| Descending efferent pathways from the hypothalamus innervate effectors, such as skeletal muscles, and stimulate them to rhythmically contract. |

↓

| Rhythmic muscle contractions, or chills, generate body heat, which helps produce fever. |

Rare causes of chills

Chills can result from disorders that are rare in the United States but may be fairly common worldwide. Remember to ask about recent foreign travel when you obtain a patient's history. Among the many rare disorders that produce chills are:
- brucellosis (undulant fever)
- dengue fever (breakbone fever)
- epidemic typhus (louse-borne typhus)
- leptospirosis
- lymphocytic choriomeningitis
- miliary TB
- plague
- Q fever
- rat bite fever (Haverhill fever, Sodoku)
- relapsing fever (bilious typhoid).
- tularemia

Anthrax, inhalation
- Early signs and symptoms include low-grade fever, chills, cough, and chest pain.
- Later signs and symptoms are characterized by abrupt development and rapid deterioration, including high fever, dyspnea, stridor, and hypotension, generally leading to death within 24 hours.

Cholangitis
- Charcot's triad of signs and symptoms includes chills with spiking fever, abdominal pain, and jaundice.
- Other signs and symptoms include pruritus, weakness, fatigue, dark urine, and light-colored stools.

Gram-negative bacteremia
- Infection causes sudden chills and fever, nausea, vomiting, diarrhea, and prostration.
- Other signs and symptoms include tachypnea, hypotension, decreased urine output, and an altered LOC.

Hemolytic anemia
- Fulminating chills develop with fever and abdominal pain.
- Other signs and symptoms may include rapidly developing jaundice, hepatomegaly, splenomegaly, and brown or red urine.

Hepatic abscess
- Signs and symptoms include chills, fever, nausea, vomiting, diarrhea, anorexia, and severe upper abdominal tenderness and pain that may radiate to the right shoulder.

Hodgkin's lymphoma
- Several days or weeks of fever and chills alternate with periods of no fever and no chills.
- Regional lymphadenopathy may progress to hepatosplenomegaly.
- Other signs and symptoms include diaphoresis, fatigue, and pruritus.

Infective endocarditis
- Intermittent, shaking chills with fever occur abruptly.
- Other signs and symptoms include petechiae, Janeway lesions on the

hands and feet, Osler's nodes on the palms and soles, murmur, hematuria, eye hemorrhage, Roth's spots, and signs of heart failure.

Influenza
- Onset of chills, high fever, malaise, headache, myalgia, and nonproductive cough is abrupt.
- Rhinitis, rhinorrhea, laryngitis, conjunctivitis, hoarseness, and sore throat may occur.
- Chills generally subside after the first few days.
- Intermittent fever, weakness, and cough may persist for up to 1 week.

Legionnaires' disease
- Within 2 to 10 days of bacterial exposure, a sudden high fever; chills; a nonproductive cough that eventually yields mucoid and then mucopurulent sputum; and possibly, hemoptysis occur.
- Other signs and symptoms include diarrhea, flushed skin, diaphoresis, prostration, anorexia, nausea, vomiting, diffuse myalgia, mild temporary amnesia, confusion, dyspnea, crackles, tachypnea, and tachycardia.

Lymphangitis
- Chills and other systemic signs and symptoms (such as fever, malaise, and headache) develop.
- Red streaks radiating from a wound and cellulitis draining toward tender, regional lymph nodes are characteristic.
- Lymph nodes along the course of drainage may be enlarged, red, and tender.

Malaria
- The paroxysmal cycle begins with a period of chills lasting 1 to 2 hours.
- Chills are then followed by a high fever lasting 3 to 4 hours and then 2 to 4 hours of profuse diaphoresis.
- Other signs and symptoms include headache, muscle pain, and hepatosplenomegaly.

Otitis media
- Acute suppurative otitis media produces chills with fever and severe deep, throbbing ear pain.

- A mild conductive hearing loss and a bulging, hyperemic tympanic membrane may also occur.
- Other signs and symptoms include dizziness, nausea, and vomiting.

Pneumonia
- A single shaking chill signals the sudden onset of pneumococcal pneumonia.
- Other types of pneumonia cause intermittent chills.
- Other signs and symptoms include fever, productive cough, pleuritic chest pain, dyspnea, tachypnea, tachycardia, diaphoresis, crackles, rhonchi, and increased tactile fremitus.

Pyelonephritis
- Chills, high fever, and possible nausea and vomiting over several hours to days occur.
- Other signs and symptoms include anorexia, fatigue, myalgia, flank pain, costovertebral angle tenderness, hematuria or cloudy urine, and urinary frequency, urgency, and burning.

Rocky Mountain spotted fever
- Sudden onset of chills, fever, malaise, excruciating headache, and muscle, bone, and joint pain occur; a petechial rash develops after a few days.
- A thick white coating that gradually turns brown develops on the tongue.
- After 2 to 6 days of fever and occasional chills, a macular or maculopapular rash occurs on the hands and feet and then becomes generalized.

Septic shock
- Early signs and symptoms include chills, fever, and possible nausea, vomiting, and diarrhea.
- Late signs and symptoms include cold, clammy skin; rapid, thready pulse; severe hypotension; oliguria or anuria; signs of respiratory failure; and coma.
- Other signs and symptoms include tachycardia; tachypnea; warm, flushed, dry skin; thirst; anxiety; restlessness; confusion; and cool, cyanotic limbs as shock progresses.

OTHER
Drugs
- Amphotericin B, I.V. bleomycin, oral antipyretics, and phenytoin may cause chills.
- Withdrawal from alcohol, analgesics, antidepressants, benzodiazepines, ecstacy (MDMA), hallucinogens, heroin, and marijuana may cause chills.

I.V. therapy
- Infection at the I.V. insertion site can cause chills, high fever, and local redness, warmth, induration, and tenderness.

Transfusion reaction
- A hemolytic reaction may cause chills during or immediately after the transfusion.

NURSING CONSIDERATIONS
- Frequently check vital signs.
- Be alert for signs of progressive septic shock.
- Obtain cultures of blood, sputum, or wound drainage to determine the cause.
- Give prescribed antibiotics.
- Keep room temperature comfortable.
- Provide adequate hydration and nutrients.
- Administer prescribed antipyretics.

PEDIATRIC POINTERS
- Infants usually don't get chills because they have poorly developed shivering mechanisms.

PATIENT TEACHING
- Explain the importance of documenting temperature to reveal patterns.
- Explain treatment and antibiotics the patient needs.
- Explain the signs and symptoms of a worsening condition and when to seek medical attention.

Chorea

- Brief, unpredictable bursts of rapid, jerky motion that interrupt normal coordinated movement
- Indicates dysfunction of the extra-pyramidal system
- Usually involves the face, head, lower arms, and hands
- Aggravated by excitement or fatigue; may disappear during sleep
- May be difficult to distinguish from athetosis (snakelike, writhing movements), although choreiform movements are generally more rapid than athetoid ones

- Ask about the onset, duration, and description of choreiform movements.
- Note a family history of choreiform movements or Huntington's disease.
- Obtain a drug history.
- Obtain an occupational history, noting prolonged exposure to manganese or other metals.

- Ask the patient to stick out his tongue and keep it out. Typically, he'll be unable to do this; instead, his tongue will dart in and out of his mouth.
- Observe arms and legs for involuntary jerky movements.
- Ask the patient to extend and flex his hand as if halting traffic, and note the choreiform movements—they'll be extremely evident in this position.
- Check for athetosis, rigidity, or tremor.
- Assess for choreoathetotic gait by asking the patient to walk. He may change the positions of his trunk and upper body parts with each step and jerk and tilt his head to one side. His legs may move slowly and awkwardly and his gait will have a dancing quality.

MEDICAL
Cerebral infarction
- If thalamic area is involved, unilateral or bilateral chorea occurs.
- Other signs and symptoms include dysarthria, tremors, rigidity, weakness, mental status change, and sensory disturbances.

Encephalitis
- Chorea may occur in the recovery phase with low-grade fever, athetosis, hemiparesis, hemiplegia, and facial droop.
- Other signs and symptoms include headache, vomiting, photophobia, stiff neck, confusion, and drowsiness.

Huntington's disease
- Chorea may be the first sign or may occur with intellectual decline of this degenerative brain disease.
- Emotional disturbances and dementia occur.
- Choreoathetotic movements may occur, accompanied by dysarthria, dystonia, prancing gait, dysphagia, and facial grimacing.

Wilson's disease
- Chorea is an early indication of this copper metabolism disorder, in addition to dystonia that affects the arms and legs.
- Dysarthria, tremors, hoarseness, dysphagia, and slowed body movements occur.
- The pathognomonic Kayser-Fleischer ring in the cornea appears as the disease progresses.
- Other signs and symptoms include emotional and behavioral disturbances, drooling, rigidity, and mental deterioration.

OTHER
Carbon monoxide poisoning
- Chorea, rigidity, dementia, impaired sensory function, masklike facies, generalized seizures, and myoclonus may occur.

Drugs
- Phenothiazines, haloperidol, thiothixene, and loxapine commonly produce chorea.
- Metoclopramide, metyrosine, hormonal contraceptives, levodopa, and phenytoin may cause chorea.

Lead poisoning
- Chorea, seizures, headache, memory lapses, and severe mental impairment occur in later stages.
- Other signs and symptoms include masklike facies, footdrop, wristdrop, dizziness, ataxia, weakness, lethargy, abdominal pain, anorexia, nausea, vomiting, constipation, lead line on the gums, and a metallic taste.

Manganese poisoning
- Chorea occurs with propulsive gait, dystonia, and rigidity.
- Masklike facies, a resting tremor, and personality changes develop initially.
- Extreme muscle weakness and lethargy occur later.

- Pad the side rails of the patient's bed.
- Keep sharp objects out of the patient's environment.
- Help minimize physical activity and emotional upset.
- Provide adequate periods of rest and sleep.

PEDIATRIC POINTERS
- Sydenham's chorea occurs in childhood as a delayed manifestation of rheumatic fever.
- Chorea can occur in children with athetoid cerebral palsy.

- Explain safety measures to reduce the risk of falls and poisoning.
- Discuss genetic counseling (for those with Huntington's disease).

Chvostek's sign

OVERVIEW

- Spasm of the facial muscles, elicited by lightly tapping the patient's facial nerve near his lower jaw (see *Eliciting Chvostek's sign*)
- Positive sign suggesting hypocalcemia
- Positive sign occurring normally in about 25% of patients

 ACTION STAT! *Test the patient for Trousseau's sign, a reliable indicator of hypocalcemia. Monitor the patient for signs of tetany and impending seizure. Obtain an electrocardiogram to check for changes associated with hypocalcemia, which can predispose the patient to arrhythmias. Connect the patient to a cardiac monitor.*

HISTORY

- Obtain a medical history, including incidence of hypoparathyroidism, hypomagnesemia, or a malabsorption disorder.
- Ask about previous surgical removal of parathyroid glands.
- Determine whether mental changes have occurred.
- Question the patient about other symptoms, including tingling sensations around the mouth and in the fingertips and feet.

PHYSICAL ASSESSMENT

- Observe the patient's behavior.
- Observe for seizures, tetany, and facial spasms.
- Check for dry and scaling skin, brittle nails, and dry hair.
- Take vital signs because an irregular pulse and hypotension suggest hypocalcemia.
- Auscultate the lungs.
- Note signs of bronchospasm, laryngospasm, and airway obstruction.

TOP TECHNIQUE

Eliciting Chvostek's sign

Begin by telling the patient to relax his facial muscles. Then stand directly in front of him and tap the facial nerve either just anterior to the earlobe and below the zygomatic arch or between the zygomatic arch and the corner of his mouth. A positive response varies from twitching of the lip at the corner of the mouth to spasm of all facial muscles, depending on the severity of hypocalcemia.

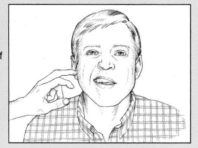

CAUSES

MEDICAL
Hypocalcemia
◆ The degree of muscle spasm elicited reflects the patient's calcium level.
◆ Paresthesia in the fingers, toes, and circumoral area that progresses to muscle tension and carpopedal spasms occur initially.
◆ Muscle weakness, muscle twitching, hyperactive deep tendon reflexes, choreiform movements, muscle cramps, fatigue, and palpitations may be present.
◆ Mental status changes; diplopia; difficulty swallowing; abdominal cramps; dry, scaly skin; brittle nails; and thin, patchy scalp hair and eyebrows occur with chronic hypocalcemia.

OTHER
Treatments
◆ Massive blood transfusion can lower calcium levels.

NURSING CONSIDERATIONS

◆ Collect blood samples for ongoing calcium studies.
◆ Administer oral or I.V. calcium supplements.
◆ Look for Chvostek's sign postoperatively.

PEDIATRIC POINTERS
◆ Because this Chvostek's sign may be observed in healthy infants, it isn't used to detect neonatal tetany.

GERIATRIC POINTERS
◆ Consider malabsorption and poor nutritional status in the elderly patient with Chvostek's sign and hypocalcemia.

PATIENT TEACHING

◆ Explain which early signs and symptoms of hypocalcemia a patient should report to the physician immediately.
◆ Teach the patient about the underlying cause of hypocalcemia and how to prevent it.

Clubbing

OVERVIEW

◆ Painless increase in soft tissue around the tips of the fingers or toes (usually on both sides) (see *Rare causes of clubbing*)
◆ Nonspecific sign of pulmonary and cyanotic cardiovascular disorders

HISTORY

◆ Obtain a thorough medical history, asking about any cardiovascular and pulmonary disorders.
◆ Ask about drug history.

PHYSICAL ASSESSMENT

◆ Perform a cardiopulmonary examination.
◆ Evaluate the extent of clubbing in the fingers and toes. (See *Checking for clubbed fingers*.)

Rare causes of clubbing

Clubbing is typically a sign of pulmonary or cardiovascular disease, but it can also result from certain hepatic and GI disorders, such as cirrhosis, Crohn's disease, and ulcerative colitis. Clubbing occurs only rarely in these disorders, however, so first check for more common signs and symptoms. For example, a patient with cirrhosis usually experiences right-upper-quadrant pain and hepatomegaly, a patient with Crohn's disease typically has abdominal cramping and tenderness, and a patient with ulcerative colitis may develop diffuse abdominal pain and blood-streaked diarrhea.

TOP TECHNIQUE

Checking for clubbed fingers

To assess the patient for chronic tissue hypoxia, check his fingers for clubbing. Normally, the angle between the fingernail and the point where the nail enters the skin is about 160 degrees. Clubbing occurs when that angle increases to 180 degrees or more, as shown below.

NORMAL FINGER

Normal angle (160 degrees)

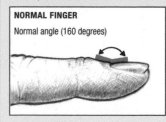

CLUBBED FINGER

Angle greater than 180 degrees

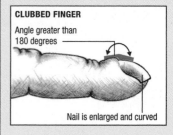

Nail is enlarged and curved

MEDICAL

Bronchiectasis
◆ Clubbing is a late sign.
◆ A cough that produces copious, foul-smelling, and mucopurulent sputum is a classic sign.
◆ Hemoptysis and coarse crackles during inspiration are also characteristic.
◆ Other signs and symptoms include weight loss, fatigue, weakness, exertional dyspnea, rhonchi, fever, malaise, and halitosis.

Bronchitis
◆ Clubbing is a late sign.
◆ Other signs and symptoms include chronic productive cough, barrel chest, dyspnea, wheezing, use of accessory muscles, cyanosis, tachypnea, crackles, scattered rhonchi, and prolonged expiration.

Emphysema
◆ Clubbing is a late sign.
◆ Other signs and symptoms include anorexia, malaise, dyspnea, tachypnea, diminished breath sounds, accessory muscle use, barrel chest, a productive cough, peripheral cyanosis, and pursed-lip breathing.

Endocarditis
◆ In subacute infective endocarditis, clubbing occurs with fever, anorexia, pallor, weakness, night sweats, fatigue, tachycardia, and weight loss.
◆ Other signs and symptoms include arthralgia, petechiae, murmurs, Osler's nodes, splinter hemorrhages, Janeway lesions, splenomegaly, and Roth's spots.

Heart failure
◆ Clubbing is a late sign with accompanying wheezing, dyspnea, and fatigue.
◆ Other signs and symptoms include jugular vein distention, hepato-
megaly, tachypnea, palpitations, dependent edema, weight gain, nausea, anorexia, chest tightness, slowed mental response, hypotension, diaphoresis, narrow pulse pressure, pallor, oliguria, a gallop rhythm, and crackles on inspiration.

Interstitial fibrosis
◆ Clubbing is a late sign.
◆ Other signs and symptoms may include intermittent chest pain, dyspnea, crackles, fatigue, weight loss, and cyanosis.

Lung abscess
◆ Clubbing occurs initially but may reverse with resolution of the abscess.
◆ Weakness, fatigue, anorexia, headache, malaise, weight loss, and fever with chills may also be present.
◆ Other signs and symptoms include pleuritic chest pain; dyspnea; crackles; productive cough with a large amount of purulent, foul-smelling, often bloody sputum; and halitosis.

Lung and pleural cancer
◆ Clubbing is common.
◆ Other signs and symptoms include hemoptysis, dyspnea, wheezing, chest pain, weight loss, anorexia, fatigue, and fever.

◆ Don't mistake curved nails for clubbing.

PEDIATRIC POINTERS
◆ Clubbing usually occurs in children with cyanotic congenital heart disease or cystic fibrosis.
◆ Surgical correction of heart defects may reverse clubbing.

GERIATRIC POINTERS
◆ Arthritic deformities of the fingers or toes may disguise clubbing.

◆ Explain that clubbing may not disappear even after the cause has been resolved.
◆ Teach the patient about the underlying diagnosis.

Cogwheel rigidity

- Cardinal sign of Parkinson's disease
- Muscle rigidity that reacts with superimposed ratchetlike movements when the muscle is passively stretched

- Determine when the patient first noticed associated signs of Parkinson's disease such as tremors, slow movements, "pill-rolling" hand movements, stiffness in his arms and legs, and handwriting becoming smaller.
- Ask which medications the patient is taking and ask if they've helped relieve some of his symptoms. If he's taking levodopa and his symptoms have worsened, find out if he has exceeded the prescribed dosage. If you suspect an overdose, withhold the drug.
- Ask if the patient has been taking a phenothiazine or another antipsychotic and has no history of Parkinson's disease as he may be having an adverse reaction. Withhold the drug, as appropriate.

- You can elicit cogwheel rigidity by stabilizing the patient's forearm and then moving his wrist through the range of motion.
- It usually appears in the arms but can sometimes be elicited in the ankle.
- You and the patient will be able to see and feel these characteristic movements, thought to be a combination of rigidity and tremor.
- Observe the patient for signs of pronounced parkinsonism, such as drooling, masklike facies, dysphagia, monotone speech, and altered gait.

MEDICAL
Parkinson's disease
◆ In this degenerative neurologic syndrome, cogwheel rigidity occurs together with an insidious tremor, which usually begins in the fingers, increases during stress or anxiety, and decreases with purposeful movement and sleep.
◆ Bradykinesia also occurs. The patient walks with short, shuffling steps; his gait lacks normal parallel motion and may be retropulsive or propulsive.
◆ Other signs and symptoms include a monotonal way of speaking, a mask-like facial expression, depression, drooling, dysphagia, dysarthria, loss of posture control causing him to walk with his body bent forward, oculogyric crisis, and blepharospasm.

OTHER
Drugs
◆ Phenothiazines and other antipsychotics (such as haloperidol, thiohixene, and loxapine). Contaminated heroin can also cause cogwheel rigidity.
◆ Metoclopramide causes it infrequently.

◆ If the patient has associated muscular dysfunction, assist him with ambulation, feeding, and other activities of daily living (ADLs), as needed.
◆ Provide symptomatic care, as appropriate. For example, if the patient develops constipation, administer a stool softener; if he experiences dysphagia, offer a soft diet with frequent small feedings.
◆ Refer the patient to the National Parkinson Foundation or the American Parkinson Disease Association, both of which provide educational materials and support.

◆ Review the disease process and prognosis with the patient and family.
◆ Instruct the patient in the appropriate use of devices to assist with ADLs, such as eating utensils and walking aids.
◆ Discuss safety precautions, such as eating a soft diet for dysphagia and using a walker or cane for ambulation safety.
◆ Review the use of medications and their side effects.

Confusion

- Refers to the inability to think quickly and coherently
- May be temporary or irreversible
- Severe: arises suddenly and is accompanied by hallucinations and psychomotor activity; also known as *delirium*
- Dementia: long-term, progressive confusion with deterioration of all cognitive functions

- Obtain a medical history, including incidence of head trauma or cardiopulmonary, metabolic, cerebrovascular, or neurologic disorders.
- Check with family members or friends about the onset and frequency of confusion.
- Ask what drugs the patient is taking and about alcohol use.
- Inquire about changes in his daily habits.

- Assess the patient for systemic disorders.
- Obtain vital signs, and watch for changes in blood pressure, temperature, and pulse.
- Perform a neurologic assessment to establish level of consciousness.

MEDICAL

Alzheimer's disease

- Primary progressive dementia with insidious onset occurs.
- Initially, it's characterized by loss of recent and remote memory, mood changes, and disorientation.
- As disease progresses, impaired cognition, inability to concentrate, confusion, and severe deterioration in memory, language, and motor function occur.

Brain tumor

- Tumor may be mild and difficult to detect in the early stages; however, confusion worsens as the tumor impinges on cerebral structures.
- Other signs and symptoms include personality changes, bizarre behavior, sensory and motor deficits, visual field deficits, headache, vomiting, and aphasia.

Decreased cerebral perfusion

- Mild confusion is an early symptom; it may be insidious and fleeting or acute and permanent.
- Other signs and symptoms include hypotension, tachycardia or bradycardia, irregular pulse, ventricular gallop, edema, and cyanosis.

Fluid and electrolyte imbalance

- The extent of imbalance determines the severity of confusion.
- Signs of dehydration may also be present.

Head trauma

- Confusion may occur at the time of injury, shortly afterward, or months or years afterward.
- Other signs and symptoms commonly include vomiting, severe headache, pupillary changes, and sensory and motor deficits.

Heat stroke

- Early findings include irritability and dizziness.
- Confusion gradually worsens as body temperature rises.

◆ Delirium, seizures, and loss of consciousness eventually occur.

Hypothermia
◆ Confusion may be an early sign of hypothermia, progressing to stupor and coma as temperature drops.
◆ Other signs and symptoms include slurred speech, cold and pale skin, hyperactive deep tendon reflexes, tachycardia, hypotension, and bradypnea.

Hypoxemia
◆ Confusion ranges from mild disorientation to delirium.
◆ In advanced stages of chronic pulmonary disorders, persistent confusion, severe dyspnea, disability, cor pulmonale, and severe respiratory failure occur.

Infection
◆ Severe generalized infection commonly produces delirium.
◆ Central nervous system (CNS) infections cause varying degrees of confusion, headache, and nuchal rigidity.

Metabolic encephalopathy
◆ Hyperglycemia and hypoglycemia can produce sudden confusion.
◆ Uremic and hepatic encephalopathies produce gradual confusion that may progress to seizures and coma.

Nutritional deficiencies
◆ Inadequate intake of thiamine, niacin, or vitamin B_{12} produces insidious, progressive confusion.
◆ Other CNS abnormalities may induce hallucinations and paranoia.

Seizure disorder
◆ Mild to moderate confusion may immediately follow a seizure, disappearing within several hours.
◆ The patient may have difficulty talking and may fall into a deep sleep after the seizures.

Thyroid hormone disorders
◆ Hyperthyroidism produces mild to moderate confusion along with nervousness, inability to concentrate, weight loss, flushed skin, and tachycardia.
◆ Hypothyroidism produces mild, insidious confusion and memory loss; weight gain; bradycardia; and fatigue.

OTHER
Alcohol
◆ Intoxication causes confusion and stupor.
◆ Alcohol withdrawal may cause delirium and seizures.

Drugs
◆ Large doses of CNS depressants produce confusion.
◆ Opioid and barbiturate withdrawal can cause confusion, possibly with delirium.
◆ Other drugs that commonly cause confusion include lidocaine, digoxin, indomethacin, atropine, chloroquine, cimetidine, and cycloserine.

Heavy metal poisoning
◆ Confusion, weakness, and drowsiness occur.
◆ Other signs and symptoms include headache, vomiting, seizures, tremors, gait disturbances, and mental deterioration.

NURSING CONSIDERATIONS
◆ Keep the patient safe from injury, such as falls and getting lost.
◆ Keep the patient calm and quiet.
◆ Plan uninterrupted rest periods for the patient.
◆ Treatment is directed at correcting the underlying cause of confusion.

PEDIATRIC POINTERS
◆ Confusion can't be determined in infants and very young children.
◆ Older children with acute febrile illnesses commonly experience transient delirium or acute confusion.

GERIATRIC POINTERS
◆ Elderly patients will typically become more confused and disoriented at the end of the day.

PATIENT TEACHING
◆ Teach the patient and family how to encourage orientation with tools such as calendars and reminder notes.
◆ Teach the family how to provide a pleasant, quiet environment.
◆ Teach the patient and family the importance of routines and uninterrupted rest periods.
◆ Discuss the underlying reason for confusion and whether confusion is acute or chronic.
◆ Teach patient and family the importance of safety precautions, such as providing close supervision while smoking (or not smoking), keeping side rails up, removing obstacles that could cause a fall, and keeping the bed in a low position.
◆ Teach about hospital procedures and tests to assist in diagnosis.

Conjunctival injection

- Common ocular sign associated with inflammation
- Nonuniform redness of the conjunctiva
- May be diffuse, localized, or peripheral or may encircle a clear cornea

◆ **ACTION STAT!** *To treat a chemical splash, first remove contact lenses (if present). Then quickly irrigate the eye with normal saline solution. Evert the lids and wipe the fornices with a cotton-tipped applicator to remove foreign-body particles and as much of the chemical as possible.*

HISTORY

- Determine the onset, location, and duration of eye pain.
- Determine whether other signs or symptoms are present.
- Ask about a history of eye disease or trauma.

PHYSICAL ASSESSMENT

- If the eyelids can be opened without applying pressure, test visual acuity.
- Determine the location and severity of injection.
- Note any discharge, edema, ocular deviation, conjunctival follicles, ptosis, or exophthalmos.
- Test pupillary reaction to light.

CAUSES

MEDICAL
Blepharitis
- Diffuse conjunctival injection occurs, and ulcerations that burn and itch appear on the eyelids.
- The patient may report a sensation of a foreign body in the eye.
- Rubbing of the eyes may lead to reddened rims or continuous blinking.

Conjunctival foreign bodies and abrasions
- Localized conjunctival injection occurs.
- Eye pain is sudden and severe.
- Increased tearing and photophobia may be present, but visual acuity usually isn't affected.

Conjunctivitis
- With allergic conjunctivitis, a milky, diffuse, usually bilateral peripheral conjunctival injection occurs.
- With bacterial conjunctivitis, diffuse peripheral conjunctival injection occurs along with a thick, purulent eye discharge that contains mucus threads.
- With fungal conjunctivitis, diffuse peripheral conjunctival injection occurs with photophobia and increased tearing, itching, and burning.
- With viral conjunctivitis, the conjunctival injection is brilliant red, diffuse, and peripheral.

Corneal abrasion
- Diffuse conjunctival injection is extremely painful, especially when the eyelids move over the abrasion.

- Other signs and symptoms include photophobia, excessive tearing, blurred vision, and a sensation of a foreign body in the eye.

Corneal erosion
- Diffuse conjunctival injection, severe, continuous pain, and photophobia develop.
- Decreased visual acuity may occur.

Corneal ulcer
- Diffuse conjunctival injection increases around the cornea.
- Corneal opacities and an abnormal pupillary response to light are associated with iritis.
- Other signs and symptoms include severe photophobia, severe pain in and around the eye, markedly decreased visual acuity, and copious and purulent eye discharge and crusting.

Dacryoadenitis
- Diffuse conjunctival injection occurs with constant tearing caused by inflammation of the tear duct.
- Other signs and symptoms include pain over the temporal part of the eye, considerable lid swelling, and purulent eye discharge.

Episcleritis
- Conjunctival injection is localized and raised and may be violet or purplish pink due to sclera inflammation.
- Other signs and symptoms include deep pain, photophobia, increased tearing, and conjunctival edema.

Glaucoma
- Conjunctival injection is typically circumcorneal with acute angle-closure glaucoma.
- Corneas appear steamy because of corneal edema.
- The pupil of the affected eye is moderately dilated and completely unresponsive to light.
- Other signs and symptoms include severe eye pain, nausea, vomiting, severely elevated intraocular pressure, blurred vision, and the percep-

tion of rainbow- colored halos around lights.

Hyphema
◆ Blood enters the anterior chamber of the eye after trauma.
◆ Diffuse conjunctival injection occurs, possibly with lid and orbital edema.
◆ Pain may be present in and around the eye.

Iritis
◆ Marked conjunctival injection is found mainly around the cornea.
◆ Other signs and symptoms include moderate to severe pain, photophobia, blurred vision, constricted pupils, and poor pupillary response to light.

Keratoconjunctivitis sicca
◆ This inflammation of the conjunctiva and cornea is associated with decreased tear production.
◆ Severe diffuse conjunctival injection occurs.
◆ Other signs and symptoms include generalized eye pain along with burning, itching, a foreign-body sensation, excessive mucus secretion from the eye, absence of tears, and photophobia.

Lyme disease
◆ This inflammatory disease is caused by bacteria transmitted by tick bite.
◆ Conjunctival injection occurs with diffuse urticaria, malaise, fatigue, headache, fever, chills, aches, and lymphadenopathy.
◆ Other ocular signs and symptoms include pain, photophobia, conjunctivitis, and blurry or double vision.

Ocular lacerations and intraocular foreign bodies
◆ Diffuse conjunctival injection may be increased in the area of injury.
◆ Impaired visual acuity and moderate to severe pain vary with the type and extent of the injury.
◆ Other signs and symptoms include lid edema, photophobia, excessive tearing, and abnormal pupillary response.

Ocular tumors
◆ If the tumor is located in the orbit behind the globe, conjunctival injection may occur with exophthalmos.
◆ Conjunctival edema, ocular deviation, and diplopia may occur with muscle involvement.

Uveitis
◆ Diffuse conjunctival injection may be increased in the circumcorneal area.
◆ Other signs and symptoms include constricted, irregularly shaped pupils; blurred vision; tenderness; photophobia; and sudden, severe ocular pain.

OTHER
Chemical burns
◆ Diffuse conjunctival injection occurs, with severe pain being the most prominent symptom.
◆ Other signs and symptoms include photophobia, blepharospasm, and decreased visual acuity in the affected eye; a grayish-appearing cornea; and differently sized pupils.

NURSING CONSIDERATIONS
◆ Obtain cultures of any eye discharge; record its appearance, consistency, and amount.
◆ If the patient has photophobia, darken his room.
◆ Administer pain medications, as prescribed.

PEDIATRIC POINTERS
◆ An infant can develop self-limited chemical conjunctivitis at birth from receiving silver nitrate eye drops.
◆ An infant may develop bacterial conjunctivitis 2 to 5 days after birth caused by contamination from the birth canal.
◆ An infant with congenital syphilis has prominent conjunctival injection and grayish pink corneas.
◆ The most common viral cause of congenital conjunctivitis is herpes simplex.

PATIENT TEACHING
◆ Teach the patient techniques for reducing photophobia.
◆ If visual acuity is impaired, help the patient to orient himself to his surroundings.
◆ Instruct the patient in ways to avoid spreading infection.

Constipation

OVERVIEW

- Refers to small, infrequent, or difficult bowel movements
- Can lead to headache, anorexia, and abdominal discomfort
- Usually occurs when the urge to defecate is suppressed and the muscles associated with bowel movements remain contracted (see *How habits and stress cause constipation*)

HISTORY

- Ask about frequency, size, and consistency of bowel movements.
- Determine the onset and location of associated pain.
- Find out about any changes in diet, eating habits, drug or alcohol use, or physical activity.
- Determine dietary fiber and fluid intake.
- Ask about recent emotional distress.
- Obtain a history of GI, rectoanal, neurologic, or metabolic disorders; abdominal surgery; or radiation therapy.
- Ask about the use of drugs, including over-the-counter preparations, such as laxatives, mineral oil, stool softeners, and enemas.

PHYSICAL ASSESSMENT

- Inspect the abdomen for distention or scars from previous surgery.
- Auscultate for bowel sounds and characterize their motility.
- Percuss all four abdominal quadrants.
- Gently palpate for abdominal tenderness, a palpable mass, and hepatomegaly.
- Examine the rectum; inspect for inflammation, lesions, scars, fissures, and external hemorrhoids.
- Palpate the anal sphincter for laxity or stricture.
- Palpate for rectal masses and fecal impaction.
- Obtain a stool specimen, and test it for occult blood.

CAUSES

MEDICAL
Anal fissure
- Acute constipation usually develops from the fear of the severe tearing or burning pain associated with bowel movements.
- A few drops of blood may be reported on toilet tissue or underwear.

Anorectal abscess
- Constipation occurs with severe, throbbing, localized pain and tenderness at the abscess site.
- Other signs and symptoms may include localized inflammation, swelling, purulent drainage, fever, and malaise.

Diverticulitis
- Constipation or diarrhea occurs with left-lower-quadrant pain and tenderness.
- A tender, fixed, firm abdominal mass may be palpable.
- Mild nausea, flatulence, and a low-grade fever may develop.

Hemorrhoids
- Constipation occurs as the patient tries to avoid the severe pain of defecation.
- Bleeding may occur during defecation.

Hepatic porphyria
- This is a metabolic disorder related to the use and storage of energy.
- Abdominal pain, which may be severe, colicky, localized, or generalized, precedes constipation.
- Areas exposed to light may develop skin lesions with itching, burning, erythema, altered pigmentation, and edema.
- If the disease is severe, delirium, coma, seizures, paraplegia, or complete flaccid paralysis may occur.
- Other signs and symptoms include fever, sinus tachycardia, labile hypertension, excessive diaphoresis, severe vomiting, photophobia, urine retention, nervousness or restlessness, disorientation, absent or diminished

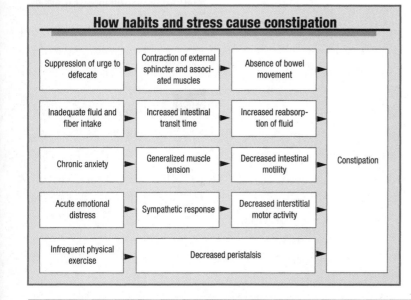

How habits and stress cause constipation

Suppression of urge to defecate → Contraction of external sphincter and associated muscles → Absence of bowel movement →

Inadequate fluid and fiber intake → Increased intestinal transit time → Increased reabsorption of fluid →

Chronic anxiety → Generalized muscle tension → Decreased intestinal motility → Constipation

Acute emotional distress → Sympathetic response → Decreased interstitial motor activity →

Infrequent physical exercise → Decreased peristalsis →

deep tendon reflexes, and visual hallucinations.

Hypercalcemia
♦ Common signs and symptoms include anorexia, nausea, vomiting, polyuria, and polydipsia.
♦ Other signs and symptoms may include arrhythmias, bone pain, muscle weakness and atrophy, hypoactive deep tendon reflexes, and personality changes.

Hypothyroidism
♦ Constipation occurs early and insidiously.
♦ Other signs and symptoms include fatigue, sensitivity to cold, anorexia with weight gain, menorrhagia, decreased memory, hearing impairment, muscle cramps, thinning hair, and paresthesia.

Intestinal obstruction
♦ With partial obstruction, constipation may alternate with leakage of liquid stools.
♦ With complete obstruction, obstipation may occur.
♦ Hyperactive bowel sounds, visible peristaltic waves, a palpable abdominal mass, and abdominal tenderness may also develop.
♦ Other signs and symptoms include episodes of colicky abdominal pain, abdominal distention, nausea, and vomiting.

Irritable bowel syndrome
♦ Alternating constipation and diarrhea, an intense urge to defecate, and feelings of incomplete evacuation usually occur.
♦ Nausea and abdominal distention and tenderness may be triggered by stress; defecation usually produces relief.
♦ Stools are hard and dry and contain visible mucus.

Mesenteric artery ischemia, acute
♦ Constipation is sudden.
♦ Initially, the abdomen is soft and nontender, progressing to severe abdominal pain, tenderness, vomiting, and anorexia.

♦ Later, abdominal guarding, rigidity, and distention; bruit; tachycardia; syncope; fever; and signs of shock may be present.

Multiple sclerosis
♦ Constipation occurs with ocular disturbances, vertigo, and sensory disturbances.
♦ Urinary urgency, frequency, and incontinence as well as emotional instability may occur.
♦ Other signs and symptoms include motor weakness, seizures, paralysis, muscle spasticity, gait ataxia, intention tremor, hyperreflexia, dysarthria, and dysphagia.

Spinal cord lesion
♦ Constipation may occur in addition to urine retention, sexual dysfunction, and pain.
♦ Motor weakness, paralysis, or sensory impairment below the level of the lesion may also occur.

Ulcerative colitis
♦ Constipation may occur in patients with chronic ulcerative colitis.
♦ Bloody diarrhea with pus, mucus, or both is the hallmark sign.
♦ Weight loss, weakness, and arthralgia are late findings.
♦ Other signs and symptoms include hyperactive bowel sounds, cramping lower abdominal pain, tenesmus, anorexia, low-grade fever, nausea, and vomiting.

OTHER
Diagnostic tests
♦ Retention of barium during certain GI studies can cause constipation.

Drugs
♦ Constipation may occur with the use of antacids containing aluminum or calcium, anticholinergics, drugs with anticholinergic effects, calcium-channel blockers, opioid analgesics, and vinca alkaloids.
♦ Overusing laxatives or enemas can lead to constipation.

Surgery and radiation therapy
♦ Rectoanal surgery can traumatize nerves, resulting in constipation.
♦ Abdominal irradiation can cause intestinal stricture and constipation.

NURSING CONSIDERATIONS

♦ If the patient has instructions for bed rest, reposition him frequently.
♦ Provide medications such as stool softeners, as ordered.
♦ Help the patient perform active or passive exercises.
♦ Give him fluids to support adequate hydration.
♦ Monitor the frequency of bowel movements and the intake and output of fluids.

PEDIATRIC POINTERS
♦ In infants, causes include inadequate fluid intake, anal fissures, Hirschsprung's disease, and casein and calcium in cow's milk.
♦ In older children, causes include inadequate fiber intake, excessive intake of milk, bowel spasm, mechanical obstruction, hypothyroidism, reluctance to stop playing for bathroom breaks, and the lack of privacy in some school bathrooms.

GERIATRIC POINTERS
♦ Acute constipation is associated with structural abnormalities.
♦ Chronic constipation is chiefly caused by lifelong bowel and dietary habits and laxative use.

PATIENT TEACHING

♦ Encourage avoidance of straining, laxatives, and enemas.
♦ Explain the role of diet and fluid intake.
♦ Encourage the patient to exercise.
♦ Train him in relaxation techniques.
♦ Discuss and encourage abdominal toning exercises.

Corneal reflex, absent

OVERVIEW

- Afferent fibers for this reflex located in ophthalmic branch of trigeminal nerve (cranial nerve [CN] V); efferent fibers located in facial nerve (CN VII)
- Unilateral or bilateral absence of reflex possibly resulting from damage to these nerves

HISTORY

- Because an absent corneal reflex may signify such progressive neurologic disorders as Guillain-Barré syndrome, ask the patient about associated symptoms—facial pain, dysphagia, and limb weakness.

PHYSICAL ASSESSMENT

- Test the corneal reflex bilaterally by drawing a fine-pointed wisp of sterile cotton from a corner of each eye to the cornea. Normally, even though only one eye is tested at a time, the patient blinks bilaterally each time either cornea is touched—this is the corneal reflex.
- When this reflex is absent, neither eyelid closes when the cornea of one is touched. (See *Eliciting the corneal reflex.*)
- If you can't elicit the corneal reflex, look for other signs of trigeminal nerve dysfunction. To test the three sensory portions of the nerve, touch each side of the patient's face on the brow, cheek, and jaw with a cotton wisp, and ask him to compare the sensations.
- If you suspect facial nerve involvement, note if the upper face (brow and eyes) and lower face (cheek, mouth, and chin) are weak bilaterally. Lower motor neuron facial weakness affects the face on the same side as the lesion, whereas upper motor neuron weakness affects the side opposite the lesion—predominantly the lower facial muscles.
- Obtain vital signs and complete physical assessment.

 TOP TECHNIQUE

Eliciting the corneal reflex

To elicit the corneal reflex, have the patient turn her eyes away from you to avoid blinking involuntarily during the procedure. Then approach the patient from the opposite side, out of her line of vision, and brush the cornea lightly with a fine wisp of sterile cotton. Repeat the procedure on the other eye.

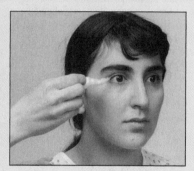

MEDICAL

Acoustic neuroma

- This benign neoplasm affects the trigeminal nerve, causing a diminished or absent corneal reflex, tinnitus, and unilateral hearing impairment.
- Facial palsy and anesthesia, palate weakness, and signs of cerebellar dysfunction (ataxia, nystagmus) may result if the tumor impinges on the adjacent cranial nerves, brain stem, and cerebellum.

Bell's palsy

- This disorder is the most common cause of diminished or absent corneal reflex and paralysis of CN VII, probably due to a viral infection.
- Other signs and symptoms include complete hemifacial weakness or paralysis; drooling on the affected side, which also sags and appears masklike; and constant tearing and inability of the eye on the affected side to close.

Brain stem infarction or injury

- An absent corneal reflex can occur on the side opposite the lesion when infarction or injury affects CN V or VII or their connection in the central trigeminal tract.
- With massive brain stem infarction or injury, the patient also displays respiratory changes, such as apneustic breathing or periods of apnea; bilateral pupillary dilation or constriction with decreased responsiveness to light; rising systolic blood pressure; a widening pulse pressure; bradycardia; and coma.
- Other signs and symptoms include a decreased level of consciousness, dysphagia, dysarthria, contralateral limb weakness, and early signs and symptoms of increased intracranial pressure, such as a headache and vomiting.

Guillain-Barré syndrome

- With this polyneuropathic disorder, a diminished or absent corneal reflex accompanies ipsilateral loss of facial muscle control.
- Muscle weakness, the dominant neurologic sign, typically starts in the legs, and then extends to the arms and facial nerves within 72 hours.
- Other signs and symptoms include dysarthria, dysphagia, paresthesia, respiratory muscle paralysis, respiratory insufficiency, orthostatic hypotension, incontinence, diaphoresis, and tachycardia.

- When the corneal reflex is absent, you'll need to take measures to protect the patient's affected eye from injury such as lubricating the eye with artificial tears to prevent drying.
- Cover the cornea with a shield and avoid excessive corneal reflex testing.
- Prepare the patient for cranial X-rays or computed tomography scanning.

PEDIATRIC POINTERS

- Brain stem lesions and injuries are usual causes of absent corneal reflexes in children; Guillain-Barré syndrome and trigeminal neuralgia are less common.
- Infants, especially those born prematurely, may have an absent corneal reflex due to anoxic damage to the brain stem.

- Teach the patient and family about the underlying diagnosis and prognosis.
- Teach the patient and family about hospital procedures and testing.
- Provide patient and family with resources for home care and follow-up care.

Costovertebral angle tenderness

OVERVIEW

- Indicates sudden distention of the renal capsule
- Accompanies unelicited, dull, constant flank pain in the costovertebral angle (CVA), just to the side of the spine and the 12th rib
- Elicited by percussing the CVA (see *Eliciting costovertebral angle tenderness*)
- Travels forward, below the ribs toward the umbilicus

HISTORY

- Find out about other signs and symptoms of renal or urologic dysfunction.
- Ask about voiding habits and the onset and description of any recent changes.
- Obtain a personal or family history of urinary tract infections, congenital anomalies, calculi, other obstructive nephropathies or uropathies, or renovascular disorders.

PHYSICAL ASSESSMENT

- Take vital signs.
- If the patient has hypertension and bradycardia, look for other autonomic effects of renal pain.
- Inspect, auscultate, and gently palpate the abdomen for clues to the underlying cause of CVA tenderness.
- Look for abdominal distention, hypoactive bowel sounds, and palpable masses.

TOP TECHNIQUE

Eliciting costovertebral angle tenderness

To elicit costovertebral angle (CVA) tenderness, have the patient sit upright facing away from you or have him lie in a prone position. Place the palm of your left hand over the left CVA, then strike the back of your left hand with the ulnar surface of your right fist (as shown). Repeat this percussion technique over the right CVA. A patient with CVA tenderness will experience intense pain.

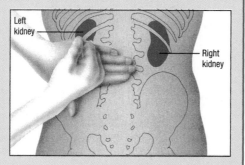

Left kidney

Right kidney

MEDICAL

Calculi
- CVA tenderness occurs with waves of waxing and waning flank pain that may radiate to the groin, testicles, suprapubic area, or labia, caused by calculi of the urinary tract system.
- Other signs and symptoms include nausea, vomiting, severe abdominal pain, abdominal distention, and decreased bowel sounds.

Perirenal abscess
- Exquisite CVA tenderness occurs with flank pain that may radiate to the groin or down the leg.
- Other signs and symptoms include dysuria, persistent high fever, chills, erythema of the skin, and a palpable abdominal mass.

Pyelonephritis, acute
- This is a bacterial infection of the renal pelvis.
- CVA tenderness occurs with persistent high fever, chills, flank pain, anorexia, nausea and vomiting, weakness, dysuria, hematuria, nocturia, urinary urgency and frequency, and tenesmus.

Renal artery occlusion
- CVA tenderness and flank pain occur.
- Other signs and symptoms include severe, continuous upper abdominal pain; nausea; vomiting; hematuria; decreased bowel sounds; and high fever.

- Give prescribed drugs for pain.
- Monitor vital signs and fluid intake and urine output.
- Collect blood samples and urine specimens, as ordered.

PEDIATRIC POINTERS
- An infant won't exhibit CVA tenderness; instead he'll display nonspecific signs and symptoms.
- In older children, CVA tenderness has the same significance as in adults.

GERIATRIC POINTERS
- Advanced age and cognitive impairment reduce an elderly patient's ability to perceive pain.

- Explain any dietary restrictions the patient needs.
- Tell the patient to drink at least 2 qt (2 L) of fluid daily unless he's instructed otherwise.
- Explain which signs and symptoms of kidney infection he should report.
- Emphasize the importance of taking the full course of prescribed antibiotics.

Cough, barking

OVERVIEW

- Resonant, brassy, and harsh cough
- Part of a complex of signs and symptoms that characterize croup syndrome
- Indicates edema of the larynx and surrounding tissue
- Can lead to airway occlusion, a life-threatening emergency (see *Managing a barking cough*)

HISTORY

- Ask about the onset of cough and other associated signs and symptoms.
- Find out about aggravating and alleviating factors.
- Determine whether the child has a history of previous episodes of croup syndrome.

PHYSICAL ASSESSMENT

- Observe the child for signs of respiratory distress.
- Note use of sternal or intercostal retractions or nasal flaring.
- Observe skin for cyanosis and diaphoresis.
- Take vital signs, noting respiratory rate and depth.
- Auscultate the lungs.

ACTION STAT!

Managing a barking cough

If the child experiences edema, quickly evaluate his respiratory status. Then take his vital signs. Be particularly alert for tachycardia and signs of hypoxemia. Also, check for a decreased level of consciousness. Try to determine if the child has been playing with a small object that he may have aspirated.

Check for cyanosis in the lips and nail beds. Observe the patient for sternal or intercostal retractions or nasal flaring. Next, note the depth and rate of his respirations; they may become increasingly shallow as respiratory distress increases. Observe the child's body position. Is he sitting up, leaning forward, struggling to breathe? Observe his activity level and facial expression. As respiratory distress increases from airway edema, the child will become restless and have a frightened, wide-eyed expression. As air hunger continues, the child will become lethargic and difficult to arouse.

If the child shows signs of severe respiratory distress, try to calm him, maintain airway patency, and provide oxygen. Endotracheal intubation or a tracheotomy may be necessary.

MEDICAL

Aspiration of foreign body

- Sudden hoarseness occurs initially with partial obstruction of the upper airway, followed by barking cough and inspiratory stridor.
- Other signs and symptoms of this life-threatening condition include gagging, tachycardia, dyspnea, decreased breath sounds, wheezing, and cyanosis.

Epiglottiditis

- A life-threatening childhood disorder, it starts with a barking cough and a high fever at night.
- The child is hoarse, dysphagic, dyspneic, and restless and appears extremely ill and panicky.
- Cough may progress to severe respiratory distress with sternal and intercostal retractions, nasal flaring, cyanosis, and tachycardia.

Laryngotracheobronchitis, acute

- Also known as viral croup.
- Fever, runny nose, poor appetite, and infrequent cough occur initially in patients age 3 months to 5 years.
- When infection descends into the laryngotracheal area, barking cough, hoarseness, and inspiratory stridor occur.
- As respiratory distress progresses, substernal and intercostal retractions, tachycardia, restlessness, cyanosis, irritability, paleness, and shallow, rapid respirations occur.

Spasmodic croup

- This occurs most often in children age 1 to 3 and may be associated with viral, allergic, and psychological factors.
- Onset of a barking cough is abrupt and usually awakens a child from sleep; the attacks subside within a few hours but tend to recur.
- The child may be hoarse, restless, and dyspneic, but without fever.
- As the condition worsens, signs and symptoms include sternal and intercostal retractions, nasal flaring, tachycardia, cyanosis, and an anxious, frantic appearance.

- Don't inspect the throat of a child with barking cough unless intubation equipment is available.
- If the child isn't in severe respiratory distress, a neck X-ray may be needed to check for epiglottal edema.
- A chest X-ray can rule out lower respiratory tract infection.
- Depending on child's age and degree of respiratory distress, oxygen may be administered.
- Rapid-acting epinephrine and a steroid may be needed.
- Observe the child frequently, and if oxygen is used, monitor the level.
- Maintain a calm, quiet environment and offer reassurance.
- Encourage the parents to stay with the child.

PEDIATRIC POINTERS

- Because a child's airway is smaller in diameter than that of an adult, edema can rapidly lead to airway occlusion, a life-threatening emergency.

- Discuss with parents or caregiver methods of relieving subsequent attacks.
- Discuss the diagnosis behind barking cough and signs and symptoms to look for.

Cough, nonproductive

- Noisy, forceful expulsion of air from the lungs, but one that doesn't yield sputum
- Can cause airway collapse or rupture of alveoli or blebs
- May occur in paroxysms and can worsen by becoming more frequent
- May be acute (self-limiting) or chronic (see *Reviewing the cough mechanism*)

Reviewing the cough mechanism

Cough receptors are thought to be located in the nose, sinuses, auditory canals, nasopharynx, larynx, trachea, bronchi, pleurae, diaphragm and, possibly, the pericardium and GI tract. When a cough receptor is stimulated, the vagus and glossopharyngeal nerves transmit the impulse to the "cough center" in the medulla. From there, the impulse is transmitted to the larynx and to the intercostal and abdominal muscles. Deep inspiration (1) is followed by closure of the glottis and the vocal cords (2), relaxation of the diaphragm, and contraction of the abdominal and intercostal muscles. The resulting increased pressure in the lungs opens the glottis to release the forceful, noisy expiration known as a cough (3).

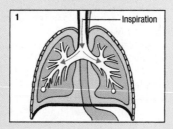

1 — Inspiration

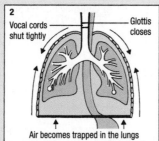

2
Vocal cords shut tightly — Glottis closes

Air becomes trapped in the lungs

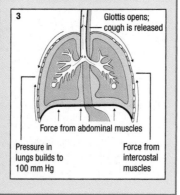

3 — Glottis opens; cough is released

Force from abdominal muscles

Pressure in lungs builds to 100 mm Hg   Force from intercostal muscles

- Ask about the onset, frequency, and description of cough.
- Ask about aggravating factors.
- Obtain a smoking history.
- Find out the onset and location of associated pain.
- Obtain a history of surgery or trauma.
- Inquire about hypersensitivity to drugs, foods, pets, dust, or pollen.
- Find out which drugs the patient is taking.
- Ask about recent changes in appetite, weight, exercise tolerance, or energy level.
- Ask about recent exposure to irritating fumes, chemicals, or smoke.

- Observe the patient, and note behavior, cyanosis, clubbed fingers, or edema.
- Take the patient's vital signs, checking the depth and rhythm of respirations; note if wheezing occurs with breathing.
- Inspect the neck for distended veins and a deviated trachea.
- Check the skin, noting whether it's cool or warm, dry or clammy.
- Check the mouth and nose for congestion, inflammation, drainage, and signs of infection.
- Examine the chest, looking for abnormal chest wall configuration and motion, such as use of accessory muscles and retraction.
- Auscultate for wheezing, crackles, rhonchi, pleural rubs, and decreased or absent breath sounds.
- Percuss for dullness, tympany, and flatness.

CAUSES

MEDICAL

Airway occlusion

- Partial occlusion of the upper airway produces a sudden onset of dry, paroxysmal coughing.
- If choking on a foreign object, the patient may clutch his throat with thumb and fingers extended.
- Other signs and symptoms include gagging, wheezing, hoarseness, stridor, tachycardia, and decreased breath sounds.

Anthrax, inhalation

- Initial signs and symptoms include low-grade fever, chills, weakness, cough, and chest pain.
- Rapid deterioration marked by fever, dyspnea, stridor, and hypotension, generally leading to death within 24 hours, occurs in the second stage.

Aortic aneurysm, thoracic

- A brassy cough occurs with dyspnea, hoarseness, wheezing, and a substernal ache in the shoulders, lower back, or abdomen.
- Other signs and symptoms include facial or neck edema, neck vein distention, dysphagia, and prominent veins over the chest, stridor, paresthesia, and neuralgia.

Asthma

- Attacks start with a nonproductive cough and mild wheezing.
- As the attack progresses, severe dyspnea, audible wheezing, chest tightness, and a cough that produces thick mucus develops.
- Other signs and symptoms include anxiety, rhonchi, prolonged expiration, intercostal and supraclavicular retractions on inspiration, accessory muscle use, flaring nostrils, tachypnea, tachycardia, diaphoresis, and flushing or cyanosis.

Atelectasis

- As lung tissue deflates, it stimulates cough receptors, causing a nonproductive cough.

- Trachea may deviate toward the affected side.
- Other signs and symptoms include pleuritic chest pain, anxiety, cyanosis, diaphoresis, dullness on percussion, inspiratory lag, substernal or intercostal retractions, decreased vocal fremitus, dyspnea, tachypnea, and tachycardia.

Bronchitis, chronic

- A nonproductive, hacking cough later becomes productive.
- Clubbing may occur in stages.
- Other signs and symptoms include prolonged expiration, wheezing, dyspnea, accessory muscle use, barrel chest, cyanosis, tachypnea, crackles, and scattered rhonchi.

Bronchogenic carcinoma

- Chronic, nonproductive cough, dyspnea, and vague chest pain are early indicators.
- Other signs and symptoms include weight loss, wheezing, hemoptysis, and stridor.

Common cold

- Nonproductive, hacking cough progresses to a mix of sneezing, headache, malaise, fatigue, rhinorrhea, myalgia, arthralgia, nasal congestion, and sore throat.

Esophageal achalasia

- Regurgitation and aspiration produce a dry cough.
- Recurrent pulmonary infections and dysphagia may develop.
- Weight loss, heartburn, and chest pain that increases after eating may be reported.

Esophageal diverticula

- Nocturnal nonproductive cough, regurgitation and aspiration, dyspepsia, and dysphagia are characteristic findings.
- Other signs and symptoms include a swollen neck, a gurgling sound, halitosis, and weight loss.

(continued)

Esophageal occlusion
♦ Immediate nonproductive coughing and gagging accompanies a sensation of something stuck in the throat.
♦ Other signs and symptoms include neck or chest pain, dysphagia, and the inability to swallow.

Esophagitis with reflux
♦ Regurgitation and aspiration produce a nonproductive nocturnal cough.
♦ Other signs and symptoms include chest pain that mimics angina pectoris; heartburn that worsens if the patient lies down soon after eating; and increased salivation, dysphagia, hematemesis, and melena.

Hodgkin's lymphoma
♦ A crowing nonproductive cough may develop.
♦ Painless swelling of cervical lymph nodes or, occasionally, the axillary, mediastinal, or inguinal nodes, is an early sign.
♦ Pruritus is also an early sign.
♦ Other signs and symptoms include dyspnea, dysphagia, hepatosplenomegaly, edema, jaundice, nerve pain, and hyperpigmentation.

Hypersensitivity pneumonitis
♦ Acute, nonproductive cough, fever, dyspnea, and malaise occur 5 to 6 hours after exposure to an antigen.
♦ Chest tightness and extreme fatigue may also occur.

Interstitial lung disease
♦ Nonproductive cough and progressive dyspnea occur.
♦ Other signs and symptoms include cyanosis, clubbing, fine crackles, fatigue, chest pain, weight loss, and dyspnea on exertion.

Laryngeal tumor
♦ Mild, nonproductive cough; minor throat discomfort; and hoarseness are early signs.
♦ Dysphagia, dyspnea, cervical lymphadenopathy, stridor, and earache occur later.

Laryngitis
♦ In acute cases, a nonproductive cough occurs with localized pain, hoarseness, fever, and malaise.

Legionnaires' disease
♦ A nonproductive cough progresses to a cough that may produce mucoid, mucopurulent, and bloody sputum.
♦ Prodromal signs and symptoms include malaise, headache, diarrhea, anorexia, diffuse myalgia, and generalized weakness.

Lung abscess
♦ Nonproductive cough, weakness, dyspnea, and pleuritic chest pain occur initially.
♦ Later, cough produces purulent, foul-smelling sputum.
♦ Other signs and symptoms include diaphoresis, fever, headache, malaise, fatigue, crackles, decreased breath sounds, anorexia, and weight loss.

Mediastinal tumor
♦ Nonproductive cough, dyspnea, and retrosternal pain occur.
♦ Snoring respirations with suprasternal retraction on inspiration, hoarseness, dysphagia, tracheal shift or tug, jugular vein distention, and facial or neck edema may develop.

Pleural effusion
♦ Pleural effusion is compression of the lung resulting from increased fluid in the pleural space.
♦ Nonproductive cough, dyspnea, pleuritic chest pain, and decreased chest motion are characteristic findings.
♦ Other signs and symptoms include pleural rub, tachycardia, tachypnea, egophony, flatness on percussion, decreased or absent breath sounds, and decreased tactile fremitus.

Pneumonia
♦ Bacterial pneumonia causes a nonproductive, hacking, painful cough that eventually becomes productive.
♦ Mycoplasmal pneumonia causes a nonproductive cough that may be paroxysmal, arising 2 to 3 days after onset of malaise, headache, and sore throat.
♦ Viral pneumonia causes a nonproductive, hacking cough and gradual onset of malaise, headache, and low-grade fever.
♦ Other signs and symptoms include shaking chills, headache, high fever, dyspnea, pleuritic chest pain, tachypnea, tachycardia, grunting respirations, nasal flaring, decreased breath sounds, fine crackles, rhonchi, and cyanosis.

Pneumothorax
♦ The patient with this life-threatening disorder exhibits dry cough and signs of respiratory distress as the lung is compressed because of free air in the pleural cavity.
♦ Other signs and symptoms include sudden, sharp chest pain that worsens with chest movement; subcutaneous crepitation; hyperresonance or tympany; decreased vocal fremitus; and decreased or absent breath sounds on the affected side.

Pulmonary edema
♦ Dry cough, exertional dyspnea, paroxysmal nocturnal dyspnea, orthopnea, tachycardia, tachypnea, dependent crackles, and ventricular gallop occur initially.
♦ Respirations become more rapid and labored, with diffuse crackles and coughing that produces frothy, bloody sputum as the condition worsens.

Pulmonary embolism
♦ This life-threatening disorder causes sudden dry cough, dyspnea, anxiety, and pleuritic or anginal chest pain.
♦ More commonly, the cough produces blood-tinged sputum.
♦ Other signs and symptoms include tachycardia, low-grade fever, pleural rub, diffuse wheezing, dullness on percussion, and decreased breath sounds.

Sarcoidosis

◆ Sarcoidosis is a multisystem, granuloma-producing disorder that especially affects the lungs.
◆ A nonproductive cough is accompanied by dyspnea, substernal pain, and malaise.
◆ Other signs and symptoms include fatigue, arthralgia, myalgia, weight loss, tachypnea, crackles, lymphadenopathy, hepatosplenomegaly, skin lesions, vision impairment, difficulty swallowing, and arrhythmias.

Severe acute respiratory syndrome

◆ In this life-threatening disorder, severe acute respiratory syndrome begins with a fever; headache, malaise, dry nonproductive cough, and dyspnea also occur.

Sinusitis, chronic

◆ Chronic nonproductive cough, which may develop from postnasal drip, is often worse in the morning.
◆ Nasal mucosa may appear inflamed; nasal congestion with profuse drainage and a musty breath odor may occur.

Tracheobronchitis, acute

◆ As secretions increase, a dry cough becomes productive.
◆ Chills, sore throat, slight fever, muscle and back pain, and substernal tightness generally precede the cough's onset.

Tularemia

◆ Tularemia is transmitted from a bite from an infected animal or blood-sucking insect.
◆ Abrupt onset of fever, chills, headache, generalized myalgia, nonproductive cough, dyspnea, pleuritic chest pain, and empyema occurs.

OTHER
Diagnostic tests

◆ Pulmonary function tests and bronchoscopy may stimulate cough receptors, triggering coughing.

Drugs

◆ Certain medications such as angiotensin-converting enzyme inhibitors may cause a cough.

Treatments

◆ Suctioning or deep endotracheal or tracheal tube placement can trigger a paroxysmal or hacking cough.
◆ Intermittent positive-pressure breathing or spirometry may cause a nonproductive cough.
◆ Inhalants, such as pentamidine, may stimulate coughing.

NURSING CONSIDERATIONS

◆ A nonproductive, paroxysmal cough may induce life-threatening bronchospasm; the patient may need a bronchodilator.
◆ Unless the patient has chronic obstructive pulmonary disease, give an antitussive and a sedative to suppress the cough.
◆ Humidify the air in the patient's room.

PEDIATRIC POINTERS

◆ Sudden onset of paroxysmal nonproductive coughing may indicate aspiration of a foreign body.
◆ Nonproductive coughing can also result from asthma, bacterial pneumonia, acute bronchiolitis, acute otitis media, measles, cystic fibrosis, airway hyperactivity, or a foreign body in the external auditory canal; it may also be psychogenic.

GERIATRIC POINTERS

◆ Nonproductive cough may indicate serious acute or chronic illness in elderly patients.

PATIENT TEACHING

◆ Explain how use a humidifier.
◆ Teach the patient to avoid respiratory irritants; encourage use of respirator mask when he must be near respiratory irritants.
◆ Explain to the patient why nonproductive coughs should be suppressed and productive coughs should be encouraged.
◆ Explain the importance of adequate fluids and nutrition.
◆ If the patient smokes, stress the importance of smoking cessation, and refer him to appropriate resources, support groups, and information to help him quit.

Cough, productive

◆ Sudden, forceful, expulsion of air from the lungs with sputum, blood, or both
◆ May be acute or chronic, causing inflammation, edema, and increased mucus production

ACTION STAT! *If the patient has acute respiratory distress from thick or excessive secretions, bronchospasm, or fatigue, take vital signs and check the rate, depth, and rhythm of respirations. Keep the airway patent, and provide supplemental oxygen if he becomes restless or confused, or if his respirations become shallow, irregular, rapid, or slow. Look for stridor, wheezing, choking, gurgling, nasal flaring, and cyanosis.*

HISTORY

◆ Ask about the onset of coughing.
◆ Find out about the amount, color, odor, and consistency of the sputum.
◆ Note time of day and what aggravates and alleviates coughing and sputum production.
◆ Ask the patient to describe the sound of the cough.
◆ Note the location and severity of pain.
◆ Ask about weight and appetite changes, smoking and alcohol use, asthma, allergies, and respiratory problems.
◆ Obtain a drug history.
◆ Review his occupational history for exposure to chemicals or respiratory irritants.

PHYSICAL ASSESSMENT

◆ Examine the patient's mouth and nose for congestion, drainage, or inflammation.
◆ Note breath odor.
◆ Inspect the neck for distended veins, and palpate for tenderness and masses or enlarged lymph nodes.
◆ Observe the chest for accessory muscle use, retractions, and uneven chest expansion.
◆ Percuss the chest for dullness, tympany, or flatness.
◆ Auscultate for pleural rub and abnormal breath sounds.

CAUSES

MEDICAL

Aspiration pneumonitis
◆ Sputum is pink, frothy, and possibly purulent.
◆ Other signs and symptoms include severe dyspnea, fever, tachypnea, fatigue, chest pain, halitosis, tachycardia, wheezing, and cyanosis.

Asthma, acute
◆ A life-threatening disorder, acute asthma may produce tenacious mucoid sputum and mucus plugs.
◆ As the attack progresses, severe dyspnea, audible wheezing, and chest tightness occur.
◆ Other signs and symptoms include apprehension, prolonged expirations, intercostal and supraclavicular retraction on inspiration, accessory muscle use, rhonchi, crackles, flaring nostrils, tachypnea, tachycardia, diaphoresis, and flushing or cyanosis.

Bronchiectasis
◆ Cough produces copious, mucopurulent, layered sputum (top: frothy; middle: clear; bottom: dense; purulent particles).
◆ Sputum is foul- or sweet-smelling.
◆ Other signs and symptoms include hemoptysis, persistent coarse crackles, wheezing, rhonchi, exertional dyspnea, weight loss, fatigue, malaise, weakness, fever, and late-stage clubbing.

Bronchitis, chronic
◆ Cough is nonproductive initially.
◆ Mucoid sputum becomes purulent.
◆ Coughing usually occurs when the patient is recumbent or rises from sleep.
◆ Other signs and symptoms include prolonged expiration, use of accessory muscles, barrel chest, tachypnea, cyanosis, wheezing, exertional dyspnea, scattered rhonchi, coarse crackles, and late-stage clubbing.

Chemical pneumonitis
◆ Cough produces purulent sputum.
◆ Other signs and symptoms include dyspnea, wheezing, orthopnea, malaise, and crackles; mucus irritation of the conjunctivae, throat, and nose; laryngitis; and rhinitis.

Common cold
◆ Cough produces sputum that's mucoid or mucopurulent.
◆ Other signs and symptoms include dry, hacking cough; sneezing; headache; malaise; fatigue; rhinorrhea; nasal congestion; sore throat; and myalgia.

Legionnaires' disease
◆ Cough produces sputum that's scant, mucoid, nonpurulent, and blood-streaked, caused by a bacterial infection.
◆ Early signs and symptoms include malaise, fatigue, weakness, anorexia, myalgia, and diarrhea.
◆ Within 12 to 48 hours, cough becomes dry, with accompanying sudden high fever and chills.
◆ Other signs and symptoms include pleuritic pain, headache, tachypnea, tachycardia, nausea, vomiting, dyspnea, crackles, and confusion.

Lung abscess, ruptured
◆ Cough produces sputum that's purulent, foul-smelling, and blood-tinged.
◆ Other signs and symptoms include diaphoresis, anorexia, clubbing, weight loss, weakness, fatigue, fever, chills, dyspnea, headache, malaise, pleuritic chest pain, and inspiratory crackles.

Lung cancer
◆ Chronic cough is an early sign, which produces small amounts of purulent (or mucopurulent), blood-streaked sputum.

- With bronchoalveolar cancer, cough produces large amounts of frothy sputum.
- Other signs and symptoms include dyspnea, anorexia, fatigue, weight loss, chest pain, fever, diaphoresis, wheezing, and clubbing.

Pneumonia
- Dry cough becomes productive as condition progresses.
- Other signs and symptoms develop suddenly and include shaking chills, high fever, myalgia, pleuritic chest pain, tachycardia, tachypnea, dyspnea, cyanosis, diaphoresis, decreased breath sounds, crackles, and rhonchi.

Pneumonic plague
- Pulmonary signs and symptoms include productive cough, chest pain, tachypnea, dyspnea, hemoptysis, and increasing respiratory distress.
- Other signs and symptoms include fever, chills, and swollen, inflamed, and tender lymph nodes.

Pulmonary edema
- A life-threatening disorder, early signs include exertional dyspnea; paroxysmal nocturnal dyspnea, followed by orthopnea; and nonproductive cough that eventually produces frothy, bloody sputum.
- Other signs and symptoms include fever, fatigue, tachycardia, tachypnea, crackles, and ventricular gallop.

Pulmonary embolism
- A life-threatening disorder, the first sign is usually severe dyspnea with angina or pleuritic chest pain.
- Cough may be nonproductive or may produce blood-tinged sputum.
- Severe anxiety, low-grade fever, tachycardia, tachypnea, and diaphoresis develop.
- Other signs and symptoms include pleural rub, wheezing, crackles, chest dullness on percussion, decreased breath sounds, and signs of circulatory collapse.

Pulmonary emphysema
- Chronic cough produces scant, mucoid, translucent, grayish-white sputum, which can become mucopurulent.
- Other signs and symptoms include thin appearance, weight loss, accessory muscle use, tachypnea, grunting expirations through pursed lips, diminished breath sounds, exertional dyspnea, rhonchi, barrel chest, anorexia, and late clubbing.

Pulmonary tuberculosis
- Cough may be mild to severe, with scant, mucoid or copious, and purulent sputum.
- Other signs and symptoms include hemoptysis, malaise, dyspnea, pleuritic chest pain, night sweats, fatigue, and weight loss.

Silicosis
- Silicosis occurs after inhalation of silica dust over a period of years, resulting in progressive fibrosis of the lungs.
- Cough with mucopurulent sputum is the first sign.
- Other signs and symptoms include exertional dyspnea, tachypnea, weight loss, fatigue, weakness, recurrent respiratory infections, and end-inspiratory crackles.

Tracheobronchitis
- After the onset of chills, sore throat, fever, muscle and back pain, and substernal tightness, cough becomes productive.
- Sputum is mucoid, mucopurulent, or purulent.
- Other signs and symptoms include rhonchi, wheezes, crackles, fever, and bronchospasm.

OTHER
Diagnostic tests
- Bronchoscopy and pulmonary function tests may cause productive coughing.

Drugs
- Expectorants increase productive coughing.

Respiratory therapy
- Incentive spirometry, intermittent positive-pressure breathing, and nebulizer therapy may cause productive coughing.

NURSING CONSIDERATIONS
- Give a mucolytic and an expectorant to increase productive coughing.
- Increase the patient's fluid intake to thin secretions.
- Give a bronchodilator to relieve bronchospasm and open airways, as prescribed.
- If an infection is present, give antibiotics, as prescribed.
- Humidify the air to relieve mucous membrane irritation and loosen secretions.
- Provide pulmonary physiotherapy to loosen secretions.
- Provide rest periods.
- Collect sputum specimens for culture and sensitivity testing.

PEDIATRIC POINTERS
- A child with a productive cough can quickly develop airway occlusion and respiratory distress.
- Causes of a productive cough in children include asthma, bronchiectasis, bronchitis, acute bronchiolitis, cystic fibrosis, and pertussis.
- High humidity can induce bronchospasm in a hyperactive child or overhydration in an infant.

PATIENT TEACHING
- Refer the patient to resources to quit smoking.
- Teach the patient coughing and deep-breathing techniques.
- Teach the patient and caregiver to use chest percussion to loosen secretions.
- Explain the importance of adequate hydration and prescribed medications to thin secretions and improve expectoration.
- Explain infection control techniques.
- Explain how the patient can avoid respiratory irritants.

Crackles

- Nonmusical clicking or rattling noises heard during auscultation of breath sounds
- May be on one or both sides, moist- or dry-sounding
- Usually occur during inspiration and recur constantly from one respiratory cycle to the next
- Indicate abnormal movement of air through fluid-filled airways
- Also known as *rales* or *crepitations*

ACTION STAT! *Take vital signs and pulse oximetry, and examine the patient for signs of respiratory distress or airway obstruction. Check the depth and rhythm of respirations. Check for increased accessory muscle use and chest-wall motion, retractions, stridor, or nasal flaring. Provide supplemental oxygen. Endotracheal intubation may be necessary.*

HISTORY

- Ask about the onset, duration, and description of cough and pain.
- Note the sputum's consistency, amount, odor, and color.
- Obtain a medical history, including incidence of cancer, respiratory or cardiovascular problems, surgery, or trauma.
- Find out about smoking and alcohol use.
- Obtain a drug and occupational history.
- Inquire about recent weight loss, anorexia, nausea, vomiting, fatigue, weakness, vertigo, hoarseness, difficulty swallowing, and syncope.
- Determine exposure to respiratory irritants.

PHYSICAL ASSESSMENT

- Examine the nose and mouth for signs of infection.
- Note breath odor.
- Check the neck for masses, tenderness, lymphadenopathy, swelling, tracheal deviation, or venous distention.
- Inspect the chest for abnormal configuration or uneven expansion.
- Percuss the chest for dullness, tympany, or flatness.
- Auscultate the lungs for other abnormal, diminished, or absent breath sounds.
- Listen for abnormal heart sounds.
- Check the hands and feet for edema or clubbing.

CAUSES

MEDICAL
Acute respiratory distress syndrome
- In this life-threatening disorder, diffuse, fine to coarse crackles are usually heard in the dependent portions of the lungs.
- Other signs and symptoms include cyanosis, nasal flaring, tachypnea, tachycardia, grunting respirations, rhonchi, dyspnea, anxiety, and decreased level of consciousness.

Asthma, acute
- Dry, whistling crackles occur.
- Dry cough and mild wheezing progress to severe dyspnea, audible wheezing, chest tightness, and productive cough.
- Other signs and symptoms include anxiety, prolonged expirations, rhonchi, intercostal and supraclavicular retractions, accessory muscle use, flaring nostrils, tachypnea, tachycardia, diaphoresis, and flushing or cyanosis.

Bronchiectasis
- Persistent, coarse crackles are heard over the affected area of the lung.
- Chronic cough that produces copious amounts of mucopurulent sputum accompanies crackles.

- Other signs and symptoms include halitosis, wheezing, exertional dyspnea, rhonchi, weight loss, fatigue, malaise, weakness, recurrent fever, and late clubbing.

Bronchitis, chronic
- Coarse crackles are usually heard at the lung base.
- Other signs and symptoms include prolonged expirations, wheezing, rhonchi, exertional dyspnea, tachypnea, cyanosis, clubbing, and persistent, productive cough.

Chemical pneumonitis
- Diffuse, fine to coarse, moist crackles can be heard.
- Other signs and symptoms include a productive cough with purulent sputum, dyspnea, wheezing, orthopnea, fever, malaise, and mucous membrane irritation.

Interstitial fibrosis of the lungs
- Cellophane-like crackles can be heard over all lobes.
- As the disease progresses, other signs and symptoms include nonproductive cough, dyspnea, fatigue, weight loss, cyanosis, pleuritic chest pain, nasal flaring, and cyanosis.

Legionnaires' disease
- Diffuse, moist crackles can be heard in patients with this acute bronchopneumonia.
- Early signs and symptoms include malaise, fatigue, weakness, anorexia, myalgia, and diarrhea.
- Within 12 to 48 hours, a dry cough develops, with accompanying sudden high fever and chills.
- Other signs and symptoms include pleuritic chest pain, headache, tachypnea, tachycardia, nausea, vomiting, dyspnea, confusion, flushing, diaphoresis, and prostration.

Lung abscess
- Fine to medium and moist inspiratory crackles occur.
- Other signs and symptoms include sweats, anorexia, weight loss, fever, fatigue, weakness, dyspnea, clubbing, pleuritic chest pain, pleural

rub, and a cough that produces large amounts of foul-smelling, purulent, bloody sputum.

Pneumonia
◆ Bacterial pneumonia produces diffuse, fine crackles.
◆ Mycoplasmal pneumonia produces medium to fine crackles.
◆ Viral pneumonia causes gradually developing, diffuse crackles.
◆ Other signs and symptoms include sudden onset of shaking chills, high fever, tachypnea, pleuritic chest pain, cyanosis, grunting respirations, nasal flaring, decreased breath sounds, myalgia, headache, tachycardia, dyspnea, diaphoresis, rhonchi, and a dry cough that becomes productive.

Pulmonary edema
◆ A life-threatening disorder, moist, bubbling crackles on inspiration are one of the first signs.
◆ Other signs and symptoms include exertional dyspnea; paroxysmal nocturnal dyspnea, then orthopnea; tachycardia; tachypnea; ventricular gallop; and a cough that's initially nonproductive, but later produces frothy, bloody sputum.

Pulmonary embolism
◆ A life-threatening disorder, fine to coarse crackles and severe dyspnea are early signs and may be accompanied by angina or pleuritic chest pain.
◆ Cough may be nonproductive or produce blood-tinged sputum.
◆ Acute anxiety, low-grade fever, tachycardia, tachypnea, and diaphoresis develop.
◆ Other signs and symptoms include pleural rub, wheezing, chest dullness on percussion, decreased breath sounds, and signs of circulatory collapse.

Pulmonary tuberculosis
◆ Fine crackles occur after coughing.
◆ Sputum may be scant, mucoid or copious, and purulent.
◆ Other signs and symptoms include hemoptysis, malaise, dyspnea, pleuritic chest pain, fatigue, night sweats, weakness, weight loss, and amphoric breath sounds.

Sarcoidosis
◆ Sarcoidosis is a multisystem, granuloma-producing disorder that especially affects the lungs.
◆ Fine, basilar, end-inspiratory crackles occur.
◆ Other signs and symptoms include malaise, fatigue, weakness, weight loss, cough, dyspnea, and tachypnea.

Silicosis
◆ End-inspiratory, fine crackles are heard at the lung bases, resulting from pulmonary fibrosis.
◆ Productive cough with mucopurulent sputum is the first sign.
◆ Other signs and symptoms include exertional dyspnea, tachypnea, weight loss, fatigue, weakness, and recurrent respiratory infections.

Tracheobronchitis
◆ Moist or coarse crackles occur.
◆ With severe disease, moderate fever and bronchospasm occur.
◆ Other signs and symptoms include productive cough, chills, sore throat, slight fever, muscle and back pain, substernal tightness, rhonchi, and wheezes.

◆ Elevate the head of the bed to ease the patient's breathing.
◆ Administer fluids and humidified air to liquefy secretions and relieve mucous membrane inflammation.
◆ Administer oxygen.
◆ If crackles result from cardiogenic pulmonary edema, give a diuretic, as prescribed.
◆ Turn the patient every 1 to 2 hours, and encourage deep breathing.
◆ Plan regular rest periods for him.

PEDIATRIC POINTERS
◆ Pneumonias produce diffuse, sudden crackles.
◆ Esophageal atresia and tracheoesophageal fistula can cause bubbling, moist crackles.
◆ Pulmonary edema causes fine crackles.
◆ Bronchiectasis produces moist crackles.
◆ Cystic fibrosis produces widespread, fine to coarse inspiratory crackles in infants.
◆ Sickle cell anemia may produce crackles with pulmonary infection or infarction.

GERIATRIC POINTERS
◆ Crackles that clear after deep breathing may indicate mild basilar atelectasis.

◆ Teach the patient effective coughing techniques.
◆ Teach him to avoid respiratory irritants.
◆ Stress the importance of quitting smoking, and refer him to appropriate resources to help him.
◆ Teach the patient energy conservation techniques, particular with chronic disorders.

Crepitation, bony

- Palpable vibration or an audible crunching sound that results when one bone grates against another
- Results from a fracture, but may also happen when bones that have been stripped of their protective articular cartilage grind against each other as they articulate—for example, in patients with advanced arthritic or degenerative joint disorders

ACTION STAT! *If you detect bony crepitation in a patient with a suspected fracture, ask him if he feels pain and if he can point to the painful area. To prevent lacerating nerves, blood vessels, or other structures, immobilize the affected area by applying a splint that includes the joints above and below the affected area. Elevate the affected area, if possible, and apply cold packs. Inspect for abrasions or lacerations. Find out how and when the injury occurred. Palpate pulses distal to the injury site; check the skin for pallor or coolness. Test motor and sensory function distal to the injury site.*

- If the patient doesn't have a suspected fracture, ask about a history of osteoarthritis or rheumatoid arthritis.
- Obtain a medication history, and ask if any medication helps ease arthritic discomfort.

- Obtain the patient's vital signs, and test his joint range of motion (ROM) if fracture isn't suspected.
- Eliciting bony crepitation can help confirm the diagnosis of a fracture, but it can also cause further soft tissue, nerve, or vessel injury. Always evaluate distal pulses and perform neurologic checks distal to the suspected fracture site before manipulating an extremity.
- Rubbing fractured bone ends together can convert a closed fracture into an open one if a bone end penetrates the skin. Therefore, after the initial detection of crepitation in a patient with a fracture, avoid subsequent elicitation of this sign.

CAUSES

MEDICAL
Fracture
◆ Crepitus occurs when broken bone segments grate against each other.
◆ A fracture typically causes acute local pain, hematoma, edema, and decreased ROM.
◆ Neurovascular damage may cause increased capillary refill time, diminished or absent pulses, mottled cyanosis, paresthesia, and decreased sensation (all distal to the fracture site).
◆ An open fracture produces an obvious skin wound.
◆ Other signs and symptoms may include deformity, point tenderness, discoloration of the limb, and loss of limb function.

Osteoarthritis
◆ In its advanced form, joint crepitation may be elicited during ROM testing.
◆ Soft fine crepitus on palpation may indicate roughening of the articular cartilage; coarse grating may indicate badly damaged cartilage.
◆ The cardinal symptom of osteoarthritis is joint pain, especially during motion and weight bearing.
◆ Other signs and symptoms include joint stiffness that typically occurs after resting and subsides within a few minutes after the patient begins moving.

Rheumatoid arthritis
◆ In its advanced form, bony crepitation is heard when the affected joint is rotated.

◆ Rheumatoid arthritis usually develops insidiously, producing nonspecific signs and symptoms, such as fatigue, malaise, anorexia, a persistent low-grade fever, weight loss, lymphadenopathy, and vague arthralgia and myalgia. Later, more specific and localized articular signs develop, commonly at the proximal finger joints.
◆ Signs usually occur bilaterally and symmetrically and may extend to the wrists, knees, elbows, and ankles.
◆ The affected joints stiffen after inactivity with increased warmth, swelling, and tenderness of affected joints as well as limited ROM.

NURSING CONSIDERATIONS

◆ If a fracture is suspected, prepare the patient for X-rays of the affected area, and reexamine his neurovascular status frequently.
◆ Keep the affected part immobilized and elevated until treatment begins.
◆ Give an analgesic to relieve pain.
◆ Keep in mind that degenerative joint changes, which usually begin by age 20 or 30, progress more rapidly after age 40 and occur primarily in weight-bearing joints, such as the lumbar spine, hips, knees, and ankles.

PEDIATRIC POINTERS
◆ Bony crepitation in a child usually occurs after a fracture. Obtain an accurate history of the injury, and be alert for the possibility of child abuse. In a teenager, bony crepitation and pain in the patellofemoral joint help diagnose chondromalacia of the patella.

PATIENT TEACHING

◆ Teach the patient about the underlying cause of bony crepitation.
◆ Inform the patient about tests and procedures.
◆ Teach the patient about prescribed medications, their use, and possible adverse effects.

Crepitation, subcutaneous

OVERVIEW

- Results from trapping of air or gas bubbles in the subcutaneous tissue
- Crackling sound on palpation
- Bubbles that feel like small, unstable nodules
- Edema usual in affected area
- If edema affects the neck or upper chest, life-threatening airway occlusion possible

 ACTION STAT! *For signs of respiratory distress, quickly test for Hamman's sign. (See* Testing for Hamman's sign.*) Endotracheal intubation, an emergency tracheotomy, or chest tube insertion will be needed. Provide supplemental oxygen, and start an I.V. line to administer fluids and medications. Connect the patient to a cardiac monitor.*

HISTORY

- Ask if the patient is having difficulty breathing.
- Ask about the onset, location, and severity of any associated pain.
- Obtain a medical and surgical history, including recent thoracic surgery, diagnostic tests, and respiratory therapy as well as trauma or chronic pulmonary disease.

PHYSICAL ASSESSMENT

- Palpate the affected skin to evaluate the location and extent of crepitus.
- Palpate frequently to determine if subcutaneous crepitation is increasing.
- Perform abbreviated cardiac, pulmonary, and GI assessments as the patient's condition allows.
- When the patient is stabilized, perform a complete physical examination.

TOP TECHNIQUE

Testing for Hamman's sign

To test for Hamman's sign, help the patient assume a left-lateral recumbent position. Then place your stethoscope over the precordium. If you hear a loud crunching sound that synchronizes with his heartbeat, the patient has a positive Hamman's sign.

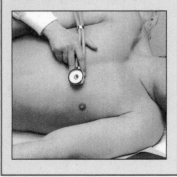

MEDICAL
Orbital fracture
◆ Subcutaneous crepitation of the eyelid and orbit develops when fracture allows air from the nasal sinus to escape into subcutaneous tissue.
◆ Periorbital ecchymosis is the most common sign.
◆ Other signs and symptoms include facial and eyelid edema, diplopia, a hyphema, impaired extraocular movements, and a dilated or unreactive pupil on the affected side.

Pneumothorax
◆ Subcutaneous crepitation occurs in the upper chest and neck in severe cases.
◆ One-sided chest pain increases on inspiration.
◆ Other signs and symptoms include dyspnea, anxiety, restlessness, tachypnea, cyanosis, tachycardia, accessory muscle use, asymmetrical chest expansion, decreased or absent breath sounds on the affected side, and a nonproductive cough.

Rupture of esophagus
◆ Subcutaneous crepitation may be palpable in the neck, chest wall, or supraclavicular fossa.
◆ With cervical esophagus rupture, signs and symptoms include excruciating pain in the neck or supraclavicular area, resistance to passive neck movement, local tenderness, soft-tissue swelling, dysphagia, odynophagia, and orthostatic vertigo.
◆ With life-threatening rupture of the intrathoracic esophagus, signs and symptoms include a positive Hamman's sign; severe retrosternal, epigastric, neck, or scapular pain; edema of the chest wall and neck; dyspnea; tachypnea; asymmetrical chest movement; nasal flaring; cyanosis; diaphoresis; tachycardia; hypotension; dysphagia; and fever.

Rupture of trachea or major bronchus
◆ A life-threatening disorder, abrupt subcutaneous crepitation of the neck and anterior chest wall occurs.
◆ Other signs and symptoms include severe dyspnea with nasal flaring, tachycardia, accessory muscle use, hypotension, cyanosis, extreme anxiety, hemoptysis, and mediastinal emphysema with a positive Hamman's sign.

OTHER
Diagnostic tests
◆ Endoscopic tests can rupture or perforate respiratory or GI organs, producing subcutaneous crepitation.

Respiratory treatments
◆ Intermittent positive-pressure breathing and mechanical ventilation can rupture alveoli, producing subcutaneous crepitation.

Thoracic surgery
◆ If air escapes into the tissue in the area of the incision, subcutaneous crepitation can occur.

◆ Monitor vital signs frequently, especially respirations.
◆ Look for signs of respiratory distress and airway obstruction.
◆ Tell the patient that the affected tissues will eventually absorb the air or gas bubbles, decreasing subcutaneous crepitation.
◆ Provide reassurance to reduce anxiety.

PEDIATRIC POINTERS
◆ Children may develop subcutaneous crepitation in the neck from ingestion of corrosive substances that perforate the esophagus.

◆ Explain diagnostic tests and procedures the patient needs.
◆ Explain the signs and symptoms of subcutaneous crepitation to report.

Cry, high-pitched (cerebral cry)

OVERVIEW

- Brief, sharp, piercing vocal sound produced by a neonate or infant
- Late sign of increased intracranial pressure (ICP), whether acute or chronic
- Change in volume of one of the brain's components—brain tissue, cerebrospinal fluid, and blood—possibly causing increased ICP
- Acute onset, demands emergency treatment to prevent permanent brain damage or death
- In neonates with increased ICP: may result from intracranial bleeding associated with birth trauma or from congenital malformations, such as craniostenosis and Arnold-Chiari deformity
- In infants with increased ICP: may result from meningitis, head trauma, or child abuse

ACTION STAT! After completing your examination, elevate the infant's head to promote cerebral venous drainage and decrease ICP. Start an I.V. line, and give a diuretic and a corticosteroid, as ordered, to decrease ICP. Be sure to keep endotracheal (ET) intubation equipment close by to secure an airway.

HISTORY

- Obtain a brief history asking if the infant fell recently or experienced even minor head trauma.
- Ask the parent about changes in the infant's behavior during the past 24 hours.
- Ask about vomiting, restlessness, diminished sucking reflex or if he cries when moved.
- Suspect child abuse if the infant's history is inconsistent with physical findings.

PHYSICAL ASSESSMENT

- Perform a neurologic examination. Remember that neurologic responses in a neonate or young infant are primarily reflex responses.
- Observe posture and examine muscle tone. Look for signs of seizure, such as tremors and twitching.
- Examine the size and shape of the infant's head. Note bulging of fontanels and signs of injury.
- Check pupillary size and response to light. Unilateral or bilateral dilation and a sluggish response to light may accompany increased ICP.
- Test the infant's reflexes; expect Moro's reflex to be diminished.

MEDICAL
Increased ICP

◆ A high-pitched cry is a late sign of increased ICP.

◆ Typically, the infant also displays bulging fontanels, increased head circumference, and widened sutures.

◆ Earlier signs and symptoms of increasing ICP include seizures, bradycardia, possible vomiting, dilated pupils, decreased level of consciousness, increased systolic blood pressure, a widened pulse pressure, and an altered respiratory pattern.

◆ The infant with increased ICP requires specialized care and monitoring in the intensive care unit.

◆ Monitor his vital signs and neurologic status to detect subtle changes in his condition.

◆ Monitor his intake and output. Monitor ICP, restrict fluids, and administer a diuretic, as prescribed.

◆ Increase the head of the bed 30 degrees, if the condition permits, and keep the head midline.

◆ Perform nursing care judiciously because procedures may cause a further increase in ICP.

◆ For an infant with severely increased ICP, ET intubation and mechanical hyperventilation may be needed to decrease serum carbon dioxide levels and constrict cerebral blood vessels.

◆ Hyperventilation is used for acute increases in ICP, the risks and benefits of which must be carefully weighed. Alternatively, barbiturate coma or hypothermia therapy may be needed to decrease the infant's metabolic rate.

◆ Avoid jostling the infant, which may aggravate increased ICP.

◆ Comfort him and maintain a calm, quiet environment because the infant's crying or exposure to environmental stimuli may also worsen increased ICP.

◆ Teach the family about the patient's diagnosis, prognosis, and treatment plan.

◆ Explain all procedures and monitoring equipment.

◆ Teach the parents how to participate in care, if possible.

◆ Explain all medications, their purpose, and possible adverse effects.

Cyanosis

OVERVIEW

- Refers to a bluish or bluish-black discoloration of the skin and mucous membranes
- Results from excessive concentration of unoxygenated hemoglobin in the blood
- Classified as central (inadequate oxygenation of systemic arterial blood) or peripheral (sluggish peripheral circulation)
- Isn't always an accurate gauge of oxygenation

   ACTION STAT! *If sudden, localized cyanosis occurs with other signs of arterial occlusion, protect the affected limb from injury, but don't massage it. If central cyanosis stems from a pulmonary disorder or shock, perform a rapid evaluation. Take immediate steps to maintain an airway, assist breathing, and monitor circulation.*

HISTORY

- Obtain a medical history, including cardiac, pulmonary, and hematologic disorders, and previous surgery.
- Evaluate the patient's mental status while obtaining his history.
- Ask about the onset, aggravating and alleviating factors, and characteristics of the cyanosis.
- Ask about other signs and symptoms.

PHYSICAL ASSESSMENT

- Take vital signs, measure oxygen saturation, and evaluate respiratory rate and rhythm.
- Check for nasal flaring and accessory muscle use.
- Inspect the skin, lips, and nail bed color and mucous membranes.
- Inspect for asymmetrical chest expansion or barrel chest.
- Inspect the abdomen for ascites.
- Palpate peripheral pulses, test capillary refill, and note edema.
- Percuss and palpate for liver enlargement and tenderness.
- Percuss the lungs for dullness or hyperresonance.
- Auscultate for decreased or adventitious breath sounds.
- Auscultate heart rate and rhythm.
- Auscultate abdominal aorta and femoral arteries for bruits.

CAUSES

MEDICAL
Arteriosclerotic occlusive disease, chronic
- Peripheral cyanosis occurs in the legs whenever they're in a dependent position.
- Leg ulcers and gangrene are late signs.
- Other signs and symptoms include intermittent claudication and burning pain at rest, paresthesia, pallor, muscle atrophy, weak leg pulses, and impotence.

Bronchiectasis
- Chronic central cyanosis develops.
- The classic sign is chronic productive cough with copious, foul-smelling, mucopurulent sputum, or hemoptysis.
- Other signs and symptoms include dyspnea, recurrent fever and chills, weight loss, malaise, clubbing, and signs of anemia.

Buerger's disease
- This is an occlusive inflammatory disorder of the lower extremity arteries.
- Exposure to cold initially causes the feet to become cold, cyanotic, and numb; later, they redden, become hot, and tingle.
- Intermittent claudication of the instep is characteristic.
- Other signs and symptoms include weak, peripheral pulses and, in later stages, ulceration, muscle atrophy, and gangrene.

Chronic obstructive pulmonary disease
- Chronic central cyanosis occurs in advanced stages.
- Exertion aggravates cyanosis.
- Barrel chest and clubbing are late signs.
- Other signs and symptoms include exertional dyspnea, productive cough with thick sputum, anorexia, weight loss, pursed-lip breathing, tachypnea, accessory muscle use, and wheezing.

Heart failure
- Acute or chronic cyanosis may occur (late sign).
- With left-sided heart failure, central cyanosis occurs with tachycardia, fatigue, dyspnea, cold intolerance, orthopnea, cough, ventricular or atrial gallop, and crackles.
- With right-sided heart failure, peripheral cyanosis occurs with fatigue, peripheral edema, ascites, jugular vein distention, and hepatomegaly.

Peripheral arterial occlusion, acute
- Acute cyanosis of the arm or leg occurs.
- Cyanosis is accompanied by sharp or aching pain that worsens with movement.
- Paresthesia, weakness, decreased or absent pulse, and pale, cool skin occur in the affected extremity.

Pneumonia
- Acute central cyanosis is usually preceded by fever, shaking chills, cough with purulent sputum, crackles, rhonchi, and pleuritic chest pain

that's exacerbated by deep inspiration.
- Other signs and symptoms include tachycardia, dyspnea, tachypnea, diminished breath sounds, diaphoresis, myalgia, fatigue, headache, and anorexia.

Pneumothorax
- Acute central cyanosis is a cardinal sign.
- Rapid, shallow respirations; weak, rapid pulse; pallor; jugular vein distention; anxiety; and absence of breath sounds over the affected lobe may also occur.
- Other signs and symptoms include sharp chest pain that's exacerbated by movement, deep breathing, and coughing; asymmetrical chest movement; and shortness of breath.

Polycythemia vera
- Ruddy complexion that can appear cyanotic is characteristic of this bone marrow disease.
- Other signs and symptoms include hepatosplenomegaly, headache, dizziness, fatigue, blurred vision, chest pain, intermittent claudication, and coagulation defects.

Pulmonary edema
- Acute central cyanosis occurs because of impaired gas exchange.
- Other signs and symptoms include dyspnea; orthopnea; frothy, blood-tinged sputum; tachycardia; tachypnea; crackles; ventricular gallop; cold, clammy skin; hypotension; weak, thready pulse; and confusion.

Pulmonary embolism
- Acute central cyanosis occurs when a large embolus obstructs pulmonary circulation.
- Other signs and symptoms include anxiety, syncope, jugular vein distention, dyspnea, chest pain, tachycardia, paradoxical pulse, dry cough or productive cough with blood-tinged sputum, fever, restlessness, and diaphoresis.

Raynaud's phenomenon
- Raynaud's disease is a vascular disorder characterized by episodes of vasospasm in the small peripheral arteries and arterioles.
- Exposure to cold or stress causes the fingers or hands to blanch, turn cold, then become cyanotic, and finally to redden with return of normal temperature.
- Numbness and tingling may also develop.

Shock
- Acute peripheral cyanosis develops in the hands and feet.
- Feet may be cold, clammy, and pale.
- Central cyanosis develops with progression of shock and organ system failures.
- Other signs and symptoms include lethargy, confusion, increased capillary refill time, tachypnea, hyperpnea, hypotension, and a rapid, weak pulse.

NURSING CONSIDERATIONS

- Provide supplemental oxygen to improve oxygenation.
- Deliver small doses of oxygen of 2 L/minute to patients with chronic obstructive pulmonary disease (COPD); use a low-flow oxygen rate for mild COPD exacerbations.
- For acute situations, a high-flow oxygen rate may be needed initially; in working with a patient who has COPD, remember to be attentive to his respiratory drive and adjust the amount of oxygen accordingly.
- Position the patient comfortably to ease breathing.
- Give a diuretic, bronchodilator, antibiotic, or cardiac drug, as prescribed.
- Provide rest periods to prevent dyspnea; encourage energy conservation.

PEDIATRIC POINTERS
- Central cyanosis may result from cystic fibrosis, asthma, airway obstruction, acute laryngotracheobronchitis, epiglottiditis, or congenital heart defects.

- Cyanosis around the mouth may precede generalized cyanosis.
- Acrocyanosis may occur in infants because of excessive crying or exposure to cold.

GERIATRIC POINTERS
- Because of reduced tissue perfusion in elderly people, peripheral cyanosis can occur even with a slight decrease in cardiac output or systemic blood pressure.

PATIENT TEACHING

- Instruct the patient to seek medical attention if cyanosis occurs.
- Discuss the safe use of oxygen in the home.
- Teach the patient and family about the medical diagnosis and treatment plan.
- Teach the importance of prescribed medications, how to administer them, and possible adverse effects.
- Discuss the importance of frequent rest periods.
- Discuss the importance of follow-up care.
- Discuss the importance of smoking cessation, and refer patient for assistance as needed.

Decerebrate posture

OVERVIEW

- Characterized by internally rotated and extended arms, pronated wrists, flexed fingers, stiffly extended legs, and forced plantar flexion of the feet (see *Differentiating decerebrate posture from decorticate posture*)
- Indicates upper brain stem damage
- May occur spontaneously or be elicited by noxious stimuli
- Also known as *decerebrate rigidity* or *abnormal extensor reflex*

 ACTION STAT! Check if the patient's airway is patent. Insert an artificial airway, if needed, to prevent aspiration. (If you suspect spinal cord injury, don't disrupt spinal alignment.) Suction, as needed. Give supplemental oxygen. Intubation and mechanical ventilation may be required. Keep emergency resuscitation equipment handy.

HISTORY

- Question family members to determine when the patient's level of consciousness (LOC) began to deteriorate.
- Ask if onset was abrupt or gradual and occurred with other signs or symptoms.
- Obtain a medical history, asking about diabetes, liver disease, cancer, blood clots, and aneurysm.
- Ask about recent trauma or accident.

PHYSICAL ASSESSMENT

- Take vital signs.
- Determine LOC using the Glasgow Coma Scale.
- Evaluate pupils for size, equality, and response to light.
- Test deep tendon reflexes and cranial nerve reflexes.
- Check for doll's eye reflex.

TOP TECHNIQUE

Differentiating decerebrate posture from decorticate posture

Decerebrate posture results from damage to the upper brain stem. In this posture, the arms are adducted and extended, with the wrists pronated and the fingers flexed. The legs are stiffly extended, with plantar flexion of the feet.

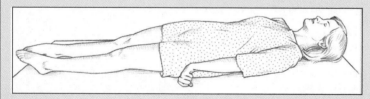

Decorticate posture results from damage to one or both corticospinal tracts. In this posture, the arms are adducted and flexed, with the wrists and fingers flexed on the chest. The legs are stiffly extended and internally rotated, with plantar flexion of the feet.

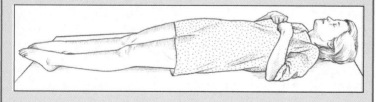

MEDICAL

Brain stem infarction
- Coma may occur with decerebrate posture.
- Absence of doll's eye sign, a positive Babinski's reflex, and flaccidity occur with deep coma.
- Other signs and symptoms vary with the severity of infarct and may include cranial nerve palsies, cerebellar ataxia, and sensory loss.

Brain stem tumor
- Decerebrate posture is a late sign that occurs with coma.
- Earlier signs and symptoms include hemiparesis or quadriparesis, cranial nerve palsies, vertigo, dizziness, ataxia, and vomiting.

Cerebral lesion
- Increased intracranial pressure (ICP) may produce decerebrate posture, a late sign.
- Other signs and symptoms include coma, abnormal pupil size and response to light, and the classic triad of increased ICP: bradycardia, increasing systolic blood pressure, and widening pulse pressure.

Hepatic encephalopathy
- A late sign in this disorder, decerebrate posture occurs with coma resulting from increased ICP and increasing serum ammonia levels.
- Other signs and symptoms include fetor hepaticus, a positive Babinski's reflex, and hyperactive deep tendon reflexes.

Hypoglycemic encephalopathy
- Decerebrate posture and coma may occur.
- Low glucose levels are characteristic.
- Muscle spasms, twitching, and seizures progress to flaccidity.
- Other signs and symptoms include dilated pupils, slow respirations, and bradycardia.

Hypoxic encephalopathy
- Decerebrate posture occurs.
- Other signs and symptoms include coma, positive Babinski's reflex, absence of doll's eye sign, hypoactive deep tendon reflexes, fixed pupils, and respiratory arrest.

Pontine hemorrhage
- In this life-threatening disorder, decerebrate posture occurs rapidly along with coma.
- Other signs and symptoms include paralysis, absence of doll's eye sign, a positive Babinski's reflex, and small, reactive pupils.

Posterior fossa hemorrhage
- Decerebrate posture occurs with vomiting, headache, vertigo, ataxia, stiff neck, drowsiness, papilledema, and cranial nerve palsies.
- Eventually, coma and respiratory arrest may occur.

OTHER

Diagnostic tests
- Removing spinal fluid during a lumbar puncture may cause the brain stem to compress, causing decerebrate posture and coma.

- Monitor neurologic status and vital signs.
- Look for symptoms of increased ICP and neurologic deterioration.

PEDIATRIC POINTERS
- Children younger than age 2 may not display decerebrate posture because of nervous system immaturity.
- In children, the most common cause of decerebrate posture is head injury.

- Explain that decerebrate posture is a reflex response.
- Provide emotional support to the patient and his family.
- Teach the patient and family about the medical diagnosis, prognosis, and treatment plan.

Decorticate posture

OVERVIEW

- Signals corticospinal damage, usually from stroke or head injury
- Characterized by adducted arms, flexion of the elbows, flexed wrists and fingers on the chest, and extended and internally rotated legs with plantar flexion of the feet
- May occur spontaneously or be elicited by noxious stimuli
- Intensity of the stimulus, the duration of the posture, and frequency of spontaneous episodes dependent on severity and location of cerebral injury
- Carries a more favorable prognosis than decerebrate posture (see *Differentiating decerebrate posture from decorticate posture,* page 158)

ACTION STAT! *Obtain vital signs and evaluate level of consciousness (LOC). Maintain a patent airway and prevent aspiration. (If you suspect spinal cord injury, don't disrupt spinal alignment.) Intubation and mechanical ventilation may be required.*

HISTORY

- Check for symptoms, such as headache, dizziness, nausea, changes in vision, numbness or tingling, and behavioral changes. If a symptom is present, ask when it began.
- Obtain a medical history, asking about cerebrovascular disease, cancer, meningitis, encephalitis, upper respiratory tract infection, bleeding or clotting disorders, or recent trauma.
- Obtain history from family members if the patient's LOC is decreased, or he's unable to communicate.

PHYSICAL ASSESSMENT

- Test motor and sensory functions.
- Evaluate pupil size, equality, and response to light.
- Test cranial nerve function and deep tendon reflexes.

CAUSES

MEDICAL
Brain abscess
- Decorticate posture may occur along with aphasia, behavioral changes, altered vital signs, decreased LOC, hemiparesis, headache, dizziness, seizures, nausea, and vomiting.

Brain tumor
- Decorticate posture results from increased intracranial pressure (ICP).
- Other signs and symptoms include headache, behavioral changes, memory loss, diplopia, blurred vision or vision loss, seizures, ataxia, apraxia, aphasia, sensory loss, paresthesia, vomiting, papilledema, and signs of hormonal imbalance.

Head injury
- Decorticate posture may result, depending on the injury.
- Other signs and symptoms include headache, nausea, vomiting, dizziness, irritability, decreased LOC, aphasia, hemiparesis, seizures, and pupillary dilation.

Stroke
- A stroke involving the cerebral cortex produces decorticate posture on one side of the body.
- Other signs and symptoms include hemiplegia, dysarthria, dysphagia, sensory loss, apraxia, agnosia, aphasia, memory loss, decreased LOC, homonymous hemianopia, and blurred vision.

NURSING CONSIDERATIONS

- Monitor neurologic status and vital signs frequently to detect signs of deterioration.
- Look for other signs of increased ICP.

PEDIATRIC POINTERS
- Decorticate posture is an unreliable sign before age 2 years because of nervous system immaturity.
- In children, decorticate posture usually results from head injury.

PATIENT TEACHING

- Explain the signs and symptoms of decreased LOC and seizures.
- Discuss the patient's or caregiver's quality-of-life concerns.
- Provide referrals, as appropriate.
- Explain to the caregiver how to keep the patient safe, especially during seizure.

Deep tendon reflexes, hyperactive

OVERVIEW

- Abnormally brisk muscle contractions in response to sudden stretch after sharp tapping of muscle's tendon of insertion (see *Tracing the reflex arc*)
- Graded as brisk or pathologically hyperactive
- Results from damage to the reflex arc sequence

HISTORY

- Obtain a medical history, including spinal cord injury, other trauma, or prolonged exposure to cold.
- Ask the female patient if she's pregnant.
- Determine the onset and progression of other signs and symptoms, including paresthesia, vomiting, and altered bladder habits.
- Obtain drug history.
- Obtain immunization history, especially tetanus vaccine.

PHYSICAL ASSESSMENT

- Evaluate level of consciousness.
- Take vital signs.
- Test motor and sensory function in the limbs.
- Check for ataxia or tremors and for speech and visual deficits.

Tracing the reflex arc

Sharply tapping a tendon initiates a sensory (afferent) impulse that travels along a peripheral nerve to a spinal nerve and then to the spinal cord. The impulse enters the spinal cord through the posterior root, synapses with a motor (efferent) neuron in the anterior horn on the same side of the spinal cord, and then is transmitted through a motor nerve fiber back to the muscle. When the impulse crosses the neuromuscular junction, the muscle contracts, completing the reflex arc.

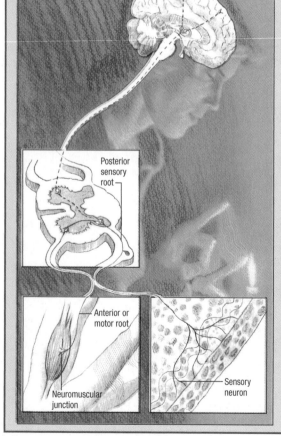

Posterior sensory root

Anterior or motor root

Neuromuscular junction

Sensory neuron

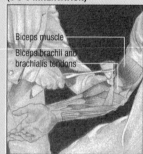

BICEPS REFLEX (C 5-6 INNERVATION)

Biceps muscle

Biceps brachii and brachialis tendons

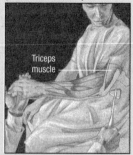

TRICEPS REFLEX (C 7-8 INNERVATION)

Triceps muscle

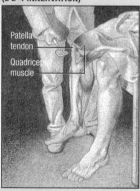

PATELLAR REFLEX (L 2-4 INNERVATION)

Patella tendon

Quadriceps muscle

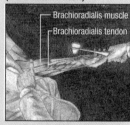

BRACHIORADIALIS REFLEX (C 5-6 INNERVATION)

Brachioradialis muscle

Brachioradialis tendon

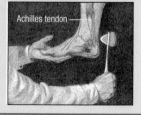

ACHILLES TENDON REFLEX (S 1-2 INNERVATION)

Achilles tendon

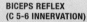

- Test for Chvostek's sign, Trousseau's sign, and carpopedal spasm.

CAUSES

MEDICAL
Amyotrophic lateral sclerosis
- Generalized, hyperactive deep tendon reflexes (DTRs) accompany weakness of the hands and forearms and spasticity of the legs in this motor neuron disease.
- Atrophy of the neck and tongue muscles, fasciculations, weakness of the legs, and bulbar signs eventually develop.

Brain tumor
- Hyperactive DTRs occur on the side opposite the lesion.
- Other signs and symptoms include one-sided paresis or paralysis, visual field deficits, spasticity, and a positive Babinski's reflex.

Gestational hypertension
- Onset of generalized hyperactive DTRs is gradual.
- If the condition progresses to eclampsia, seizures may occur.
- Other signs and symptoms include abnormal weight gain; edema of the face, fingers, and abdomen; albuminuria; oliguria; severe headache; blurred or double vision; epigastric pain; nausea and vomiting; irritability; cyanosis; shortness of breath; and crackles.

Hepatic encephalopathy
- Generalized hyperactive DTRs occur late in comatose stage.
- Other signs and symptoms include a positive Babinski's reflex, fetor hepaticus, and coma.

Hypocalcemia
- Onset of generalized hyperactive DTRs may be gradual or sudden.
- Other signs and symptoms include paresthesia, muscle twitching and cramping, positive Chvostek's and Trousseau's signs, carpopedal spasm, tetany, abdominal and muscle cramps, arrhythmias, and diarrhea.

Hypomagnesemia
- Onset of generalized hyperactive DTRs is gradual.
- Other signs and symptoms include muscle cramps, hypotension, tachycardia, paresthesia, ataxia, tetany, seizures, positive Chvostek's sign, confusion, and arrhythmias.

Hypothermia
- Mild hypothermia produces generalized hyperactive DTRs.
- Other signs and symptoms include shivering, fatigue, weakness, lethargy, slurred speech, ataxia, muscle stiffness, arrhythmias, diuresis, hypotension, and cold, pale skin.

Multiple sclerosis
- This progressive disease is caused by demyelination of the white matter of the brain and spinal cord.
- Hyperactive DTRs are preceded by weakness and paresthesia in arms and legs.
- Ataxia, diplopia, vertigo, vomiting, and urine retention or incontinence occur later.
- Other signs and symptoms include clonus and a positive Babinski's reflex.

Spinal cord lesion
- Incomplete lesions cause hyperactive DTRs below the lesion.
- In a traumatic lesion, hyperactive DTRs follow resolution of spinal shock.
- In a neoplastic lesion, hyperactive DTRs gradually occur.
- A lesion at or above T6 may produce autonomic hyperreflexia with diaphoresis and flushing above the lesion, headache, nasal congestion, nausea, hypertension, and bradycardia.
- Other signs and symptoms include paralysis and sensory loss below the level of the lesion, urine retention and overflow incontinence, and alternating constipation and diarrhea.

Stroke
- If the origin of the corticospinal tracts is affected, hyperactive DTRs

on the side opposite the lesion suddenly occur.
- Other signs and symptoms include anesthesia, visual field deficits, spasticity, a positive Babinski's reflex, and one-sided paresis or paralysis.

Tetanus
- Sudden onset of generalized hyperactive DTRs occurs.
- Other signs and symptoms include tachycardia, diaphoresis, low-grade fever, painful and involuntary muscle contractions, trismus (lockjaw), and *risus sardonicus* (a masklike grin).

NURSING CONSIDERATIONS

- If motor weakness is present, perform range-of-motion exercises.
- Reposition the patient frequently, provide a special mattress, massage his back, and ensure adequate nutrition.
- Give a muscle relaxant and a sedative to relieve severe muscle contractions, as prescribed.
- Keep emergency resuscitation equipment on hand.
- Provide a quiet, calm atmosphere to reduce neuromuscular excitability.
- Assist with activities of daily living.

PEDIATRIC POINTERS
- Cerebral palsy typically causes hyperactive DTRs in children.
- Stage II Reye's syndrome causes generalized hyperactive DTRs; in stage V, DTRs are absent.
- Hyperreflexia may be normal in neonates.

PATIENT TEACHING

- Explain to the caregiver the procedures and treatments that the patient may need.
- Discuss safety measures that need to be taken.
- Provide emotional support.

Deep tendon reflexes, hypoactive

OVERVIEW

- Abnormally diminished muscle contractions in response to sudden stretch after sharp tapping of the muscle's tendon of insertion
- Result from damage to the reflex arc involving the specific muscle, the peripheral nerve, the nerve roots, or the spinal cord
- Important sign of many disorders, especially when they appear with other neurologic signs

HISTORY

- Obtain a medical history.
- Ask about other signs and symptoms.
- Take a family and drug history.

PHYSICAL ASSESSMENT

- Assess level of consciousness and speech.
- Test motor function in the limbs.
- Palpate for muscle atrophy or increased mass.
- Test sensory function, assessing for paresthesia.
- Observe gait and coordination.
- Check for Romberg's sign.
- Check for signs of vision and hearing loss.
- Take vital signs and note increased heart rate and blood pressure.
- Inspect the skin for pallor, dryness, flushing, and diaphoresis.
- Auscultate for hypoactive bowel sounds.
- Palpate for bladder distention.
- Document the muscles in which deep tendon reflexes (DTRs) are lessened. (See *Documenting deep tendon reflexes*.)

Documenting deep tendon reflexes

To record the patient's deep tendon reflex scores, draw a stick figure and enter the rating on the drawing for each reflex. The figure shown here indicates hypoactive deep tendon reflexes in the legs; the other reflexes are normal.

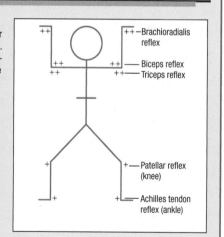

KEY:
- 0 = absent
- + = hypoactive (diminished)
- ++ = normal
- +++ = brisk (increased)
- ++++ = hyperactive (clonus may be present)

MEDICAL
Botulism

- This life-threatening paralytic illness is caused by ingestion of contaminated food or, rarely, by a wound infection.
- Generalized hypoactive DTRs accompany progressive descending muscle weakness.
- Respiratory distress and severe constipation may also develop.
- Other signs and symptoms include blurred vision, double vision, anorexia, nausea, vomiting, vertigo, hearing loss, dysarthria, and dysphagia.

Cerebellar dysfunction

- Hypoactive DTRs occur with other findings depending on the cause and location of the dysfunction.

Guillain-Barré syndrome

- This syndrome is an acute, rapidly progressing, and potentially fatal form of polyneuritis.
- Hypoactive DTRs progress rapidly from hypotonia to areflexia.
- Muscle weakness begins in the legs and then extends to the arms and, possibly, to the trunk and neck, peaking in 10 to 14 days and then resolving.
- Weakness may progress to total paralysis.
- Other signs and symptoms include cranial nerve palsies, pain, paresthesia, and signs of autonomic dysfunction.

Peripheral neuropathy

- Progressive hypoactive DTRs occur.
- Other signs and symptoms include motor weakness, sensory loss, paresthesia, tremors, and possible autonomic dysfunction.

Polymyositis

- Hypoactive DTRs occur with accompanying muscle weakness, pain, stiffness, spasms and, possibly, increased size or atrophy.

Spinal cord lesions

- Transient hypoactive DTRs or areflexia occur below the lesion.
- Quadriplegia or paraplegia, flaccidity, loss of sensation, and pale, dry skin occur below the level of the lesion.
- Other signs and symptoms include urine retention with overflow incontinence, hypoactive bowel sounds, constipation, and genital reflex loss.

OTHER
Drugs

- Barbiturates and paralyzing drugs, such as pancuronium, propofol (Diprivan), and curare, may cause hypoactive DTRs.

NURSING CONSIDERATIONS

- If the patient has sensory deficits, protect him from heat, cold, and pressure.
- Keep the skin clean and dry.
- Reposition the patient frequently.
- Encourage range-of-joint-motion exercises.
- Provide a balanced diet with increased protein and fluids.

PEDIATRIC POINTERS

- Hypoactive DTRs commonly occur in children with muscular dystrophy, Friedreich's ataxia, syringomyelia, and spinal cord injury.
- Hypoactive DTRs accompany progressive muscular atrophy, which affects preschoolers and adolescents.

GERIATRIC POINTERS

- Hypoactive DTRs occur because of a decrease in the number of nerve axons and demyelination of axons in elderly patients.

PATIENT TEACHING

- Teach skills that can help the patient be as independent as possible in his daily life.
- Discuss safety measures, including walking with assistance.
- Discuss the underlying condition, diagnostic tests, and treatment options.

Depression

- Mood disturbance characterized by feelings of sadness, despair, loss of interest or pleasure in activities, and thoughts of death, suicide, or injuring oneself
- May be accompanied by somatic complaints, such as changes in appetite, sleep disturbances, restlessness or lethargy, and decreased concentration
- Clinical depression: must be distinguished from "the blues," periodic bouts of dysphoria that are less persistent and severe than the clinical disorder
- Major depression: one or more episodes of depressed mood or decreased interest or ability to take pleasure in all or most activities, lasting at least 2 weeks; strikes 10% to 15% of adults, affecting all racial, ethnic, age, and socioeconomic groups; twice as common in women as in men and is especially prevalent among adolescents

- Obtain a complete history, including onset, duration, and if the patient has had previous bouts with depression.
- Ask the patient about her family—its patterns of interaction and characteristic responses to success and failure. Find out if other family members have been depressed and whether anyone important to her has been sick or has died in the past year.
- Ask about a support network in order to determine if the patient has had one in the past and if it's still in place.
- Ask about the patient's lifestyle and if it has changed recently.

- Complete a psychological and physical examination to rule out possible medical causes.
- Obtain a description of how the patient feels about herself, her family, and her environment with the goal of exploring the nature of the depression and the extent to which other factors affect it.
- Obtain information about coping mechanisms.
- Determine patterns of drug and alcohol use. Listen for clues that she may be suicidal. (See *Suicide: Caring for the high-risk patient.*)

Suicide: Caring for the high-risk patient

One of the most common factors contributing to suicide is hopelessness, an emotion that many depressed patients experience. The patient may also provide specific clues about her intentions. For example, you may notice her talking frequently about death or the futility of life, concealing potentially harmful items (such as knives and belts), hoarding medications, giving away personal belongings, or getting her legal and financial affairs in order. If you suspect that a patient is suicidal, follow these guidelines:

- First, try to determine the patient's suicide potential. Find out how upset she is. Does she have a simple, straightforward suicide plan that's likely to succeed? Does she have a strong support system (family, friends, a therapist)? A patient with low to moderate suicide potential is noticeably depressed but has a support system. She may have thoughts of suicide, but no specific plan. A patient with high suicide potential feels profoundly hopeless and has a minimal or no support system. She thinks about suicide frequently and has a plan that's likely to succeed.

- Next, observe precautions. Ensure the patient's safety by removing any objects she could use to harm herself, such as knives, scissors, razors, belts, electric cords, shoelaces, and drugs. Know her whereabouts and what she's doing at all times; this may require one-on-one surveillance and placing the patient in a room that's close to your station. Always have someone accompany her when she leaves the unit.

- Be alert for in-hospital suicide attempts, which typically occur when there's a low staff-to-patient ratio—for example, between shifts, during evening and night shifts, or when a critical event such as a code draws attention away from the patient.

- Finally, arrange for follow-up counseling. Recognize suicidal ideation and behavior as a desperate cry for help. Contact a mental health professional for a referral.

CAUSES

MEDICAL
Organic disorders
- Organic disorders and chronic illnesses produce mild, moderate, or severe depression.
- Other causes include metabolic and endocrine disorders, such as hypothyroidism, hyperthyroidism, and diabetes; infectious diseases, such as influenza, hepatitis, and encephalitis; degenerative diseases, such as Alzheimer's disease, multiple sclerosis, and multi-infarct dementia; and neoplastic disorders, such as cancer.

Postpartum period
- Postpartum depression occurs in about 1 in every 2,000 to 3,000 women who have given birth.
- Symptoms range from mild postpartum blues to an intense, suicidal, depressive psychosis.

Psychiatric disorders
- Affective disorders are typically characterized by abrupt mood swings from depression to elation (mania) or by prolonged episodes of either mood.
- Severe depression may last from weeks to months without treatment.
- Moderate depression occurs in cyclothymic disorders and usually alternates with moderate mania.
- Moderate depression that's more or less constant over a 2-year period typically results from dysthymic disorders.
- Chronic anxiety disorders, such as panic and obsessive-compulsive disorder, may be accompanied by depression.

OTHER
Alcohol abuse
- Long-term alcohol use, intoxication, or withdrawal commonly produces depression.

Drugs
- Various drugs cause depression as an adverse effect.

- More common depression-causing drugs include barbiturates; chemotherapeutic drugs, such as asparaginase; anticonvulsants, such as diazepam; and antiarrhythmics, such as disopyramide.
- Other depression-inducing drugs include centrally acting antihypertensives, such as reserpine (common with high doses), methyldopa, and clonidine; beta-adrenergic blockers, such as propranolol; levodopa; indomethacin; cycloserine; corticosteroids; and hormonal contraceptives.

NURSING CONSIDERATIONS

- Be aware of your own vulnerability to feelings of despair that can stem from interacting with a depressed patient.
- Help the patient set realistic goals.
- Promote feelings of self-worth by encouraging expression of opinions and decision making.
- Determine suicide potential, and take steps to help ensure patient safety. Provide close surveillance to prevent a suicide attempt, if necessary.
- Provide a calm, unconditional environment for the patient to verbalize her feelings.
- Make sure the patient receives adequate nourishment and rest, and keep environment free from stress and excessive stimulation.
- Arrange for ordered diagnostic tests to determine if depression has an organic cause, and administer prescribed drugs.
- Arrange for follow-up counseling, or contact a mental health professional for a referral.

PEDIATRIC POINTERS
- Because emotional lability is normal in adolescence, depression can be difficult to assess and diagnose in teenagers.
- Clues to underlying depression may include somatic complaints, sexual promiscuity, poor grades, and abuse of alcohol or drugs.

- Use of a family systems model usually helps determine the cause of depression in adolescents.
- Once family roles are determined, family therapy or group therapy with peers may help the patient overcome her depression.
- In severe cases, an antidepressant may be required.

GERIATRIC POINTERS
- Many elderly patients have physical complaints, somatic complaints, agitation, or changes in intellectual functioning (memory impairment), making the diagnosis of depression difficult in these patients.
- Depressed older adults who are age 85 and older, who have low self-esteem, and who need to be in control have the highest risk of suicide.

PATIENT TEACHING

- Discuss patient's condition, prognosis, and treatment with patient and family members.
- Teach patient about specific medication use, adverse effects, and the importance of avoiding alcohol when taking most antidepressants.
- Discuss the importance of follow-up counseling with a mental health professional.
- Provide information about group/community activities and other resources the patient can use after discharge.

Diaphoresis

OVERVIEW

- Characterized by profuse sweating (see *Understanding diaphoresis*)
- Can produce more than 1 L of sweat per hour
- Represents an autonomic nervous system response to physical or psychogenic stress or to fever or high environmental temperature

HISTORY

- Ask the patient to describe his chief complaint and quickly rule out the possibility of a life-threatening cause. (See *When diaphoresis spells crisis.*)
- Note when diaphoresis occurs (day or night).
- Investigate other signs and symptoms.
- Find out about recent travel or exposure to high environmental temperatures or to pesticides.
- Ask about recent insect bites.
- Obtain a medical history, asking about partial gastrectomy or drug or alcohol abuse.
- Take a medication history.

PHYSICAL ASSESSMENT

- Inspect the trunk, extremities, palms, soles, and forehead to determine the extent of diaphoresis.
- Observe for flushing, abnormal skin texture or lesions, and an increased amount of coarse body hair.
- Note poor skin turgor and dry mucous membranes.
- Look for splinter hemorrhages and Plummer's nails.
- Evaluate mental status.
- Take vital signs.
- Observe for fasciculations and flaccid paralysis.
- Assess for seizures.
- Note the patient's facial expression and examine the eyes.
- Auscultate breath sounds.
- Palpate for lymphadenopathy and hepatosplenomegaly.

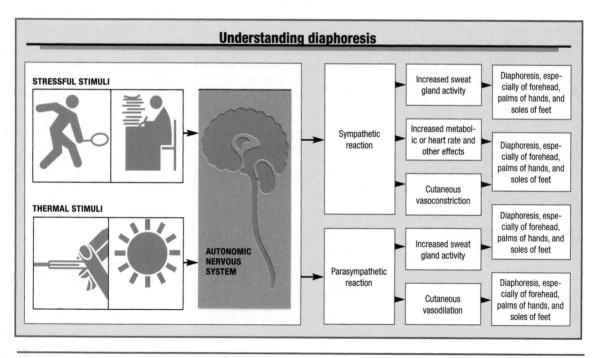

Understanding diaphoresis

MEDICAL

Acquired immunodeficiency syndrome
- Night sweats may occur early as a manifestation of the disease or from an opportunistic infection.
- Other signs and symptoms include fever, fatigue, lymphadenopathy, anorexia, weight loss, diarrhea, and a persistent cough.

Acromegaly
- Diaphoresis measures disease activity, which involves hypersecretion of growth hormone and increased metabolic rate.
- Other signs and symptoms include a hulking appearance; an enlarged supraorbital ridge and thickened ears and nose; warm, oily skin; enlarged hands, feet, and jaw; joint pain; weight gain; hoarseness; increased coarse body hair; elevated blood pressure; and visual field deficits or blindness.

Anxiety disorders
- Diaphoresis occurs on the palms, soles, and forehead.
- Fear, difficulty concentrating, and behavior changes occur.
- Other signs and symptoms include palpitations, tachycardia, tachypnea, tremors, and GI distress.

Autonomic hyperreflexia
- Profuse diaphoresis above the level of injury, pounding headache, blurred vision, and dramatically elevated blood pressure occur after resolution of spinal shock in spinal cord injury above T6.
- Other signs and symptoms include flushing, restlessness, nausea, nasal congestion, and bradycardia.

Heart failure
- In left-sided heart failure, diaphoresis follows fatigue, dyspnea, orthopnea, and tachycardia.
- In right-sided heart failure, diaphoresis follows jugular vein distention, muffled heart sounds, and dry cough.
- Other signs and symptoms include tachypnea, cyanosis, edema, crackles, ventricular gallop, and anxiety.

Heat exhaustion
- Profuse diaphoresis, fever, fatigue, weakness, and anxiety may occur initially.
- Other later signs and symptoms include ashen gray appearance, dilated pupils, and normal or abnormally low temperature; condition may progress to circulatory collapse and shock.

Hodgkin's lymphoma
- Initial sign is usually a painless swelling of a cervical lymph node.
- Other signs and symptoms may include night sweats, fever, fatigue, pruritus, and weight loss.

ACTION STAT!

When diaphoresis spells crisis

Diaphoresis is an early sign of certain life-threatening disorders. These guidelines will help you promptly detect such disorders and intervene to minimize harm to the patient.

HYPOGLYCEMIA

If you observe diaphoresis in a patient who complains of blurred vision, ask him about increased irritability and anxiety. Has the patient been unusually hungry lately? Does he have tremors? Take the patient's vital signs, noting hypotension and tachycardia. Then ask about a history of type 2 diabetes or antidiabetic therapy. If you suspect hypoglycemia, evaluate the patient's blood glucose level using a glucose reagent strip, or send a serum sample to the laboratory. Administer I.V. glucose 50%, as ordered, to return the patient's glucose level to normal. Monitor his vital signs and cardiac rhythm. Ensure a patent airway, and be prepared to assist with breathing and circulation, if necessary.

HEATSTROKE

If you observe profuse diaphoresis in a weak, tired, and apprehensive patient, suspect heatstroke, which can progress to circulatory collapse. Take vital signs, noting a normal or subnormal temperature. Check for ashen gray skin and dilated pupils. Was the patient recently exposed to high temperatures and humidity? Was he wearing heavy clothing or performing strenuous physical activity at the time? Also, ask if he takes a diuretic, which interferes with normal sweating.

   Then take the patient to a cool room, remove his clothing, and use a fan to direct cool air over his body. Obtain I.V. access, and prepare for electrolyte and fluid replacement. Monitor the patient for signs of shock. Check his urine output carefully along with other sources of output (such as tubes, drains, and ostomies).

AUTONOMIC HYPERREFLEXIA

If you observe diaphoresis in a patient with a spinal cord injury above T6 or T7, ask if he has a pounding headache, restlessness, blurred vision, or nasal congestion. Take the patient's vital signs, noting bradycardia or extremely elevated blood pressure. If you suspect autonomic hyperreflexia, quickly rule out its common complications. Examine the patient for eye pain associated with intraocular hemorrhage and for facial paralysis, slurred speech, or limb weakness associated with intracerebral hemorrhage.

   Quickly reposition the patient to remove any pressure stimuli. Also, check for a distended bladder or fecal impaction. Remove any kinks from the urinary catheter if necessary, and administer a suppository or manually remove impacted feces. If you can't locate and relieve the causative stimulus, ensure I.V. access. Prepare to administer hydralazine for hypertension, as prescribed.

MYOCARDIAL INFARCTION OR HEART FAILURE

If the diaphoretic patient complains of chest pain and dyspnea, or has arrhythmias or electrocardiogram changes, suspect a myocardial infarction or heart failure. Connect the patient to a cardiac monitor, ensure a patent airway, and administer supplemental oxygen. Insert an I.V. catheter, and administer an analgesic and nitrates, as prescribed. Prepare the patient for cardiac catheterization and percutaneous coronary intervention, if necessary. Be prepared to begin emergency resuscitation if cardiac or respiratory arrest occurs.

(continued)

Hypoglycemia

◆ Rapidly induced hypoglycemia may cause diaphoresis, irritability, tremors, hypotension, blurred vision, tachycardia, hunger, and loss of consciousness.
◆ Confusion, motor weakness, hemiplegia, seizures, or coma may also occur.

Infective endocarditis, subacute

◆ Generalized night sweats occur early.
◆ A sudden change in a murmur or a new murmur is a classic sign.
◆ Other signs and symptoms include intermittent low-grade fever, weakness, fatigue, petechiae, splinter hemorrhages, weight loss, anorexia, and arthralgia.

Liver abscess

◆ Diaphoresis, right-upper-quadrant pain, weight loss, fever, chills, nausea, vomiting, and anemia commonly occur.
◆ Other signs and symptoms include possible jaundice, chalk-colored stools, and dark urine.

Lung abscess

◆ Commonly, drenching night sweats occur.
◆ Cough produces copious purulent, foul-smelling, bloody sputum.
◆ Other signs and symptoms include fever with chills, pleuritic chest pain, dyspnea, weakness, anorexia, weight loss, headache, malaise, clubbing, tubular or amorphic breath sounds, and dullness on percussion.

Malaria

◆ This acute infectious disease is transmitted by mosquitoes in tropical and subtropical climates.
◆ Profuse diaphoresis marks the third stage of paroxysmal malaria, after chills (first stage) and high fever (second stage).
◆ Headache, arthralgia, and hepatosplenomegaly may occur.
◆ Severe malaria may progress to delirium, seizures, and coma.

Myocardial infarction

◆ Diaphoresis with acute, substernal, radiating chest pain occurs in this life-threatening condition.
◆ Anxiety, dyspnea, nausea, vomiting, tachycardia, blood pressure change, crackles, pallor, and clammy skin may also occur.

Opioid and alcohol withdrawal syndromes

◆ Generalized diaphoresis occurs with dilated pupils, tachycardia, tremors, and altered mental status.
◆ Other findings include severe muscle cramps, paresthesia, tachypnea, altered blood pressure, nausea, vomiting, and seizures.

Pheochromocytoma

◆ This tumor of the adrenal medulla results in severe hypertension, increased metabolism, diaphoresis, and hyperglycemia.
◆ Headache, palpitations, tachycardia, anxiety, tremors, paresthesia, abdominal pain, tachypnea, nausea, vomiting, and orthostatic hypotension may also be present.

Pneumonia

◆ Intermittent, generalized diaphoresis accompanies fever and chills.
◆ Other findings include pleuritic pain, tachypnea, dyspnea, productive cough, headache, fatigue, myalgia, abdominal pain, anorexia, and cyanosis.

Relapsing fever

◆ Profuse diaphoresis marks resolution of the crisis stage of relapsing fever, which produces attacks of high fever, myalgia, headache, arthralgia, diarrhea, vomiting, coughing, and eye or chest pain.
◆ Febrile attack abruptly terminates in chills with tachycardia and tachypnea.
◆ Diaphoresis, flushing, and hypotension may then lead to circulatory collapse and death.

Tetanus

◆ Profuse sweating is accompanied by low-grade fever, tachycardia, and hyperactive deep tendon reflexes.
◆ Early restlessness, pain, and stiffness in the jaw, abdomen, and back progresses to spasms from lockjaw, risus sardonicus, dysphagia, and opisthotonos.

Thyrotoxicosis

◆ Diaphoresis with heat intolerance, weight loss despite increased appetite, tachycardia, palpitations, an enlarged thyroid gland, dyspnea, nervousness, diarrhea, tremors, Plummer's nails, and exophthalmos may occur.

Tuberculosis

◆ Night sweats may occur in patients with primary tuberculosis infection, as well as low-grade fever, fatigue, weakness, anorexia, and weight loss.
◆ In reactivation phase, mucopurulent productive cough, occasional hemoptysis, and chest pain may also be present.

OTHER
Alcohol and opioid withdrawal

◆ Generalized diaphoresis occurs with dilated pupils, tachycardia, tremors, and altered mental status.
◆ Other findings include severe muscle cramps, paresthesia, tachypnea, altered blood pressure, nausea, vomiting, and seizures.

Drugs

◆ Aspirin or acetaminophen poisoning causes diaphoresis.
◆ Sympathomimetics, antipyretics, thyroid hormones, corticosteroids, and certain antipsychotics may cause diaphoresis.

Dumping syndrome

◆ This syndrome results from rapid emptying of gastric contents into the small intestine after partial gastrectomy.

◆ Diaphoresis, palpitations, profound weakness, epigastric distress, nausea, and explosive diarrhea occur soon after eating.

Pesticide poisoning
◆ Toxic effects of pesticide poisoning are diaphoresis, nausea, vomiting, diarrhea, blurred vision, miosis, and excessive lacrimation and salivation.

NURSING CONSIDERATIONS

◆ Sponge the face and body.
◆ Change wet clothes and sheets, as needed
◆ To prevent skin irritation, dust skin folds in the groin and axillae and under pendulous breasts with cornstarch.
◆ Replace fluids and electrolytes.
◆ Monitor fluid intake and urine output.
◆ Encourage oral fluids high in electrolytes.
◆ Keep the room temperature moderate.

PEDIATRIC POINTERS
◆ Diaphoresis in children commonly results from environmental heat, overdressing, drug withdrawal from the mother's addiction, heart failure, thyrotoxicosis, and the effects of such drugs as antihistamines, ephedrine, haloperidol, and thyroid hormone.
◆ Sweat glands function immaturely in infants.

GERIATRIC POINTERS
◆ In tuberculosis, fever and night sweats may not occur in elderly patients, who instead may exhibit a change in activity or weight.
◆ Elderly patients may not exhibit diaphoresis because of a decreased sweating mechanism, increasing the risk for developing heatstroke.

PATIENT TEACHING

◆ Explain proper skin care.
◆ Explain the causative disease process.
◆ Discuss the importance of fluid replacement and how to make sure fluid intake is adequate.

Diarrhea

OVERVIEW

- Increase in the volume of stools
- May be acute or chronic
- May be caused by one or more pathophysiologic mechanisms (see *What causes diarrhea*)
- Can cause life-threatening fluid and electrolyte imbalances

ACTION STAT! If diarrhea is profuse, check for signs of shock. If they occur, place the patient in the supine position and elevate his legs 20 degrees. Insert an I.V. catheter for fluid replacement and monitor for electrolyte imbalances. Keep emergency resuscitation equipment readily available.

HISTORY

- Ask about frequency and duration.
- Check for other signs and symptoms, such as pain, cramps, difficulty breathing, weakness, and fatigue.
- Find out about his drug history.
- Ask about recent GI surgery or radiation therapy.
- Review his diet and ask about food allergies.
- Ask about possible stress factors.

PHYSICAL ASSESSMENT

- Check skin turgor and mucous membranes; observe for rash.
- Take orthostatic blood pressure measurements.
- Inspect the abdomen for distention, and palpate for tenderness.
- Percuss the abdomen for tympany.
- Auscultate bowel sounds.
- Take the patient's temperature and note any chills.

CAUSES

MEDICAL
Anthrax, GI
- Initial signs and symptoms include decreased appetite, nausea, vomiting, and fever.
- Later signs and symptoms include severe bloody diarrhea, abdominal pain, ascites, and hematemesis.

Clostridium difficile infection
- This infection commonly occurs after antibiotic treatment.
- Soft, unformed stools or watery diarrhea may occur that may be foul-smelling or bloody.
- Toxic megacolon, colonic perforation, or peritonitis may develop in severe cases.
- Other signs and symptoms include abdominal pain, cramping, and tenderness; fever; and a white blood cell count as high as 20,000/μl.

Crohn's disease
- This is an inflammation of the GI tract that extends through all layers of the intestinal wall.
- Diarrhea is accompanied by abdominal pain, with guarding and tenderness and nausea.
- Other signs and symptoms may include fever, chills, anorexia, weakness, and weight loss.

Escherichia coli *0157:H7* infection
- This strain of *E. coli* has been associated with animals and with eating undercooked meat.
- Watery or bloody diarrhea, nausea, vomiting, fever, and abdominal cramps occur.

Infections
- Acute viral, bacterial, and protozoan infections cause sudden onset of watery diarrhea with abdominal pain, cramps, nausea, vomiting, and fever.
- Chronic tuberculosis and fungal and parasitic infections produce a less severe but more persistent diarrhea, along with epigastric distress, vomiting, weight loss, and passage of blood and mucus.

Intestinal obstruction
- Partial intestinal obstruction increases intestinal motility, resulting in diarrhea along with abdominal pain with tenderness and guarding, nausea and, possibly, distention.

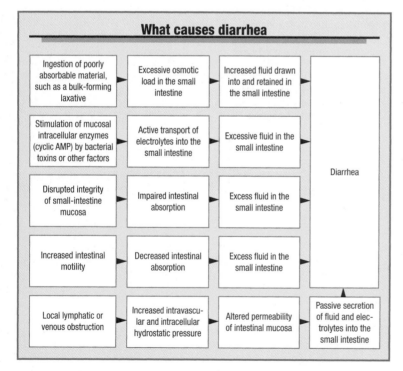

What causes diarrhea

Ingestion of poorly absorbable material, such as a bulk-forming laxative → Excessive osmotic load in the small intestine → Increased fluid drawn into and retained in the small intestine

Stimulation of mucosal intracellular enzymes (cyclic AMP) by bacterial toxins or other factors → Active transport of electrolytes into the small intestine → Excessive fluid in the small intestine

Disrupted integrity of small-intestine mucosa → Impaired intestinal absorption → Excess fluid in the small intestine

Increased intestinal motility → Decreased intestinal absorption → Excess fluid in the small intestine

Local lymphatic or venous obstruction → Increased intravascular and intracellular hydrostatic pressure → Altered permeability of intestinal mucosa → Passive secretion of fluid and electrolytes into the small intestine

→ Diarrhea

- Other signs and symptoms include borborygmi and rushes on auscultation and vomiting of fecal material.

Irritable bowel syndrome
- Diarrhea alternates with constipation or normal bowel function.
- Other signs and symptoms include abdominal pain, tenderness, and distention; flatus; dyspepsia; passage of mucus and pasty pencil-like stools; and nausea.

Ischemic bowel disease
- In this life-threatening disorder, bloody diarrhea occurs with abdominal pain.
- Other signs and symptoms include abdominal distention, nausea, vomiting and, if severe, shock.

Lactose intolerance
- Diarrhea occurs within hours of ingesting milk or milk products.
- Other signs and symptoms include cramps, abdominal pain, borborygmi, bloating, nausea, and flatus.

Large-bowel cancer
- Bloody diarrhea is seen with a partial obstruction.
- Other signs and symptoms include abdominal pain, anorexia, weight loss, weakness, fatigue, and exertional dyspnea.

Listeriosis
- This infection is caused by ingestion of contaminated food, primarily affecting people with weakened immune systems.
- Diarrhea occurs along with fever, myalgias, abdominal pain, nausea and vomiting.
- If infection spreads to the nervous system, meningitis, fever, headache, nuchal rigidity, and altered level of consciousness may occur.

Malabsorption syndrome
- Diarrhea occurs after meals along with steatorrhea, abdominal distention, and muscle cramps.
- Other signs and symptoms include anorexia, weight loss, bone pain, anemia, weakness, fatigue, bruising, and night blindness.

Pseudomembranous enterocolitis
- In this life-threatening disorder, copious watery, green, foul-smelling, bloody diarrhea rapidly precipitates signs of shock.
- Other signs and symptoms include colicky abdominal pain, distention, fever, and dehydration.

Rotavirus gastroenteritis
- Diarrhea occurs before fever, nausea, and vomiting.

Thyrotoxicosis
- Diarrhea accompanies diaphoresis, dyspnea, tachycardia, nervousness, tremors, palpitations, heat intolerance, weight loss despite increased appetite, and, possibly, exophthalmos.

Ulcerative colitis
- Recurrent bloody diarrhea with pus or mucus is a characteristic sign.
- Weight loss, anemia, and weakness are late findings.
- Other signs and symptoms include tenesmus, hyperactive bowel sounds, cramping, lower abdominal pain, low-grade fever, anorexia, nausea, and vomiting.

OTHER
Drugs
- Many antibiotics, herbal remedies, and laxative abuse cause diarrhea.
- Other drugs that may cause diarrhea include antacids containing magnesium, colchicine, guanethidine, lactulose, dantrolene, ethacrynic acid, mefenamic acid, methotrexate, metyrosine and, in high doses, cardiac glycosides and quinidine.

Lead poisoning
- Diarrhea alternates with constipation.
- Other signs and symptoms include abdominal pain, anorexia, nausea, vomiting, a metallic taste, headache, dizziness, and a bluish gingival lead line.

Treatments
- Gastrectomy, gastroenterostomy, or pyloroplasty may produce diarrhea as part of dumping or postgastrectomy syndrome.
- High-dose radiation therapy may produce enteritis, leading to diarrhea.

NURSING CONSIDERATIONS
- Administer an analgesic and an opiate as prescribed to decrease intestinal motility, unless the patient has a possible or confirmed stool infection.
- Clean the perineum thoroughly to prevent skin breakdown.
- Quantify the amount of liquid stools and monitor intake and output.
- Monitor electrolyte levels and hematocrit.
- Administer I.V. fluid replacements as prescribed.

PEDIATRIC POINTERS
- Diarrhea in children commonly results from infection.
- Chronic diarrhea may result from malabsorption syndrome, an anatomic defect, or allergies.
- Diarrhea can quickly cause life-threatening dehydration in children.
- Obtain stool specimens as needed to assess for blood, and to send for further testing.

PATIENT TEACHING
- Emphasize the importance of maintaining adequate hydration.
- Explain foods or liquids the patient should avoid.
- Explain infection control techniques.
- Discuss stress-reduction techniques.
- Refer for counseling, as needed.
- Discuss the importance of medical follow-up with inflammatory bowel disease.

Diplopia

OVERVIEW

- Refers to double vision or seeing one object as two
- Results when extraocular muscles fail to work together, causing images to fall on the wrong parts of the retinas
- Can occur in one eye or in both eyes

HISTORY

- Ask about other symptoms, including severe headache, neurologic symptoms, and eye pain.
- Ask about the onset and ask for a description of the diplopia.
- Obtain a medical history, asking about hypertension; diabetes mellitus; allergies; thyroid, neurologic, or muscular disorders; extraocular muscle disorders; trauma; or eye surgery.

PHYSICAL ASSESSMENT

- Evaluate level of consciousness (LOC); pupil size, equality, and response to light; and motor and sensory function.
- Take vital signs.
- Observe the patient for ocular deviation, ptosis, proptosis, lid edema, and conjunctival injection.
- Distinguish monocular from binocular diplopia.
- Test visual acuity and extraocular muscles. (See *Testing extraocular muscles.*)

CAUSES

MEDICAL
Brain tumor
- Diplopia may be an early symptom.
- Other signs and symptoms vary with tumor size and location but may include eye deviation, emotional lability, decreased LOC, headache, vomiting, seizures, hearing loss, visual field defects, abnormal pupillary responses, nystagmus, motor weakness, and paralysis.

Diabetes mellitus
- Sudden diplopia with intense periorbital pain or head pain may be a long-term effect.

Encephalitis
- A brief episode of diplopia and eye deviation may occur initially.
- Sudden onset of high fever, severe headache, and vomiting are also early findings.
- As inflammation progresses, decreased LOC, seizures, ataxia, and paralysis indicate meningeal irritation.

Head injury
- Diplopia may occur in potentially life-threatening head injuries depending on the site and extent of injury.
- Other signs and symptoms include eye deviation, pupillary changes, headache, decreased LOC, altered vital signs, nausea, vomiting, and motor weakness or paralysis.

Intracranial aneurysm
- In this life-threatening condition, diplopia and eye deviation occur initially, possibly with ptosis and a dilated pupil on the affected side.
- A recurrent, severe, one-sided, frontal headache develops.
- Other signs and symptoms include neck and spinal pain and rigidity, decreased LOC, tinnitus, dizziness, nausea, vomiting, and muscle weakness or paralysis on one side.

TOP TECHNIQUE

Testing extraocular muscles

The coordinated action of six muscles controls eyeball movements. To test the function of each muscle and the cranial nerve (CN) that innervates it, ask the patient to look in the direction you indicate (each of which you select as shown below). The six directions you can test make up the cardinal positions of gaze. The patient's inability to turn the eye in the designated direction indicates muscle weakness or paralysis.

KEY:
SR – superior rectus (CN III)
IR – inferior rectus (CN III)
MR – medial rectus (CN III)
LR – lateral rectus (CN VI)
IO – inferior oblique (CN III)
SO – superior oblique (CN IV)

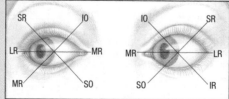

Multiple sclerosis

◆ Multiple sclerosis is a progressive disease caused by demyelination of the white matter of the brain and spinal cord.
◆ Diplopia is a common early symptom and is usually accompanied by blurred vision and paresthesia.
◆ As the disease progresses, other signs and symptoms include nystagmus, constipation, muscle weakness, paralysis, spasticity, hyperreflexia, intention tremor, gait ataxia, dysphagia, dysarthria, impotence, emotional lability, and urinary frequency, urgency, and incontinence.

Myasthenia gravis

◆ This progressive disorder causes failure in transmission of nerve impulses.
◆ Diplopia and ptosis occur initially and may worsen throughout the day.
◆ As the disorder progresses, other muscles are involved, resulting in blank facial expression; nasal voice; difficulty making fine hand movements, chewing, and swallowing; and, possibly, life-threatening respiratory muscle weakness.

Ophthalmologic migraine

◆ Diplopia occurs and persists for days after the headache.
◆ Other signs and symptoms include severe, one-sided pain; ptosis; irritability; depression; slight confusion; and extraocular muscle palsies.

Orbital blowout fracture

◆ Monocular diplopia affecting the upward gaze usually occurs.
◆ With marked periorbital edema, diplopia may affect other directions of gaze.
◆ Periorbital ecchymoses occurs, but visual acuity is unaffected.
◆ Other signs and symptoms include eyelid edema, subcutaneous crepitation of the eyelid and orbit, dilated and unreactive pupil, and hyphema.

Orbital cellulitis

◆ Diplopia develops suddenly.
◆ Other signs and symptoms include eye deviation and pain, purulent drainage, lid edema, chemosis and redness, proptosis, nausea, and fever.

Orbital tumors

◆ Diplopia may occur, possibly with proptosis and blurred vision.
◆ One or both eyes may appear prominent with accompanying pain, redness, and swelling of the affected eye.

Stroke

◆ If stroke affects the vertebrobasilar artery, diplopia occurs.
◆ Other signs and symptoms include one-sided motor weakness or paralysis, ataxia, decreased LOC, dizziness, aphasia, visual field deficits, slurred speech, and dysphagia.

Thyrotoxicosis

◆ Diplopia beginning in the upper field of gaze accompanies exophthalmos.
◆ Impaired eye movement, excessive tearing, lid edema, and inability to close the lids occur.
◆ Other signs and symptoms include tachycardia, palpitations, weight loss, diarrhea, tremors, an enlarged thyroid gland, dyspnea, nervousness, diaphoresis, and heat intolerance.

Transient ischemic attack

◆ Diplopia, dizziness, tinnitus, hearing loss, and numbness may occur.

NURSING CONSIDERATIONS

◆ Monitor vital signs and neurologic status.
◆ Provide a safe environment.
◆ Institute seizure precautions, if needed.

PEDIATRIC POINTERS

◆ School-age children who complain of double vision require a careful examination to rule out serious disorders, such as a brain tumor.

PATIENT TEACHING

◆ Explain the safety measures that are needed.
◆ Teach the patient skills of ambulation with assistance.
◆ Provide orientation to room and meal tray.
◆ Teach the patient about underlying cause, diagnostic tests, and treatments.

Dizziness

- Sensation of imbalance or faintness
- May be associated with giddiness, weakness, confusion, and blurred or double vision
- Commonly results from inadequate blood flow and oxygen supply to the cerebrum and spinal cord
- Commonly confused with vertigo, a sensation of revolving in space—or of surroundings revolving about oneself—with associated nausea, vomiting, nystagmus, staggering gait, and tinnitus or hearing loss

◆ *ACTION STAT! Ensure the patient's safety and prevent falls. Determine the severity and onset of the dizziness and ask if he has a headache or blurred vision. Take his blood pressure, and check for orthostatic hypotension. Determine if he's at risk for hypoglycemia. Have him lie down, and recheck vital signs every 15 minutes. Start an I.V. catheter; give prescribed drugs, as needed.*

- Obtain a medical history, noting diabetes mellitus, head injury, anxiety disorders, and cardiovascular, pulmonary, and kidney disease.
- Take a drug history and determine whether the patient is taking antihypertensives.
- Determine the onset and characteristics of dizziness.
- Ask about emotional stress.
- Ask about other signs and symptoms, such as palpitations, chest pain, diaphoresis, shortness of breath, and chronic cough.

- Check neurologic status, including level of consciousness, motor and sensory functions, and reflexes.
- Inspect for poor skin turgor and dry mucous membranes.
- Auscultate heart rate and rhythm.
- Inspect for barrel chest, clubbing, cyanosis, and accessory muscle use.
- Auscultate breath and heart sounds.
- Check for orthostatic hypotension.
- Palpate for edema and capillary refill time.

MEDICAL

Anemia
- Dizziness is aggravated by postural changes or exertion.
- Other signs and symptoms include pallor, dyspnea, fatigue, tachycardia, and bounding pulse.

Cardiac arrhythmias
- Dizziness lasts for several seconds or longer and may precede fainting.
- Other signs and symptoms include palpitations; irregular, rapid, or thready pulse; hypotension; weakness; blurred vision; paresthesia, and confusion.

Carotid sinus hypersensitivity
- Brief episodes of dizziness that usually progress to fainting.
- Episode is preceded by stimulation of one or both carotid arteries.
- Other signs and symptoms include sweating, nausea, and pallor.

Generalized anxiety disorder
- Continuous dizziness may intensify as the disorder worsens.
- Other signs and symptoms include persistent anxiety, insomnia, difficulty concentrating, fidgeting, cold and clammy hands, dry mouth, frequent urination, tachycardia, tachypnea, diaphoresis, palpitations, and irritability.

Hypertension
- Dizziness may precede fainting or may be relieved by rest.
- Other signs and symptoms include headache, blurred vision, and retinal changes.

Hyperventilation syndrome
- Dizziness lasts a few minutes.
- With frequent hyperventilation, dizziness occurs between episodes.
- Other signs and symptoms include apprehension, diaphoresis, pallor, dyspnea, chest tightness, palpitations, trembling, fatigue, and peripheral and circumoral paresthesia.

Hypoglycemia
- Dizziness, headache, clouding of vision, restlessness, and mental status changes can result from fasting hypoglycemia.
- Other signs and symptoms include irritability, trembling, hunger, cold sweats, and tachycardia.

Hypovolemia
- Dizziness results from lack of circulating volume.
- Other signs and symptoms include orthostatic hypotension, thirst, poor skin turgor, and flattened neck veins.

Orthostatic hypotension
- Dizziness may terminate in fainting or disappear with rest after position change.
- Other signs and symptoms include dim vision, spots before the eyes, pallor, diaphoresis, hypotension, tachycardia, and signs of dehydration.

Panic disorder
- Dizziness may accompany acute panic attacks.
- Other signs and symptoms include anxiety, dyspnea, palpitations, chest pain, a choking or smothering sensation, vertigo, paresthesia, hot and cold flashes, diaphoresis, and trembling or shaking.

Postconcussion syndrome
- Dizziness, headache, emotional lability, alcohol intolerance, fatigue, anxiety and, possibly, vertigo occur 1 to 3 weeks after a head injury.
- Dizziness or other symptoms are intensified by physical or mental stress.

Transient ischemic attack
- Dizziness of varying severity, diplopia, blindness or visual field deficits, ptosis, tinnitus, hearing loss, paresis, and numbness occur.

OTHER

Drugs
- Antihistamines, antihypertensives, anxiolytics, central nervous system depressants, decongestants, opioids, and vasodilators commonly cause dizziness.
- Herbal remedies such as St. John's wort can produce dizziness.

NURSING CONSIDERATIONS

- If the patient is dizzy, provide for his safety.
- Monitor vital signs, neurologic status, and intake and output.

PEDIATRIC POINTERS
- If you suspect dizziness, assess for vertigo, a more common symptom in children.

PATIENT TEACHING

- Teach the patient how to control dizziness.
- Teach the patient safety measures for when dizziness happens in the future.
- Teach the patient about underlying disease process and treatment.

Doll's eye reflex, absent

OVERVIEW

- Indicator of injury to the midbrain or pons, involving cranial nerves III and VI, possibly indicating brain death
- Tested by rapid, gentle turning of patient's head from side to side, noting the position of the eyes with each head turn if cervical spinal injury isn't suspected
- Normal reflex: eyes deviate in the direction opposite the head turn, and then return to the middle gaze
- Negative reflex: eyes remain fixed in the center (see *Testing for doll's eye sign*)
- Also known as *negative oculocephalic reflex*

HISTORY

- Obtain a medical history from the patient's family.
- Ask about a drug history.

PHYSICAL ASSESSMENT

- Evaluate level of consciousness using the Glasgow Coma Scale.
- Note decerebrate or decorticate posture.
- Examine the pupils for size, equality, and response to light.
- Check for signs of increased intracranial pressure (ICP).

TOP TECHNIQUE

Testing for doll's eye sign

To evaluate the patient's oculocephalic reflex, hold the upper eyelids open and quickly (but gently) turn the head from side to side, noting eye movements with each head turn.
  With absent doll's eye sign, the eyes remain fixed in midposition.

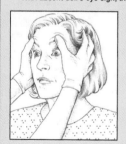 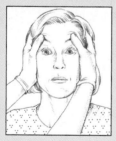 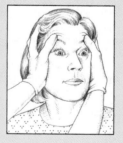

MEDICAL

Brain stem infarction
- Absent doll's eye sign accompanies coma.
- Other signs and symptoms include limb paralysis, cranial nerve palsies, cerebellar ataxia, variable sensory loss, a positive Babinski's reflex, decerebrate posture, and muscle flaccidity.

Brain stem tumors
- Absent doll's eye sign accompanies coma.
- Coma may be preceded by hemiparesis, nystagmus, extraocular nerve palsies, facial pain or sensory loss, facial paralysis, diminished corneal reflex, tinnitus, hearing loss, dysphagia, drooling, vertigo, ataxia, and vomiting.

Central midbrain infarction
- Coma, Weber's syndrome (oculomotor palsy with contralateral hemiplegia), contralateral ataxic tremor, nystagmus, and pupillary abnormalities may accompany absent doll's eye sign.

Cerebellar lesion
- If the lesion progresses to coma, absent doll's eye sign occurs.
- Coma may be preceded by headache, nystagmus, ocular deviation to the side of the lesion, unequal pupils, dysarthria, dysphagia, ipsilateral facial paresis, cerebellar ataxia, and signs of increasing ICP.

Pontine hemorrhage
- In this life-threatening disorder, absent doll's eye sign and coma develop within minutes.
- Other ominous signs, such as complete paralysis, decerebrate posture, a positive Babinski's reflex, and small, reactive pupils, may then accompany rapid progression to death.

Posterior fossa hematoma
- Absent doll's eye sign and coma occur, preceded by headache, vomiting, drowsiness, confusion, unequal pupils, dysphagia, cranial nerve palsies, stiff neck, and cerebellar ataxia.

OTHER

Drugs
- Barbiturates may produce severe central nervous depression, resulting in coma and absent doll's eye sign.

- To reduce the risk of spinal cord damage, don't attempt to elicit doll's eye sign in a comatose patient with suspected cervical spine injury. Instead, use the cold caloric test by injecting cold water into the ear. The eyes move slowly to the irrigated ear in a normal response.
- Monitor vital signs and neurologic status.
- Provide emotional support to the family.

PEDIATRIC POINTERS
- Doll's eye sign isn't present for the first 10 days after birth and may be irregular until age 2.
- Absent doll's eye sign in children may accompany coma from head injury, near-drowning or suffocation, or brain stem astrocytoma.

- Discuss medical diagnosis and treatment plan with patient's family.
- Teach family about all hospital procedures and tests to be performed on the patient.

Drooling

- Results from a failure to swallow or retain saliva or from excess salivation
- May be scant or copious (up to 1 L daily) and may cause circumoral irritation
- Warns of potential aspiration

HISTORY

- Determine the amount of drooling and when it began.
- Ask about associated signs and symptoms such as sore throat; difficulty swallowing, chewing, speaking, or breathing; pain or stiffness in the face and neck; and muscle weakness in the face and extremities.
- Ask about mental status changes, such as drowsiness or agitation and changes in vision, hearing, and sense of taste.
- Ask about anorexia, weight loss, fatigue, nausea, vomiting, altered bowel or bladder habits, recent cold or infection, recent animal bite or pesticide exposure.
- Obtain a complete drug history.

PHYSICAL ASSESSMENT

- Take the patient's vital signs.
- Inspect for signs of facial paralysis or abnormal expression.
- Examine the mouth and neck for swelling, the throat for edema and redness, and the tonsils for exudate; note foul breath odor.
- Examine the tongue for bilateral furrowing (trident tongue). Look for pallor and skin lesions and for frontal baldness. Carefully assess any bite or puncture marks.
- Assess cranial nerves II through VII, IX, and X and pupillary size and response to light.
- Assess speech, gag reflex, and ability to swallow.
- Palpate for lymphadenopathy, especially in the cervical area.
- Test for poor balance, hyperreflexia, and a positive Babinski's reflex.
- Assess sensory function for paresthesia.

CAUSES

MEDICAL

Bell's palsy

- Drooling accompanies the gradual onset of facial hemiplegia.
- The affected side of the face sags and is expressionless, the nasolabial fold flattens, and the palpebral fissure (the distance between the upper and lower eyelids) widens.
- The patient usually complains of pain in or behind the ear.
- Other signs and symptoms include unilateral, diminished or absent corneal reflex, decreased tear production, Bell's phenomenon (upward deviation of the eye with attempt at lid closure), and partial loss of taste or abnormal taste sensation.

Esophageal tumor

- Copious and persistent drooling is typically preceded by weight loss and progressively severe dysphagia.
- Other signs and symptoms include substernal, back, or neck pain and blood-flecked regurgitation.

Ludwig's angina

- Ludwig's angina is a bacterial infection of the sublingual and submandibular spaces.
- Moderate to copious drooling stems from dysphagia and local swelling of the floor of the mouth, causing tongue displacement.
- Submandibular swelling of the neck and signs of respiratory distress may also occur.

Myotonic dystrophy

- Facial weakness and a sagging jaw account for constant drooling in this disorder.
- Other signs and symptoms include myotonia (inability to relax a muscle after its contraction), muscle wasting, cataracts, testicular atrophy, frontal baldness, ptosis, and a nasal, monotone voice.

Peritonsillar abscess

◆ Severe sore throat causes dysphagia with moderate to copious drooling in this abscess.
◆ Palpation may reveal cervical lymphadenopathy.
◆ Other signs and symptoms include high fever, rancid breath, and enlarged, reddened, edematous tonsils that may be covered by a soft, gray exudate.

Rabies

◆ When this acute central nervous system infection advances to the brain stem, it produces drooling, or "foaming at the mouth."
◆ Rabies is accompanied by hydrophobia in about 50% of cases.
◆ Seizures and hyperactive deep tendon reflexes may also occur before the patient develops generalized flaccid paralysis and coma.

Seizures, generalized

◆ Tonic-clonic muscular reactions that cause excessive salivation and frothing at the mouth accompanied by loss of consciousness and cyanosis occur.
◆ In the unresponsive postictal state, the patient may still drool.

OTHER

Pesticide poisoning

◆ Toxic effects of pesticides may include excess salivation with drooling.
◆ Other signs and symptoms include diaphoresis, nausea and vomiting, involuntary urination and defecation, blurred vision, miosis, increased lacrimation, fasciculations, weakness, flaccid paralysis, signs of respiratory distress, and coma.

NURSING CONSIDERATIONS

◆ Be alert for aspiration in the drooling patient. Position him upright or on his side.
◆ Provide frequent mouth care, and suction, as necessary, to control drooling.
◆ Be prepared for tracheostomy and intubation. Also be prepared to administer oxygen or to execute an abdominal thrust.
◆ Help the patient cope with drooling by providing a covered, opaque collecting jar to decrease odor and prevent possible transmission of infection. Keep tissues handy and drape a towel across his chest at mealtime.
◆ Encourage oral hygiene.

PEDIATRIC POINTERS

◆ Normally, an infant can't control saliva flow until about age 1, when muscular reflexes that initiate swallowing and lip closure mature.
◆ Salivation and drooling typically increase with teething, which begins at about the fifth month and continues until about age 2.
◆ Excessive salivation and drooling may also occur in response to hunger or anticipation of feeding and in association with nausea.
◆ Common causes of drooling include epiglottiditis, retropharyngeal abscess, severe tonsillitis, stomatitis, herpetic lesions, esophageal atresia, cerebral palsy, mental deficiency, and drug withdrawal in neonates of addicted mothers. It may also result from a foreign body in the esophagus, causing dysphagia.

PATIENT TEACHING

◆ Teach the patient exercises to help strengthen facial muscles, if appropriate.
◆ Show him how to perform meticulous skin care, especially around the mouth and in the neck area, to prevent skin breakdown. Cornstarch may be placed on the neck to reduce the risk of maceration.
◆ Teach the patient and family members the importance of positioning upright to avoid aspiration.
◆ Teach the patient about the underlying disease process and treatment.

Dysarthria

OVERVIEW

- Characterized by poorly articulated speech, resulting in slurring and labored, irregular rhythm
- Results from damage to brain stem that affects cranial nerves IX, X, or XII

ACTION STAT! Assess the patient for difficulty swallowing. Withhold food and fluids. Determine respiratory rate and depth and measure vital capacity. Assess blood pressure and heart rate. Ensure a patent airway and place the patient in Fowler's position. Suction his mouth and oropharynx, and administer oxygen, as necessary. Keep emergency resuscitation equipment readily available. If progressive respiratory muscle weakness occurs, intubation and mechanical ventilation may be necessary.

HISTORY

- Ask about the onset and characteristics of dysarthria.
- Obtain a drug and alcohol history.
- Obtain a medical history, including incidence of seizures.

PHYSICAL ASSESSMENT

- If the patient wears dentures, check them for proper fit.
- Have the patient produce a few simple sounds and words.
- Compare muscle strength and tone in the limbs on one side of the body with the other.
- Assess the patient's tactile sense.
- Test deep tendon reflexes, and note gait ataxia.
- Assess cerebellar function.
- Test visual fields and ask about double vision.
- Check for signs of facial weakness.
- Determine level of consciousness (LOC) and mental status.

CAUSES

MEDICAL

Alcoholic cerebellar degeneration

- Chronic, progressive dysarthria occurs.
- Other signs and symptoms include ataxia, diplopia, ophthalmoplegia, hypotension, and altered mental status.

Amyotrophic lateral sclerosis

- This motor neuron disease causes muscle atrophy.
- Dysarthria occurs and worsens as the disease progresses.
- Other signs and symptoms include dysphagia; difficulty breathing; muscle atrophy and weakness, especially in the hands and feet; fasciculations; spasticity; hyperactive deep tendon reflexes in the legs; and excessive drooling.

Basilar artery insufficiency

- This disorder causes random, brief episodes of bilateral brain stem dysfunction.
- Dysarthria accompanies diplopia, vertigo, facial numbness, ataxia, paresis, and visual field loss, lasting from minutes to hours.

Botulism

- This life-threatening paralytic illness is caused by ingestion of contaminated food or, rarely, a wound infection.
- Dysarthria, dysphagia, diplopia, and ptosis are characteristic signs.
- Initial signs and symptoms include dry mouth, sore throat, weakness, vomiting, and diarrhea.
- As the disorder progresses, descending weakness or paralysis of muscles in the extremities and trunk causes hyporeflexia and dyspnea.

Multiple sclerosis

- This progressive disease is caused by demyelination of the white matter of the brain and spinal cord.
- Dysarthria may occur with nystagmus, blurred or double vision, dysphagia, ataxia, and intention tremor.

◆ Other signs and symptoms include paresthesia, spasticity, hyperreflexia, muscle weakness or paralysis, constipation, emotional lability, and urinary frequency, urgency, and incontinence.

Myasthenia gravis
◆ This progressive disorder causes failure in the transmission of nerve impulses.
◆ Dysarthria, associated with a nasal voice, worsens during the day but may temporarily improve with short rest periods.
◆ Other signs and symptoms include dysphagia, drooling, facial weakness, diplopia, ptosis, dyspnea, and muscle weakness.

Olivopontocerebellar degeneration
◆ Dysarthria, a major sign of this genetic neurologic disease, accompanies cerebellar ataxia and spasticity.
◆ Other signs and symptoms include abnormal eye movement, sexual dysfunction, bowel and bladder problems, and difficulty swallowing.

Parkinson's disease
◆ Dysarthria and a monotone voice occur in this degenerative neurologic syndrome.
◆ Other signs and symptoms include muscle rigidity, bradykinesia, involuntary tremor usually beginning in the fingers, difficulty walking, muscle weakness, stooped posture, masklike facies, dysphagia, and drooling.

Stroke, brain stem
◆ Dysarthria that's most severe at onset of the stroke occurs with dysphonia and dysphagia.
◆ Other signs and symptoms include facial weakness, diplopia, hemiparesis, spasticity, drooling, dyspnea, and decreased LOC.

Stroke, cerebral
◆ Weakness produces dysarthria that's most severe at onset of the stroke.
◆ Other signs and symptoms include dysphagia, drooling, dysphonia, hemianopsia, aphasia, spasticity, and hyperreflexia.

OTHER
Drugs
◆ Large doses of anticonvulsants and barbiturates can cause dysarthria.

Manganese poisoning
◆ Progressive dysarthria is accompanied by weakness, fatigue, confusion, hallucinations, drooling, hand tremors, limb stiffness, spasticity, gross rhythmic movements of the trunk and head, and propulsive gait.

Mercury poisoning
◆ Progressive dysarthria is accompanied by fatigue, depression, lethargy, irritability, confusion, ataxia, tremors, and changes in vision, hearing, and memory.

NURSING CONSIDERATIONS

◆ Consult with a speech pathologist, as needed.
◆ Give prescribed drugs and treatments, as needed.
◆ Assess swallow and gag reflexes before feeding the patient.
◆ Give the patient time to express himself and encourage the use of gestures.

PEDIATRIC POINTERS
◆ Dysarthria usually results from brain stem glioma; it may also result from cerebral palsy.
◆ Because dysarthria is difficult to detect in infants and young children, look for other neurologic deficits.

PATIENT TEACHING

◆ Encourage the patient to express his feelings by providing different ways in which he can communicate.
◆ Teach the patient about the underlying condition and treatment.

Dysmenorrhea

- Characterized by mild to severe cramping or colicky pain in the pelvis or lower abdomen that may radiate to the thighs and lower sacrum
- Precedes menstruation by several days or may accompany it, with pain gradually subsiding as bleeding tapers off
- Affects more than 50% of menstruating women and is the leading cause of lost time from school and work among women of childbearing age
- Stress and poor health possible aggravating factors

- Obtain a thorough menstrual and sexual history.
- Get a full description of the intensity and type of pain, where it's located, when it begins and ends, and how long the patient has been experiencing it.
- Ask about associated signs and symptoms, such as nausea and vomiting, altered elimination habits, bloating, water retention, pelvic or rectal pressure, and unusual fatigue, irritability, or depression.
- Ask about signs and symptoms of urinary system obstruction, such as pyuria, urine retention, or incontinence.

- Take vital signs, noting fever and accompanying chills.
- Inspect the abdomen for distention, and palpate for tenderness and masses.
- Note costovertebral angle tenderness.

MEDICAL

Adenomyosis
- Endometrial tissue invades the myometrium, resulting in severe dysmenorrhea with pain radiating to the back or rectum, menorrhagia, and a symmetrically enlarged, globular uterus that's usually softer on palpation than a uterine myoma.

Cervical stenosis
- Dysmenorrhea occurs with scant or absent menstrual flow.

Endometriosis
- Steady, aching pain typically begins before menses and peaks at the height of menstrual flow, but it may also occur between menstrual periods.
- Pain may arise at the endometrial deposit site or may radiate to the perineum or rectum.
- A tender, fixed adnexal mass is usually palpable on bimanual examination.
- Other signs and symptoms include premenstrual spotting, dyspareunia, infertility, nausea and vomiting, painful defecation, and rectal bleeding and hematuria during menses.

Pelvic inflammatory disease
- This chronic infection produces dysmenorrhea accompanied by fever; malaise; a foul-smelling, purulent vaginal discharge; menorrhagia; dyspareunia; severe abdominal pain; nausea and vomiting; and diarrhea.
- A pelvic examination may reveal cervical motion tenderness and bilateral adnexal tenderness.

Premenstrual syndrome
- Cramping pain usually begins with menstrual flow and persists for several hours or days, diminishing as flow decreases.
- Abdominal bloating, breast tenderness, palpitations, diaphoresis, flushing, depression, and irritability commonly precede menses by several days to 2 weeks.

- Other signs and symptoms include nausea, vomiting, diarrhea, and headache.

Primary dysmenorrhea, idiopathic
- Increased prostaglandin secretion intensifies uterine contractions, causing mild to severe spasmodic cramping pain in the lower abdomen, which radiates to the sacrum and inner thighs.
- The pain peaks a few hours before menses.
- Other signs and symptoms include nausea and vomiting, fatigue, diarrhea, and headache.

Uterine leiomyomas
- If these tumors twist or degenerate after circulatory occlusion or infection or if the uterus contracts in an attempt to expel them, they may cause constant or intermittent lower abdominal pain that worsens with menses.
- Palpation may reveal the tumor mass, which is almost always nontender, and an enlarged uterus.
- Other signs and symptoms include backache, constipation, menorrhagia, and urinary frequency or retention.

OTHER
Intrauterine devices
- These devices may cause severe cramping and heavy menstrual flow.

NURSING CONSIDERATIONS

- Historically, incidence of dysmenorrhea was viewed as idiopathic in origin. However, current research suggests that prostaglandins do play a large role; therefore, encourage the patient to view dysmenorrhea as a real medical problem, not as a sign of maladjustment.

PEDIATRIC POINTERS
- Dysmenorrhea is rare during the first year of menstruation, before the menstrual cycle becomes ovulatory.
- Incidence is generally higher among adolescents than older women.

PATIENT TEACHING

- Teach the adolescent about dysmenorrhea.
- Encourage good hygiene, nutrition, and exercise.
- Advise the patient to place a heating pad on her abdomen to relieve the pain. This therapy reduces abdominal muscle tension and increases blood flow.

- Teach the patient effleurage, a light circular massage with the fingertips, which may provide relief.
- Teach comfort measures including drinking warm beverages, taking a warm shower, performing waist-bending and pelvic-rocking exercises, and walking.
- Inform the patient that increasing aerobic exercise and dietary intake of vitamin B_1 and fish oil capsules have also proved effective in relieving dysmenorrhea.
- Teach the patient that taking a nonsteroidal anti-inflammatory drug (NSAID) 1 to 2 days before the onset of menses is usually helpful. If she isn't trying to get pregnant, taking monophasic birth control pills is also beneficial. However, warn the patient that both of these treatments may reduce menstrual flow and duration. So, be sure to rule out the possibility of pregnancy before starting either of these therapies. Explain the actions and adverse effects of these drugs. (See *Relief for dysmenorrhea*.)

Relief for dysmenorrhea

To relieve cramping and other symptoms caused by primary dysmenorrhea or an intrauterine device, the patient may receive a prostaglandin inhibitor, such as aspirin, ibuprofen, indomethacin, or naproxen. These nonsteroidal anti-inflammatory drugs block prostaglandin synthesis early in the inflammatory reaction, thereby inhibiting prostaglandin action at receptor sites. They also have analgesic and antipyretic effects.

Make sure you and your patient are informed about the adverse effects and cautions associated with these drugs.

ADVERSE EFFECTS
Alert the patient to the possible adverse effects of prostaglandin inhibitors. Central nervous system effects include dizziness, headache, and vision disturbances. GI effects include nausea, vomiting, heartburn, and diarrhea. Advise the patient to take the drug with milk or after meals to reduce gastric irritation.

CONTRAINDICATIONS
Because prostaglandin inhibitors are potentially teratogenic, be sure to rule out the possibility of pregnancy before starting the patient on this therapy. Advise any patient who suspects she's pregnant to delay therapy until menses begins.

OTHER CAUTIONS
If the patient has cardiac decompensation, hypertension, renal dysfunction, an ulcer, or a coagulation defect (and is receiving ongoing anticoagulant therapy), use caution when administering a prostaglandin inhibitor. Because a patient who is hypersensitive to aspirin may also be hypersensitive to other prostaglandin inhibitors, watch for signs of gastric ulceration and bleeding.

Dyspareunia

OVERVIEW

- Pain that occurs with attempted penetration or during or after coitus

HISTORY

- Obtain a description of the pain including its location, how long it lasts, if it occurs with attempted penetration or deep thrusting, if it's always during intercourse, or if it's relieved by changing coital position or using a vaginal lubricant.
- Obtain a history of pelvic, vaginal, or urinary tract infection.
- Obtain a sexual and menstrual history.
- Try to determine her attitude toward sexual intimacy.
- Ask about a history of rape, incest, or sexual abuse as a child.

PHYSICAL ASSESSMENT

- Take vital signs.
- Palpate the abdomen for tenderness, pain, or masses and for inguinal lymphadenopathy.
- Inspect the genitalia for lesions and vaginal discharge.

CAUSES

MEDICAL

Allergies
- Allergic reactions to diaphragms or condoms may result in dyspareunia.

Atrophic vaginitis
- In postmenopausal and breast-feeding women, decreased estrogen secretion may lead to inadequate vaginal lubrication and dyspareunia, which intensifies as intercourse continues.
- Patients may complain of a watery discharge at the same time that they're feeling "dry."
- Other signs and symptoms include pruritus, burning, bleeding, and vaginal tenderness.

Bartholinitis
- This inflammatory disorder may produce throbbing pain accompanied by vulvar tenderness during intercourse.
- The patient may also complain of pain with walking or sitting.
- Chronic inflammation causes a purulent discharge from the infected cyst.

Cervicitis
- This inflammatory disorder causes pain with deep penetration.
- Other signs and symptoms include dull lower abdominal pain, a purulent vaginal discharge, backache, and metrorrhagia.

Condylomata acuminata
- Papular, mosaic, warty growths occur on the vulva, vaginal and cervical walls, and perianal area.
- During and after intercourse, they may bleed, itch, cause burning or paresthesia in the vaginal introitus, and become tender.
- A profuse, odorless vaginal discharge may also occur.

Cystitis
- Dyspareunia may occur if the patient has inflammation or infection of the bladder.
- Other signs and symptoms include dysuria; urinary urgency, frequency, or incontinence; pyuria; and, after coitus, hematuria.

Endometriosis
- Causes intense pain during deep coital penetration, but may be relieved by changing position.
- Aching pain may occur during gentle thrusting or during a pelvic examination.
- Pain is usually in the lower abdomen or behind the uterus and may be worse on one side.
- Typically, a tender, fixed adnexal mass is palpable on bimanual examination.
- Other signs and symptoms include dysmenorrhea, irregular menses, infertility, painful urination or defecation, and rectal bleeding and hematuria during menses.

Episiotomy
- If the episiotomy scar constricts the vaginal introitus or narrows the vaginal barrel, the patient may experience perineal pain with coitus.

Herpes genitalis
- During intercourse, friction against lesions on the labia, vulva, vagina, or perianal skin causes pain and itching. The lesions are fluid-filled and usually painless at first, but may rupture and form shallow, painful ulcers with erythema and edema.
- Other signs and symptoms include leukorrhea, fever, malaise, headache, inguinal lymphadenopathy, myalgia, and dysuria.

Occlusive or rigid hymen
- Dyspareunia may prevent penetration in this condition.

Ovarian cyst or tumor
- Lower abdominal pain accompanies deep penetration during intercourse.
- Other signs and symptoms include chronic lower back pain; a tender, palpable abdominal mass; constipation; urinary frequency; menstrual irregularities; and hirsutism.

Pelvic inflammatory disease
- Deep penetration causes severe pain that's unrelieved by changing coital positions.
- Uterine tenderness may also occur with gentle thrusting or during a pelvic examination.
- Other signs and symptoms include fever; malaise; a foul-smelling, purulent vaginal discharge; menorrhagia; dysmenorrhea; a soft, enlarged uterus; severe abdominal pain; nausea and vomiting; cervical motion tenderness; and diarrhea.

Pelvic irradiation
- Radiation therapy for pelvic cancer may cause pelvic and vaginal scarring, resulting in dyspareunia.

Psychological factors

◆ Dyspareunia may result from guilty feelings about sex, fear of pregnancy or of injury to the fetus during pregnancy, and anxiety caused by a disrupted sexual relationship or by a new sexual partner.
◆ Inadequate vaginal lubrication associated with insufficient foreplay and mental or physical fatigue may also cause dyspareunia.
◆ Repeated episodes of painful coitus condition the patient to anticipate pain, causing fear, which prevents sexual arousal and adequate vaginal lubrication.

Uterine prolapse

◆ Sharp or aching pain occurs when the penis strikes the descended cervix of a patient with uterine prolapse.
◆ Other signs and symptoms include dysmenorrhea, pelvic pressure, leukorrhea, urine retention and urinary incontinence, and chronic lower back pain.

Vaginitis

◆ Infection produces dyspareunia along with vulvar pain, burning, and itching during and for several hours after coitus.
◆ Symptoms may be aggravated by sexual arousal aside from intercourse.
◆ Vaginal discharge varies with the causative organism. *Candida albicans* produces a curdlike, odorless to musty-smelling discharge; *Trichomonas vaginalis* produces a yellow-green, frothy, fish-smelling discharge; bacterial vaginosis and *Neisseria gonorrhoeae* produce a profuse, whitish-yellow, foul-smelling discharge.
◆ Pruritus and dysuria may also occur.

OTHER

Aging

◆ Diminished vaginal lubrication occurs.

Contraceptive and hygienic products

◆ Some spermicidal jellies, douches, and vaginal creams and deodorants cause irritation and edema, resulting in dyspareunia.
◆ An ill-fitting diaphragm may produce dyspareunia during intercourse.
◆ An incorrectly placed intrauterine device may cause dyspareunia during orgasm.

Drugs

◆ Antihistamines, decongestants, and nonsteroidal anti-inflammatory drugs decrease lubrication, resulting in dyspareunia.

NURSING CONSIDERATIONS

◆ Prepare the patient for a pelvic examination. Explain that it involves inspection of the vagina and cervix and bimanual palpation of the uterus, fallopian tubes, and ovaries. Remind her to breathe deeply and evenly during the examination to aid relaxation.
◆ Encourage the patient to discuss dyspareunia openly. A woman may hesitate to report dyspareunia because of embarrassment and modesty.

PEDIATRIC POINTERS

◆ Dyspareunia can also be an adolescent problem.
◆ Although about 40% of adolescents are sexually active by age 19, most are reluctant to initiate a frank sexual discussion.
◆ Obtain a thorough sexual history by asking the patient direct but non-judgmental questions.

GERIATRIC POINTERS

◆ In postmenopausal women, the absence of estrogen reduces vaginal diameter and elasticity, which causes tearing of the vaginal mucosa during intercourse. These tears as well as inflammatory reactions to bacterial invasion cause fibrous adhesions that occlude the vagina.

PATIENT TEACHING

◆ If an antimicrobial or anti-inflammatory drug is prescribed, teach the patient how to apply the cream or insert the vaginal suppository.
◆ To minimize dyspareunia, advise the patient to apply a vaginal lubricant before intercourse, to attempt different coital positions, and to increase foreplay time.
◆ Teach her Kegel exercises to reduce muscle tension. (See *How to do Kegel exercises.*)

How to do Kegel exercises

Kegel exercises are isometric exercises that strengthen the pubococcygeal (PC) muscle to regain voluntary control of it. These steps will teach your patient how to perform Kegel exercises.

◆ Begin by sitting on the toilet with your legs spread. Then, without moving your legs, start and stop the flow of urine. The PC muscle is the one that contracts to help control urine flow.
◆ Now that you've identified the PC muscle, you can exercise it regularly. Like most isometric exercises, Kegel exercises can be performed almost anywhere—while sitting at your desk, lying in bed, standing in line, and especially while urinating. As you perform these exercises, remember to breathe naturally—don't hold your breath.
◆ Now, periodically contract the PC muscle as you did to stop the urine flow. Count slowly to three and then relax the muscle.
◆ Next, contract and relax the PC muscle as quickly as possible, without using your stomach or buttock muscles.
◆ Finally, slowly contract the entire vaginal area. Then bear down, using your abdominal muscles and your PC muscle.

For the first week, repeat each exercise 10 times (1 set) for 5 sets daily. Then each week, add 5 repetitions of each exercise (15, 20, and so forth). Keep doing 5 sets daily. After about 2 weeks of practice, you'll notice improvement.

Dyspepsia

- Feeling of uncomfortable fullness after meals
- Associated with belching, heartburn, nausea, and, possibly, cramping and abdominal distention
- Results from altered gastric secretions leading to excess stomach acidity
- Aggravated by spicy, fatty, or high-fiber foods and by excessive caffeine intake

- Ask about the onset, duration, and description of dyspepsia.
- Ask about alleviating and aggravating factors.
- Ask the patient about nausea, vomiting, melena, hematemesis, cough, chest pain, or urine changes.
- Obtain a drug and surgical history.
- Obtain a medical history, including renal, cardiovascular, or pulmonary disorders.
- Ask about an unusual or overwhelming amount of emotional stress.

- Inspect the abdomen for distention, ascites, scars, obvious hernias, jaundice, uremic frost, and bruising.
- Auscultate for bowel sounds and characterize their motility.
- Percuss then palpate the abdomen, noting any tenderness, pain, organ enlargement, or tympany.
- Auscultate for gallops and crackles.
- Percuss the lungs to detect consolidation.
- Note peripheral edema and swelling of lymph nodes.

MEDICAL

Cholelithiasis
- Dyspepsia may occur, typically after intake of fatty foods.
- Other signs and symptoms include diaphoresis, tachycardia, chills, low-grade fever, petechiae, bleeding tendencies, jaundice with pruritus, dark urine, clay-colored stools, and biliary colic.

Cirrhosis
- Dyspepsia occurs because of the inflammatory process and impaired bile production.
- Dyspepsia is relieved by ingestion of an antacid.
- Other signs and symptoms include anorexia, nausea, vomiting, flatulence, weight loss, jaundice, hepatomegaly, ascites, diarrhea, constipation, abdominal distention, and epigastric or right-upper-quadrant pain.

Duodenal ulcer
- Dyspepsia ranges from a vague fullness or pressure to a boring or aching sensation.
- Symptom occurs 1½ to 3 hours after eating and is relieved by ingestion of food or antacids.
- Pain may awaken the patient at night with heartburn and fluid regurgitation.

Gastric dilation, acute
- In this life-threatening disorder, dyspepsia is an early symptom.
- Nausea, vomiting, upper abdominal distention, succussion splash, and apathy occur.
- Dehydration and gastric bleeding may also occur.

Gastric ulcer
- Dyspepsia and heartburn occur after eating.
- Epigastric pain is a characteristic symptom that may occur with vomiting, fullness, weight loss, GI bleeding, and abdominal distention and may not be relieved by food.

Gastritis, chronic

◆ Dyspepsia is relieved by antacids; lessened by smaller, more frequent meals; and aggravated by spicy foods or excessive caffeine.
◆ Other signs and symptoms include anorexia, a feeling of fullness, vague epigastric pain, belching, nausea, and vomiting.

GI cancer

◆ Chronic dyspepsia occurs along with anorexia, fatigue, jaundice, melena, hematemesis, constipation, weight loss, weakness, syncope, and abdominal pain.

Heart failure

◆ In right-sided heart failure, transient dyspepsia may occur with chest tightness and pain or ache in the right upper quadrant because of vascular congestion.
◆ Other signs and symptoms include hepatomegaly, anorexia, nausea, vomiting, bloating, ascites, tachycardia, jugular vein distention, tachypnea, dyspnea, orthopnea, edema, and fatigue.

Hepatitis

◆ Before an attack, moderate to severe dyspepsia along with fever, malaise, arthralgia, coryza, myalgia, nausea, vomiting, an altered sense of taste or smell, and hepatomegaly occur.
◆ Jaundice marks the onset of an attack with continuing dyspepsia, anorexia, irritability, and severe pruritus.
◆ As jaundice clears, dyspepsia and other GI effects also diminish.

Hiatal hernia

◆ Dyspepsia occurs when gastric reflux through the hernia causes esophagitis, esophageal ulceration, or stricture.
◆ Dyspepsia is accompanied by heartburn and retrosternal or substernal chest pain.

Pancreatitis, chronic

◆ A feeling of fullness or dyspepsia may occur with epigastric pain that radiates to the back or through the abdomen.

◆ Other signs and symptoms include anorexia, nausea, vomiting, jaundice, dramatic weight loss, Turner's or Cullen's sign, hyperglycemia, and steatorrhea.

Uremia

◆ Dyspepsia may be the earliest and most important GI complaint.
◆ As the disease progresses, edema, pruritus, pallor, hyperpigmentation, uremic frost, ecchymoses, irritability, drowsiness, muscle twitching, seizures, and oliguria may occur.
◆ Other signs and symptoms include anorexia, nausea, vomiting, bloating, diarrhea, abdominal cramps, epigastric pain, and weight gain.

OTHER
Drugs

◆ Antibiotics, antihypertensives, corticosteroids, diuretics, and nonsteroidal anti-inflammatory drugs may cause dyspepsia.

Pregnancy

◆ Hormone changes slow the digestive process and relax the cardiac sphincter, allowing gastric reflux.
◆ This problem may increase in later pregnancy because of the pressure of the fetus on the mother's internal organs.

Surgery

◆ After GI surgery, postoperative gastritis can cause dyspepsia.

NURSING CONSIDERATIONS

◆ Give an antacid 30 minutes before or 1 hour after a meal.
◆ Provide food to relieve dyspepsia.
◆ If drugs cause dyspepsia, give them after meals.

PEDIATRIC POINTERS

◆ Dyspepsia may occur in adolescents with peptic ulcer disease, but it isn't relieved by food.
◆ Dyspepsia may occur with congenital pyloric stenosis, but projectile vomiting after meals is more common.
◆ Lactose intolerance may also cause dyspepsia.

GERIATRIC POINTERS

◆ Most elderly patients with chronic pancreatitis have less severe pain than younger adults, and some have no pain at all.

PATIENT TEACHING

◆ Discuss the importance of small, frequent meals.
◆ Describe foods or liquids the patient should avoid.
◆ Discuss stress reduction techniques the patient can use.
◆ Instruct the patient to avoid lying down for 2 to 3 hours after eating and to avoid tight or constrictive clothing.

Dysphagia

- Refers to difficulty swallowing, the most common symptom of esophageal disorders
- Factors that interfere with swallowing: severe pain, obstruction, abnormal peristalsis, impaired gag reflex, and excessive, scanty, or thick oral secretions
- Classified by three phases: transfer of chewed food to back of throat (phase 1), transport of food into the esophagus (phase 2), or entrance of food into stomach (phase 3)
- Increases the risk of choking and aspiration and may lead to malnutrition and dehydration

ACTION STAT! *If the patient has signs of respiratory distress, such as dyspnea and stridor, suspect an airway obstruction and quickly perform abdominal thrusts. Administer oxygen and insert an endotracheal tube.*

HISTORY

- Obtain a medical and surgical history.
- Ask about the onset and description of pain, if present.
- Determine aggravating and alleviating factors.
- Ask about recent vomiting, regurgitation, weight loss, anorexia, hoarseness, dyspnea, or cough.

PHYSICAL ASSESSMENT

- Evaluate swallowing and cough reflexes.
- If a sufficient swallow or cough reflex is present, check the gag reflex.
- Listen to the patient's speech for signs of muscle weakness.
- Check the mouth for dry mucous membranes and thick, sticky secretions.
- Observe for tongue and facial weakness and obstructions.
- Assess for disorientation.

CAUSES

MEDICAL
Achalasia

- Gradually developing phase 3 dysphagia occurs and is precipitated or exacerbated by stress.
- Regurgitation of undigested food, especially at night, causes wheezing, coughing, choking, and halitosis.
- Other signs and symptoms include weight loss, cachexia, hematemesis, and heartburn.

Airway obstruction

- Phase 2 dysphagia occurs with gagging and dysphonia.
- When hemorrhage obstructs the trachea, dysphagia is sudden in onset, but painless.
- When inflammation causes the obstruction, dysphagia is slow in onset and painful.
- Signs of respiratory distress occur with life-threatening upper airway obstruction.

Amyotrophic lateral sclerosis

- Dysphagia occurs with accompanying muscle weakness and atrophy, fasciculations, dysarthria, dyspnea, shallow respirations, tachypnea, slurred speech, hyperactive deep tendon reflexes, and emotional lability in this motor neuron disease.

Botulism

- Phase 1 dysphagia and dysuria usually begin within 36 hours of toxin ingestion.
- Blurred or double vision, dry mouth, sore throat, nausea, vomiting, and diarrhea occurs, with gradual symmetrical descending weakness or paralysis.

Esophageal cancer

- Painless dysphagia (phases 2 and 3) with weight loss are the earliest and most common findings.
- As the cancer advances, dysphagia becomes painful and is accompanied by steady chest pain, hemoptysis, hoarseness, and sore throat.

- Other signs and symptoms include nausea, vomiting, fever, hiccups, hematemesis, melena, and halitosis.

Esophageal diverticulum

- Phase 3 dysphagia occurs when the enlarged diverticulum obstructs the esophagus.
- Other signs and symptoms include regurgitation, chronic cough, hoarseness, chest pain, and halitosis.

Esophageal obstruction by foreign body

- Sudden onset of phase 2 or 3 dysphagia occurs with gagging, coughing, and esophageal pain.
- If the obstruction compresses the trachea, dyspnea occurs.

Esophageal spasm

- Phase 2 dysphagia occurs along with substernal chest pain.
- Pain that radiates may be relieved by drinking water.
- Bradycardia may also occur.

Esophageal stricture

- Phase 3 dysphagia occurs, possibly with drooling, tachypnea, and gagging.
- With chemical ingestion, burns, ulcers, or erythema of the lips and mouth may develop.

Esophagitis

- Corrosive esophagitis, resulting from ingestion of alkalis or acids, causes severe phase 3 dysphagia with marked salivation, hematemesis, tachypnea, fever, and intense pain in the mouth and chest that's aggravated by swallowing.
- Candidal esophagitis causes phase 2 dysphagia, sore throat and, possibly, retrosternal pain on swallowing.
- Reflux esophagitis causes phase 3 dysphagia (late symptom) with heartburn; regurgitation; vomiting; a dry, nocturnal cough; and substernal chest pain.

Hypocalcemia

- Phase 1 dysphagia with numbness and tingling in the nose, ears, fingertips, and toes, and around the mouth occurs.

Other signs and symptoms include tetany with carpopedal spasms, muscle twitching, and laryngeal spasms.

Laryngeal cancer, extrinsic
- Phase 2 dysphagia and dyspnea develop late.
- Other signs and symptoms include muffled voice, stridor, pain, halitosis, weight loss, ipsilateral otalgia, chronic cough, and cachexia.

Lower esophageal ring
- Phase 3 dysphagia occurs with feeling of a foreign body in the lower esophagus that may be relieved by drinking water or vomiting.

Myasthenia gravis
- This progressive disorder causes failure in nerve impulse transmission.
- Painless phase 1 dysphagia develops after ptosis and diplopia.
- Other signs and symptoms include masklike facies, nasal voice, nasal regurgitation, shallow respirations, dyspnea, and head bobbing.

Oral cavity tumor
- Painful phase 1 dysphagia occurs with hoarseness and ulcers.
- Other signs and symptoms include abnormal taste or bleeding in the mouth or dentures that no longer fit.

Parkinson's disease
- Late, painless progressive phase 1 dysphagia causes choking in this degenerative neurologic disorder.
- Other signs and symptoms include bradykinesia, tremors, muscle rigidity, dysarthria, masklike facies, muffled voice, increased salivation and lacrimation, constipation, stooped posture, propulsive gait, and incontinence.

Pharyngitis, chronic
- Painful phase 2 dysphagia occurs with a dry, sore throat; cough; and thick mucus and sensation of fullness in the throat.

Progressive systemic sclerosis
- This diffuse connective tissue disease, also known as *scleroderma*, is

preceded by Raynaud's phenomenon. Mild dysphagia becomes so severe that only liquids can be swallowed.
- Heartburn, weight loss, abdominal distention, diarrhea, and malodorous, and floating stools occur.
- Other signs and symptoms include joint pain and stiffness, masklike facies, and thickening of the skin that becomes taut and shiny.

Rabies
- In this life-threatening disorder, phase 2 dysphagia of liquids results in pharyngeal muscle spasms.
- Other signs and symptoms include dehydration, drooling, hydrophobia, and progressive flaccid paralysis that leads to vascular collapse, coma, and death.

Tetanus
- Phase 1 dysphagia occurs about 1 week after the unimmunized patient receives a puncture wound.
- Other signs and symptoms include marked muscle hypotonicity, hyperactive deep tendon reflexes, tachycardia, diaphoresis, drooling, trismus (lockjaw), risus sardonicus, opisthotonos, boardlike abdominal rigidity, seizures, and low-grade fever.

OTHER
Lead poisoning
- Painless, progressive dysphagia occurs.
- Other signs and symptoms include a lead line on the gums, metallic taste, papilledema, ocular palsy, footdrop or wristdrop, mental impairment, seizures, and signs of hemolytic anemia.

Procedures
- Recent tracheostomy or repeated or prolonged intubation may cause temporary dysphagia.

Radiation therapy
- Radiation therapy for oral cancer may cause scant salivation and temporary dysphagia.

Dyspnea

- Shortness of breath
- Indicates cardiopulmonary dysfunction
- May arise suddenly or slowly and subside rapidly or persist for years (see *Grading dyspnea*)

◆◆ **ACTION STAT!** *Look for signs of respiratory distress. Give oxygen, if needed. Ensure patent I.V. access and begin cardiac and oxygen saturation monitoring. Insertion of a chest tube for severe pneumothorax and for continuous positive airway pressure, intubation, and mechanical ventilation may be needed.*

HISTORY

- Ask about onset and progression, and determine aggravating and alleviating factors.
- Ask the patient if he has a cough.
- Include trauma, upper respiratory tract infection, deep vein phlebitis, orthopnea, paroxysmal nocturnal dyspnea, fatigue, smoking, or exposure to occupational hazards.

PHYSICAL ASSESSMENT

- Look for pursed-lip exhalation, clubbing, peripheral edema, barrel chest,

Grading dyspnea

- *Grade 0:* not troubled by breathlessness except with strenuous exercise
- *Grade 1:* troubled by shortness of breath when hurrying on a level path or walking up a slight hill
- *Grade 2:* walks more slowly on a level path than people of the same age because of breathlessness or has to stop to breathe when walking on a level path at his own pace
- *Grade 3:* stops to breathe after walking about 100 yards (91 m) on a level path
- *Grade 4:* too breathless to leave the house or breathless when dressing or undressing

diaphoresis, jugular vein distention, and edema.
- Take vital signs.
- Auscultate lung and heart sounds.
- Palpate the abdomen for hepatomegaly.

CAUSES

MEDICAL

Acute respiratory distress syndrome
- In this life-threatening condition, acute dyspnea is usually the first complaint.
- Progressive respiratory distress with restlessness, anxiety, decreased mental acuity, tachycardia, and crackles and rhonchi occur.
- Other signs and symptoms include cyanosis, tachypnea, motor dysfunction, intercostal and suprasternal retractions, and shock.

Amyotrophic lateral sclerosis
- Dyspnea slowly worsens over time, in this motor neuron disease.
- Other signs and symptoms include dysphagia, dysarthria, muscle weakness and atrophy, fasciculations, shallow respirations, tachypnea, and emotional lability.

Anemia
- Dyspnea is gradual in onset.
- Fatigue, weakness, syncope, tachycardia, tachypnea, restlessness, and anxiety occur.
- Other signs and symptoms include pallor, inability to concentrate, irritability, dysphagia, smooth tongue, and spoon-shaped and brittle nails.

Anthrax, inhalation
- Dyspnea occurs in the second stage of this life-threatening disorder, with fever, stridor, and hypotension.
- Other signs and symptoms include fever, chills, weakness, cough, and chest pain.

Asthma
- Dyspneic attacks occur with audible wheezing, dry cough, accessory muscle use, nasal flaring, intercostal and supraclavicular retractions, tachy-

pnea, tachycardia, diaphoresis, prolonged expiration, flush or cyanosis, and anxiety.

Cor pulmonale
- This serious chronic heart disorder is caused by lung diseases.
- Chronic dyspnea begins gradually with exertion and progressively worsens until it occurs even at rest.
- Other signs and symptoms include chronic productive cough, wheezing, tachypnea, jugular vein distention, edema, fatigue, weakness, and hepatomegaly.

Emphysema
- Progressive exertional dyspnea occurs.
- Other signs and symptoms include barrel chest, accessory muscle use, diminished breath sounds, anorexia, weight loss, malaise, peripheral cyanosis, tachypnea, pursed-lip breathing, prolonged expiration, a chronic and productive cough, and late clubbing.

Flail chest
- Sudden dyspnea is accompanied by paradoxical chest movement, severe chest pain, hypotension, tachypnea, tachycardia, and cyanosis.
- Bruising and decreased or absent breath sounds occur over the affected side.

Guillain-Barré syndrome
- Slowly worsening dyspnea occurs with fatigue and ascending muscle weakness and paralysis following a fever and upper respiratory tract infection.
- Other signs and symptoms include facial diplegia, dysphagia or dysarthria and, less commonly, weakness of the muscles supplied by cranial nerve XI.

Heart failure
- Dyspnea occurs gradually with orthopnea, tachypnea, tachycardia, palpitations, ventricular gallop, fatigue, dependent edema, jugular vein distention, paroxysmal nocturnal

dyspnea, hepatosplenomegaly, cough, and weight gain.

Inhalation injury
◆ Dyspnea may be sudden or gradual (over several hours) with sooty or bloody sputum, persistent cough, and oropharyngeal edema.
◆ Other signs and symptoms include orofacial burns, singed nasal hairs, crackles, rhonchi, wheezing, and signs of respiratory distress.

Lung cancer
◆ Dyspnea develops slowly, progressively worsening over time.
◆ Other signs and symptoms include fever, hemoptysis, productive cough, wheezing, clubbing, pain, weight loss, anorexia, and pleural rub.

Myasthenia gravis
◆ This progressive disorder causes failure in nerve impulse transmission.
◆ Bouts of dyspnea occur with difficulty chewing and swallowing.
◆ With myasthenic crisis, acute respiratory distress with shallow respirations and tachypnea occur.

Myocardial infarction
◆ Dyspnea occurs suddenly with crushing substernal chest pain that may radiate to the back, neck, jaw, and arms.
◆ Other signs and symptoms include nausea, vomiting, diaphoresis, vertigo, tachycardia, anxiety, and pale, cool, clammy skin.

Pleural effusion
◆ Dyspnea develops slowly and progressively worsens over time.
◆ Initial signs and symptoms include pleural friction rub and pleuritic pain that worsens with cough and deep breathing.
◆ Other signs and symptoms include dry cough, dullness on percussion, tachycardia, tachypnea, weight loss, fever, and decreased breath sounds.

Pneumonia
◆ Dyspnea occurs suddenly with fever, shaking chills, pleuritic chest pain, and a productive cough.

◆ Other signs and symptoms include fatigue, headache, myalgia, anorexia, abdominal pain, crackles, rhonchi, tachycardia, tachypnea, cyanosis, decreased breath sounds, and diaphoresis.

Pneumothorax
◆ Acute dyspnea occurs that's unrelated to the severity of pain.
◆ Sudden, stabbing chest pain radiates to the arms, face, back, or abdomen.
◆ Other signs and symptoms include anxiety, restlessness, dry cough, cyanosis, tachypnea, decreased or absent breath sounds on the affected side, splinting, and accessory muscle use.

Pulmonary edema
◆ Acute dyspnea is preceded by signs of heart failure.
◆ Other signs and symptoms include tachycardia, tachypnea, crackles, ventricular gallop, thready pulse, hypotension, diaphoresis, cyanosis, marked anxiety, and a cough that's dry or produces copious amounts of pink, frothy sputum.

Pulmonary embolism
◆ Acute dyspnea occurs in this life-threatening disorder, usually with sudden pleuritic chest pain.
◆ Other signs and symptoms include tachycardia, low-grade fever, tachypnea, pleural rub, crackles, diffuse wheezing, dullness on percussion, nonproductive cough or productive cough with blood-tinged sputum, decreased breath sounds, diaphoresis, anxiety and, with a massive embolism, signs of shock.

Severe acute respiratory syndrome
◆ This life-threatening acute infectious disorder produces fever with headache; malaise; a dry, nonproductive cough; and dyspnea.

Shock
◆ In this life-threatening disorder, sudden dyspnea progressively worsens over time.
◆ Other signs and symptoms include severe hypotension, tachypnea,

tachycardia, decreased peripheral pulses, decreased mental acuity, restlessness, anxiety, and cool, clammy skin.

Tuberculosis
◆ Dyspnea occurs with chest pain, crackles, and productive cough.
◆ Other signs and symptoms include night sweats, fever, anorexia, weight loss, palpitations on mild exertion, and dullness on percussion.

NURSING CONSIDERATIONS

◆ Monitor the patient closely.
◆ Position the patient comfortably, usually in high- or forward-leaning position.
◆ Administer oxygen, if needed.

PEDIATRIC POINTERS
◆ Suspect dyspnea in an infant who breathes costally, an older child who breathes abdominally, or any child who uses his neck or shoulder muscles to help him breathe.
◆ Acute epiglottiditis and laryngotracheobronchitis can cause severe dyspnea in a child.

GERIATRIC POINTERS
◆ An older patient with dyspnea from chronic illness may not be aware of a change in his breathing pattern.

PATIENT TEACHING

◆ Teach the patient about the underlying condition, diagnostic tests, and treatment.
◆ Teach the patient about pursed-lip, diaphragmatic breathing, chest splinting, and energy conservation.
◆ Instruct the patient to avoid chemical irritants, pollutants, and people with respiratory infections.
◆ Teach the patient with chronic dyspnea about oxygen use, if prescribed.

Dystonia

OVERVIEW

- Slow, involuntary movements of large-muscle groups in the limbs, trunk, and neck
- May involve flexion of the foot, hyperextension of the legs, extension and pronation of the arms, arching of the back, and extension and rotation of the neck (spasmodic torticollis)
- Aggravated by walking and emotional stress and relieved by sleep
- May be intermittent—lasting just a few minutes—or continuous and painful
- Occasionally causes permanent contractures, resulting in a grotesque posture

HISTORY

- If possible, include the patient's family in the history taking; they may be more aware of behavior changes than the patient is.
- Obtain a history of when dystonia occurs and what aggravates it.
- Find out if there's a family history of dystonia.
- Obtain a drug history, noting especially if the patient takes a phenothiazine or an antipsychotic. Dystonia is a common adverse effect of these drugs, and the dosage may need to be adjusted to minimize this effect.

PHYSICAL ASSESSMENT

- Examine the patient's coordination and voluntary muscle movement. Observe his gait as he walks across the room; then have him squeeze your fingers to assess muscle strength. (See *Recognizing dystonia*.)
- Check coordination by having him touch your fingertip and then his nose repeatedly.
- Test gross motor movement of the leg: Have him place his heel on one knee, slide it down his shin to the top of his great toe, and then return it to his knee.
- Assess fine-motor movement by asking him to touch each finger to his thumb in succession.

Recognizing dystonia

Dystonia, chorea, and athetosis may occur simultaneously. To differentiate among these three, keep the following points in mind:

- *Dystonic movements* are slow and twisting and involve large-muscle groups in the head, neck (as shown below), trunk, and limbs. They may be intermittent or continuous.
- *Choreiform movements* are rapid, highly complex, and jerky.
- *Athetoid movements* are slow, sinuous, and writhing, but always continuous; they typically affect the hands and extremities.

DYSTONIA OF THE NECK (SPASMODIC TORTICOLLIS)

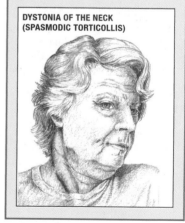

MEDICAL
Alzheimer's disease
◆ Dystonia is late sign of Alzheimer's disease, which is marked by slowly progressive dementia.
◆ Other signs and symptoms include decreased attention span, amnesia, agitation, an inability to carry out activities of daily living, dysarthria, and emotional lability.

Dystonia musculorum deformans
◆ Prolonged, generalized dystonia is the hallmark sign of this disorder, which usually develops in childhood and worsens with age.
◆ Initially, it causes foot inversion, which is followed by growth retardation and scoliosis.
◆ Late signs include twisted, bizarre postures, limb contractures, and dysarthria.

Hallervorden-Spatz disease
◆ Dystonic trunk movements accompanied by choreoathetosis, ataxia, myoclonus, and generalized rigidity occur.
◆ The patient also exhibits a progressive intellectual decline and dysarthria.

Huntington's disease
◆ Dystonic movements mark the preterminal stage of Huntington's disease.
◆ Characterized by progressive intellectual decline, this disorder leads to dementia and emotional lability.
◆ Other signs and symptoms include horeoathetosis accompanied by dysarthria, dysphagia, facial grimacing, and a wide-based, prancing gait.

Parkinson's disease
◆ Dystonic spasms are common with Parkinson's disease.
◆ Other signs and symptoms include uniform or jerky rigidity, pill-rolling tremor, bradykinesia, dysarthria, dysphagia, drooling, masklike facies, monotone voice, stooped posture, and propulsive gait.

Wilson's disease
◆ Progressive dystonia and chorea of the arms and legs mark Wilson's disease, an inherited metabolic disorder.
◆ Other signs and symptoms include hoarseness, bradykinesia, behavior changes, dysphagia, drooling, dysarthria, tremors, and Kayser-Fleischer rings (rusty brown rings at the periphery of the cornea).

OTHER
Drugs
◆ Piperazine phenothiazines, such as acetophenazine and carphenazine, can cause dystonia; aliphatics, such as chlorpromazine, cause it less commonly; and piperidines cause it rarely.
◆ Haloperidol, loxapine, and other antipsychotics usually produce acute facial dystonia as well as antiemetic doses of metoclopramide, risperidone, metyrosine, and excessive doses of levodopa.

◆ Encourage the patient to obtain adequate sleep and avoid emotional upset.
◆ Avoid range-of-motion exercises, which can aggravate dystonia.
◆ If dystonia is severe, protect the patient from injury by raising and padding his bed rails. Provide an uncluttered environment if he's ambulatory.

PEDIATRIC POINTERS
◆ Children don't exhibit dystonia until after they can walk. Even so, it rarely occurs until after age 10.
◆ Common causes include Fahr's syndrome, dystonia musculorum deformans, athetoid cerebral palsy, and the residual effects of anoxia at birth.

◆ Teach the patient and family about the underlying diagnosis and treatment plan.
◆ Teach the importance of adequate sleep and avoiding emotional upset.
◆ Discuss the patient's home environment and what safety measures can be taken.

Dysuria

- Painful or difficult urination commonly accompanied by urinary frequency, urgency, or hesitancy
- Usually reflects irritation or inflammation from a lower urinary tract infection (UTI), which stimulates nerve endings in the bladder and urethra (see *Preventing urinary tract infections*)
- Pain just before voiding: usually indicates bladder irritation or distention
- Pain at start of voiding: typically results from bladder outlet irritation
- Pain at end of voiding: may signal bladder spasms; in women, may indicate vaginal candidiasis

- Obtain a description of the severity, location, and what precipitates it and what alleviates or aggravates the pain.
- Ask about previous urinary or genital tract infections or if the patient has recently undergone an invasive procedure, such as cystoscopy or urethral dilatation.
- Ask about a history of intestinal disease, menstrual disorders, vaginal discharge or pruritus, or use of products that irritate the urinary tract, such as bubble bath salts, feminine deodorants, contraceptive gels, or perineal lotions.

- Inspect the urethral meatus for discharge, irritation, or other abnormalities.
- A pelvic or rectal examination may be necessary.

MEDICAL
Appendicitis
- Dysuria may occur that persists throughout voiding and is accompanied by bladder tenderness.
- Other signs and symptoms include periumbilical abdominal pain that shifts to McBurney's point, anorexia, nausea, vomiting, constipation, a slight fever, abdominal rigidity and rebound tenderness, and tachycardia.

Bladder cancer
- In this predominantly male disorder, dysuria occurs throughout voiding and is a late symptom associated with urinary frequency and urgency, nocturia, hematuria, and perineal, back, or flank pain.

Cystitis
- Dysuria throughout voiding is common in all types of cystitis, as are urinary frequency, nocturia, straining to void, and hematuria.
- Bacterial cystitis, the most common cause of dysuria in women, may also produce urinary urgency, perineal and lower back pain, suprapubic discomfort, fatigue and, possibly, a low-grade fever.
- With chronic interstitial cystitis, dysuria is most acute at the end of voiding.
- With tubercular cystitis, symptoms may also include urinary urgency, flank pain, fatigue, and anorexia.
- With viral cystitis, severe dysuria occurs with gross hematuria, urinary urgency, and a fever.

Preventing urinary tract infections

Teach the patient these guidelines to prevent recurrent urinary tract infections:

- Drink at least 10 glasses of fluid, especially water, daily. This helps flush bacteria from the urinary tract.
- Empty your bladder completely every 2 to 3 hours or as soon as you feel the urge to urinate.
- Wipe your perineum from front to back after urinating or defecating to prevent contamination with fecal material.
- Wear cotton underpants, which allow better ventilation and absorption than synthetic ones.
- Take showers instead of baths. If you must bathe, don't use bubble bath salts, bath oil, perfume, or other chemical irritants in the water. Also, avoid using feminine deodorants, douches, and similar irritants. Avoid using menstrual pads, which may also act as irritants.
- Urinate before and after intercourse.
- Follow an acid-ash diet, which includes meats, eggs, cheese, nuts, prunes, plums, whole grains and, especially, cranberry juice in your daily intake. These foods acidify the urine, which helps decrease bacterial growth. Avoid foods containing baking soda or powder, such as most baked goods.
- Avoid coffee, tea, and alcohol, which tend to irritate the bladder.
- Seek medical help for any unusual vaginal discharge, which suggests infection.

Paraurethral gland inflammation
◆ Dysuria throughout voiding occurs with urinary frequency and urgency, a diminished urine stream, mild perineal pain and, occasionally, hematuria.

Prostatitis
◆ Acute prostatitis commonly causes dysuria throughout or toward the end of voiding as well as a diminished urine stream, urinary frequency and urgency, hematuria, suprapubic fullness, fever, chills, fatigue, myalgia, nausea, vomiting, and constipation.
◆ With chronic prostatitis, urethral narrowing causes dysuria throughout voiding.
◆ Other signs and symptoms include urinary frequency and urgency; a diminished urine stream; perineal, back, and buttock pain; urethral discharge; nocturia; and, at times, hematospermia and ejaculatory pain.

Pyelonephritis, acute
◆ More common in females, dysuria is present throughout voiding.
◆ Other signs and symptoms include a persistent high fever with chills, costovertebral angle tenderness, unilateral or bilateral flank pain, weakness, urinary urgency and frequency, nocturia, straining on urination, hematuria, nausea, vomiting, and anorexia.

Reiter's syndrome
◆ Most cases of this syndrome follow venereal or enteric infection, but the cause is unknown.
◆ More common in males, dysuria occurs 1 to 2 weeks after sexual contact.
◆ Initially signs and symptoms include mucopurulent discharge, urinary urgency and frequency, meatal swelling and redness, suprapubic pain, anorexia, weight loss, and a low-grade fever.
◆ Hematuria, conjunctivitis, arthritic symptoms, a papular rash, and oral and penile lesions may follow.

Urethritis
◆ In sexually active men, dysuria occurs throughout voiding and is accompanied by a reddened meatus and copious, yellow, purulent discharge (gonorrheal infection) or white or clear mucoid discharge (nongonorrheal infection).

Urinary obstruction
◆ Outflow obstruction by urethral strictures or calculi produces dysuria throughout voiding.
◆ With complete obstruction, bladder distention develops and dysuria precedes voiding.
◆ Other signs and symptoms include diminished urine stream, urinary frequency and urgency, and a sensation of fullness or bloating in the lower abdomen or groin.

Vaginitis
◆ Dysuria occurs throughout voiding along with urinary frequency and urgency, nocturia, hematuria, perineal pain, and vaginal discharge and odor.

OTHER
Chemical irritants
◆ Bubble bath, bath salts, feminine deodorants, and spermicides can cause dysuria.

Drugs
◆ Monoamine oxidase inhibitors and metyrosine can cause dysuria.

NURSING CONSIDERATIONS
◆ Monitor vital signs and intake and output.
◆ Give medications, as prescribed.
◆ Obtain urine samples for testing, as ordered.

GERIATRIC POINTERS
◆ Elderly patients may underreport urinary-related symptoms.
◆ Older men have an increased incidence of nonsexual urinary tract infections.
◆ Postmenopausal women have an increased incidence of noninfectious dysuria.

PATIENT TEACHING
◆ Explain the importance of increased fluid intake.
◆ Emphasize the importance of frequent urination.
◆ Teach the patient to perform proper perineal care.
◆ Discourage the use of bubble baths and vaginal deodorants.
◆ Discuss the importance of taking prescribed drugs as instructed.

Earache

OVERVIEW

- Caused by disorders of the external and middle ear from allergies, infection, obstruction, or trauma
- Ranges from a feeling of fullness or blockage to deep, boring pain
- Also known as *otalgia*

HISTORY

- Ask about the onset and description of the pain.
- Inquire about recent head cold or problems with mouth, sinuses, or throat.
- Find out about aggravating and alleviating factors.
- Ask about itching, drainage, ringing noises, dizziness, vertigo, nausea, vomiting, and fever, and whether he has pain when he opens his mouth.
- Ask about recent airplane travel, travel to high altitudes, or scuba diving.
- Obtain a medical history, including incidence of head colds or problems with the eyes, mouth, teeth, jaw, sinuses, and throat.
- Obtain a drug history including over-the-counter medications.

PHYSICAL ASSESSMENT

- Inspect external ear for redness, drainage, swelling, or deformity.
- Apply pressure to mastoid process and tragus to check for tenderness.
- Using an otoscope, examine external auditory canal for lesions, bleeding or other discharge, impacted cerumen, foreign bodies, tenderness, or swelling. (See *Using an otoscope*.)
- Examine the tympanic membrane.
- Perform tests for hearing loss.
- Obtain vital signs.
- Obtain sample of drainage for testing.

 TOP TECHNIQUE

Using an otoscope

When the patient reports an earache, use an otoscope to inspect the ear structures closely. Follow these techniques to obtain the best view and ensure the patient's safety.

CHILD YOUNGER THAN AGE 3

To inspect a young child's ear, grasp the lower part of the auricle and pull it down and back to straighten the upward S curve of the external canal. Then gently insert the speculum into the canal no more than ½" (1.3 cm).

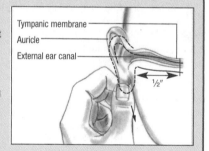

ADULT

To inspect an adult's ear, grasp the upper part of the auricle and pull it up and back to straighten the external canal. Then insert the speculum about 1" (2.5 cm). Also use this technique for children age 3 and older.

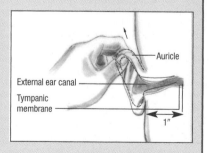

CAUSES

MEDICAL

Abscess, extradural

- Severe earache is accompanied by persistent ipsilateral headache, malaise, hearing loss, and recurrent mild fever.

Barotrauma, acute

- Earache ranges from mild pressure to severe pain with hearing loss and dizziness.
- Tympanic membrane ecchymoses or bleeding into the tympanic cavity may also occur.

Cerumen impaction

- Signs and symptoms include a blockage or a sensation of fullness in the ear accompanied by partial hearing loss, itching, dizziness, and ringing in the ear.

Chondrodermatitis nodularis chronica

- Small, painful, indurated areas develop along the upper rim of the auricle.
- Lesion may have a central core with scaly discharge.

Frostbite

- Burning or tingling pain may occur in the ear, followed by numbness.
- Ear appears mottled and gray or white and turns purplish as it warms.

Furunculosis

- Infected hair follicles in the outer ear canal may produce severe, localized ear pain from a pus-filled furuncle.
- Pain is aggravated by jaw movement and relieved by rupture or incision of the furuncle.
- Other signs and symptoms include pinna tenderness, swelling of the auditory meatus, partial hearing loss, and a feeling of fullness in the ear canal.

Herpes zoster oticus

- Burning or stabbing pain typically occurs with the ear vesicles.
- Other signs and symptoms include hearing loss; vertigo; transitory, ipsilateral, facial paralysis; partial loss of taste; tongue vesicles; and nausea and vomiting.

Mastoiditis, acute

- Dull ache behind the ear is accompanied by low-grade fever and purulent discharge.
- Eardrum appears dull and edematous and may perforate, and soft tissue near the eardrum may sag.

Ménière's disease

- An inner-ear disorder that may cause a sensation of fullness in the affected ear, severe vertigo, tinnitus, and sensorineural hearing loss.
- Other signs and symptoms include nausea, vomiting, diaphoresis, and nystagmus.

Middle ear tumor

- Deep, boring ear pain and facial paralysis are late signs.
- Hearing loss and facial nerve dysfunction may develop.

Otitis externa, acute

- Initially, pain is mild to moderate and occurs with tragus manipulation.
- Later, ear pain intensifies, causing the affected side of the head to ache.
- Other signs and symptoms include fever; sticky yellow or purulent discharge; partial hearing loss; a feeling of blockage; swelling of the tragus, external meatus, and external ear canal; reddened eardrum; lymphadenopathy; dizziness; and malaise.

Otitis media, acute

- Acute serous otitis media may cause a feeling of fullness in the ear, hearing loss, and a vague sensation of top-heaviness.
- Acute suppurative otitis media involves severe, deep, throbbing ear pain, hearing loss, and fever.

Petrositis

- Infection, resulting from acute otitis media, produces deep ear pain with headache and pain behind the eye.
- Other signs and symptoms include diplopia, loss of lateral gaze, vomiting, sensorineural hearing loss, vertigo, and, possibly, nuchal rigidity.

Temporomandibular joint infection

- Ear pain is referred from the jaw joint.
- Pain is aggravated by pressure on the joint with jaw movement and may radiate to the temporal area or entire side of the head.

NURSING CONSIDERATIONS

- Give an analgesic, as prescribed.
- Apply heat to relieve discomfort.
- Instill eardrops, as prescribed.

PEDIATRIC POINTERS

- Common causes of earache in children are acute otitis media and insertion of foreign bodies that become lodged or cause infection.
- In a child not old enough to speak, ear tugging and crying may indicate an earache.

PATIENT TEACHING

- Teach the patient or caregiver how to instill eardrops correctly.
- Explain the importance of taking prescribed antibiotics correctly and for the full term.
- Explain ways to avoid vertigo.
- Instruct the patient or caregiver about ways to avoid ear trauma.

Edema, generalized

OVERVIEW

- Excessive accumulation of interstitial fluid throughout the body (see *Understanding fluid balance.*)
- May be chronic or acute and progressive

 ACTION STAT! *If the patient has severe edema, take his vital signs and determine the degree of pitting. (See* Edema: Pitting or nonpitting?*) Check for jugular vein distention and cyanotic lips. Auscultate the lungs and heart. Look for signs of heart failure or pulmonary conges-tion. Place the patient in Fowler's position and prepare to administer oxygen and an I.V. diuretic, as prescribed. Have emergency resuscitation equipment readily available.*

HISTORY

- Note the onset, location, and description of edema.
- Ask about shortness of breath or pain.
- Obtain a medical history, including incidence of previous burns and cardiac, renal, hepatic, endocrine, and GI disorders.
- Obtain a surgical and trauma history.
- Find out about recent weight gain and urine output changes.
- Ask the patient to describe his diet.
- Obtain a drug history.

Understanding fluid balance

Normally, fluid moves freely between the interstitial and intravascular spaces to maintain homeostasis. Four basic types of pressure control fluid shifts across the capillary membrane that separates these spaces:

- capillary hydrostatic pressure (internal fluid pressure on the capillary membrane)
- interstitial fluid pressure (external fluid pressure on the capillary membrane)
- osmotic pressure (fluid-attracting pressure from protein concentration within the capillary)
- interstitial osmotic pressure (fluid-attracting pressure from protein concentration outside the capillary).

Here's how these pressures maintain homeostasis. Normally, capillary hydrostatic pressure is greater than plasma osmotic pressure at the capillary's arterial end, forcing fluid out of the capillary. At the capillary's venous end, the reverse is true: The plasma osmotic pressure is greater than the capillary hydrostatic pressure, drawing fluid into the capillary. Normally, the lymphatic system transports excess interstitial fluid back to the intravascular space.

Edema results when this balance is upset by increased capillary permeability, lymphatic obstruction, persistently increased capillary hydrostatic pressure, decreased plasma osmotic or interstitial fluid pressure, or dilation of precapillary sphincters.

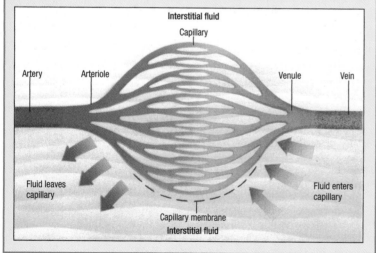

TOP TECHNIQUE

Edema: Pitting or nonpitting?

To differentiate pitting from nonpitting edema, press your finger against a swollen area for 5 seconds, and then quickly remove it.

In pitting edema, pressure forces fluid into the underlying tissues, causing an indentation that fills slowly. To determine the severity of pitting edema, estimate the indentation's depth in centimeters: 1+ (1 cm), 2+ (2 cm), 3+ (3 cm), or 4+ (4 cm).

In nonpitting edema, pressure leaves no indentation because fluid has coagulated in the tissues. Typically, the skin feels unusually tight and firm.

PITTING EDEMA (4+)

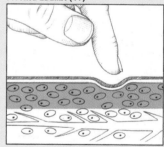

NONPITTING EDEMA

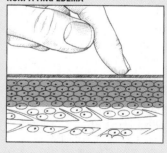

- Compare the patient's arms and legs for symmetrical edema.
- Note ecchymoses and cyanosis.
- Assess the back, sacrum, and hips of a bedridden patient for dependent edema.
- Palpate peripheral pulses, noting any coolness in hands and feet.
- Perform complete cardiac and respiratory assessments.

CAUSES

MEDICAL

Angioneurotic edema or angioedema

- Recurrent attacks of acute, painless, nonpitting edema involving the skin and mucous membranes may result from food or drug allergy, heredity, or emotional stress.
- May be the result of food or drug allergy, heredity, or emotional stress.
- Abdominal pain, nausea, vomiting, and diarrhea accompany visceral edema.
- Dyspnea and stridor accompany life-threatening laryngeal edema.

Burns

- Severe generalized edema may occur within 2 days of a major burn.
- Depending on the degree of edema, signs and symptoms of reduced or absent local circulation and airway obstruction may occur.

Cirrhosis

- Edema is a late sign.
- Other signs and symptoms include abdominal pain, anorexia, nausea, vomiting, hepatomegaly, ascites, jaundice, pruritus, bleeding tendencies, musty breath, lethargy, mental changes, and asterixis.

Heart failure

- Severe, generalized pitting edema may follow leg edema.
- Edema may improve with exercise or elevation of limbs and is worst at the end of day.

- Other classic, late signs and symptoms include hemoptysis, cyanosis, clubbing, crackles, marked hepatosplenomegaly, and a ventricular gallop.

Myxedema

- Myxedema is a form of hypothyroidism characterized by generalized nonpitting edema with dry, flaky, inelastic, waxy, pale skin; puffy face; and upper eyelid droop.
- Other signs and symptoms include masklike facies, hair loss or coarsening, hoarseness, weight gain, fatigue, cold intolerance, bradycardia, constipation, abdominal distention, menorrhagia, impotence, and infertility.

Nephrotic syndrome

- Edema is initially localized around the eyes, and then becomes generalized and pitting.
- Anasarca develops in severe cases.
- Other signs and symptoms include ascites, anorexia, fatigue, malaise, depression, and pallor.

Pericardial effusion

- Generalized pitting edema may be most prominent in arms and legs.
- Other signs and symptoms include chest pain, dyspnea, orthopnea, nonproductive cough, pericardial friction rub, jugular vein distention, dysphagia, fatigue, and fever.

Renal failure

- Generalized pitting edema occurs as a late sign.
- With chronic renal failure, edema is less likely to become generalized; its severity depends on the degree of fluid overload.
- Other signs and symptoms include oliguria, anorexia, nausea, vomiting, drowsiness, confusion, hypertension, dyspnea, crackles, dizziness, and pallor.

Septic shock

- A late sign of this life-threatening disorder, generalized edema typically develops rapidly.
- Edema becomes pitting and moderately severe.

- Other signs and symptoms include cool skin, hypotension, oliguria, anxiety, and signs of respiratory failure.

OTHER

Drugs

- Drugs that cause sodium retention—such as antihypertensives, corticosteroids, androgenic and anabolic steroids, estrogens, and nonsteroidal anti-inflammatory drugs—may aggravate or cause generalized edema.
- In patients with cardiac or renal disease, I.V. saline solution infusions and enteral feedings may cause sodium and fluid overload, resulting in generalized edema.

Treatments

- Enteral feedings and I.V. saline solution infusions may cause sodium and fluid overload.

NURSING CONSIDERATIONS

- Position the patient with his limbs above heart level to promote drainage.
- If the dyspnea develops, lower the patient's limbs, elevate the head of the bed, and administer oxygen.
- Restrict fluids and sodium, and administer a diuretic or I.V. albumin, as prescribed.
- Monitor intake and output, daily weight, and abdominal girth.
- Monitor electrolyte and coagulation levels.

PEDIATRIC POINTERS

- Renal failure typically causes generalized edema; kwashiorkor causes massive generalized edema.

GERIATRIC POINTERS

- Use caution when giving I.V. fluids or drugs that can raise sodium levels.

PATIENT TEACHING

- Explain signs and symptoms of edema that the patient should report.
- Discuss foods and fluids the patient should avoid.

Edema of the arm

OVERVIEW

- Results from excess interstitial fluid in the arm
- Signals localized fluid imbalance between the vascular and interstitial spaces

ACTION STAT! *Remove rings, bracelets, and watches from the affected arm. With neuromuscular compromise, elevate the arm.*

HISTORY

- Ask when the edema began.
- Find out about arm pain, numbness, or tingling.
- Find out what alleviates and aggravates the edema.
- Take a medical history, noting incidence of recent injury, I.V. therapy, surgery, or radiation therapy.

PHYSICAL ASSESSMENT

- Compare the size and symmetry of arms, and test for pitting.
- Examine and compare the color and temperature of both arms.
- Look for erythema, ecchymoses, and wounds.
- Palpate both arms, and compare their pulses.
- Look for arm tenderness and decreased sensation or mobility.

MEDICAL

Angioneurotic edema or angioedema

◆ Recurrent attacks of acute, painless, nonpitting edema involving the skin and mucous membranes may result from food or drug allergy, heredity, or emotional stress.
◆ If the edema spreads to the larynx, signs of respiratory distress may occur.

Arm trauma

◆ Severe edema affects the entire arm.
◆ Other signs and symptoms include ecchymoses or superficial bleeding, pain or numbness, deformity if the arm is fractured, and possibly, paralysis.

Burns

◆ Within 2 days of injury, mild to severe edema, pain, and tissue damage may develop.
◆ Depending on the burn degree, the arm may exhibit erythema; blisters; white, brown, or leathery tissue; or charring.

Envenomation

◆ Initially, edema may develop around the bite or sting and quickly spreads to the entire arm.
◆ Pain, erythema, pruritus, and paresthesia may occur.
◆ Later, nausea, vomiting, weakness, muscle cramps, fever, chills, hypotension, and headache develop.
◆ In severe cases, dyspnea, seizures, and paralysis occur.

Superior vena cava syndrome

◆ Edema in both arms usually progresses slowly and is accompanied by edema in the face and neck.
◆ Other signs and symptoms include dilated veins over edematous area, headache, vertigo, and vision disturbances.

Thrombophlebitis

◆ Arm edema with accompanying pain and warmth may occur.
◆ With deep vein thrombosis, cyanosis, fever, chills, and malaise occur.
◆ With superficial vein thrombosis, redness, tenderness, and induration along the vein occur.

OTHER

Treatments

◆ Infiltration of I.V. fluid into the interstitial tissue may cause localized arm edema.
◆ Axillary node dissection and mastectomy that disrupts lymphatic drainage may cause edema of the entire arm.
◆ Radiation therapy for breast cancer may cause arm edema.

◆ Elevate the arm and frequently reposition the patient.
◆ Use bandages and dressings, as needed, to promote drainage.
◆ Care for the patient's skin to prevent breakdown of skin and formation of pressure ulcers.
◆ Give an analgesic and anticoagulant, as needed and prescribed.
◆ Monitor neurovascular status frequently.

PEDIATRIC POINTERS

◆ Arm edema rarely occurs in children, but it may result from burns or crush injuries.

◆ Instruct the patient in postoperative arm care.
◆ Teach the patient arm exercises that will help to prevent lymphedema.
◆ Teach the patient about the underlying condition and treatment plan.

Edema of the face

OVERVIEW

♦ Involves localized or generalized facial swelling
♦ May extend to neck and upper arms

ACTION STAT! *If a patient has facial edema from burns or recent exposure to an allergen, quickly assess his respiratory system. If you detect respiratory distress, give epinephrine as ordered. For patients with absent breath sounds and cyanosis, tracheal intubation, cricothyroidotomy, or tracheotomy may be needed to maintain a patent airway. Always administer oxygen.*

HISTORY

♦ Ask about the onset (sudden or gradual) and description of facial edema.
♦ Ask about changes in urine color or output and weight gain.
♦ Note changes in appetite.
♦ Obtain a drug and allergy history.
♦ Ask about recent facial trauma.

PHYSICAL ASSESSMENT

♦ Observe and note the severity, extent of pitting, and location of edema. (See *Recognizing angioneurotic edema.*)
♦ Take vital signs.
♦ Assess neurologic condition.
♦ Examine the oral cavity.
♦ Visualize the oropharynx and look for soft-tissue swelling.
♦ Assess ability to swallow.

Recognizing angioneurotic edema

Most dramatic in the lips, eyelids, and tongue, angioneurotic edema commonly results from an allergic reaction. It's characterized by rapid onset of painless, nonpitting, subcutaneous swelling that usually resolves in 1 to 2 days. This type of edema may also involve the hands, feet, genitalia, and viscera; laryngeal edema may cause life-threatening airway obstruction.

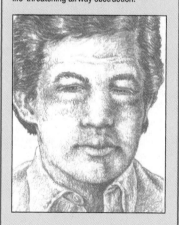

CAUSES

MEDICAL

Abscess, periodontal
♦ Edema of the side of the face, pain, warmth, erythema, and purulent discharge around the affected tooth occur.
♦ Gums may be bright red and inflamed.

Abscess, peritonsillar
♦ Facial edema with severe throat pain, neck swelling, drooling, cervical adenopathy, fever, chills, and malaise occur.

Allergic reaction
♦ Facial edema may develop.
♦ With life-threatening anaphylaxis, angioneurotic facial edema may occur with urticaria and flushing.
♦ Airway edema causes hoarseness, stridor, bronchospasm, dyspnea, tachypnea, and, possibly, signs of shock.

Chalazion
♦ This disorder is a chronic inflammatory granuloma in the eyelid.
♦ Localized swelling and tenderness of the affected eyelid occurs with a small red lump on the conjunctiva.
♦ Other signs and symptoms include tearing and photophobia.

Conjunctivitis
♦ Eyelid edema occurs with accompanying excessive tearing, and itchy, burning eyes.
♦ Other signs and symptoms include thick purulent discharge, crusty eyelids, conjunctival injection, and, with corneal involvement, photophobia and pain.

Corneal ulcers, fungal
♦ Eyelids are red and edematous with accompanying conjunctival injection, intense pain, photophobia, severely impaired visual acuity, and copious, purulent eye discharge.
♦ A dense, central ulcer grows slowly, is whitish gray, and is surrounded by progressively clearer rings.

Dacryocystitis
◆ Prominent eyelid edema occurs with accompanying excessive tearing, pain, tenderness, and purulent discharge.

Facial burns
◆ Extensive edema may develop, impairing respiration.
◆ Other signs and symptoms include singed nasal hairs and eyebrows, red mucosa, sooty sputum, and signs of respiratory distress.

Facial trauma
◆ Extent of edema and other findings vary with the type of injury.
◆ Contusion may cause localized edema; nasal or maxillary fractures cause more generalized edema.

Herpes zoster ophthalmicus
◆ Eyelids are red and edematous with accompanying excessive tearing and a serous discharge.
◆ Severe facial pain occurs several days before vesicles erupt along with fever and malaise.

Hordeolum (stye)
◆ Localized eyelid edema, erythema, photophobia, foreign-body sensation, and pain occurs.

Malnutrition
◆ Facial edema is followed by swelling of the feet and legs.
◆ Other signs and symptoms include muscle atrophy and weakness; anorexia; diarrhea; lethargy; dry, wrinkled skin; sparse, brittle hair; and slowed pulse and respiratory rates.

Myxedema
◆ Generalized facial edema occurs with accompanying waxy, dry skin; hair loss or coarsening; upper eyelid drooping; and other signs of hypothyroidism.

Nephrotic syndrome
◆ Periorbital edema is typically the first sign and precedes dependent and abdominal edema.

◆ Other signs and symptoms include weight gain, nausea, anorexia, lethargy, fatigue, and pallor.

Orbital cellulitis
◆ Periorbital edema is sudden in onset.
◆ Other signs and symptoms include purulent discharge, hyperemia, exophthalmos, conjunctival injection, impaired extraocular movements, fever, and extreme orbital pain.

Preeclampsia
◆ Edema of the face, hands, and ankles is an early sign of pregnancy-induced hypertension.
◆ Other signs and symptoms include excessive weight gain, severe headache, blurred vision, and midepigastric pain.

Rhinitis, allergic
◆ Red, edematous eyelids are accompanied by paroxysmal sneezing, itchy nose and eyes, and profuse, watery rhinorrhea.
◆ Other signs and symptoms include nasal congestion, excessive tearing, headache, sinus pain, malaise, and fever.

Sinusitis
◆ Frontal sinusitis causes edema of the forehead and eyelids.
◆ Maxillary sinusitis produces edema in the maxillary area as well as malaise, gingival swelling, and trismus (lockjaw).
◆ Signs and symptoms common to both include facial pain, fever, nasal congestion, purulent nasal discharge, and red, swollen nasal mucosa.

Superior vena cava syndrome
◆ Gradually developing facial and neck edema occurs with thoracic vein or jugular vein distention.
◆ Other signs and symptoms include headache, vision disturbances, and vertigo.

OTHER
Diagnostic tests
◆ Allergic reaction to contrast media may produce facial edema.

Drugs
◆ Long-term use of glucocorticoids and allergic reactions to drugs (such as aspirin, antipyretics, penicillin, and sulfa preparations) may produce facial edema.
◆ Ingestion of the fruit pulp of ginkgo biloba can cause severe erythema and edema and the rapid formation of vesicles.

Surgery and transfusion
◆ Cranial, nasal, or jaw surgery may cause facial edema.
◆ A blood transfusion that causes an allergic reaction may cause facial edema.

NURSING CONSIDERATIONS
◆ Administer an analgesic for pain, as prescribed.
◆ Apply a topical drug to reduce itching, as prescribed.
◆ Apply cold compresses to the eyes.
◆ Elevate the head of the bed to help drain the accumulated fluid.
◆ Monitor the patient for signs of respiratory distress.

PEDIATRIC POINTERS
◆ Children are more likely to develop periorbital edema because of lower periorbital tissue pressure.

PATIENT TEACHING
◆ Explain the risks of delayed treatment of allergy symptoms.
◆ Explain which signs and symptoms the patient or caregiver should report.
◆ Discuss ways to avoid allergens and insect bites or stings.
◆ Emphasize the importance of having an anaphylaxis kit, and instruct in its use.
◆ Discuss importance of medical identification bracelet.

Edema of the leg

- Results when excess interstitial fluid accumulates in one or both legs
- May be slight or dramatic, pitting or nonpitting, and affect just the foot or extend to the thigh

HISTORY

- Ask about the onset (gradual or sudden) and description of edema.
- Find out about recent leg injury, surgery, or illness.
- Obtain a drug history.
- Inquire about a history of cardiovascular disease.

PHYSICAL ASSESSMENT

- Examine legs for pitting edema.
- Palpate or auscultate peripheral pulses.
- Observe leg color and look for unusual vein patterns.
- Palpate for warmth, tenderness, and cords, and gently squeeze the calf muscle against the tibia to check for deep pain.
- If edema is only in one leg, look for Homans' sign.
- Note skin thickening, drainage, odors, unusual growths, or ulceration in edematous areas.

CAUSES

MEDICAL

Burns

- Two days or less after injury, mild to severe edema, pain, and tissue damage may occur.
- Depending on the degree of the burn, the leg may have erythema; blisters; white, brown, or leathery tissue; or charring.

Cellulitis

- Pitting edema occurs with accompanying orange peel skin with erythema, warmth, and tenderness in the infected area.

Envenomation

- Mild to severe localized edema may develop suddenly at the site of the bite or sting.
- Late signs include nausea, vomiting, weakness, muscle cramps, fever, chills, hypotension, headache and, in severe cases, dyspnea, seizures, and paralysis.
- Other signs and symptoms include erythema, pain, urticaria, pruritus, and a burning sensation.

Heart failure

- Edema in both legs is an early sign of right-sided heart failure.
- Pitting ankle edema signals more advanced heart failure.
- Other signs and symptoms include weight gain, anorexia, nausea, chest tightness, hypotension, pallor, tachypnea, exertional dyspnea, orthopnea, paroxysmal nocturnal dyspnea, palpitations, ventricular gallop, and crackles.

Hypoproteinemia

- Edema in both legs occurs with accompanying muscle weakness; lethargy; anorexia; diarrhea; apathy; dry, wrinkled skin; and signs of anemia.

Leg trauma

◆ Mild to severe localized edema may form at the site of the trauma.
◆ Ecchymoses or bleeding, pain or numbness, and paralysis may occur.
◆ Deformity may be present if a fracture has occurred.

Nephrotic syndrome

◆ Edema in both legs occurs with polyuria and eyelid edema.
◆ Generalized pitting edema may occur as well as ascites, fatigue, malaise, depression, and pallor.

Osteomyelitis

◆ Edema follows fever, localized tenderness, and muscle spasms, and pain that increases with leg movement.
◆ If the lower leg is affected, localized, mild to moderate edema develops and may spread to the adjacent joint.

Rupture of popliteal cyst

◆ Onset of calf pain and edema is sudden, usually occurring after walking or exercising.

Thrombophlebitis

◆ Mild to moderate edema occurs.
◆ With deep vein thrombosis, severe pain, warmth, and cyanosis in the affected leg as well as fever, chills, and malaise occur.
◆ With superficial thrombophlebitis, pain, warmth, redness, tenderness, and induration along the affected vein occur.

Venous insufficiency, chronic

◆ Moderate to severe edema in one or both legs occurs; initially, edema is soft and pitting; later, it's hard.
◆ Other signs include darkened skin and painless stasis ulcers around the ankles.

OTHER
Drugs

◆ Hormonal contraceptives, lithium, nonsteroidal anti-inflammatory drugs, vasodilators, and drugs that cause sodium retention can cause leg edema.

Surgery

◆ Venous insufficiency and leg edema may follow saphenous vein retrieval for coronary artery bypass and other vascular surgeries.

NURSING CONSIDERATIONS

◆ Have the patient avoid prolonged sitting or standing.
◆ Elevate his legs, as needed.
◆ Give an analgesic and antibiotic, as prescribed.
◆ Monitor intake and output, and check weight and leg circumference daily to detect changes.
◆ Monitor the patient for skin breakdown.

PEDIATRIC POINTERS

◆ Leg edema is uncommon but may result from osteomyelitis, leg trauma, or heart failure.

PATIENT TEACHING

◆ Teach the proper application of antiembolism stockings or bandages.
◆ Instruct the patient in appropriate leg exercises.
◆ Explain the foods or fluids the patient should avoid.

Enuresis

- Night-time urinary incontinence in girls age 5 and older and boys age 6 and older; most common in boys
- Rarely continues into adulthood but may occur in some adults with sleep apnea
- Primary enuresis: child has never achieved bladder control
- Secondary enuresis: child who achieved bladder control for at least 3 months has lost it

- Obtain information from the parents as well as the child.
- Determine the number of nights each week or month that the child wets the bed, if there's a family history of enuresis, what the child's fluid intake is, and what are his typical sleep and voiding patterns.
- Ask if the child has ever had control of his bladder and if so, try to pinpoint what may have precipitated enuresis, such as an organic disorder or psychological stress.
- Ask if bed-wetting occurs both at home and away from home and how the parents have tried to manage the problem.
- Observe the child's and parents' attitudes toward bed-wetting.
- Ask about pain with urination.

- Perform a physical examination to detect signs of neurologic or urinary tract disorders.
- Observe the child's gait to check for motor dysfunction, and test sensory function in the legs.
- Inspect the urethral meatus for erythema, and obtain a urine specimen.
- A rectal examination to evaluate sphincter control may also be required.

MEDICAL

Detrusor muscle hyperactivity

◆ Involuntary detrusor muscle contractions may cause primary or secondary enuresis associated with urinary urgency, frequency, and incontinence.
◆ Signs and symptoms of urinary tract infection (UTI) are also common.

UTI

◆ In children, most UTIs produce secondary enuresis.
◆ Low back pain, fever, fatigue, and suprapubic discomfort may also occur.
◆ Other signs and symptoms include urinary frequency and urgency, dysuria, straining to urinate, and hematuria.

Urinary tract obstruction

◆ Although it usually causes daytime incontinence, this disorder may also produce primary or secondary enuresis as well as flank and lower back pain; upper abdominal distention; urinary frequency, urgency, hesitancy, and dribbling; dysuria; diminished urine stream; hematuria; and variable urine output.

OTHER

Psychological stress

◆ Commonly results from the birth of a sibling; the death of a parent or loved one; divorce; or premature, rigorous toilet training.
◆ The child may be too embarrassed or ashamed to discuss his bed-wetting, which intensifies psychological stress and makes enuresis more likely, thus creating a vicious cycle.

◆ Provide emotional support to the child and his family.
◆ Encourage the parents to accept and support the child.
◆ Bladder training may help control enuresis caused by detrusor muscle hyperactivity.
◆ An alarm device may be useful for children ages 8 and older. This moisture-sensitive device fits in his mattress and triggers an alarm when moistened, waking the child. The alarm conditions him to avoid bed-wetting and should be used only in cases in which enuresis is having adverse psychological effects on the child.
◆ Pharmacologic treatment with imipramine, desmopressin, or an anticholinergic may be helpful.

◆ Teach parents how to manage enuresis at home. (See *Helping your child have dry nights*.)

Helping your child have dry nights

Although no single treatment for bed-wetting is always effective, by following these recommendations, the child's parents can help him achieve bladder control:
◆ Restrict the child's intake of fluids—especially colas—after supper.
◆ Make sure the child urinates before bedtime. In addition, wake him once during the night to go to the bathroom.
◆ Reward the child after each dry night with praise and encouragement. Keep a progress chart, marking each dry night with a sticker.
◆ Reward the child with a book, a small toy, or a special activity for a certain number of consecutive dry nights.
◆ Always give the child emotional support. Never punish him if he wets the bed; instead, reassure him that he'll learn to achieve bladder control. Remember that most children simply outgrow bed-wetting. However, wet and dry nights will alternate before your child develops a constant pattern of dryness.

Epistaxis

- Also called *nosebleed;* occurs in the anteriorinferior nasal septum (most commonly) or at the point where the inferior turbinates meet the nasopharynx
- Usually from only one nostril, bleeding may be mild to severe or even life-threatening

✦ **ACTION STAT!** *If the patient has severe epistaxis, quickly take vital signs and look for signs of hypovolemic shock. Insert a large-gauge I.V. catheter for fluid and blood replacement. Unless you suspect a nasal fracture, control bleeding by pinching the nares closed, then place gauze under the nose. Have a hypovolemic patient lie down and turn his head to the side to prevent aspiration. If the patient isn't hypovolemic, have him sit upright and tilt his head forward. Check airway patency. If the patient is unstable, begin cardiac monitoring and give oxygen.*

HISTORY

- Ask about recent trauma or surgery.
- Obtain a description of past nosebleeds.
- Take a medical history, including incidence of hypertension, bleeding or liver disorders, and other recent illnesses.
- Find out what drugs the patient is taking, especially anti-inflammatory drugs and anticoagulants.

PHYSICAL ASSESSMENT

- Inspect for other signs of bleeding.
- Look for trauma injuries.

CAUSES

MEDICAL
Aplastic anemia
- Nosebleeds are accompanied by ecchymoses, retinal hemorrhages, menorrhagia, petechiae, and signs of GI bleeding.
- Other signs and symptoms may include fatigue, dyspnea, headache, tachycardia, and pallor.

Biliary obstruction
- Epistaxis occurs along with other bleeding tendencies.
- Other signs and symptoms include colicky right-upper-quadrant pain after eating fatty food, nausea, vomiting, fever, flatulence, and jaundice.

Cirrhosis
- Epistaxis and other bleeding tendencies are late signs.
- Other late findings include ascites, abdominal pain, shallow respirations, hepatomegaly or splenomegaly, and fever.
- Other signs and symptoms include muscle atrophy, pruritus, dry skin, abnormal pigmentation, and central nervous system disturbances.

Coagulation disorders
- Epistaxis, ecchymoses, petechiae, menorrhagia, GI bleeding, and bleeding from the oral mucosa.

Glomerulonephritis, chronic
- Nosebleeds occur with accompanying hypertension, proteinuria, hematuria, headache, edema, oliguria, hemoptysis, nausea, vomiting, pruritus, dyspnea, malaise, and fatigue.

Hepatitis
- Epistaxis occurs with accompanying jaundice, clay-colored stools, pruritus, hepatomegaly, abdominal pain, fever, fatigue, dark amber urine, anorexia, nausea, and vomiting.

Hypertension
- Severe hypertension can produce extreme epistaxis with accompanying dizziness, headache, anxiety, peripheral edema, nocturia, nausea, vomiting, drowsiness, and confusion.

Infectious mononucleosis
- Blood may ooze from the nose.
- Other signs and symptoms include include sore throat, cervical lymphadenopathy, and a fluctuating fever that peaks in the evening.

Influenza
- A slow, oozing nosebleed may occur with dry cough, chills, fever, malaise, myalgia, sore throat, hoarseness, conjunctivitis, facial flushing, headache, rhinitis, and rhinorrhea.

Leukemia
- With acute leukemia, sudden epistaxis is accompanied by high fever and other types of abnormal bleeding tendencies.
- With chronic leukemia, epistaxis is a late sign that may be accompanied by other bleeding tendencies, extreme fatigue, weight loss, hepatosplenomegaly, bone pain, macular or nodular skin lesions, pallor, weakness, dyspnea, tachycardia, palpitations, and headache.

Maxillofacial injury
- Severe epistaxis may occur with accompanying pain from facial structure damage; swelling; diplopia; conjunctival hemorrhage; lip edema; and buccal, mucosal, and soft palatal ecchymoses.

Nasal fracture
- One or both nostrils may bleed.
- Other signs and symptoms include nasal swelling, periorbital ecchymoses and edema, pain, nasal deformity, and crepitation of the nasal bones.

Polycythemia vera
- Spontaneous epistaxis is a common sign of this bone marrow disorder.
- Other signs and symptoms include bleeding gums; ecchymoses; ruddy cyanosis of the face, nose, ears, and lips; headache; dizziness; vision disturbances; hypertension; chest pain; splenomegaly; epigastric pain; pruritus; and dyspnea.

Renal failure
- Epistaxis can occur with accompanying oliguria or anuria, weight loss, anorexia, abdominal pain, diarrhea, nausea, vomiting, tissue wasting, dry

mucous membranes, uremic breath, Kussmaul's respirations, deteriorating mental condition, and tachycardia.

Sarcoidosis
◆ Oozing epistaxis may occur along with extensive nasal mucosal lesions, a nonproductive cough, substernal pain, malaise, and weight loss.
◆ Other signs and symptoms include tachycardia, arrhythmias, parotid enlargement, cervical lymphadenopathy, skin lesions, hepatosplenomegaly, and arthralgia.

Sinusitis, acute
◆ Bloody or blood-tinged nasal discharge may become purulent and copious 48 hours after onset.
◆ Other signs and symptoms include nasal congestion, pain, and tenderness; malaise; headache; low-grade fever; and red, edematous nasal mucosa.

Skull fracture
◆ Epistaxis is direct or indirect, depending on the type of fracture.
◆ With a severe skull fracture, signs and symptoms include severe headache, decreased level of consciousness, hemiparesis, dizziness, seizures, projectile vomiting, and decreased pulse and respirations.

Systemic lupus erythematosus
◆ Oozing epistaxis occurs.
◆ Other signs and symptoms include butterfly rash, lymphadenopathy, joint pain and stiffness, anorexia, nausea, vomiting, myalgia, and weight loss.

OTHER
Chemical irritants
◆ Some chemicals, such as phosphorus, sulfuric acid, ammonia, printer's ink, and chromates, irritate the nasal mucosa, producing epistaxis.

Drugs
◆ Anti-inflammatories or anticoagulants can cause or worsen epistaxis.
◆ Frequent cocaine use may also cause epistaxis.

Vigorous nose blowing
◆ Vigorous nose blowing may rupture superficial blood vessels and cause epistaxis.

NURSING CONSIDERATIONS

◆ Monitor for signs of hypovolemic shock.
◆ If external pressure doesn't control the bleeding, insert cotton saturated with a vasoconstrictor and local anesthetic into the nose, as prescribed.
◆ If bleeding persists, anterior or posterior nasal packing may be needed. (See *Controlling epistaxis with nasal packing.*)
◆ Administer humidified oxygen by face mask to a patient with posterior packing.

PEDIATRIC POINTERS
◆ Causes of epistaxis include nose picking, allergic rhinitis, biliary atresia, cystic fibrosis, hereditary afibrinogenemia, nasal trauma from foreign body, and rubeola.

PATIENT TEACHING

◆ Teach the patient or caregiver pinching pressure techniques.
◆ Discuss ways to prevent nosebleeds.

Controlling epistaxis with nasal packing

When direct pressure and cautery fail to control epistaxis, nasal packing may be required. Anterior packing may be used if the patient has severe bleeding in the anterior nose. This involves inserting horizontal layers of petroleum jelly gauze strips into the nostrils near the turbinates.

Posterior packing may be needed if the patient has severe bleeding in the posterior nose or if blood from anterior bleeding starts flowing backward. This type of packing consists of a gauze pack secured by three strong silk sutures. After the nose is anesthetized, sutures are pulled through the nostrils with a soft catheter, and the pack is positioned behind the soft palate. Two of the sutures are tied to a gauze roll under the patient's nose, which keeps the pack in place. The third suture is taped to his cheek. Instead of a gauze pack, an indwelling urinary or nasal epistaxis catheter may be inserted through the nose into the area behind the soft palate and inflated with 10 ml of water to compress the bleeding point.

PRECAUTIONS
If the patient has nasal packing, follow these guidelines:
◆ Watch for signs of respiratory distress, such as dyspnea, which may occur if the packing slips and obstructs the airway.
◆ Keep emergency equipment (flashlights, scissors, and hemostat) at the patient's bed-

side. Expect to cut the cheek suture (or deflate the catheter) and remove the pack at the first sign of airway obstruction.
◆ Avoid tension on the cheek suture, which could cause the posterior pack to slip out of place.
◆ Keep the call bell within easy reach.
◆ Monitor vital signs frequently. Watch for signs of hypoxia, such as tachycardia and restlessness.
◆ Elevate the head of the patient's bed, and remind him to breathe through his mouth.
◆ Administer humidified oxygen, as needed.
◆ Instruct the patient not to blow his nose for 48 hours after the packing is removed.

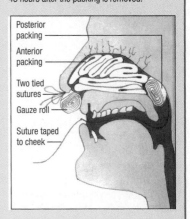

Posterior packing
Anterior packing
Two tied sutures
Gauze roll
Suture taped to cheek

Erectile dysfunction

OVERVIEW

- Inability to achieve and maintain penile erection sufficient to complete satisfactory sexual intercourse
- May be primary or secondary
- Occurs with psychological, vascular, neurologic, or hormonal dysfunction

HISTORY

- Find out about onset, quality, aggravating and alleviating factors, and progression of impotence.
- Obtain a psychosocial history.
- Review the patient's medical history, noting incidence of diabetes mellitus, hypertension, heart disease, urologic disease, and neurologic disease.
- Ask about the patient's surgical history, including neurologic, hormonal, vascular, and urologic surgery.
- Find out about recent trauma and its severity, other findings, and treatment.
- Ask about alcohol and drug use or abuse.
- Ask about diet, smoking, and exercise.

PHYSICAL ASSESSMENT

- Inspect and palpate the genitalia and prostate for structural abnormalities.
- Assess sensory function in the perineum.
- Test motor strength and deep tendon reflexes.
- Note neurologic deficits.
- Take vital signs.
- Palpate pulses for quality.
- Note cyanosis and cool extremities.
- Auscultate for abdominal, aortic, femoral, carotid, or iliac bruits.
- Palpate for thyroid gland enlargement.

MEDICAL
Central nervous system disorders
◆ Spinal cord lesions from trauma produce sudden impotence.
◆ Complete lesion above S2 causes loss of voluntary erectile control but not reflex erection and reflex ejaculation.
◆ Complete lesion in the lumbosacral spinal cord causes loss of reflex ejaculation and reflex erection.
◆ Degenerative disease of the brain and spinal cord cause progressive impotence.

Endocrine disorders
◆ Testicular or pituitary dysfunction may cause impotence from deficient androgens.
◆ Adrenocortical and thyroid disease and chronic hepatitis may cause impotence by affecting hormone regulation.

Penile disorders
◆ In Peyronie's disease, a bent penis makes erection painful and penetration difficult.
◆ Phimosis prevents erection until circumcision releases constricted foreskin.
◆ Other inflammatory, infectious, or destructive diseases of the penis may cause impotence.

Peripheral neuropathy
◆ Progressive impotence occurs.
◆ Other signs and symptoms include bladder distention with overflow incontinence, orthostatic hypotension, syncope, paresthesia and other sensory disturbances, muscle weakness, and leg atrophy.

Vascular disorders
◆ Advanced atherosclerosis, Leriche's syndrome, and arteriosclerosis, thrombosis, or embolization of smaller vessels supplying the penis can result in impotence.

OTHER
Alcohol and drugs
◆ Alcoholism and drug abuse are linked to erectile dysfunction, as are many prescription drugs, especially antihypertensives.

Psychological distress
◆ Diverse psychological causes can result in impotence.

Surgery
◆ Surgical injury to the penis, bladder neck, urinary sphincter, rectum, or perineum can cause impotence, as can injury to local nerves or blood vessels.

Trauma
◆ Traumatic injury involving the penis, urethra, prostate, perineum, or pelvis can cause sudden impotence.

NURSING CONSIDERATIONS

◆ Help the patient feel comfortable about discussing his sexuality.
◆ Discuss counseling for the patient and his partner.
◆ Provide care for treatments, such as surgical revascularization, drug-induced erection, surgical repairs, and penile prosthesis.
◆ Provide emotional support, and encourage the patient to talk about his feelings.

GERIATRIC POINTERS
◆ Keep in mind that sexual performance doesn't normally decline with aging and that elderly patients can be capable of and interested in sexual activity.

PATIENT TEACHING

◆ Explain which treatment options are available to the patient.
◆ Explain the importance of routine follow-up for treatment of medical conditions.
◆ Discuss with the patient the importance of communicating with his sexual partner.

Erythema

◆ Refers to red skin caused by dilated or congested blood vessels
◆ Common sign of skin inflammation or irritation
◆ Color ranging from bright red, in acute conditions, to pale violet or brown, in chronic conditions
◆ Blanches momentarily when pressure is applied, distinguishing it from purpura (redness from bleeding into the skin)

ACTION STAT! *If the patient has sudden erythema with rapid pulse, dyspnea, hoarseness, and agitation, quickly take his vital signs and treat him for anaphylactic shock. Provide respiratory support and give epinephrine, as ordered.*

◆ Ask about the onset and duration of erythema.
◆ Obtain a medical history, including incidence of recent fever, upper respiratory tract infection, skin disease, allergies, or asthma.
◆ Ask about pain or itching.
◆ Note recent falls or injury.
◆ Ask about exposure to anyone with a rash.
◆ Take a drug history, including recent immunizations.
◆ Review food intake and exposure to chemicals.

◆ Assess the extent, distribution, and intensity of erythema.
◆ Look for edema and other skin lesions.
◆ Examine the affected area for warmth.
◆ Gently palpate the affected area to check for tenderness or crepitus.

MEDICAL

Allergic reactions
◆ Localized reaction produces erythema, hivelike eruptions, and edema.
◆ With life-threatening anaphylaxis, erythema is sudden and accompanied by flushing; facial edema; diaphoresis; weakness; bronchospasm with tachypnea and dyspnea; shock; and airway edema with hoarseness and stridor.

Burns
◆ With thermal burns, erythema and swelling appear first, possibly followed by blisters.
◆ Burns from ultraviolet rays cause delayed erythema and tenderness.

Candidiasis
◆ If the skin is affected, erythema and a scaly, papular rash under breasts or at axillae, neck, umbilicus, or groin develop.
◆ Small pustules occur at the periphery of the rash.

Cellulitis
◆ Erythema, tenderness, and edema occur with accompanying pain and warmth at the site of the infection.

Dermatitis
◆ With atopic dermatitis, erythema and intense pruritus precede the development of small papules that may redden, weep, scale, and lichenify.
◆ With contact dermatitis, erythema appears with vesicles, blisters, or ulcerations.
◆ With seborrheic dermatitis, erythema appears with dull-red or yellow lesions that are sharply marginated and may be ring-shaped and covered with greasy scales.

Erysipelas
◆ Streptococcal pharyngitis usually precedes this infection.
◆ Reddish, well-demarcated, tender, warm areas occur most commonly on the face and neck.

◆ Other signs and symptoms include fever, chills, local adenopathy, malaise, headache, and sore throat.

Erythema annulare centrifugum
◆ Small, pink, infiltrated papules appear on the trunk, buttocks, and inner thighs, slowly spreading at the margins and clearing in the center.
◆ Other signs and symptoms include itching, scaling, and tissue hardening.

Erythema marginatum rheumaticum
◆ Erythematous lesions caused by rheumatic fever are superficial, flat, and slightly hardened.
◆ Lesions shift, spread rapidly, and may last for hours or days.

Erythema multiforme
◆ This condition may be caused by herpes simplex infection or to an allergic reaction.
◆ In minor form, urticarial red-pink, iris-shaped, localized lesions that burn or itch typically occur on flexor surfaces of extremities.
◆ Early signs and symptoms include mild fever, cough, and sore throat.
◆ In major form, blisters on the lips, tongue, and buccal mucosa and sore throat precede development of widespread erythematous, symmetrical, bullous lesions.
◆ Early signs and symptoms include cough, vomiting, diarrhea, coryza, and epistaxis.
◆ Late signs and symptoms include fever, prostration, conjunctivitis, vulvitis, balanitis, and difficulty with oral intake because of oral lesions.

Erythema nodosum
◆ This condition may be caused by drug sensitivity, sarcoidosis, or various infections.
◆ Tender erythematous nodules develop suddenly in crops on the shins, knees, and ankles.
◆ Other signs and symptoms include mild fever, chills, malaise, muscle and joint pain, and swollen feet and ankles.

Gout
◆ Tight, erythematous skin is seen over inflamed, edematous joint.
◆ The metatarsophalangeal joint of the great toe usually becomes inflamed first, followed by the instep, ankle, heel, knee, or wrist joint.

Liver disease, chronic
◆ Local vasodilation and palmar erythema occur along with jaundice, pruritus, spider angiomas, xanthomas, and characteristic systemic signs.

Lupus erythematosus
◆ Characteristic erythematous butterfly rash develops.
◆ Rash may range from a blush with swelling to a scaly, sharply demarcated, macular rash with plaques that may spread to the forehead, chin, ears, chest, and other sun-exposed body parts.
◆ With systemic lupus erythematosus, acute onset of erythema may accompany photosensitivity and mucous membrane ulcers.

Psoriasis
◆ Silvery white scales with a thickened erythematous base affect the elbows, knees, chest, scalp, and intergluteal folds.
◆ Fingernails become thick and pitted.

Rheumatoid arthritis
◆ During flare-ups, erythema, heat, swelling, pain, and stiffness occur at affected joints.
◆ Early signs and symptoms include malaise, fatigue, myalgia, and morning stiffness.
◆ As the disease progresses, other signs and symptoms include muscle atrophy, palmar erythema, edema, mottled skin, and structural deformities.

Rosacea
◆ Scattered erythema develops across the center of the face, followed by superficial telangiectases, papules, pustules, and nodules.

(continued)

Rubella

- Flat solitary lesions form a blotchy pink erythematous rash that spreads rapidly to the trunk and extremities, clearing in 4 to 5 days.
- Small red lesions may appear on the soft palate.
- Other signs and symptoms include fever, headache, malaise, sore throat, a gritty eye sensation, lymphadenopathy, joint pain, and coryza.

Staphylococcal scalded skin syndrome

- Occurring mainly in infants and small children, erythema and widespread exfoliation of superficial epidermal layers occur.
- Other signs and symptoms include low-grade fever and irritability.

Thrombophlebitis

- Erythema may develop over the inflamed vein.
- Fever, chills, and malaise may accompany severe, localized pain, warmth, and induration; distal edema; and a positive Homans' sign.

OTHER

Drugs

- Many drugs commonly cause erythema. (See *Drugs associated with erythema.*)

Radiation therapy

- Radiation therapy may produce dull erythema and edema within 24 hours.

Rare causes

- A number of rare disorders cause erythema. (See *Rare causes of erythema.*)

- Monitor and replace fluids and electrolytes, as ordered.
- Certain drugs may be withheld until the cause of erythema is identified.
- Give an antibiotic and topical or systemic corticosteroid, as prescribed.
- To relieve itching skin, give soothing baths or apply open wet dressings containing starch, bran, or sodium bicarbonate.
- Give an antihistamine and an analgesic, as prescribed.
- Keep erythematous legs elevated above heart level.
- For a burn patient with erythema, immerse the affected area in cold water, or apply a sheet soaked in cold water.

PEDIATRIC POINTERS

- Neonates may develop a pink papular rash during the first 4 days after birth, which spontaneously disappears.
- Infections and other disorders can cause erythema in neonates and infants.

Drugs associated with erythema

Suspect drug-induced erythema in any patient who develops this sign within 1 week of starting a drug. Erythematous lesions can vary in size, shape, type, and amount, but they almost always appear suddenly and symmetrically on the trunk and inner arms. The following drugs can produce erythematous lesions:

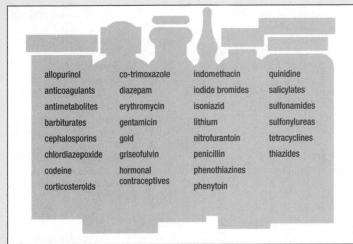

allopurinol	co-trimoxazole	indomethacin	quinidine
anticoagulants	diazepam	iodide bromides	salicylates
antimetabolites	erythromycin	isoniazid	sulfonamides
barbiturates	gentamicin	lithium	sulfonylureas
cephalosporins	gold	nitrofurantoin	tetracyclines
chlordiazepoxide	griseofulvin	penicillin	thiazides
codeine	hormonal contraceptives	phenothiazines	
corticosteroids		phenytoin	

Some drugs—particularly barbiturates, hormonal contraceptives, salicylates, sulfonamides, and tetracycline—can cause a "fixed" drug eruption. In this type of reaction, lesions can appear in any body part and flake off after a few days, leaving a brownish purple pigmentation. Repeated drug administration causes the original lesions to recur and new ones to develop.

Rare causes of erythema

In exceptional cases, your patient's erythema may be caused by one of these rare disorders:

- acute febrile neutrophilic dermatosis, which produces erythematous lesions on the face, neck, and extremities after a high fever
- erythema abigne, which produces lacy erythema and telangiectases after exposure to radiant heat
- erythema chronicum migrans, which produces erythematous macules and papules on the trunk, upper arms, or thighs after a tick bite
- erythema gyratum repens, which produces wavy bands of erythema and is commonly associated with internal malignancy
- toxic epidermal necrolysis, which causes severe, widespread erythema, tenderness, bullae formation, and exfoliation; this disorder is usually caused by medications and may be fatal because of epidermal destruction and its consequences.

- Roseola, rubeola, scarlet fever, granuloma annulare, and cutis marmorata cause erythema in children.

GERIATRIC POINTERS
- Well-defined purple macules or patches, usually on the back of the hands and on the forearms, may result from blood leaking through fragile capillaries.

PATIENT TEACHING
- Teach the patient to recognize the signs and symptoms of flare-ups of disease.
- Stress the avoidance of sun exposure and use of sunblock.
- Teach the patient methods to relieve itching.
- Teach the patient infection control techniques, as appropriate.

Exophthalmos

OVERVIEW

- Abnormal protrusion of one or both eyeballs
- May be sudden or gradual, mild or dramatic
- Also known as *proptosis*

HISTORY

- Ask about the onset of exophthalmos.
- Find out if the patient has pain and its quality, quantity, and duration.
- Inquire about recent sinus infection or vision problems.
- Obtain a medical history, including incidence of thyroid disease.
- Ask about recent injury or trauma.

PHYSICAL ASSESSMENT

- Take vital signs, noting fever.
- Evaluate severity of exophthalmos with exophthalmometer and assess for unilateral exophthalmos. (See *Detecting unilateral exophthalmus*.)
- If eyes bulge severely, look for cloudiness on the cornea, which may indicate ulcer formation.
- Observe for and describe any eye discharge, noting presence of ptosis.
- Check visual acuity, with and without correction.
- Palpate the thyroid for enlargement or goiter.

 TOP TECHNIQUE

Detecting unilateral exophthalmos

If one of the patient's eyes seems more prominent than the other, examine both eyes from above the patient's head. Look down across his face, gently draw his lids up, and compare the relationship of the corneas to the lower lids. Abnormal protrusion of one eye suggests unilateral exophthalmos.

Don't perform this test if you suspect eye trauma.

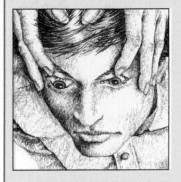

CAUSES

MEDICAL

Foreign body in eye
- Exophthalmos may accompany eye pain, redness, and tearing.
- Loss of vision or blurred vision occurs in the affected eye.

Hemangioma
- Exophthalmos is progressive and may be mild or severe, as proliferation of blood vessels leads to a mass.
- Other signs and symptoms include ptosis, limited extraocular movements, and blurred vision.

Lacrimal gland tumor
- Exophthalmos usually develops slowly in one eye, displacing it downward toward the nose.
- Other signs and symptoms may include ptosis, eye deviation, and pain.

Optic nerve meningioma
- Exophthalmos in one eye and a swollen temple are common.
- Other signs and symptoms may include impaired visual acuity, visual field deficits, and headache.

Orbital cellulitis
- Acute infection of the orbital tissues and eyelids leads to exophthalmos as edema progresses and should be treated promptly.
- Untreated, the infection can spread to the sinuses, meninges, or brain, where it can be life-threatening.
- Other signs and symptoms include fever, eye pain, headache, malaise, conjunctival injection, tearing, eyelid edema and erythema, purulent discharge, and impaired extraocular movements.

Orbital choristoma
- Progressive exophthalmos may occur with diplopia and blurred vision.
- A mass may be visible in the orbital area.

Orbital emphysema

◆ Exophthalmos in one eye, crepitation on palpation of the globe, and orbital pressure occur from an air leak into the orbit from the sinus.

Parasite infestation

◆ Painless, progressive exophthalmos develops in one eye and may spread to the other eye.
◆ Other signs and symptoms include limited extraocular movement, diplopia, eye pain, and impaired visual acuity.

Scleritis, posterior

◆ Onset of mild to severe exophthalmos in one eye is gradual.
◆ Other signs and symptoms include severe eye pain, diplopia, papilledema, limited extraocular movement, and impaired visual acuity.

Thyrotoxicosis

◆ Exophthalmos is a hallmark sign and is usually in both eyes, progressive, and severe.
◆ Ptosis, increased tearing, lid lag and edema, photophobia, conjunctival injection, diplopia, and decreased visual acuity occur.
◆ Other signs and symptoms include enlarged thyroid gland, nervousness, heat intolerance, weight loss despite increased appetite, sweating, diarrhea, tremors, palpitations, and tachycardia.

NURSING CONSIDERATIONS

◆ Provide privacy and emotional support.
◆ Protect the eye from trauma, especially drying of the cornea.
◆ Don't place a gauze eye pad or other objects over the affected eye.
◆ If a slit-lamp examination is needed, explain the procedure to the patient.
◆ If needed, refer the patient to an ophthalmologist for a complete examination.

PEDIATRIC POINTERS

◆ Rhabdomyosarcoma produces rapid onset of exophthalmos.
◆ In Hand-Schüller-Christian syndrome, exophthalmos typically accompanies signs of diabetes insipidus and bone destruction.

PATIENT TEACHING

◆ Explain ways to protect the eye from trauma, wind, and dust.
◆ Explain the proper application of eye drops or ointments to the eye, if prescribed.

Eye discharge

OVERVIEW

- Excretion of any substance other than tears
- Usually occurs with conjunctivitis

HISTORY

- Determine the onset and description of eye drainage.
- Assess the location and description of pain, if needed.
- Inquire about additional signs and symptoms, including burning, tearing, sensitivity to light, and the sensation of something foreign in the eye.

PHYSICAL ASSESSMENT

- Take vital signs.
- Inspect the eye discharge, noting the amount, color, consistency, and source. (See *Assessing the source of eye discharge.*)
- Test visual acuity, with and without correction.
- Examine external eye structures, beginning with the unaffected eye, to prevent cross-contamination.
- Observe for eyelid edema, entropion, crusts, lesions, and trichiasis.
- Ask the patient to blink, watching for impaired lid movement.
- If eyes seem to bulge, measure them with an exophthalmometer.
- Test the six fields of gaze.
- Examine for conjunctival injection and follicles and for corneal cloudiness or white lesions.

 TOP TECHNIQUE

Assessing the source of eye discharge

Eye discharge can come from the tear sac, punctum, meibomian glands, or canaliculi. If the patient reports a discharge that isn't immediately apparent, you can express a sample by pressing your fingertip lightly over these structures. Then characterize the discharge, note its source, and send a specimen for culture, if needed.

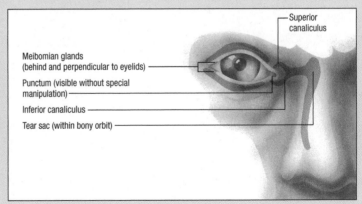

Meibomian glands (behind and perpendicular to eyelids)

Punctum (visible without special manipulation)

Inferior canaliculus

Tear sac (within bony orbit)

Superior canaliculus

MEDICAL

Conjunctivitis

- *Allergic:* With itching and tearing, both eyes excrete a ropy discharge.
- *Bacterial:* Moderate, greenish white purulent or mucopurulent discharge may form sticky crusts on the eyelids during sleep.
- *Viral:* A serous, clear discharge and preauricular adenopathy are usually present.
- *Fungal:* Copious, thick, purulent discharge makes the eyelids crusty and sticky.
- *Inclusion:* Scant mucoid discharge in both eyes is accompanied by pseudoptosis and conjunctival follicles.

Corneal ulcers

- Copious, purulent eye discharge from one eye occurs along with crusty, sticky eyelid.
- Severe pain, photophobia, conjunctival injection, and impaired visual acuity may occur.
- A bacterial corneal ulcer may cause an irregular gray-white area on the cornea, blurred vision, and pupil constriction.
- Fungal corneal ulcers also result in eyelid edema and erythema; and a painless, dense, whitish gray central ulcer that develops slowly and may be surrounded by progressively clearer rings.

Dacryocystitis

- Scant but continuous purulent discharge is produced that's easily expressed from the tear sac.
- Other signs and symptoms include excessive eye tearing, and pain, tenderness, and erythema near the tear sac.

Herpes zoster ophthalmicus

- Moderate to copious serous eye discharge accompanies excessive tearing.
- Other signs and symptoms include eyelid edema and erythema; conjunctival injection, eye pain, and severe facial pain that occurs several days before vesicles erupt; and a white, cloudy cornea.

Keratoconjunctivitis sicca

- Excessive, continuous mucoid discharge due to insufficient tearing occurs.
- Other signs and symptoms include eye pain, itching, burning, a foreign-body sensation, corneal abrasions, dramatic conjunctival injection, and difficulty closing the eye.

Meibomianitis

- A continuous frothy, foul-smelling, cheesy yellow eye discharge may be produced by inflamed eyelid glands.
- The eye appears chronically red, with inflamed lid margins.

Orbital cellulitis

- A purulent eye discharge may be present, but eyelid edema is the obvious sign.
- Other signs and symptoms include exophthalmos, conjunctival injection, headache, orbital pain, impaired visual acuity, limited extraocular movement, and fever.

Psoriasis vulgaris

- Substantial mucous discharge and redness occur in both eyes.
- Lesions occur on the eyelids but may extend to the conjunctiva, causing irritation, excessive tearing, and a foreign-body sensation.

- Apply warm soaks to soften crusts on the eyelids and lashes.
- Gently wipe the eyes with a soft gauze pad.
- Carefully dispose of used dressings, tissues, and cotton swabs.
- Sterilize ophthalmic equipment after use.

PEDIATRIC POINTERS

- In children, eye discharge usually results from eye trauma, eye infection, or upper respiratory tract infection.
- In infants, prophylactic eye drops (silver nitrate) commonly cause eye irritation and discharge.

- Instruct the patient or caregiver about measures to prevent the spread of infection.
- Instruct the patient or caregiver how to give eyedrops, if prescibed.
- Teach about the underlying diagnosis and treatment plan.

Eye pain

OVERVIEW

- Burning, throbbing, aching, stabbing, or foreign-body sensation in eye

 ACTION STAT! *If the patient has eye pain caused by a chemical burn, remove contact lenses and irrigate the eye with at least 1 L of normal saline solution. Evert lids and wipe fornices. If the patient has eye pain from acute angle-closure glaucoma, intervene to decrease intraocular pressure (IOP). If drug treatment doesn't reduce IOP, the patient needs laser iridotomy or surgical peripheral iridectomy to preserve vision.*

HISTORY

- Ask about the onset, description, and duration of pain.
- Find out about other symptoms, such as burning, itching, or discharge.
- Ask about recent trauma, surgery, or headaches.

PHYSICAL ASSESSMENT

- If you suspect trauma, don't manipulate the eye.
- Carefully assess the lids and conjunctivae for redness, inflammation, and swelling.
- Examine the eyes for ptosis and exophthalmos.
- Test visual acuity, with and without correction
- Assess extraocular movements.
- Characterize any discharge. (See *Examining the external eye.*)

CAUSES

MEDICAL
Blepharitis
- Burning pain in both eyelids, itching, sticky discharge, and conjunctival injection occur.

- Other signs and symptoms include foreign-body sensation, lid ulcerations, and loss of eyelashes.

Burns
- With chemical burns, sudden and severe eye pain may occur with erythema and blistering of the face and lids, photophobia, miosis, conjunctival injection, and blurred vision.
- With ultraviolet radiation burns, moderate to severe pain occurs about 12 hours after exposure along with photophobia and vision changes.

Chalazion
- Localized pain, tenderness, redness, conjunctival injection, swelling, and a small red lump develop on the eyelid.
- Other signs and symptoms include tearing and photophobia.

Conjunctivitis
- *Allergic:* Mild, burning pain occurs in both eyes with itching, conjunctival injection, and a ropy discharge.

- *Bacterial:* Pain occurs when it affects the cornea along with burning, a foreign-body sensation, conjunctival injection, and a purulent discharge.
- *Fungal:* Pain occurs when it affects the cornea along with itching, burning, conjunctival injection, photophobia, and a thick, purulent discharge.
- *Viral:* Pain occurs along with itching, red eyes, foreign-body sensation, visible conjunctival follicles, and eyelid edema.

Corneal abrasions
- Eye pain is characterized by a foreign-body sensation.
- Other signs and symptoms include excessive tearing, photophobia, and conjunctival injection.

Corneal erosion, recurrent
- Severe pain occurs on waking and continues during the day along with conjunctival injection and photophobia.

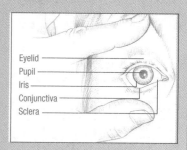

TOP TECHNIQUE

Examining the external eye

For patients with eye pain or other ocular symptoms, examination of the external eye forms an important part of the ocular assessment. Here's how to examine the external eye.

First, inspect the eyelids for ptosis and incomplete closure. Also, observe the lids for edema, erythema, cyanosis, hematoma, and masses. Evaluate skin lesions, growths, swelling, and tenderness by gross palpation. Are the lids everted or inverted? Do the eyelashes turn inward? Have some of them been lost? Do the lashes adhere to one another or contain a discharge? Next, examine the lid margins, noting especially any debris, scaling, lesions, or unusual secretions. Also, watch for eyelid spasms.

Now gently retract the eyelid with your thumb and forefinger, and assess the conjunctiva for redness, cloudiness, follicles, and blisters or other lesions. Check for chemosis by pressing the lower lid against the eyeball and noting any bulging above this compression point. Observe the sclera, noting any change from its normal white color.

Next, shine a light across the cornea to detect scars, abrasions, or ulcers. Note any color changes, dots, or opaque or cloudy areas. Also, assess the anterior eye chamber, which should be clean, deep, shadow-free, and filled with clear aqueous humor.

Inspect the color, shape, texture, and pattern of the iris. Then assess the pupils' size, shape, and equality. Finally, evaluate their response to light. Are they sluggish, fixed, or unresponsive? Does pupil dilation or constriction occur only on one side?

Eyelid
Pupil
Iris
Conjunctiva
Sclera

Corneal ulcers
◆ Severe eye pain may occur with purulent eye discharge, sticky eyelids, photophobia, conjunctival injection, and impaired visual acuity.
◆ Bacterial corneal ulcers produce a grayish white, irregularly shaped ulcer on the cornea, and pupil constriction.
◆ Fungal corneal ulcers produce eyelid edema and erythema, and a dense, cloudy, central ulcer surrounded by progressively clearer rings.

Dacryocystitis
◆ Pain and tenderness occur near the infected tear sac.
◆ Other signs and symptoms include excessive tearing, a purulent discharge, eyelid edema, and swelling of the lacrimal punctum area.

Foreign body in cornea or conjunctiva
◆ Sudden severe pain is common, but vision usually remains intact.
◆ Other signs and symptoms include excessive tearing, photophobia, miosis, a foreign-body sensation, a dark speck on the cornea, and dramatic conjunctival injection.

Glaucoma
◆ *Open-angle glaucoma* may cause mild aching in the eyes as well as halo vision, loss of peripheral vision, and reduced visual acuity that's uncorrected with glasses.
◆ *Angle-closure glaucoma* is characterized by blurred vision and sudden, excruciating pain in and around the eye that may be accompanied by nausea, vomiting, halo vision, rapidly decreasing visual acuity, and a fixed, nonreactive pupil.

Herpes zoster ophthalmicus
◆ Ocular and facial pain occur days before vesicles erupt.
◆ Other signs and symptoms include red, swollen eyelids; excessive tearing; a serous eye discharge; conjunctival injection; and a white, cloudy cornea.

Hordeolum (stye)
◆ Localized eye pain, burning, and discomfort increases as the stye grows.

◆ Eyelid erythema and edema are also common signs.

Hyphema
◆ Sudden pain in and around the eye occurs after eye injury or surgery, when blood enters the anterior eye chamber.
◆ Orbital and lid edema, conjunctival injection, nausea, and visual impairment may develop.

Keratoconjunctivitis sicca
◆ Chronic burning pain occurs in both eyes because of inadequate tear formation.
◆ Other signs and symptoms include itching, a foreign-body sensation, photophobia, dramatic conjunctival injection, difficulty moving the eyelids, and excessive mucoid discharge.

Lacrimal gland tumor
◆ Tumor produces eye pain, impaired visual acuity, and some degree of exophthalmos.

Migraine headache
◆ Migraines can produce head pain so severe that the eyes also ache.
◆ Other signs and symptoms include nausea, vomiting, blurred vision, and light and noise sensitivity.

Optic cellulitis
◆ Dull, aching pain occurs in the affected eye.
◆ Other signs and symptoms include exophthalmos, eyelid edema and erythema, purulent discharge, impaired extraocular movement, and, possibly, decreased visual acuity and fever.

Optic neuritis
◆ Pain in and around the eye occurs with eye movement.
◆ Severe vision loss, tunnel vision, and sluggish pupillary response may develop.

Orbital floor fracture
◆ Eye pain and dramatic eyelid edema occur, possibly with exophthalmos and diplopia.

◆ Other signs and symptoms include reduced vision, ecchymosis, and ptosis.

Uveitis
◆ With anterior uveitis, onset of severe pain is sudden with dramatic conjunctival injection, photophobia, and a small, nonreactive pupil.
◆ With posterior uveitis, onset of pain is insidious, with gradual blurring of vision and distorted pupil shape.
◆ With lens-induced uveitis, moderate eye pain occurs with conjunctival injection, pupil constriction, and impaired visual acuity.

OTHER
Treatments
◆ Contact lenses may cause eye pain and a foreign-body sensation.
◆ Ocular surgery may produce eye pain, ranging from a mild ache to a severe pounding or stabbing sensation.

NURSING CONSIDERATIONS

◆ To reduce eye pain, provide a darkened, quiet environment and have the patient close his eyes.
◆ Give prescribed pain medications, as needed.

PEDIATRIC POINTERS
◆ Trauma and infection are the most common causes of eye pain in children.
◆ Tightly shutting or frequently rubbing the eyes may be nonverbal clues to eye pain.

PATIENT TEACHING

◆ Stress the importance of following instructions for drug therapy.
◆ Instruct the patient about infection control techniques.
◆ Give the patient careful instructions about eye protection.
◆ Explain that the patient should seek medical attention for eye pain.

Facial pain

OVERVIEW

- May result from various neurologic, vascular, or infectious disorders
- May be referred from the ears, nose, paranasal sinuses, teeth, neck, and jaw
- Typically paroxysmal and intense

HISTORY

- Ask about onset, description, location, and duration.
- Determine what alleviates or aggravates the pain.
- Ask about sensitivity to hot, cold, or sweet liquids or foods.
- Obtain a medical and dental history, noting incidence of previous head trauma, dental disease, and infection.

PHYSICAL ASSESSMENT

- Inspect the ear for vesicles and changes in the tympanic membrane.
- Inspect the nose for deformity or asymmetry and characterize any secretions.
- Palpate the sinuses for tenderness and swelling.
- Evaluate oral hygiene.
- Have the patient open and close his mouth as you palpate the temporomandibular joint for tenderness, spasm, locking, and crepitus.
- Assess cranial nerves V and VII. (See *Major nerve pathways of the face.*)

Major nerve pathways of the face

Cranial nerve V has three branches. The *oph-thalmic branch* supplies sensation to the anterior scalp, forehead, upper nose, and cornea. The *maxillary branch* supplies sensation to the midportion of the face, lower nose, upper lip, and mucous membrane of the anterior palate. The *mandibular branch* supplies sensation to the lower face, lower jaw, mucous membrane of the cheek, and base of the tongue.

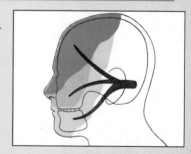

Cranial nerve VII innervates the facial muscles. Its motor branch controls the muscles of the forehead, eye orbit, and mouth.

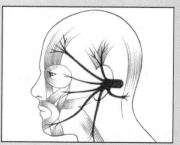

CAUSES

MEDICAL

Angina pectoris
◆ Jaw pain may be described as burning, squeezing, or as feeling tight.
◆ Pain may radiate to the left arm, neck, and shoulder blade.

Dental caries
◆ Caries in the mandibular molars can produce ear, preauricular, and temporal pain.
◆ Caries in the maxillary teeth can produce maxillary, orbital, retro-orbital, and parietal pain.

Herpes zoster oticus
◆ Severe pain localizes around the ear, followed by the appearance of vesicles in the ear.
◆ Eye pain may occur with corneal and scleral damage and impaired vision.

Multiple sclerosis
◆ Facial pain may resemble that of trigeminal neuralgia.
◆ Pain is accompanied by jaw and facial weakness.
◆ Other signs and symptoms include visual blurring, diplopia, and nystagmus; sensory impairment; generalized muscle weakness and gait abnormalities; urinary disturbances; and emotional lability.

Ocular glaucoma
◆ Periorbital pain appears late.
◆ Other signs and symptoms include loss of peripheral vision, reduced visual acuity (especially at night), and seeing halos around lights.

Postherpetic neuralgia
◆ Burning, itching, prickly pain occurs that worsens with contact or movement and persists along any of the three trigeminal nerve divisions.
◆ Mild hypoesthesia or paresthesia and vesicles affect the area before the onset of pain.

Sinusitis, acute
◆ Acute maxillary sinusitis produces pressure, fullness, or burning pain over the cheekbone and upper teeth and around the eyes that worsens with bending over.
◆ Acute frontal sinusitis produces severe pain above or around the eyes that worsens when the patient is in a supine position.
◆ Acute ethmoid sinusitis produces pain at or around the inner corner of the eye.
◆ Acute sphenoid sinusitis produces a persistent, deep-seated pain behind the eyes or nose or on the top of the head that increases with bending forward.

Sinusitis, chronic
◆ Chronic maxillary sinusitis produces a chronic toothache or a feeling of pressure below the eyes.
◆ Chronic frontal sinusitis produces a persistent low-grade pain above the eyes.
◆ Chronic ethmoid sinusitis is characterized by nasal congestion and discharge and discomfort at medial corners of the eyes.
◆ Chronic sphenoid sinusitis produces a persistent low-grade, diffuse headache or retro-orbital discomfort.

Sphenopalatine neuralgia
◆ Deep, boring pain occurs below the ear and may radiate to the eye, the other ear, cheek, nose, palate, maxillary teeth, temple, neck, shoulder, or back of head.
◆ Attacks bring increased tearing and salivation, rhinorrhea, a sensation of fullness in the ear, tinnitus, vertigo, taste disturbance, pruritus, and shoulder stiffness or weakness.

Temporal arteritis
◆ Pain occurs behind one eye or in the scalp, jaw, tongue, or neck.
◆ A typical episode consists of a severe throbbing or boring temporal headache with redness, swelling, and nodulation of the temporal artery.

Temporomandibular joint syndrome
◆ An intermittent severe, dull ache or intense spasm, usually on one side, radiates to the cheek, temple, lower jaw, or ear.
◆ Other signs and symptoms include trismus (lockjaw); malocclusion; and clicking, crepitus, and tenderness of the joint.

Trigeminal neuralgia
◆ Paroxysms of intense pain shoot along the three branches of the trigeminal nerve.
◆ May be triggered by touching the nose, cheek, or mouth; exposure to hot or cold; consuming hot or cold foods or beverages; or even smiling and talking.

NURSING CONSIDERATIONS

◆ Give drugs for pain, as prescribed.
◆ Apply direct heat or give a muscle relaxant, as prescribed.
◆ Provide a humidifier, vaporizer, or decongestant to relieve nasal or sinus congestion.

PEDIATRIC POINTERS
◆ Look for subtle signs of pain, such as facial rubbing, irritability, or poor eating habits.

PATIENT TEACHING

◆ Teach the patient about triggers to avoid.
◆ Explain which signs and symptoms to report.
◆ Teach patient about prescribed medications, dosage, and possible adverse effects.

Fasciculations

OVERVIEW

- Local, painless muscle contractions representing the spontaneous discharge of a muscle fiber bundle innervated by a single motor nerve filament
- Causes visible dimpling or wavelike twitching of the skin, but not strong enough to cause a joint to move
- Occur once every several seconds to two or three times per second
- Benign, nonpathologic fasciculations: common and normal; often occur in tense, anxious, or overtired people and typically affect the eyelid, thumb, or calf
- May also indicate a severe neurologic disorder, most notably a diffuse motor neuron disorder
- Occasionally occurring, myokymia—continuous, rapid fasciculations that cause a rippling effect of muscles at rest

ACTION STAT! *If the onset was sudden, ask about any precipitating events, such as exposure to pesticides. Pesticide poisoning, although uncommon, is a medical emergency requiring prompt and vigorous intervention. You may need to maintain airway patency, monitor vital signs, give oxygen, and perform gastric lavage or induce vomiting.*

HISTORY

- Obtain a history of sensory changes, such as paresthesia, or any difficulty speaking, swallowing, breathing, or controlling bowel or bladder function or pain.
- Ask about a history of neurologic disorders, cancer, recent infections, or stress.
- Ask about dietary habits and for a recall of recent food and fluid intake because electrolyte imbalances may also cause muscle twitching.

PHYSICAL ASSESSMENT

- Perform a physical examination, looking for fasciculations while the affected muscle is at rest.
- Observe and test for motor and sensory abnormalities, particularly muscle atrophy and weakness, and decreased deep tendon reflexes. If you note these signs and symptoms, suspect motor neuron disease, and perform a comprehensive neurologic examination.

MEDICAL

Amyotrophic lateral sclerosis

◆ In this progressive neurologic disorder, coarse fasciculations usually begin in the small muscles of the hands and feet, and then spread to the forearms and legs.

◆ Widespread, symmetrical muscle atrophy and weakness may result in dysarthria; difficulty chewing, swallowing, and breathing; and, occasionally, choking and drooling.

Bulbar palsy

◆ Fasciculations of the face and tongue commonly appear early in bulbar palsy.

◆ Progressive signs and symptoms include dysarthria, dysphagia, hoarseness, and drooling.

◆ Eventually, weakness spreads to the respiratory muscles.

Guillain-Barré syndrome

◆ Fasciculations may occur, but the cardinal neurologic symptom is muscle weakness, which typically begins in the legs and spreads quickly to the arms and face.

◆ Other signs and symptoms include paresthesia, incontinence, footdrop, tachycardia, dysphagia, and respiratory insufficiency.

Herniated disk

◆ Fasciculations of the muscles innervated by compressed nerve roots may be widespread and profound, but the hallmark of a herniated disk is severe lower back pain that may radiate unilaterally to the leg.

◆ Coughing, sneezing, bending, and straining exacerbate the pain.

◆ Other signs and symptoms include muscle weakness, atrophy, and spasms; paresthesia; footdrop; steppage gait; and hypoactive deep tendon reflexes in the leg.

Poliomyelitis, spinal paralytic

◆ Coarse fasciculations, usually transient but occasionally persistent, accompany progressive muscle weakness, spasms, and atrophy.

◆ Other signs and symptoms include decreased reflexes, paresthesia, coldness and cyanosis in the affected limbs, bladder paralysis, dyspnea, elevated blood pressure, and tachycardia.

Spinal cord tumor

◆ Fasciculations, muscle atrophy, and cramps may develop asymmetrically at first and then bilaterally as cord compression progresses.

◆ Motor and sensory changes distal to the tumor include weakness or paralysis, areflexia, paresthesia, and a tightening band of pain.

◆ Bowel and bladder control may also be lost.

Syringomyelia

◆ Fasciculations may occur along with Charcot's joints, areflexia, muscle atrophy, and deep, aching pain in this spinal cord disease.

◆ Other signs and symptoms include thoracic scoliosis and loss of pain and temperature sensation over the neck, shoulders, and arms.

OTHER

Pesticide poisoning

◆ Ingestion of organophosphate or carbamate pesticides commonly produces acute onset of long, wavelike fasciculations and muscle weakness that rapidly progresses to flaccid paralysis.

◆ Seizures, vision disturbances (pupillary constriction or blurred vision), and increased secretions (tearing, salivation, pulmonary secretions, or diaphoresis) may also occur.

◆ Other signs and symptoms include nausea, vomiting, diarrhea, loss of bowel and bladder control, hyperactive bowel sounds, and abdominal cramping. Cardiopulmonary signs and symptoms include bradycardia, dyspnea or bradypnea, and pallor or cyanosis.

◆ Prepare the patient for diagnostic studies, such as spinal X-rays, myelography, computed tomography scan, magnetic resonance imaging, and electromyography with nerve conduction velocity tests.

◆ Prepare the patient for laboratory tests such as serum electrolyte levels.

◆ Help the patient with progressive neuromuscular degeneration perform activities of daily living, and provide appropriate assistive devices.

PEDIATRIC POINTERS

◆ Fasciculations, particularly of the tongue, are an important early sign of Werdnig-Hoffmann disease also known as spinal muscular atrophy.

◆ Teach effective stress management techniques to the patient with stress-induced fasciculations.

◆ Teach about the underlying diagnosis, treatment regimen, and prognosis.

◆ Teach the patient with pesticide poisoning ways to prevent it in the future.

Fatigue

OVERVIEW

- Feeling of excessive tiredness, lack of energy, or exhaustion, with strong desire to rest or sleep
- Reflects hypermetabolic and hypometabolic states in which nutrients needed for cellular energy and growth are lacking

HISTORY

- Review the pattern, onset, and duration of fatigue.
- Ask if the patient has other symptoms.
- Inquire about viral or bacterial illness or stress.
- Ask about nutrition and appetite or weight changes.
- Review the medical and psychiatric history for disorders that produce fatigue.
- Ask about a family history of chronic disorders.
- Obtain a drug and alcohol history.
- Ask about carbon monoxide exposure.

PHYSICAL ASSESSMENT

- Observe the patient's general appearance for overt signs of depression or organic illness.
- Evaluate mental status.
- Take vital signs.
- Perform a complete physical examination.

CAUSES

MEDICAL
Acquired immunodeficiency syndrome
- Fatigue, fever, night sweats, weight loss, diarrhea, and a cough may develop.
- Signs of opportunistic infection and malnutrition may also be apparent.

Adrenocortical insufficiency
- Mild fatigue initially appears after exertion and stress; later, it becomes more severe and persistent.
- Other signs and symptoms include weakness, weight loss, nausea, vomiting, anorexia, abdominal pain, chronic diarrhea, hyperpigmentation, orthostatic hypotension, and a weak, irregular pulse.

Anemia
- Fatigue after mild activity is a common initial symptom.
- Other signs and symptoms include listlessness, irritability, inability to concentrate, pallor, tachycardia, and dyspnea.

Anxiety
- Chronic anxiety invariably produces fatigue characterized as nervous exhaustion.
- Other signs and symptoms include apprehension, indecisiveness, restlessness, insomnia, trembling, and increased muscle tension.

Cancer
- Unexplained fatigue is typically the earliest sign.
- Other signs and symptoms vary with the type of cancer and may include pain, nausea, vomiting, anorexia, weight loss, abnormal bleeding, and a palpable mass.

Carbon monoxide poisoning
- Fatigue occurs with headache, dyspnea, and confusion and can progress to unconsciousness and apnea.

Chronic fatigue syndrome
- Fatigue is incapacitating.
- Other signs and symptoms include sore throat, myalgia, low-grade fever, painful lymph nodes, sleep disturbances, and cognitive dysfunction.

Chronic obstructive pulmonary disease
- Progressive fatigue and dyspnea are the earliest symptoms.
- Other signs and symptoms include a chronic and productive cough, weight loss, barrel chest, cyanosis, slight dependent edema, and poor exercise tolerance.

Depression
- Persistent fatigue unrelated to exertion accompanies chronic depression.
- Other somatic complaints include headache, anorexia, constipation, and sexual dysfunction.
- Other signs and symptoms include insomnia, slowed speech, agitation or bradykinesia, irritability, loss of concentration, feelings of worthlessness, and persistent thoughts of death.

Diabetes mellitus
- Insidious or abrupt fatigue is the most common symptom of this disorder.
- Other signs and symptoms include weight loss, blurred vision, polyuria, polydipsia, and polyphagia.

Heart failure
- Persistent fatigue and lethargy are characteristic.
- Left-sided heart failure produces exertional and paroxysmal nocturnal dyspnea, orthopnea, and tachycardia.
- Right-sided heart failure produces jugular vein distention and, possibly, a slight but persistent nonproductive cough.

Hypercortisolism (Cushing's syndrome)
- Fatigue occurs from sleep disturbances.
- Other signs and symptoms include truncal obesity with slender extremities, buffalo hump, moon face, purple striae, acne, hirsutism, increased blood pressure, and muscle weakness.

Hypopituitarism
- Slowly developing fatigue, lethargy, and weakness occurs.
- Other signs and symptoms include irritability, anorexia, amenorrhea or impotence, decreased libido, hypotension, dizziness, headache, vision disturbances, and cold intolerance.

Hypothyroidism
◆ Fatigue occurs early, along with forgetfulness, cold intolerance, weight gain, metrorrhagia, and constipation.
◆ Other signs and symptoms include coarse hair and alopecia; anorexia; edema; dry, flaky skin; and thinning nails.

Infection
◆ With chronic infection, fatigue is typically the most prominent symptom.
◆ With acute infection, brief fatigue typically accompanies headache, anorexia, arthralgia, chills, and fever.

Lyme disease
◆ Fatigue, malaise, headache, fever, chills, expanding red rash, and muscle and joint aches occur in this tick-borne inflammatory disease.
◆ In later stages, arthritis, fluctuating meningoencephalitis, and cardiac abnormalities may occur.

Malnutrition
◆ Easy fatigability, lethargy, and apathy occur.
◆ Other signs and symptoms include weight loss, muscle wasting, pallor, edema, cold sensation, and dry, flaky skin.

Myasthenia gravis
◆ Easy fatigability and muscle weakness, which worsen as the day progresses, are classic symptoms of this neuromuscular disease.
◆ Symptoms worsen with exertion and subside with rest.

Myocardial infarction
◆ Fatigue can be severe but is typically overshadowed by chest pain.
◆ Other signs and symptoms include dyspnea, anxiety, pallor, cold sweat, increased or decreased blood pressure, and abnormal heart sounds.

Narcolepsy
◆ This sleep disorder commonly causes hypersomnia, hypnagogic hallucinations, cataplexy, sleep paralysis, insomnia, and fatigue.

Renal failure
◆ Acute renal failure causes sudden fatigue with drowsiness and lethargy.
◆ Chronic renal failure causes insidious fatigue and lethargy with marked changes in all body systems.
◆ Other signs and symptoms include oliguria, ammonia breath odor, nausea, vomiting, diarrhea or constipation, dry skin and mucous membranes, muscle twitching, changes in personality and level of consciousness, seizures, and coma.

Restrictive lung disease
◆ Chronic fatigue may accompany dyspnea, cough, cyanosis, and rapid, shallow respirations.

Rheumatoid arthritis
◆ Fatigue, weakness, and anorexia precede joint pain, tenderness, warmth, swelling, and morning stiffness.
◆ Other signs and symptoms include enlarged lymph nodes, fever, leukopenia, subcutaneous nodules, pericarditis, and Raynaud's phenomenon.

Systemic lupus erythematosus
◆ In patients with this inflammatory connective tissue disease, fatigue occurs with generalized aching, malaise, low-grade fever, headache, and irritability.
◆ Other signs and symptoms include joint pain and stiffness, butterfly rash, photosensitivity, Raynaud's phenomenon, patchy alopecia, and mucous membrane ulcers.

Thyrotoxicosis
◆ Fatigue may occur with enlarged thyroid gland, tachycardia, palpitations, tremors, weight loss despite increased appetite, diarrhea, dyspnea, nervousness, diaphoresis, heat intolerance, amenorrhea, and exophthalmos.

Valvular heart disease
◆ Progressive fatigue and a cardiac murmur are accompanied by exertional dyspnea, cough, and hemoptysis.

OTHER
Drugs
◆ Antihypertensives and sedatives may cause fatigue.
◆ In the patient taking digoxin, fatigue may signal toxicity.

NURSING CONSIDERATIONS
◆ Help the patient determine and pace activities.
◆ Encourage rest periods.
◆ Take measures to reduce pain and nausea.
◆ If fatigue results from a psychogenic cause, refer the patient for psychological counseling.

PEDIATRIC POINTERS
◆ Fatigue occurs normally during accelerated growth phases but can also signal depression.
◆ In a pubescent child, consider drug abuse.

GERIATRIC POINTERS
◆ Fatigue may be insidious and mask more serious underlying conditions in this age group.

PATIENT TEACHING
◆ Teach the patient about the underlying disease and treatment plan.
◆ Educate the patient about lifestyle modifications, including diet and exercise.
◆ Stress the importance of pacing his activities and planning rest periods.
◆ Discuss stress management techniques.

Fecal incontinence

- Refers to the involuntary passage of feces
- Follows any loss or impairment of external anal sphincter control
- May be temporary or permanent, with sudden or gradual onset

HISTORY

- Ask about the onset, duration, and severity of fecal incontinence and presence of abdominal pain.
- Note a discernible pattern.
- Note the frequency, consistency, and volume of stools.
- Obtain a medical and surgical history, focusing on incidence of GI, neurological, and psychological disorders.

PHYSICAL ASSESSMENT

- If a brain or spinal cord lesion is the suspected cause, perform a neurologic examination. (See *How the nervous system controls defecation*.)
- If a GI disturbance seems likely, inspect, auscultate, percuss, and palpate the abdomen.
- Inspect the anal area for excoriation or infection.
- Check for fecal impaction.

CAUSES

MEDICAL
Dementia
- Fecal as well as urinary incontinence may occur as the result of any chronic degenerative brain disease.
- Other signs and symptoms include impaired judgment and abstract thinking, amnesia, emotional lability, hyperactive deep tendon reflexes (DTRs), aphasia or dysarthria, and diffuse choreoathetoid movements.

Gastroenteritis
- Temporary fecal incontinence may occur with explosive diarrhea.
- Other signs and symptoms include nausea, vomiting, headache, myalgia, hyperactive bowel sounds, and colicky, peristaltic abdominal pain.

Head trauma
- Fecal incontinence can occur because of neurologic damage.
- Other signs and symptoms depend on the location and severity of the injury and may include decreased level of consciousness, seizures, vomiting, and motor and sensory impairments.

Inflammatory bowel disease
- Nocturnal fecal incontinence may occur with diarrhea.
- Other signs and symptoms include abdominal pain, anorexia, weight loss, blood in stool, and hyperactive bowel sounds.

Multiple sclerosis
- Fecal incontinence varies depending on size and location of plaque within the nervous system.
- Other signs and symptoms include muscle weakness, ataxia, and paralysis; gait disturbances; sensory impairment; blurred vision, diplopia, or nystagmus; urinary disturbances; and emotional lability.

How the nervous system controls defecation

Three neurologic mechanisms normally control defecation: the intrinsic defecation reflex in the colon, the parasympathetic defecation reflex involving sacral segments of the spinal cord, and voluntary control. Here's how they interact. When the rectum is distended by feces, this activates the relatively weak intrinsic reflex, causing afferent impulses to spread through the myenteric plexus, starting peristalsis in the descending and sigmoid colon and in the rectum. The feces move toward the anus, causing receptive relaxation of the internal anal sphincter.

To complete defecation, the parasympathetic reflex magnifies the intrinsic reflex. Stimulation of afferent nerves in the rectal wall sends impulses through the spinal cord and back to the descending and sigmoid colon, rectum, and anus to intensify peristalsis. (See illustration.)

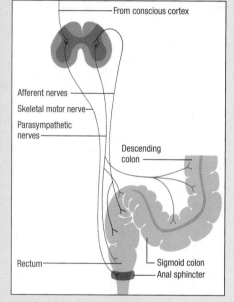

From conscious cortex

Afferent nerves
Skeletal motor nerve
Parasympathetic nerves

Descending colon

Rectum
Sigmoid colon
Anal sphincter

However, when the feces move and the sphincter relaxes, this may cause the external anal sphincter to immediately contract and the feces to be temporarily retained. At this point, conscious control of the external sphincter either prevents or permits defecation. Except in infants or neurologically impaired patients, this voluntary mechanism further contracts the sphincter to prevent defecation at inappropriate times, or relaxes it and allows defecation to occur.

Rectovaginal fistula
◆ Fecal incontinence occurs with uninhibited passage of flatus via the vagina.

Spinal cord lesions
◆ Fecal incontinence occurs that may be permanent, depending on the severity of the lesion.
◆ Other signs and symptoms include motor and sensory disturbances below the level of the lesion.

Stroke
◆ Temporary fecal incontinence occurs that resolves when muscle tone and DTRs are restored.
◆ Persistent fecal incontinence reflects extensive neurologic damage.
◆ Other signs and symptoms include urinary incontinence, hemiplegia, dysarthria, aphasia, sensory losses, reflex changes, and visual field deficits.

Tabes dorsalis
◆ This late sign of syphilis may result in fecal incontinence.
◆ Other signs and symptoms include urinary incontinence, ataxic gait, paresthesia, loss of DTRs and temperature sensation, severe flashing pain, Charcot's joints, Argyll Robertson pupils, and impotence.

OTHER
Drugs
◆ Chronic laxative abuse may cause insensitivity to a fecal mass or loss of the colonic defecation reflex.

Surgery
◆ Pelvic, prostate, or rectal surgery occasionally produces temporary fecal incontinence.

NURSING CONSIDERATIONS

◆ Maintain proper hygiene, including control of odors.
◆ Take measures to allay the patient's embarrassment.
◆ Encourage Kegel exercises to strengthen abdominal and perirectal muscles for the patient with intermittent or temporary incontinence.
◆ Provide bowel retraining for the neurologically capable patient. (See *Bowel retraining tips*.)

PEDIATRIC POINTERS
◆ Fecal incontinence is normal in infants and may occur temporarily in young children who experience psychological regression from stress or a physical illness with diarrhea.
◆ Fecal incontinence may also result from myelomeningocele.

Bowel retraining tips

You can help your patient control fecal incontinence by instituting a bowel retraining program. Here's how:
◆ Begin by establishing a specific time for defecation. A typical schedule is once a day or once every other day after a meal, usually breakfast. However, be flexible when establishing a schedule, and consider the patient's normal habits and preferences.
◆ If necessary, help ensure regularity by administering a suppository, either glycerin or bisacodyl, about 30 minutes before the scheduled defecation time. Avoid the routine use of enemas or laxatives because they can cause dependence.
◆ Provide privacy and a relaxed environment to encourage regularity. If "accidents" occur, assure the patient that they're normal and don't mean that he has failed in the program.
◆ Adjust the patient's diet to provide adequate bulk and fiber; encourage him to eat more raw fruits and vegetables and whole grains. Ensure a fluid intake of at least 1 qt (1 L)/day.
◆ If appropriate, encourage the patient to exercise regularly to help stimulate peristalsis.
◆ Be sure to keep accurate intake and elimination records.

GERIATRIC POINTERS
◆ Age-related changes affecting smooth muscle cells of the colon may change GI motility and lead to fecal incontinence, but disease must still be ruled out.

PATIENT TEACHING

◆ Instruct the patient in the essential techniques of bowel retraining. Give written instructions, if appropriate.
◆ Explain how to do Kegel exercises.
◆ Teach the patient how to maintain proper hygiene.

Fetor hepaticus

OVERVIEW

- Distinctive musty, sweet breath odor that occurs with hepatic encephalopathy, a life-threatening complication of severe liver disease
- Results from the damaged liver's inability to metabolize and detoxify mercaptans produced by bacterial degradation of methionine, a sulfurous amino acid, resulting in circulation in the blood, expulsion by the lungs, and flavoring of the breath

ACTION STAT! *If you detect fetor hepaticus, quickly determine the patient's level of consciousness. If he's comatose, evaluate his respiratory status, including arterial blood gas analysis. Prepare him for intubation, and provide ventilatory support, if necessary. Start I.V. access for fluid administration, begin cardiac monitoring, and insert an indwelling urinary catheter to monitor output. Obtain venous samples for analysis of ammonia, liver function studies, and electrolytes.*

HISTORY

- Obtain a complete medical history, relying on the patient's family, if necessary.
- Focus on any factors that may have precipitated liver disease or coma, such as a recent severe infection; overuse of sedatives, analgesics (especially acetaminophen), alcohol, or diuretics; excessive protein intake; or recent blood transfusion, surgery, or GI bleeding.

PHYSICAL ASSESSMENT

- If the patient is conscious, closely observe him for signs of impending coma.
- Evaluate deep tendon reflexes, and test for asterixis and Babinski's reflex.
- Look for for signs of GI bleeding and shock, common complications of end-stage liver failure, and watch for increased anxiety, restlessness, tachycardia, tachypnea, hypotension, oliguria, hematemesis, melena, or cool, moist, pale skin.
- Evaluate the degree of jaundice and abdominal distention, and palpate the liver to assess the degree of enlargement.

CAUSES

MEDICAL
Hepatic encephalopathy

◆ Fetor hepaticus usually occurs in the final, comatose stage of this disorder but it may occur earlier.
◆ Tremors progress to asterixis in the impending stage, which is also marked by lethargy, aberrant behavior, and apraxia.
◆ Hyperventilation and stupor mark the stuporous stage, during which the patient acts agitated when aroused.
◆ Seizures and coma herald the final stage, along with decreased pulse and respiratory rates, positive Babinski's reflex, hyperactive reflexes, decerebrate posture, and opisthotonos.

NURSING CONSIDERATIONS

◆ Effective treatment of hepatic encephalopathy reduces blood ammonia levels by eliminating ammonia from the GI tract. You may have to administer neomycin or lactulose to suppress bacterial production of ammonia, give sorbitol solution to induce osmotic diarrhea, give potassium supplements to correct alkalosis, provide continuous gastric aspiration of blood, or maintain the patient on a low-protein diet. If these methods prove unsuccessful, hemodialysis or exchange transfusions may be performed.
◆ During treatment, closely monitor the patient's level of consciousness, intake and output, and fluid and electrolyte balance.
◆ Place the patient in a supine position with the head of the bed at 30 degrees. Administer oxygen, if necessary.
◆ Be prepared to draw blood samples for liver function tests, serum electrolyte levels, hepatitis panel, blood alcohol count, a complete blood cell count, typing and crossmatching, a clotting profile, and ammonia level.
◆ Intubation, ventilation, or cardiopulmonary resuscitation may be necessary.

PEDIATRIC POINTERS
◆ A child who is slipping into a hepatic coma may cry, be disobedient, or become preoccupied with an activity.

PATIENT TEACHING

◆ Advise the patient to restrict his intake of dietary protein to as little as 40 g/day. Recommend that he eat vegetable protein rather than animal protein sources.
◆ Inform the patient that medications used to treat and prevent hepatic encephalopathy do so by causing diarrhea, so he shouldn't stop taking the drug when diarrhea occurs.
◆ Teach the patient about all hospital procedures and the purpose of diagnostic tests and blood samples.

Fever

OVERVIEW

- Classified as low (oral reading of 99° to 100.4° F [37.2° to 38° C]), moderate (100.5° to 104° F [38.1° to 40° C]), or high (above 104° F)
- May also be classified as remittent, intermittent, sustained, relapsing, or undulant
- Also called *pyrexia*

  ◆ **ACTION STAT!** *If a patient's fever is higher than 106° F (41.1° C), take the other vital signs and determine level of consciousness (LOC). Give an antipyretic and begin rapid cooling measures. To prevent an exaggerated cooling response, constantly monitor the patient's rectal temperature.*

HISTORY

- Ask about the onset of fever, temperature pattern, highest reading, and treatment attempts.
- Inquire about other symptoms, such as chills, fatigue, or pain.
- Obtain a medical history, including immunosuppressive treatments or disorders, infection, trauma, surgery, diagnostic testing, and use of anesthesia or other drugs.
- Ask about recent travel.

PHYSICAL ASSESSMENT

- Take vital signs.
- Let the history findings direct your physical examination, which may range from brief evaluation of one body system to comprehensive review of all systems. (See *How fever develops*.)

CAUSES

MEDICAL

Anthrax, cutaneous
- Fever may occur with lymphadenopathy, malaise, and headache.
- A small, painless or pruritic, macular or papular lesion develops, changing to a vesicle in 1 to 2 days, and then into a painless ulcer with a characteristic black, necrotic center.

Anthrax, GI
- Fever, loss of appetite, nausea, and vomiting occur after eating contaminated food.
- Abdominal pain, severe bloody diarrhea, and hematemesis may also develop.

Anthrax, inhalation
- Initially, fever, chills, weakness, cough, and chest pain occur.
- Abrupt deterioration—marked by fever, dyspnea, stridor, and hypotension—occurs in the second stage, generally leading to death within 24 hours.

Escherichia coli *0157:H7*
- Fever, bloody diarrhea, nausea, vomiting, and abdominal cramps occur after eating contaminated food.

Immune complex dysfunction
- Fever usually remains low and may be remittent, intermittent, or sustained, relative to the underlying disease.
- Other signs and symptoms also depend on the underlying disease.

Infectious and inflammatory disorders
- Fever varies depending on the disorder and may be remittent, intermittent, sustained, or relapsing.
- Fever may occur abruptly or insidiously.
- Other signs and symptoms involve every body system.

Neoplasms
- Prolonged fever of varying elevations occurs.

How fever develops

Body temperature is regulated by the hypothalamic thermostat, which has a specific set point under normal conditions. Fever can result from a resetting of this set point or from an abnormality in the thermoregulatory system itself, as shown in this flowchart.

Disruption of hypothalamic thermostat by:	*Increased production of heat from:*	*Decreased loss of heat from:*
◆ central nervous system disease ◆ inherited malignant hyperthermia	◆ strenuous exercise or other stress ◆ chills (skeletal muscle response) ◆ thyrotoxicosis	◆ anhidrotic asthenia (heatstroke) ◆ heart failure ◆ skin conditions, such as ichthyosis and congenital absence of sweat glands ◆ drugs that impair sweating

Failure of the body's temperature-regulating mechanisms

FEVER

Elevation of hypothalamic set point

Production of endogenous pyrogens

Entrance of exogenous pyrogens, such as bacteria, viruses, or immune complexes, into the body

---

- Other signs and symptoms include nocturnal diaphoresis, anorexia, fatigue, malaise, and weight loss.

Plague
- Bubonic form causes fever, chills, and swollen, inflamed, and tender lymph nodes near the bite.
- Pneumonic form manifests as a sudden onset of chills, fever, headache, and myalgia.
- Other signs and symptoms of pneumonic form include productive cough, chest pain, tachypnea, dyspnea, hemoptysis, increasing respiratory distress, and cardiopulmonary insufficiency.

Rhabdomyolysis
- This muscle disorder is characterized by fever, muscle weakness or pain, nausea, vomiting, malaise, or dark reddish-brown urine, leading to kidney damage and possible failure.

Severe acute respiratory syndrome
- Disease generally begins with fever greater than 100.4° F (38° C).
- Other symptoms include headache, malaise, a dry nonproductive cough, and dyspnea.

Smallpox
- Initial signs and symptoms include high fever, malaise, prostration, severe headache, backache, and abdominal pain.
- A maculopapular rash develops on the mucosa of the mouth, pharynx, face, and forearms and then spreads to the trunk and legs.
- Within 2 days, the rash becomes vesicular and later pustular; by day 8 or 9, crusts form that later separate, leaving a scar.

Thermoregulatory dysfunction
- Sudden onset of fever that rises rapidly and remains as high as 107° F (41.7° C) occurs in life-threatening disorders.
- Low or moderate fever appears in dehydrated patients.
- Prolonged high fever produces vomiting, anhidrosis, decreased LOC, and hot, flushed skin.

Tularemia
- This infectious disease, also known as *rabbit fever,* causes abrupt onset of fever, chills, headache, generalized myalgia, nonproductive cough, dyspnea, pleuritic chest pain, and empyema.

West Nile encephalitis
- Fever, headache, body aches, skin rash, and swollen lymph nodes occur.
- Severe infection is marked by high fever, headache, neck stiffness, stupor, disorientation, coma, tremors, seizures, and paralysis.

OTHER
Drugs
- Fever can accompany chemotherapy.
- Drugs that impair sweating, such as anticholinergics, phenothiazines, and monoamine oxidase inhibitors, can result in fever.
- Hypersensitivity to antifungals, sulfonamides, penicillins, cephalosporins, tetracyclines, barbiturates, phenytoin, quinidine, iodides, phenolphthalein, methyldopa, procainamide, and some antitoxins can cause fever and rash.
- Muscle relaxants and inhaled anesthetics can trigger malignant hyperthermia.
- Toxic doses of salicylates, amphetamines, and tricyclic antidepressants can cause fever.

TREATMENTS
- A low-grade fever may occur for several days after surgery.
- Transfusion reactions typically produce an abrupt onset of fever and chills.

NURSING CONSIDERATIONS
- Regularly monitor and record temperature.
- Increase fluid and nutritional intake.
- Maintain stable room temperature.
- Provide frequent bedding and clothing changes for diaphoretic patients.
- Give antipyretics according to a regular dosage schedule to minimize chills and diaphoresis.

PEDIATRIC POINTERS
- Infants and young children experience higher and more prolonged fevers, more rapid temperature increases, and greater temperature fluctuations.
- Common pediatric causes of fever include varicella, croup syndrome, dehydration, meningitis, mumps, otitis media, pertussis, roseola infantum, rubella, rubeola, tonsillitis, and adverse reactions to immunizations and antibiotics.
- Be aware that seizures commonly accompany extremely high fever in children.

GERIATRIC POINTERS
- Elderly patients may have impaired thermoregulatory mechanisms, making temperature change a much less reliable measure of disease severity than other measures.

PATIENT TEACHING
- Instruct the patient about the proper way to take oral temperature measurement at home.
- Emphasize the importance of increased fluid intake (unless contraindicated).
- Discuss the use of antipyretics.
- Discuss infection control techniques.

Flank pain

OVERVIEW

- Indicates renal and upper urinary tract disease or trauma
- May range from a dull ache to a severe stabbing or throbbing pain
- May be in one or both flanks, constant or intermittent
- Unaffected by position changes and typically responds to analgesics or treatment of underlying disorder

ACTION STAT! *If the patient has suffered trauma, quickly look for a visible or palpable flank mass, other injuries, costovertebral angle (CVA) tenderness, hematuria, Turner's sign, and signs of shock. If one or more signs of shock are present, insert an I.V. catheter to allow fluid or drug infusion. Insert an indwelling urinary catheter to monitor urine output and evaluate hematuria.*

HISTORY

- Ask about the onset, location, intensity, pattern, and duration of pain.
- Ask what alleviates or aggravates the pain.
- Explore precipitating events to pain.
- Ask about the patient's normal fluid intake and urine output and recent changes.
- Obtain a medical history, including incidence of urinary tract infection (UTI), obstruction, renal disease, or recent streptococcal infection.

PHYSICAL ASSESSMENT

- Obtain vital signs.
- Palpate the flank area and percuss the CVA.
- Obtain a urine sample.

CAUSES

MEDICAL

Bladder cancer

- Dull, constant flank pain radiates to the legs, back, and perineum.
- Initial signs include gross, painless, intermittent hematuria, usually with clots.
- Other signs and symptoms include urinary frequency and urgency, nocturia, dysuria, or pyuria; bladder distention; pain in the bladder, rectum, pelvis, back, or legs; diarrhea; vomiting; and sleep disturbances.

Calculi

- Other signs and symptoms include intense nausea, vomiting, CVA tenderness, hematuria, hypoactive bowel sounds, and signs and symptoms of UTI.

Cystitis, bacterial

- Flank pain occurs along with perineal, lower back, and suprapubic pain.
- Other signs and symptoms include dysuria, nocturia, hematuria, urinary frequency and urgency, tenesmus, fatigue, and low-grade fever.

Glomerulonephritis, acute

- Constant and moderately intense flank pain occurs.
- Classic signs and symptoms include moderate facial and generalized edema, hematuria, oliguria or anuria, and fatigue.
- Other signs and symptoms include low-grade fever, malaise, nausea, vomiting, dyspnea, tachypnea, and crackles.

Obstructive uropathy

- With acute obstruction, flank pain may be excruciating.
- With gradual obstruction, pain is typically a dull ache.
- A palpable abdominal mass, CVA tenderness, and bladder distention vary with the site and cause of the obstruction.
- Other signs and symptoms include nausea, vomiting, abdominal disten-

tion, anuria alternating with periods of oliguria and polyuria, and hypoactive bowel sounds.

Pancreatitis, acute
- Flank pain may develop as severe epigastric or left-upper-quadrant pain that radiates to the back.
- A severe attack causes extreme pain, nausea, persistent vomiting, abdominal tenderness and rigidity, hypoactive bowel sounds, restlessness, low-grade fever, tachycardia, hypotension, and positive Turner's and Cullen's signs.

Papillary necrosis, acute
- Intense flank pain occurs with renal colic, CVA tenderness, and abdominal pain and rigidity.
- Other signs and symptoms include oliguria or anuria, hematuria, and pyuria, with fever, chills, vomiting, and hypoactive bowel sounds.

Perirenal abscess
- Intense pain in one flank and CVA tenderness accompany dysuria, persistent high fever, and chills.

Polycystic kidney disease
- Dull, aching, pain in both flanks is an early symptom.
- Pain may become severe and colicky if cysts rupture and clots migrate or cause obstruction.
- Early signs and symptoms include polyuria, increased blood pressure, and signs of UTI.
- Late signs and symptoms include hematuria, and perineal, lower back, and suprapubic pain.

Pyelonephritis, acute
- Intense, constant flank pain develops.
- Typical signs and symptoms include dysuria, nocturia, hematuria, urgency, frequency, and tenesmus.
- Other common signs and symptoms include persistent high fever, chills, anorexia, weakness, fatigue, myalgia, abdominal pain, and CVA tenderness.

Renal cancer
- Classic signs and symptoms include pain in one flank that's dull and vague, gross hematuria, and a palpable flank mass.
- Signs of advanced disease include weight loss, leg edema, nausea, and vomiting.
- Other signs and symptoms include fever, increased blood pressure, and urine retention.

Renal infarction
- Constant, severe pain in one flank and tenderness typically accompany persistent, severe upper abdominal pain.
- Other signs and symptoms include CVA tenderness, anorexia, nausea, vomiting, fever, hypoactive bowel sounds, hematuria, and oliguria or anuria.

Renal trauma
- Variable flank pain is common.
- A visible or palpable flank mass and CVA or abdominal pain, which may be severe and radiate to the groin, may also develop.
- Other signs and symptoms include hematuria, oliguria, abdominal distention, Turner's sign, hypoactive bowel sounds, nausea, vomiting and, with severe injury, signs of shock.

Renal vein thrombosis
- Severe pain in one flank and lower back pain with CVA and epigastric tenderness are typical.
- Other signs and symptoms include fever, hematuria, and leg edema.

NURSING CONSIDERATIONS

- Give drugs for pain, as prescribed.
- Continue to monitor vital signs.
- Maintain a precise record of intake and output.
- If renal calculi are suspected, strain the patient's urine and send collected sediment for analysis.

PEDIATRIC POINTERS
- Transillumination of the abdomen and flanks may help in assessment of bladder distention and identification of masses in children.
- Common causes of flank pain in children include obstructive uropathy, acute poststreptococcal glomerulonephritis, infantile polycystic kidney disease, and nephroblastoma.

PATIENT TEACHING

- Explain the importance of increased fluid intake (unless contraindicated).
- Explain the patient's underlying condition, treatment plan, and signs and symptoms to report.
- Stress the importance of taking drugs as prescribed.
- Stress the importance of keeping follow-up appointments.

Flatulence

- Sensation of gaseous abdominal fullness
- Reflects slowed intestinal motility, excessive swallowing of air, or increased intraluminal gas production

- Determine the duration and amount of flatulence.
- Ask about other signs, including belching, snoring, and overly rapid speech.
- Inquire about unusual emotional stress.
- Obtain a medical history, including incidence of GI disorders and systemic illnesses.

- Inspect the abdomen for distention.
- Auscultate for abnormal bowel sounds.
- Percuss for increased tympany from gas accumulation.
- Palpate for tenderness and masses.

MEDICAL

Abdominal surgery

◆ When peristalsis resumes, gas accumulation produces flatulence.

Cirrhosis

◆ Early and insidious flatulence occurs.
◆ Other signs and symptoms include anorexia, dyspepsia, nausea, vomiting, diarrhea or constipation, dull right-upper-quadrant pain, hepatomegaly, splenomegaly, fatigue, and malaise.

Colon cancer

◆ Flatulence may be accompanied by abdominal distention and tympany on percussion.
◆ Other signs and symptoms include abdominal pain, anorexia, weight loss, malaise, and altered bowel habits.

Crohn's disease

◆ Flatulence accompanies abdominal pain, cramps, and tenderness; diarrhea; low-grade fever; nausea; and melena in this inflammatory bowel disease.

Irritable bowel syndrome

◆ Chronic flatulence, belching, and excessive flatus occurs.
◆ Chronic constipation, but diurnal diarrhea may occur, and intermittent lower abdominal pain occurs that abates with defecation or passage of flatus.

Lactose intolerance

◆ Flatulence develops within several hours after the ingestion of dairy products.
◆ Other signs and symptoms include cramping, abdominal pain, and diarrhea.

Malabsorption syndromes

◆ Flatulence may occur.
◆ With severe malabsorption, muscle wasting and weakness, skeletal pain, edema, ecchymoses, and ulceration of the tongue may occur.

◆ Other signs and symptoms include abdominal pain, anorexia, weight loss, and passage of bulky, oily, malodorous, or watery stools.

OTHER

Abdominal surgery

◆ When peristalsis resumes, gas accumulation produces flatulence.

Herbal products

◆ Some herbal products, such as garlic, can cause flatulence.

NURSING CONSIDERATIONS

◆ Encourage frequent repositioning, ambulation, and normal fluid intake, as permitted, to prevent gas buildup.
◆ Position the patient on his left side to aid expulsion of gas.
◆ Insert rectal tube, if needed.
◆ Give an enema, suppository, antiflatulent, or anticholinergic.
◆ Provide a diet that excludes gaseous foods.

PEDIATRIC POINTERS

◆ Stomachache commonly results from flatulence.
◆ Children may be more sensitive to flatus-producing foods and aerophagia.

GERIATRIC POINTERS

◆ Increased flatulence may result from poor dentition, leading to poor mastication of food, poor dietary intake, and decreased GI motility.

PATIENT TEACHING

◆ Explain ways to reduce flatulence.
◆ If the patient is lactose intolerant, explain which foods he should avoid.
◆ Teach the patient about an antiflatulence diet. Give written materials, if appropriate. (See *Teaching a patient to follow an antiflatulence diet.*)

Teaching a patient to follow an antiflatulence diet

To help the patient reduce gas, tell him to follow these dietary suggestions:

◆ Avoid these vegetables and fruits: broccoli, brussels sprouts, cabbage, cauliflower, cucumbers, dried beans, green peppers, kohlrabi, lettuce, lima beans, melons, onions, peas, prunes, radishes, and raw apples.
◆ Avoid all fatty foods, such as red meats, fried foods, and pastries.
◆ Avoid foods and beverages that contain excess air, including soufflés, carbonated drinks, and milk shakes.
◆ If you have lactose intolerance, avoid milk, cheese, ice cream, and all other dairy products.
◆ Don't overeat, eat too rapidly, or eat while under emotional stress.
◆ Don't drink large amounts of liquids with meals.
◆ Don't take laxatives.

Fontanel, bulging

OVERVIEW

- Fontanel that is characteristically widened and tense, with marked pulsations
- A cardinal sign of meningitis, associated with increased intracranial pressure (ICP), a medical emergency
- Also may indicate encephalitis, fluid overload, or trauma

◆✦ *ACTION STAT!* *If you detect a bulging fontanel, measure its size and the head circumference, and note the overall shape of the head. Take the infant's vital signs, and determine his level of consciousness (LOC) by observing spontaneous activity, postural reflex activity, and sensory responses. Note whether the infant assumes a normal, flexed posture or one of extreme extension, opisthotonos, or hypotonia. Observe arm and leg movements; excessive tremulousness or frequent twitching may herald the onset of a seizure. Look for other signs of increased ICP: abnormal respiratory patterns and a distinctive, high-pitched cry.*

Ensure airway patency, and have size-appropriate emergency equipment readily available. Provide oxygen, establish I.V. access, and if the infant is having a seizure, stay with him to prevent injury and administer an anticonvulsant, as ordered. Administer an antibiotic, antipyretic, and osmotic diuretic, as ordered, to help reduce cerebral edema and decrease ICP. If these measures fail to reduce ICP, neuromuscular blockade, intubation, mechanical ventilation, and, in rare cases, barbiturate coma and total body hypothermia may be necessary.

HISTORY

- Investigate the underlying cause of increased ICP.
- Obtain the child's medical history from a parent or caretaker, paying particular attention to a recent infection, rash or trauma, including birth trauma.
- Ask about changes in the infant's behavior, such as frequent vomiting, lethargy, or disinterest in feeding.

PHYSICAL ASSESSMENT

- Because prolonged coughing, crying, or lying down can cause transient, physiologic bulging, the infant's head should be observed and palpated while the infant is upright and relaxed to detect pathologic bulging.
- Obtain vital signs and weight.
- Perform a complete physical examination.

CAUSES

MEDICAL

Increased ICP

- Besides a bulging fontanel and increased head circumference, other early signs and symptoms are usually subtle and difficult to discern but may include behavioral changes, irritability, fatigue, and vomiting.
- As ICP rises, the infant's pupils may dilate, and his LOC may decrease to drowsiness and eventual coma.
- Seizures commonly occur.

NURSING CONSIDERATIONS

- Closely monitor the infant's condition, including urine output (via an indwelling urinary catheter, if necessary), and continue to observe him for seizures.
- Restrict fluids, and place the infant in the supine position, with his body tilted 30 degrees and his head up, to enhance cerebral venous drainage and reduce intracranial blood volume.

PATIENT TEACHING

- Explain the purpose and procedure of diagnostic tests to the infant's parents or caretaker. Such tests may include an intracranial computed tomography scan or skull X-ray, cerebral angiography, and a full sepsis workup, including blood studies and urine cultures.
- Explain the purpose of medications, dosages, and possible adverse effects.
- Teach the family about the underlying condition, its treatment, and prognosis.

Fontanel depression

OVERVIEW

◆ Characterized by depression of the anterior fontanel below the surrounding bony ridges of the skull and is a sign of dehydration
◆ Common disorder of infancy and early childhood
◆ May result from insufficient fluid intake, but typically reflects excessive fluid loss from severe vomiting or diarrhea
◆ May also reflect insensible water loss, pyloric stenosis, or tracheoesophageal fistula

ACTION STAT! If you detect a markedly depressed fontanel, take vital signs, weigh the infant, and check for signs and symptoms of shock: tachycardia, tachypnea, and cool, clammy skin. Insert an I.V. catheter and administer fluids, as ordered. Have size-appropriate emergency equipment readily available. Anticipate oxygen administration. Monitor urine output by weighing the wet diapers.

HISTORY

◆ Obtain a thorough patient history from a parent or caregiver, focusing on recent fever, vomiting, diarrhea, feeding routine, and behavioral changes.
◆ Ask about the infant's fluid intake and urine output over the previous 24 hours, including the number of wet diapers during that time.
◆ Ask about the child's pre-illness weight, and compare it with his current weight; weight loss in an infant reflects water loss.

PHYSICAL ASSESSMENT

◆ Obtain vital signs and weight.
◆ Assess the fontanel when the infant is in an upright position and isn't crying.
◆ The anterior fontanel usually closes by age 18 to 20 months.

MEDICAL
Dehydration

◆ In mild dehydration (5% weight loss), the anterior fontanel appears slightly depressed along with pale, dry skin and mucous membranes; decreased urine output; a normal or slightly elevated pulse rate; and possibly irritability.

◆ Moderate dehydration (10% weight loss) causes slightly more pronounced fontanel depression along with gray skin with poor turgor, dry mucous membranes, decreased tears, and decreased urine output. The infant has normal or decreased blood pressure and an increased pulse rate; he may also be lethargic.

◆ Severe dehydration (15% or greater weight loss) may result in a markedly sunken fontanel along with extremely poor skin turgor, parched mucous membranes, marked oliguria or anuria, lethargy, and signs of shock, such as rapid, thready pulse, very low blood pressure, and obtundation.

◆ Monitor the infant's vital signs and intake and output, and watch for signs of worsening dehydration.

◆ Obtain serum electrolyte values to check for an increased or decreased sodium, chloride, or potassium level.

◆ If the patient has mild dehydration, provide small amounts of clear fluids frequently or provide an oral rehydration solution. If the infant can't ingest sufficient fluid, begin I.V. parenteral nutrition, as ordered.

◆ If the patient has moderate to severe dehydration, your first priority is rapid restoration of extracellular fluid volume to treat or prevent shock. Continue to administer the I.V. solution with sodium bicarbonate added, as ordered, to combat acidosis. As renal function improves, administer I.V. potassium replacements, as ordered. Once the infant's fluid status has stabilized, begin to replace depleted fat and protein stores through diet.

◆ Teach the parents about tests to evaluate dehydration such as urinalysis for specific gravity and possibly blood tests to determine blood urea nitrogen and serum creatinine levels, osmolality, and acid-base status.

◆ Teach the parents about dehydration, its causes, and how to prevent it in the future.

◆ Teach the parents how to monitor the infant's fluid intake and output.

Footdrop

- Plantar flexion of foot with the toes bent toward the instep
- Results from weakness or paralysis of dorsiflexor muscles of foot and ankle
- Characteristic sign of certain peripheral nerve or motor neuron disorders; may also result from prolonged immobility when inadequate support, improper positioning, or infrequent passive exercise produces shortening of the Achilles tendon

HISTORY

- Obtain complete medical history.
- Ask about the onset, duration, and character of footdrop.
- Determine what alleviates or aggravates footdrop.
- Ask about weakness or tiredness.

PHYSICAL ASSESSMENT

- Assess muscle tone and strength in feet and legs; compare findings on both sides.
- Assess deep tendon reflexes (DTRs) in both legs.
- Assess the patient's gait.

CAUSES

MEDICAL
Guillain-Barré syndrome
- Footdrop and steppage gait result from profound muscle weakness.
- Weakness begins in the legs and extends to the arms and face within 72 hours, possibly progressing to total motor paralysis and respiratory failure.
- Other signs and symptoms include transient paresthesia, hypoactive DTRs, hypernasality, dysphagia, diaphoresis, tachycardia, orthostatic hypotension, and incontinence.

Herniated lumbar disk
- Footdrop and steppage gait may result from leg muscle weakness and atrophy.
- The most pronounced symptom is lower back pain that may radiate to the buttocks, legs, and feet.
- Other signs and symptoms include sciatic pain, muscle spasms, sensorimotor loss, paresthesia, hypoactive DTRs, and fasciculations.

Multiple sclerosis
- Footdrop may develop suddenly or gradually, producing steppage gait; just as with other multiple sclerosis signs and symptoms, periodic worsening and remission may occur.
- Muscle weakness ranges from minor fatigability to paraparesis with urinary urgency and constipation, depending on size and location of nervous system plaque formation.
- Other signs and symptoms include facial pain, vision disturbances, paresthesia, lack of coordination, and loss of vibration and position sensation in the ankles and toes.

Myasthenia gravis
- Footdrop and limb weakness are common in this neuromuscular disorder.
- Typically, muscle function worsens throughout the day and with exercise and improves with rest; condition may progress to skeletal and respiratory muscle paralysis.

◆ Weak eye closure, ptosis, and diplopia may also develop.

Peroneal muscle atrophy
◆ Footdrop, ankle instability, and steppage gait occur.
◆ Foot, peroneal, and ankle dorsiflexor muscles are affected first.
◆ Other early signs and symptoms include paresthesia, aching, and cramping in the feet and legs, with coldness, swelling, and cyanosis.
◆ As the disease progresses, leg muscles become weak with hypoactive or absent DTRs.
◆ Later, atrophy and sensory loss spread to the arms.

Peroneal nerve trauma
◆ Sudden footdrop resolves with the release of peroneal nerve compression.
◆ Other signs and symptoms include ipsilateral steppage gait, muscle weakness, and sensory loss over the lateral surface of the calf and foot.

Poliomyelitis
◆ Footdrop produces a steppage gait.
◆ Other signs and symptoms include fever, asymmetrical muscle weakness, paresthesia, hypoactive or absent DTRs, and permanent muscle paralysis and atrophy.

Polyneuropathy
◆ Footdrop and steppage gait with muscle weakness progresses to flaccid paralysis.
◆ Other signs and symptoms include muscle atrophy; hypoactive or absent DTRs; paresthesia, hyperesthesia, or anesthesia and loss of vibration sensation in the hands and feet; glossy skin; and anhidrosis.

Spinal cord trauma
◆ Footdrop is sudden in onset and possibly permanent.
◆ Other signs and symptoms include neck and back pain; paresthesia, sensory loss, and muscle weakness, atrophy, or paralysis distal to the injury; asymmetrical or absent DTRs; and fecal and urinary incontinence.

Stroke
◆ Footdrop occurs with arm and leg weakness or paralysis.
◆ Other signs and symptoms include paresthesia, dysphagia, visual field defects, diplopia, bowel and bladder changes, personality changes, amnesia, aphasia, dysarthria, and decreased level of consciousness.

NURSING CONSIDERATIONS

◆ Anticipate physical therapy, in-shoe splints, or leg braces.
◆ Perform range-of-motion exercises and use positioning aids to help prevent footdrop in the immobilized patient.

PEDIATRIC POINTERS
◆ Common causes of footdrop in children include spinal birth defects and degenerative disorders.

PATIENT TEACHING

◆ Explain the use of assistive devices.
◆ Emphasize the safety measures the patient should take—such as asking for assistance with activities.

Gag reflex abnormalities

OVERVIEW

- Normal gag reflex (protective mechanism that prevents aspiration of food, fluid, and vomitus): may be elicited by touching the posterior wall of the oropharynx with a tongue blade or by suctioning the throat; characterized by prompt elevation of the palate, constriction of the pharyngeal musculature, and a sensation of retching
- Abnormal gag reflex (either decreased or absent): interferes with the ability to swallow and, more important, increases susceptibility to life-threatening aspiration

ACTION STAT! *If you detect an abnormal gag reflex, immediately stop the patient's oral intake to prevent aspiration. Quickly evaluate his level of consciousness (LOC). If it's decreased, place him in a side-lying position to prevent aspiration; if not, place him in Fowler's position. Have suction equipment readily available.*

HISTORY

- Ask the patient (or a family member if the patient can't communicate) about the onset and duration of swallowing difficulties and if it's more difficult to swallow liquids than solids.
- If the patient also has trouble chewing, suspect more widespread neurologic involvement because chewing involves different cranial nerves.
- Explore the patient's medical history for vascular and degenerative disorders.

PHYSICAL ASSESSSMENT

- Assess the patient's respiratory status for evidence of aspiration.
- Perform a neurologic examination.

MEDICAL
Basilar artery occlusion
◆ This disorder may suddenly diminish or obliterate the gag reflex.
◆ Other signs and symptoms include sensory loss, dysarthria, facial weakness, extraocular muscle palsies, quadriplegia, and decreased LOC.

Brain stem glioma
◆ This lesion causes gradual loss of the gag reflex.
◆ Involvement of the corticospinal pathways causes spasticity and paresis of the arms and legs as well as gait disturbances.
◆ Other signs and symptoms reflect bilateral brain stem involvement and include diplopia and facial weakness.

Bulbar palsy
◆ Loss of the gag reflex reflects temporary or permanent paralysis of muscles supplied by cranial nerves IX and X.
◆ Other signs and symptoms of this paralysis include jaw and facial muscle weakness, dysphagia, loss of sensation at the base of the tongue, increased salivation, fasciculations, and, possibly, difficulty articulating and breathing.

Myasthenia gravis
◆ In severe myasthenia, the motor limb of the gag reflex is reduced.
◆ Weakness worsens with repetitive use and may also involve other muscles.

Wallenberg's syndrome
◆ Paresis of the palate and an impaired gag reflex usually develop within hours to days of stroke of the brain stem.
◆ Other signs and symptoms may include analgesia and thermanesthesia, occurring ipsilaterally on the face and contralaterally on the body, as well as vertigo, nystagmus, ipsilateral ataxia of the arm and leg, signs of Horner's syndrome (unilateral ptosis and miosis, hemifacial anhidrosis), and uncontrollable hiccups.

OTHER
Anesthesia
◆ General and local (throat) anesthesia can produce temporary loss of the gag reflex.

◆ Continually assess the patient's ability to swallow.
◆ If his gag reflex is absent, provide tube feedings, as ordered; if it's merely diminished, try pureed foods.
◆ Stay with him while he eats and observe for choking.
◆ Remember to keep suction equipment handy in case of aspiration.
◆ Keep accurate intake and output records, and assess the patient's nutritional status daily.
◆ Refer the patient to a speech pathologist to determine his aspiration risk and develop an exercise program to strengthen specific muscles.

PEDIATRIC POINTERS
◆ Brain stem glioma is an important cause of abnormal gag reflex in children.

◆ Advise the patient to avoid thin liquids, take small amounts, and eat slowly while sitting or in high Fowler's position.
◆ Teach the patient about scheduled diagnostic studies, such as swallow studies, computed tomography scan, magnetic resonance imaging, EEG, lumbar puncture, and arteriography.
◆ Teach the patient about the underlying diagnosis.

Gait, bizarre

◆Produced unconsciously by a person with a somatoform disorder (such as hysterical neurosis) or consciously by a malingerer
◆Has no consistent pattern
◆May mimic an organic impairment but characteristically has a more theatrical or bizarre quality with key elements missing, such as a spastic gait without hip circumduction, or leg "paralysis" with normal reflexes and motor strength
◆Manifestations may include wild gyrations, exaggerated stepping, leg dragging, or mimicking unusual walks, such as that of a tightrope walker

◆If you suspect that the patient's gait impairment has no organic cause, begin to investigate other possibilities such as emotional distress.
◆Ask when the gait first developed and whether it coincided with any stressful period or event, such as the death of a loved one or loss of a job.
◆Ask about associated symptoms, and explore any reports of frequent unexplained illnesses and multiple physician's visits.
◆Subtly try to determine if he'll gain anything from malingering, for instance, added attention or an insurance settlement.

◆Test the patient's reflexes and sensorimotor function, noting any abnormal response patterns.
◆To quickly check his reports of leg weakness or paralysis, perform a test for Hoover's sign: Place the patient in the supine position and stand at his feet. Cradle a heel in each of your palms, and rest your hands on the table. Ask the patient to raise the affected leg. In true motor weakness, the heel of the other leg will press downward; in hysteria, this movement will be absent.
◆Observe the patient for normal movements when he's unaware of being watched.

MEDICAL

Conversion disorder

◆ In this rare somatoform disorder, bizarre gait or paralysis may develop after severe stress and is not accompanied by other symptoms.

◆ The patient typically shows indifference toward his impairment.

Malingering

◆ In this rare cause of bizarre gait, the patient may also complain of headache and chest and back pain.

Somatization disorder

◆ Bizarre gait is one of many possible somatic complaints.

◆ Other pseudoneurologic signs and symptoms include fainting, weakness, memory loss, dysphagia, visual problems (diplopia, vision loss, blurred vision), loss of voice, seizures, and bladder dysfunction.

◆ The patient may also report pain in the back, joints, and extremities (most commonly the legs) and complaints in almost any body system.

◆ The patient's reflexes and motor strength remain normal, but he may exhibit peculiar contractures and arm or leg rigidity.

◆ The patient may claim that he can't stand (astasia) or walk (abasia), remaining bedridden although still able to move his legs in bed.

◆ A full neurologic workup may be necessary to completely rule out an organic cause of the patient's abnormal gait.

◆ Remember, even though a bizarre gait has no organic cause, it's real to the patient (unless, of course, he's malingering).

◆ Avoid expressing judgment on the patient's actions or motives; you'll need to be supportive and reinforce positive progress.

◆ Because muscle atrophy and bone demineralization can develop in bedridden patients, encourage range-of-motion exercises, ambulation, and resumption of normal activities.

◆ Consider a referral for physical therapy and psychiatric counseling, as appropriate.

PEDIATRIC POINTERS

◆ Bizarre gait is rare in patients younger than age 8. More common in prepubescence, it usually results from conversion disorder.

◆ Instruct the patient in the use of assistive devices, as necessary.

◆ Review the components of a safe environment, such as establishing a clear path to the bathroom and using proper footwear.

Gait, propulsive

◆ Characterized by a stooped, rigid posture, with head and neck bent forward; flexed, stiffened arms held away from the body; fingers extended; and knees and hips stiffly bent
◆ During ambulation, results in a forward shifting of the body's center of gravity and consequent impairment of balance, causing increasingly rapid, short, shuffling steps with involuntary acceleration (festination) and lack of control over forward motion (propulsion) or backward motion (retropulsion) (see *Identifying gait abnormalities*)
◆ Cardinal sign of advanced Parkinson's disease, resulting from progressive degeneration of the ganglia, which are primarily responsible for smooth muscle movement
◆ Commonly goes unnoticed or unreported until severe disability results, due to being wrongly attributed to normal aging process

◆ Obtain a history of when his gait impairment first developed and whether it has recently worsened. Because he may have difficulty remembering, include family members or friends when gathering information.
◆ Obtain a thorough drug history, including dosages. Ask about tranquilizers, especially phenothiazines.
◆ For the patient with Parkinson's disease, ask about levodopa dosage because an overdose can cause acute worsening of signs and symptoms.
◆ Ask the patient if he has been acutely or routinely exposed to carbon monoxide or manganese.

◆ Begin the physical examination by testing the patient's reflexes and sensorimotor function, noting any abnormal response patterns.

Identifying gait abnormalities

SPASTIC GAIT   SCISSORS GAIT   PROPULSIVE GAIT   STEPPAGE GAIT

MEDICAL
Parkinson's disease
- The characteristic and permanent propulsive gait associated with Parkinson's disease begins early as a shuffle; as the disease progresses, the gait slows.
- Besides the gait, akinesia also typically produces a monotone voice; drooling; masklike facies; stooped posture; and dysarthria, dysphagia, or both.
- Occasionally, it also causes an oculogyric crisis or blepharospasm.
- Other signs and symptoms include progressive muscle rigidity, which may be uniform (lead-pipe rigidity) or jerky (cogwheel rigidity); and an insidious tremor that begins in the fingers, increases during stress or anxiety, and decreases with purposeful movement and sleep.

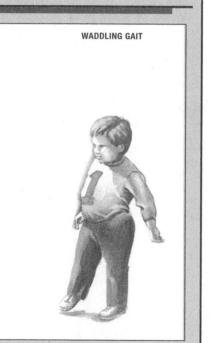

WADDLING GAIT

OTHER
Carbon monoxide poisoning
- Propulsive gait commonly appears several weeks after acute carbon monoxide intoxication.
- Earlier signs and symptoms include muscle rigidity, choreoathetoid movements, generalized seizures, myoclonic jerks, masklike facies, and dementia.

Drugs
- Propulsive gait and other extrapyramidal effects can result from the use of phenothiazines, other antipsychotics (notably haloperidol, thiothixene, and loxapine) and, infrequently, metoclopramide and metyrosine.
- Such effects are usually temporary, disappearing within a few weeks after therapy is discontinued.

Manganese poisoning
- Chronic overexposure to manganese can cause an insidious, usually permanent, propulsive gait.
- Typical early signs and symptoms include fatigue, muscle weakness and rigidity, dystonia, resting tremor, choreoathetoid movements, masklike facies, and personality changes.
- Those at risk for manganese poisoning are welders, railroad workers, miners, steelworkers, and workers who handle pesticides.

- The patient may have problems performing activities of daily living; therefore, assist him as appropriate, while at the same time encouraging his independence, self-reliance, and confidence.
- Encourage the patient to maintain ambulation; for safety reasons, remember to stay with him while he's walking, especially if he's on unfamiliar or uneven ground.
- Refer him to a physical therapist for exercise therapy and gait retraining.

PEDIATRIC POINTERS
- Propulsive gait, usually with severe tremors, typically occurs in juvenile parkinsonism, a rare form.
- Other rare causes include Hallervorden-Spatz disease secondary to loss of muscle control.

- Teach the patient and family about the underlying diagnosis and prevention, if appropriate.
- For the patient with Parkinson's disease, advise the patient and his family to allow plenty of time for activities, especially walking, because festination and poor balance make him more susceptible to falls; also teach them about safety measures.
- Teach the patient about prescribed medication administration, dosage, and possible adverse effects.

Gait, scissors

OVERVIEW

- Results from bilateral spastic paresis (diplegia), affects both legs, and has little or no effect on the arms
- Legs flexed slightly at the hips and knees, giving the appearance of crouching
- With each step, thighs adducting and knees bumping together or crossing in a scissorslike movement (see *Identifying gait abnormalities,* pages 250 and 251)
- Steps short, regular, and laborious, as if wading through waist-deep water
- Feet plantarflexed and turned inward, with a shortened Achilles tendon; results in walking on toes or on balls of feet and, possibly, scraping toes on the ground

HISTORY

- Ask the patient (or a family member if the patient can't answer) about the onset and duration of the gait and whether it has progressively worsened or remained constant.
- Ask about a history of trauma, including birth trauma, and neurologic disorders.

PHYSICAL ASSESSMENT

- Thoroughly evaluate motor and sensory function and deep tendon reflexes (DTRs) in the legs.

CAUSES

MEDICAL
Cerebral palsy
- In the spastic form of this central nervous system disorder, patients walk on their toes with a scissors gait.
- Other signs and symptoms include hyperactive DTRs, increased stretch reflexes, rapid alternating muscle contraction and relaxation, muscle weakness, underdevelopment of affected limbs, and a tendency toward contractures.

Cervical spondylosis with myelopathy
- Scissors gait develops in the late stages of this degenerative disease and steadily worsens.
- Related findings mimic those of a herniated disk: severe lower back pain, which may radiate to the buttocks, legs, and feet; muscle spasms; sensorimotor loss; and muscle weakness and atrophy.

Hepatic failure
- Scissors gait may appear several months before the onset of hepatic failure due to altered glycogen metabolism.
- Other signs and symptoms may include asterixis, generalized seizures, jaundice, purpura, dementia, and fetor hepaticus.

Multiple sclerosis
- Progressive scissors gait usually develops gradually, with periodic remissions typical of this degenerative neurologic disorder.
- Characteristic muscle weakness, usually in the legs, ranges from minor fatigability to paraparesis with urinary urgency and constipation.
- Other signs and symptoms include facial pain, visual disturbances, paresthesia, incoordination, and loss of proprioception and vibration sensation in the ankle and toes.

Pernicious anemia

◆ Scissors gait sometimes occurs as a late sign in untreated pernicious anemia's neurologic complications.
◆ Besides this disorder's classic triad of symptoms—weakness, sore tongue, and numbness and tingling in the extremities—the patient may exhibit pale lips, gums, and tongue; faintly jaundiced sclerae and pale to bright yellow skin; impaired proprioception; incoordination; and vision disturbances (diplopia, blurring).

Spinal cord trauma

◆ Scissors gait may develop during recovery from partial spinal cord compression, particularly with an injury below C6.
◆ Other signs and symptoms may include sensory loss or paresthesia, muscle weakness or paralysis distal to the injury, and bladder and bowel dysfunction.

Spinal cord tumor

◆ Scissors gait can develop gradually from a thoracic or lumbar tumor.
◆ Other signs and symptoms reflect the location of the tumor and may include radicular, subscapular, shoulder, groin, leg, or flank pain; muscle spasms or fasciculations; muscle atrophy; sensory deficits, such as paresthesia and a girdle sensation of the abdomen and chest; hyperactive DTRs; bilateral Babinski's reflex; spastic neurogenic bladder; and sexual dysfunction.

Stroke

◆ Scissors gait occasionally develops during the late recovery stage of bilateral occlusion of the anterior cerebral artery.
◆ Other signs and symptoms may include leg muscle paraparesis and atrophy, incoordination, numbness, urinary incontinence, confusion, and personality changes.

Syphilitic meningomyelitis

◆ Scissors gait appears late in this inflammatory disorder and may improve with treatment.
◆ Other signs and symptoms include sensory ataxia, changes in proprioception and vibration sensation, optic atrophy, and dementia.

Syringomyelia

◆ Scissors gait usually occurs late in this spinal cord disorder along with analgesia and thermanesthesia, muscle atrophy and weakness, and Charcot's joints.
◆ Skin in the affected areas is typically dry, scaly, and grooved.
◆ Other signs and symptoms may include loss of fingernails, fingers, or toes; Dupuytren's contracture of the palms; scoliosis; and clubfoot.

NURSING CONSIDERATIONS

◆ Because of the sensory loss associated with scissors gait, provide meticulous skin care to prevent skin breakdown and pressure ulcer formation.
◆ Promote daily active and passive range-of-motion exercises.
◆ Refer the patient to a physical therapist, if appropriate, for gait retraining and for possible application of in-shoe splints or leg braces to maintain proper foot alignment for standing and walking.

PEDIATRIC POINTERS

◆ The major causes of scissors gait in children are cerebral palsy, hereditary spastic paraplegia, and spinal injury at birth.
◆ If spastic paraplegia is present at birth, scissors gait becomes apparent when the child begins to walk, which is usually later than normal.

PATIENT TEACHING

◆ Give the patient and his family complete skin care instructions to prevent skin breakdown.
◆ If appropriate, provide bladder and bowel retraining.
◆ Teach the patient and family about the underlying diagnosis, lifestyle changes, and adaptations.
◆ Teach about prescribed medication administration, dosage, and possible adverse effects.

Gait, spastic

- Stiff, foot-dragging walk caused by unilateral leg muscle hypertonicity
- Indicates focal damage to the corticospinal tract
- Affected leg rigid, with a marked decrease in flexion at the hip and knee and, possibly, plantar flexion and equinovarus deformity of the foot
- Inability to swing leg normally at hip or knee, therefore, foot drags or shuffles, causing toes to scrape on the ground (see *Identifying gait abnormalities,* pages 250 and 251); pelvis on affected side compensates in attempt to lift toes, causing leg to abduct and circumduct
- Arm swing hindered on same side as the affected leg
- Usually develops after a period of flaccidity (hypotonicity) in affected leg
- Usually permanent

HISTORY

- Obtain a history of when the patient first noticed the gait impairment and whether it developed suddenly or gradually.
- Ask if it waxes and wanes or if it has worsened progressively and if fatigue, hot weather, or warm baths or showers worsen the gait. Such worsening typically occurs in multiple sclerosis.
- Focus your medical history questions on neurologic disorders, recent head trauma, and degenerative diseases.

PHYSICAL ASSESSMENT

- Test and compare strength, range of motion, and sensory function in all limbs.
- Observe and palpate for muscle flaccidity or atrophy.
- Test for Babinski's reflex and deep tendon reflexes.

CAUSES

MEDICAL

Brain abscess

- In this disorder, spastic gait generally develops slowly after a period of muscle flaccidity and fever.
- Early signs and symptoms reflect increased intracranial pressure (ICP), including headache, nausea, vomiting, and focal or generalized seizures.
- Later, site-specific signs and symptoms may include hemiparesis, tremors, visual disturbances, nystagmus, and pupillary inequality.
- The level of consciousness may range from drowsiness to stupor.

Brain tumor

- Depending on the site and type of tumor, spastic gait usually develops gradually and worsens over time.
- Other signs and symptoms may include signs of increased ICP, papilledema, sensory loss on the affected side, dysarthria, ocular palsies, aphasia, and personality changes.

Head trauma

- Spastic gait typically follows the acute stage of head trauma.
- The patient may also experience focal or generalized seizures, personality changes, headache, and focal neurologic signs, such as aphasia and visual field deficits.

Multiple sclerosis

- Spastic gait begins insidiously and follows this neurologic disorder's characteristic cycle of worsening and remission.
- Like other signs and symptoms of multiple sclerosis, the gait commonly worsens in warm weather or after a warm bath or shower.
- Characteristic weakness, usually affecting the legs, ranges from minor fatigability to paraparesis with urinary urgency and constipation.

- Other signs and symptoms include vision disturbances, facial pain, paresthesia, incoordination, and loss of proprioception and vibration sensation in the ankle and toes.

Stroke

- Spastic gait usually appears after a period of muscle weakness and hypotonicity on the affected side.
- Other signs and symptoms may include unilateral muscle atrophy, facial droop, sensory loss, and footdrop; aphasia; dysarthria; dysphagia; visual field deficits; diplopia; and ocular palsies.

NURSING CONSIDERATIONS

- Because leg muscle contractures are commonly associated with spastic gait, promote daily exercise and range of motion—both active and passive.
- The patient may have poor balance and a tendency to fall to the paralyzed side, so stay with him while he's walking.
- Provide a cane or a walker, if indicated.
- Refer the patient to a physical therapist, if appropriate, for gait retraining and possible application of in-shoe splints or leg braces to maintain proper foot alignment for standing and walking.

PEDIATRIC POINTERS

- Causes of spastic gait in children include sickle cell crisis, cerebral palsy, porencephalic cysts, and arteriovenous malformation that causes hemorrhage or ischemia.

PATIENT TEACHING

- Teach the patient how to use a cane or walker, if appropriate.
- Teach the patient and family safety measures to reduce risk of falling.
- Teach the patient about the underlying diagnosis and treatment options.

Gait, steppage

OVERVIEW

- Typically results from footdrop caused by weakness or paralysis of pretibial and peroneal muscles, usually from lower motor neuron lesions
- Characterized by foot hanging with toes pointing down, causing the toes to scrape the ground during ambulation; hip rotated outward to compensate with exaggerated hip and knee flexion to lift the advancing leg off the ground
- Foot hurls forward, with toes hitting the ground first, producing an audible slap (see *Identifying gait abnormalities,* pages 250 and 251)
- Has a regular rhythm, with even steps and normal upper body posture and arm swing
- May be unilateral or bilateral and permanent or transient, depending on the site and type of neural damage

HISTORY

- Begin by asking the patient about the onset of the gait and any recent changes in its character.
- Ask about family history of gait disturbance, traumatic injury to the buttocks, hips, legs, or knees, or chronic disorders that may be associated with polyneuropathy, such as diabetes mellitus, polyarteritis nodosa, and alcoholism.

PHYSICAL ASSESSMENT

- Observe whether the patient crosses his legs while sitting because this may put pressure on the peroneal nerve.
- Inspect and palpate the patient's calves and feet for muscle atrophy and wasting.
- Using a pin, test for sensory deficits along the entire length of both legs.

CAUSES

MEDICAL
Guillain-Barré syndrome

- Typically occurring after recovery from the acute stage of this neurologic disorder, steppage gait can be mild or severe and unilateral or bilateral; it's invariably permanent.
- Muscle weakness usually begins in the legs, extends to the arms and face within 72 hours, and can progress to total motor paralysis and respiratory failure.
- Other signs and symptoms include footdrop, transient paresthesia, hypernasality, dysphagia, diaphoresis, tachycardia, orthostatic hypotension, and incontinence.

Herniated lumbar disk

- Unilateral steppage gait and footdrop commonly occur with late-stage weakness and atrophy of leg muscles.
- The most pronounced symptom of a herniated lumbar disk is severe lower back pain, which may radiate to the buttocks, legs, and feet, usually unilaterally.
- Sciatic pain follows, often accompanied by muscle spasms and sensorimotor loss. Paresthesia and fasciculations may also occur.

Multiple sclerosis

- Steppage gait and footdrop follow a characteristic cycle of periodic worsening and remission in this neurologic disorder.
- Muscle weakness, usually affecting the legs, can range from minor fatigability to paraparesis with urinary urgency and constipation.
- Other signs and symptoms include facial pain, visual disturbances, paresthesia, incoordination, and sensory loss in the ankle and toes.

Peroneal muscle atrophy

◆ Bilateral steppage gait and footdrop begin insidiously in this disorder.
◆ Other early signs and symptoms include paresthesia, aching, cramping, coldness, swelling, and cyanosis in the feet and legs. Foot, peroneal, and ankle dorsiflexor muscles are affected first.
◆ As the disorder progresses, all leg muscles become weak and atrophic, with hypoactive or absent deep tendon reflexes (DTRs). Later, atrophy and sensory loss spread to the hands and arms.

Peroneal nerve trauma

◆ Temporary ipsilateral steppage gait occurs suddenly but resolves with the release of peroneal nerve pressure.
◆ Steppage gait is associated with footdrop, muscle weakness, and sensory loss over the lateral surface of the calf and foot.

Poliomyelitis

◆ Steppage gait, usually permanent and unilateral, commonly develops after the acute stage of poliomyelitis.
◆ Fever typically occurs first, accompanied by such signs and symptoms as asymmetrical muscle weakness, coarse fasciculations, paresthesia, hypoactive or absent DTRs, and permanent muscle paralysis and atrophy.
◆ Dysphagia, urine retention, and respiratory difficulty may also occur.

Polyneuropathy

◆ Diabetic polyneuropathy is a rare cause of bilateral steppage gait, which appears as a late but permanent effect.
◆ This sign is preceded by burning pain in the feet and is accompanied by leg weakness, sensory loss, and skin ulcers.

◆ In polyarteritis nodosa with polyneuropathy, unilateral or bilateral steppage gait is a late finding.
◆ Other signs and symptoms include vague leg pain, abdominal pain, hematuria, fever, and increased blood pressure.
◆ In alcoholic polyneuropathy, steppage gait appears 2 to 3 months after the onset of vitamin B deficiency. The gait may be bilateral, and it resolves with treatment of the deficiency. Early signs and symptoms include paresthesia in the feet, leg muscle weakness, and, possibly, sensory ataxia.

Spinal cord trauma

◆ In an ambulatory patient, spinal cord trauma may cause steppage gait.
◆ Paresthesia, sensory loss, asymmetrical or absent DTRs, and muscle weakness or paralysis may occur distal to the injury.
◆ Fecal and urinary incontinence may also occur.
◆ Other signs and symptoms vary with the severity of injury and may include unilateral or bilateral footdrop, neck and back pain, and vertebral tenderness and deformity.

NURSING CONSIDERATIONS

◆ The patient with steppage gait may tire rapidly when walking because of the extra effort he must expend to lift his feet off the ground. Help the patient recognize his exercise limits, and encourage him to get adequate rest.
◆ Refer patient to a physical therapist, if appropriate, for gait retraining and possible application of in-shoe splints or leg braces to maintain correct foot alignment.

PATIENT TEACHING

◆ Teach the patient about safety measures he can take at home to prevent falls.
◆ Teach patient about the underlying diagnosis and treatment options.

Gait, waddling

OVERVIEW

- Distinctive ducklike walk that's an important sign of muscular dystrophy, spinal muscle atrophy or, rarely, congenital hip displacement
- May be present when the child begins to walk or may appear later in life
- Results from deterioration of the pelvic girdle muscles—primarily the gluteus medius, hip flexors, and hip extensors—which results in instability of the weight-bearing hip during walking, thus causing the opposite hip to drop and the trunk to lean toward that side in an attempt to maintain balance (see *Identifying gait abnormalities,* pages 250 and 251)
- Typical wide stance, with trunk thrown back to further improve stability, exaggerating lordosis and abdominal protrusion
- In severe cases, may cause equinovarus deformity of the foot combined with circumduction or bowing of the legs

HISTORY

- Ask the patient (or a family member if the patient is a young child) when the gait first appeared and if it has recently worsened.
- To determine the extent of pelvic girdle and leg muscle weakness, ask if the patient falls frequently or has difficulty climbing stairs, rising from a chair, or walking; also find out if he was late in learning to walk or holding his head upright.
- Obtain a family history, focusing on problems of muscle weakness and gait and on congenital motor disorders.

PHYSICAL ASSESSMENT

- Inspect and palpate leg muscles, especially in the calves, for size and tone.
- Check for a positive Gowers' sign, which indicates pelvic muscle weakness. (See *Identifying Gowers' sign.*)
- Assess motor strength and function in the shoulders, arms, and hands, looking for weakness or asymmetrical movements.

  TOP TECHNIQUE

Identifying Gowers' sign

To check for Gowers' sign, place the patient in the supine position and ask him to rise. A positive Gowers' sign—an inability to lift the trunk without using the hands and arms to brace and push—indicates pelvic muscle weakness, as occurs in muscular dystrophy and spinal muscle atrophy.

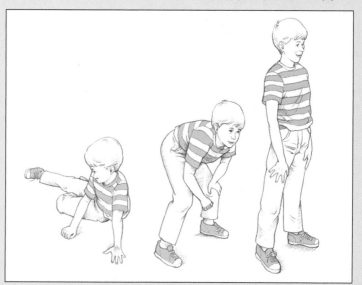

CAUSES

MEDICAL

Developmental dysplasia of the hip

◆ Bilateral hip dislocation produces a waddling gait with lordosis and pain.

Muscular dystrophy

◆ In *Duchenne's muscular dystrophy*, waddling gait becomes clinically evident by ages 3 to 5. The gait worsens as the disease progresses, until the child loses the ability to walk and needs a wheelchair, usually between ages 10 and 12.

– Early signs are usually subtle and include a delay in learning to walk, frequent falls, gait or posture abnormalities, and intermittent calf pain.

– Common later signs and symptoms include lordosis with abdominal protrusion, a positive Gowers' sign, and equinovarus foot position.

– As the disease progresses, its signs and symptoms become more prominent; they commonly include rapid muscle wasting beginning in the legs and spreading to the arms (although calf and upper arm muscles may become hypertrophied, firm, and rubbery), muscle contractures, limited dorsiflexion of the feet and extension of the knees and elbows, obesity and, possibly, mild mental retardation.

– If kyphoscoliosis develops, it may lead to respiratory dysfunction and, eventually, death from cardiac or respiratory failure.

◆ In *Becker's muscular dystrophy*, waddling gait typically becomes apparent in late adolescence, slowly worsens during the third decade, and culminates in total loss of ambulation. Muscle weakness first appears in the pelvic and upper arm muscles. Progressive wasting with selected muscle hypertrophy produces lordosis with abdominal protrusion, poor balance, a positive Gowers' sign and, possibly, mental retardation.

◆ In *facioscapulohumeral muscular dystrophy*, which usually occurs late in childhood or during adolescence, waddling gait appears after muscle wasting has spread downward from the face and shoulder girdle to the pelvic girdle and legs.

– Early signs and symptoms include progressive weakness and atrophy of facial, shoulder, and arm muscles; slight lordosis; and pelvic instability.

Spinal muscle atrophy

◆ In *Kugelberg-Welander syndrome*, waddling gait occurs early (usually after age 2) and typically progresses slowly, culminating in total loss of ambulation up to 20 years later.

– Other signs and symptoms may include muscle atrophy in the legs and pelvis, progressing to the shoulders; a positive Gowers' sign; ophthalmoplegia; and tongue fasciculations.

◆ In *Werdnig-Hoffmann disease*, waddling gait typically begins when the child learns to walk. Reflexes may be absent. The gait progressively worsens, culminating in complete loss of ambulation by adolescence.

– Other signs and symptoms include lordosis with abdominal protrusion and muscle weakness in the hips and thighs.

NURSING CONSIDERATIONS

◆ Although there's no cure for waddling gait due to muscle diseases, daily passive and active muscle-stretching exercises should be performed for both arms and legs.

◆ If possible, have the patient walk at least 3 hours each day (with leg braces if necessary) to maintain muscle strength, reduce contractures, and delay further gait deterioration.

◆ Stay with the patient when he's walking, especially if he's on unfamiliar or uneven ground.

◆ Provide a balanced diet to maintain energy levels and prevent obesity.

◆ Because of the grim prognosis associated with muscular dystrophy and spinal muscle atrophy, provide emotional support for the patient and his family.

PATIENT TEACHING

◆ Caution the patient against long, unbroken periods of bed rest, which accelerate muscle deterioration.

◆ Refer him to a local chapter of the Muscular Dystrophy Association.

◆ Teach the parents about genetic testing and counseling if they're considering having another child.

Gallop, atrial (S₄)

OVERVIEW

◆ Refers to a fourth (S$_4$) heart sound heard or palpated before the S$_1$
◆ Low-pitched sound that originates from left atrial contraction
◆ Best heard with the bell of the stethoscope pressed lightly against the cardiac apex (see *Locating heart sounds* and *Interpreting atrial gallop*)
◆ Also known as *presystolic gallop*

ACTION STAT! *If the patient has chest pain, suspect myocardial ischemia. Take vital signs and assess for signs of heart failure. Connect the patient to the cardiac monitor, obtain an electrocardiogram, and administer oxygen and an antianginal, as prescribed. If the patient has dyspnea, elevate the head of the bed. If you detect coarse crackles, give oxygen and diuretics, as prescribed. If the patient has symptomatic bradycardia, he may need atropine and a pacemaker. Have temporary external pacemaker and emergency equipment readily available.*

HISTORY

◆ Obtain a medical history, including incidence of hypertension, angina, cardiomyopathy, or valvular stenosis.
◆ Ask about the frequency and severity of anginal attacks.

PHYSICAL ASSESSMENT

◆ Take vital signs.
◆ Perform a complete cardiopulmonary examination.
◆ Obtain blood samples for testing.
◆ Obtain ECG.

TOP TECHNIQUE

Interpreting atrial gallop

Detecting subtle variations in heart sounds requires both concentration and practice. Once you recognize normal heart sounds, the abnormal sounds, such as atrial gallop, become more obvious.

HEART SOUND AND CAUSE

Atrial gallop (S$_4$)
Vibrations produced by an increased resistance to sudden, forceful ejection of atrial blood

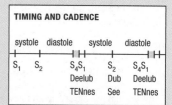

TIMING AND CADENCE					
systole	diastole		systole		diastole
S$_1$	S$_2$	S$_4$ S$_1$		S$_2$	S$_4$ S$_1$
		Deelub		Dub	Deelub
		TENnes		See	TENnes

AUSCULTATION TIPS

◆ Best heard through the bell of the stethoscope at the apex with the patient in the left semilateral position
◆ May be visible in late diastole at the midclavicular line between the fourth and fifth intercostal spaces
◆ May also be palpable in the midclavicular area with the patient in the left lateral decubitus position

---

TOP TECHNIQUE

Locating heart sounds

When auscultating for heart sounds, remember that certain sounds are heard best in specific areas. Use the auscultatory points shown here to locate heart sounds quickly and accurately. Then expand your auscultation to nearby areas.

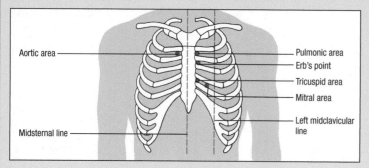

Aortic area
Midsternal line
Pulmonic area
Erb's point
Tricuspid area
Mitral area
Left midclavicular line

MEDICAL

Anemia

◆ An atrial gallop may accompany compensatory increased cardiac output.
◆ Other signs and symptoms may include fatigue, pallor, dyspnea, tachycardia, a bounding pulse, crackles, jugular vein distention, and a systolic bruit over the carotid arteries.

Angina

◆ An intermittent atrial gallop typically occurs during an attack.
◆ The gallop may be accompanied by paradoxical S_2 or a new murmur.
◆ Other signs and symptoms include chest tightness, pressure, aching, or burning that radiates to the neck, jaw, left shoulder, and arm; dyspnea; tachycardia; increased blood pressure; diaphoresis; dizziness; nausea; and vomiting.

Aortic insufficiency, acute

◆ Atrial gallop is accompanied by a soft, short diastolic murmur along the left sternal border.
◆ S_2 may be soft or absent and a soft, short midsystolic murmur may be heard over the second right intercostal space.
◆ Other signs and symptoms include tachycardia, dyspnea, jugular vein distention, crackles, cool extremities, and angina.

Aortic stenosis

◆ Atrial gallop occurs with severe valvular obstruction.
◆ Auscultation reveals a harsh, crescendo-decrescendo (louder-then-softer), systolic-ejection murmur.
◆ Angina and syncope on exertion are principal symptoms.
◆ Other signs and symptoms include crackles, orthopnea, palpitations, fatigue, and diminished carotid pulses.

Atrioventricular block

◆ First-degree atrioventricular (AV) block may cause an atrial gallop accompanied by a faint S_1, but the patient remains asymptomatic.
◆ Second-degree AV block produces an atrial gallop.
◆ Third-degree AV block produces an atrial gallop that varies in intensity with S_1.
◆ Other signs and symptoms include hypotension, light-headedness, dizziness, angina, and syncope.

Cardiomyopathy

◆ Atrial gallop is accompanied with such signs and symptoms as dyspnea, orthopnea, crackles, fatigue, syncope, chest pain, palpitations, edema, jugular vein distention, S_3, and tachycardia-bradycardia syndrome.

Hypertension

◆ Atrial gallop is an early symptom.
◆ Other signs and symptoms include headache, weakness, epistaxis, tinnitus, dizziness, and fatigue.

Mitral insufficiency

◆ Atrial gallop occurs with an S_3.
◆ Other signs and symptoms include a harsh holosystolic murmur, fatigue, dyspnea, tachypnea, orthopnea, tachycardia, crackles, and jugular vein distention.

Myocardial infarction

◆ Atrial gallop signifies a life-threatening myocardial infarction and may persist after the infarction heals.
◆ Crushing substernal chest pain may radiate to the back, neck, jaw, shoulder, and left arm.
◆ Other signs and symptoms include dyspnea, restlessness, anxiety, a feeling of impending doom, diaphoresis, pallor, clammy skin, nausea, vomiting, and increased or decreased blood pressure.

Pulmonary embolism

◆ A life-threatening disorder, right-sided atrial gallop is heard along the lower left sternal border with a loud pulmonic closure sound.
◆ Other signs and symptoms include tachycardia, tachypnea, fever, chest pain, diaphoresis, syncope, cyanosis, and a nonproductive or productive cough with blood-tinged sputum.

Thyrotoxicosis

◆ Atrial gallop occurs with an S_3.
◆ Other signs and symptoms include tachycardia, bounding pulse, widened pulse pressure, palpitations, weight loss despite increased appetite, diarrhea, tremors, an enlarged thyroid gland, dyspnea, nervousness, difficulty concentrating, heat intolerance, exophthalmos, weakness, fatigue, and muscle atrophy.

◆ Monitor for signs and symptoms of heart failure.
◆ Give drugs and oxygen, as prescribed.

PEDIATRIC POINTERS

◆ Atrial gallop may occur normally in children, especially after exercise, or may result from congenital heart disease.

GERIATRIC POINTERS

◆ Atrial gallop may occur normally in elderly patients.

◆ Discuss with the patient ways to reduce his cardiac risk.
◆ Teach the patient the correct way to measure his pulse rate.
◆ Emphasize conditions that require medical attention.
◆ Stress the importance of follow-up appointments.

Gallop, ventricular (S₃)

- Refers to a third heart sound (S₃) after the S₂
- May be physiologic or pathologic; normal S₃ may occur in children and adults up to age 40 and during the third trimester of pregnancy
- Associated with rapid ventricular filling in early diastole
- Best heard along the lower left sternal border or over the xiphoid region on inspiration (right-sided) or at the apex on expiration (left-sided)

- Ask about location, frequency, and duration of chest pain, if present, and what aggravates and alleviates it.
- Ask about palpitations, dizziness, syncope, difficulty breathing, or cough.
- Obtain a medical history, including incidence of cardiac disorders.
- Obtain a drug history.

- Auscultate for murmurs or abnormalities in S₁ and S₂. (See *Auscultating the heart* and *Interpreting ventricular gallop.*)
- Listen for pulmonary crackles.
- Assess peripheral pulses.
- Palpate the liver.
- Assess for jugular vein distention abdominal distension, and peripheral edema.

TOP TECHNIQUE

Auscultating the heart

Follow these tips when you auscultate a patient's heart:

◆ Until you become proficient at auscultation and can examine a patient quickly, explain to him that even though you may listen to his chest for a long period, it doesn't mean that anything is wrong.

◆ Concentrate as you listen for each sound.

◆ Avoid auscultating through clothing or wound dressings because they can block sound.

◆ Avoid picking up extraneous sounds by keeping the stethoscope tubing off the patient's body and other surfaces.

◆ Ask the patient to breathe normally and to hold his breath periodically to enhance sounds that may be difficult to hear.

TOP TECHNIQUE

Interpreting ventricular gallop

Detecting subtle variations in heart sounds requires both concentration and practice. Once you recognize normal heart sounds, the abnormal sounds, such as ventricular gallop, become more obvious.

HEART SOUND AND CAUSE

Ventricular gallop (S₃)
Vibrations produced by rapid blood flow into the ventricles

TIMING AND CADENCE				
systole	diastole	systole	diastole	
S₁	S₂S₃	S₁	S₂S₃	S₁
lub	dubDEE	lub	dubDEE	
ken	tucKY	ken	tucKY	

AUSCULTATION TIPS

◆ Best heard through the bell of the stethoscope at the apex with the patient in the left lateral position

◆ May be visible and palpable during early diastole at the midclavicular line between the fourth and fifth intercostal spaces

---

MEDICAL

Aortic insufficiency
◆ In acute cases, ventricular and atrial gallops may occur with a soft, short diastolic murmur.
◆ Other signs and symptoms include tachycardia, dyspnea, jugular vein distention, and crackles.
◆ In chronic cases, a ventricular gallop and a high-pitched, blowing, decrescendo diastolic murmur occur.
◆ Other signs and symptoms include tachycardia, palpitations, angina, fatigue, dyspnea, orthopnea, and crackles.

Cardiomyopathy
◆ Ventricular gallop is a common symptom.
◆ When associated with fluctuating pulse and altered S_1 and S_2, it signals advanced heart disease.
◆ Other signs and symptoms include fatigue, dyspnea, orthopnea, chest pain, palpitations, syncope, crackles, peripheral edema, jugular vein distention, and an atrial gallop.

Heart failure
◆ Ventricular gallop is a classic symptom.
◆ Sinus tachycardia occurs with left-sided heart failure.
◆ Other signs and symptoms of left-sided heart failure include fatigue, exertional dyspnea, paroxysmal nocturnal dyspnea, orthopnea, and a dry cough.
◆ Jugular vein distention occurs with right-sided heart failure.
◆ Other late signs and symptoms of right-sided heart failure include tachypnea, chest tightness, palpitations, anorexia, nausea, dependent edema, weight gain, slowed mental response, hepatomegaly, and pallor.

Mitral insufficiency
◆ In acute cases, ventricular gallop may be accompanied by an early or holosystolic decrescendo murmur at the apex, an atrial gallop, and a widely split second heart sound.

◆ Other signs and symptoms of acute valvular disease include tachycardia, tachypnea, orthopnea, dyspnea, crackles, jugular vein distention, peripheral edema, hepatomegaly, and fatigue.
◆ In chronic cases, ventricular gallop is progressively severe and accompanied by fatigue, exertional dyspnea, and palpitations.

Thyrotoxicosis
◆ Ventricular and atrial gallops may occur.
◆ Other signs and symptoms include an enlarged thyroid gland, weight loss despite increased appetite, heat intolerance, diaphoresis, nervousness, tremors, tachycardia, palpitations, diarrhea, and dyspnea.

◆ Assess for tachycardia, dyspnea, crackles, and jugular vein distention.
◆ To prevent pulmonary edema, give oxygen, diuretics, and other drugs, such as digoxin and angiotensin-converting enzyme inhibitors, as prescribed.

PEDIATRIC POINTERS
◆ Ventricular gallop is normally heard in children, but may accompany congenital abnormalities associated with heart failure or result from sickle cell anemia.

◆ Explain dietary and fluid restrictions the patient needs.
◆ Stress the importance of scheduled rest periods.
◆ Explain signs and symptoms of fluid overload that the patient should report.
◆ Teach the patient how to measure and monitor his daily weight.
◆ Teach the patient about the underlying condition and treatment options.

Genital lesions, male

- Include warts, papules, ulcers, scales, and pustules
- May be painful or painless, singular or multiple
- May result from infection, neoplasms, parasites, allergy, or drugs

HISTORY

- Ask about the onset and description of lesions.
- Obtain a description of drainage, itching, or pain.
- Take a sexual history, including frequency of relations, number of sexual partners, and pattern of condom use.

PHYSICAL ASSESSMENT

- Observe the patient for tight clothing and history of circumcision.
- Examine the skin, noting location, size, color, and pattern of lesions. (See *Recognizing common genital lesions in males.*)
- Palpate for nodules, masses, and tenderness.
- Look for bleeding, edema, or signs of infection.
- Take vital signs.

CAUSES

MEDICAL

Balanitis and balanoposthitis

- Painful ulceration on the glans, foreskin, or penile shaft occurs as a result of infection.
- Prepuce irritation and soreness precede ulceration by 2 to 3 days, followed by a foul discharge and edema.
- Other signs and symptoms include fever with chills, malaise, and dysuria.

Bowen's disease

- Painless, premalignant lesion appears as a brownish red, raised, scaly, indurated plaque with well-defined borders, usually on the penis or scrotum.

Candidiasis

- With this infection, erythematous, weepy, circumscribed lesions usually appear under the prepuce.
- Vesicles and pustules and ulcerations of the glans penis may also develop.

Chancroid

- One or more lesions erupt on the groin, inner thigh, or penis in this sexually transmitted disease (STD).
- Lesions progress from a reddened area to a small papule, then to a pustule that ulcerates.
- Ulcer is painful, deep, bleeds easily, and has a purulent gray or yellow exudate.

Recognizing common genital lesions in males

Various lesions may affect male genitalia. Some of the more common lesions and their causes appear below.

A *fixed drug eruption* causes a bright red to purplish lesion on the glans penis.

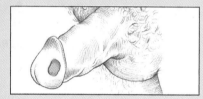

Genital warts are marked by clusters of flesh-colored papillary growths that may be barely visible or several inches in diameter.

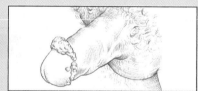

Genital herpes begins as a swollen, slightly pruritic wheal and later becomes a group of small vesicles or blisters on the foreskin, glans, or penile shaft.

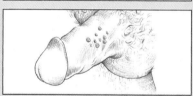

Tinea cruris (commonly known as "jock itch") produces itchy patches of well-defined, slightly raised, scaly lesions that usually affect the inner thighs and groin.

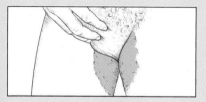

A *chancroid* causes a painful ulcer that's usually less than ¾" (2 cm) in diameter and bleeds easily. The lesion may be deep and covered by a gray or yellow exudate at its base.

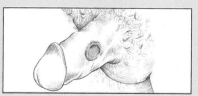

◆ Inguinal lymph nodes enlarge, become tender, and may drain pus.

Folliculitis and furunculosis
◆ Folliculitis may cause red, pointed lesions that are tender and swollen with central pustules.
◆ If folliculitis progresses to furunculosis, lesions become hard, painful nodules that may enlarge and rupture.

Genital herpes
◆ Fluid-filled vesicles develop on the glans penis, foreskin, or shaft.
◆ Vesicles are painless at first but may rupture into shallow, painful ulcers with redness, edema, and dysuria.

Genital warts
◆ Tiny red or pink painless swellings develop on the subpreputial sac or urethral meatus and spread to the perineum and perianal area.
◆ Warts may grow, become pedunculated, cauliflower-like, and malodorous.

Lichen planus
◆ Small, shiny, polygonal, violet papules with white, lacy, milky striations develop on the glans penis, after initial lesions on the arms or legs.
◆ Papules may be linear or coalesce into plaques.
◆ Other signs include pruritus, distorted nails, buccal mucosal lesions, and alopecia.

Pediculosis pubis
◆ In this parasitic infestation, erythematous, itching papules develop in the pubic area and around the anus, abdomen, and thigh.
◆ Other signs include grayish white specks (lice eggs) attached to hair shafts, and skin irritation.

Psoriasis
◆ Red, raised, scaly plaques may develop on the penis.
◆ Other signs and symptoms include itching; pain from dry, cracked, encrusted lesions; nail pitting; and joint stiffness.

Scabies
◆ Mite infestation causes crusted lesions or large papules on the glans and shaft of the penis and on the scrotum.
◆ Nocturnal itching is typical, causing excoriation.

Seborrheic dermatitis
◆ Erythematous, dry or moist greasy scaling papules and yellow crusts that form annular plaques develop on the shaft of the penis, scrotum, groin, scalp, chest, eyebrows, back, axillae, and umbilicus.

Syphilis
◆ Small, red, fluid-filled chancres may erupt on the genitalia 2 to 4 weeks after exposure to this infectious STD.
◆ Chancres erode to form painless, firm, indurated, shallow ulcers with clear bases and scant, yellow serous discharge.
◆ Early treatment is important to avoid long-term, multiorgan system dysfunction.

Tinea cruris
◆ In this superficial fungal infection, also known as *jock itch,* sharply defined, slightly raised, scaling patches typically develop on the inner thigh or groin.
◆ Pruritus may be severe.

Urticaria
◆ Pruritic hives may appear on the genitalia, especially on foreskin or shaft of penis.

OTHER
Drugs
◆ Phenolphthalein, barbiturates, and certain broad-spectrum antibiotics may cause a fixed drug eruption.

NURSING CONSIDERATIONS
◆ Screen every patient with penile lesions for STDs.
◆ Provide emotional support, especially if cancer is suspected.

PEDIATRIC POINTERS
◆ The spirochete that causes syphilis can pass through the placenta, producing congenital syphilis.
◆ In infants, contact dermatitis may cause red, weepy, excoriated lesions.
◆ In children, impetigo may cause pustules with thick, yellow, weepy crusts.
◆ Children with STDs must be evaluated for sexual abuse.
◆ Adolescents ages 15 to 19 have a high incidence of STDs.

GERIATRIC POINTERS
◆ Older patients may have different symptoms of STDs from younger patients because of other disease, decreased immunity, poor hygiene, and poor symptom reporting.

PATIENT TEACHING
◆ Explain the use of ointments and creams.
◆ Explain methods to relieve crusting and itching.
◆ Emphasize the lesion changes the patient should report.
◆ Discuss and teach the proper use of condoms for STD prevention.
◆ Discuss proper hygiene and infection control methods.

Gum bleeding

- Usually results from dental disorders but may stem from blood dyscrasias or effects of certain drugs
- Ranges from slight oozing to life-threatening hemorrhage

🔷 **ACTION STAT!** *If the patient has profuse bleeding in his mouth, check for airway patency and look for signs of cardiovascular collapse. Apply suction to remove pooled blood. Apply direct pressure to the bleeding site. Prepare to insert an airway, administer I.V. fluids, and collect serum samples, as needed.*

HISTORY

- Ask about the onset and description of the bleeding.
- Obtain a personal or family history of bleeding tendencies.
- Obtain a dental history and assess oral hygienic practices.
- Obtain a medical history, including heart, liver, or spleen disease.
- Review diet and alcohol use.
- Obtain a drug history.

PHYSICAL ASSESSMENT

- Have the patient remove his dentures.
- Examine the gums.
- Check for inflammation, pockets around teeth, swelling, retraction, hypertrophy, discoloration, and gum hyperplasia.
- Note obvious decay, discoloration, foreign material, and absence of teeth.

CAUSES

MEDICAL
Agranulocytosis
- Spontaneous gum bleeding and other systemic hemorrhages may occur in this blood disorder.
- Signs of infection, such as fever and chills, may develop.
- Oral and perianal lesions are rough-edged with a gray or black membrane.

Aplastic anemia
- Profuse or scant gum bleeding may follow trauma.
- Eventually, tachycardia and signs of heart failure develop.
- Other signs and symptoms include other signs of bleeding, weakness, fatigue, shortness of breath, headache, pallor, and fever.

Cirrhosis
- Gum bleeding, epistaxis, and other bleeding tendencies occur because of prolonged bleeding times.

- Ascites, hepatomegaly, pruritus, and jaundice develop.
- Other signs and symptoms include abdominal pain, anorexia, fatigue, nausea, vomiting, and weakness.

Gingivitis
- Gums become bulbous, reddened, and edematous and bleed easily with slight trauma.
- With acute necrotizing ulcerative gingivitis, bleeding is spontaneous, and gums are painful.
- A characteristic grayish-yellow pseudomembrane develops over punched-out gum erosions.
- Other signs and symptoms include halitosis, headache, malaise, fever, and cervical adenopathy.

Hemophilia
- Mild hemophilia causes easy bruising, hematomas, epistaxis, bleeding gums, and prolonged bleeding during and after surgery.
- Moderate disease produces more frequent episodes of abnormal bleeding.
- Severe disease causes spontaneous or severe bleeding after minor trauma, resulting in painful joints, peripheral neuropathies, anemia, shock, and even death.

Leukemia
- Early signs and symptoms include easy gum bleeding with gum swelling, necrosis, and petechiae; late signs and symptoms include confusion, headaches, vomiting, seizures, papilledema, and nuchal rigidity.
- Acute leukemia produces severe prostration marked by high fever, bleeding tendencies, dyspnea, tachycardia, palpitations, and abdominal or bone pain.
- Chronic leukemia produces less-severe bleeding tendencies.

Periodontal disease
- Gum bleeding typically occurs after chewing, toothbrushing, or gum probing but may also occur spontaneously.

Other signs and symptoms include unpleasant taste with halitosis, facial pain, loose teeth, pus-filled pockets around the teeth, and dental calculi and plaque.

Pernicious anemia
◆ Gum bleeding and a sore tongue make eating painful.
◆ Other signs and symptoms include weakness, paresthesia, altered bowel and bladder habits, personality changes, ataxia, tinnitus, dyspnea, and tachycardia.

Polycythemia vera
◆ Engorged gums ooze blood after even slight trauma.
◆ The gums and tongue are a deep red-violet.
◆ Other signs and symptoms include headache, dyspnea, dizziness, fatigue, paresthesia, tinnitus, double or blurred vision, aquagenic pruritus, epigastric distress, weight loss, ruddy cyanosis, ecchymoses, and hepatosplenomegaly.

Thrombocytopenia
◆ Blood oozes between the teeth and gums.
◆ Severe bleeding may follow minor trauma.
◆ Other signs and symptoms include large blood-filled bullae in the mouth, petechiae, ecchymoses, epistaxis, hematuria, malaise, fatigue, weakness, and lethargy.

Thrombocytopenic purpura, idiopathic
◆ Profuse gum bleeding occurs.
◆ Spontaneous hemorrhagic skin lesions range from pinpoint petechiae to massive hemorrhages.
◆ Other signs and symptoms include the tendency to bruise easily, petechiae on the oral mucosa, melena, epistaxis, and hematuria.

Vitamin K deficiency
◆ In this deficiency, which affects the clotting process, gums bleed when the teeth are brushed.
◆ Other signs and symptoms include ecchymoses, epistaxis, hematuria, hematemesis, melena, and focal neurologic deficits.

OTHER
Chemical irritants
◆ Occupational exposure to benzene may irritate the gums, resulting in bleeding.

Drugs
◆ Anticoagulants and antiplatelet drugs alter blood clotting and may cause gum bleeding.
◆ Abuse of aspirin and nonsteroidal anti-inflammatory drugs may alter platelets, causing bleeding gums.

NURSING CONSIDERATIONS

◆ Anticipate a blood or blood-product transfusion.
◆ When providing mouth care, avoid using lemon-glycerin swabs, which may burn or dry the gums.

PEDIATRIC POINTERS
◆ In neonates, bleeding gums may result from vitamin K deficiency.
◆ In infants who primarily drink cow's milk and don't receive vitamin supplements, bleeding gums can result from vitamin C deficiency.

GERIATRIC POINTERS
◆ In patients who have no teeth, constant gum trauma and bleeding may result from using a dental prosthesis.

PATIENT TEACHING

◆ Instruct the patient in proper mouth and gum care. (See *Preventing bleeding gums.*)
◆ Discuss situations that require medical attention.
◆ Emphasize the importance of seeking regular dental care.
◆ Discuss the underlying condition.

Preventing bleeding gums

Teach your patient to follow these tips to improve oral hygiene and prevent his gums from bleeding:
◆ Eliminate between-meal snacks and reduce carbohydrate intake to help prevent plaque formation on your teeth.
◆ Visit the dentist once every 6 months for thorough plaque removal.
◆ Avoid citrus fruits and juices, rough or spicy food, alcohol, and tobacco if they irritate mouth ulcers or sore gums and cause bleeding. Be sure to take vitamin C supplements if you can't consume citrus fruits and juices.
◆ Avoid using toothpicks, which may cause gum injury and infection.
◆ Brush your teeth gently after every meal, using a soft-bristled toothbrush held at a 45-degree angle to the gum line.
◆ If dentures make your gums bleed, have them evaluated for proper fit by the dentist.
◆ If the dentist tells you not to brush your teeth, rinse your mouth with salt water or hydrogen peroxide and water. Avoid using commercial mouthwashes, which contain irritating alcohol.
◆ Floss your teeth daily to remove plaque, unless flossing causes pain or bleeding.
◆ Use a Water Pik on the low-pressure setting to massage your gums.
◆ Use aspirin sparingly for toothaches or general pain relief.
◆ Control gum bleeding by applying direct pressure to the area with a gauze pad soaked in ice water.

Gynecomastia

- Increased breast size in men from excessive mammary gland development; hormonal imbalance is usually a contributing factor
- Usually bilateral and may be associated with breast tenderness and milk secretion

- Ask about the onset of breast enlargement.
- Inquire about change in appearance of nipples, tenderness, discharge, testicular mass or pain, loss of libido, decreased potency, and loss of chest, axillary, or facial hair.
- Ask about recent nipple piercing.
- Obtain a drug history.

PHYSICAL ASSESSMENT

- Examine the breasts for asymmetry, dimpling, abnormal pigmentation, or ulceration.
- Observe the testicles for size and symmetry; palpate to detect nodules, tenderness, or unusual consistency.
- Look for normal penile development after puberty, and note hypospadias.

CAUSES

MEDICAL
Adrenal carcinoma
- Estrogen production by an adrenal tumor may produce a feminizing syndrome in men characterized by gynecomastia, loss of libido, impotence, testicular atrophy, and reduced facial hair growth.

Breast cancer
- Painful gynecomastia develops rapidly in the affected breast.
- A hard, stony breast lump may be palpated.
- Other signs and symptoms include changes in breast symmetry, skin thickening, peau d'orange, nipple changes, and a watery, bloody, or purulent discharge.

Cirrhosis
- Gynecomastia, a late sign, is accompanied by testicular atrophy, decreased libido, and loss of facial, chest, and axillary hair.
- Other late signs and symptoms include mental changes, bleeding tendencies, spider angiomas, palmar erythema, severe pruritus, dry skin, fetor hepaticus, enlarged superficial abdominal veins, jaundice, and hepatomegaly.

Hypothyroidism
- Gynecomastia is accompanied by bradycardia, cold intolerance, weight gain despite anorexia, and mental dullness.
- Other signs and symptoms include periorbital edema; puffy face, hands, and feet; brittle, sparse hair; and dry, pale, cool, doughy skin.

Klinefelter's syndrome
- Painless gynecomastia first appears during adolescence.
- Before puberty, abnormally small testicles and slight mental deficiency appear.
- After puberty, sparse facial hair, a small penis, decreased libido, and impotence occur.

Malnutrition
◆ Painful gynecomastia in one breast may occur when the malnourished patient begins to take nourishment again.
◆ Other signs and symptoms include apathy; muscle wasting; weakness; limb paresthesia; anorexia; nausea; vomiting; diarrhea; dull, sparse, dry hair; brittle nails; dark, swollen cheeks and lips; dry, flaky skin; edema; and hepatomegaly.

Pituitary tumor
◆ Gynecomastia occurs with galactorrhea, impotence, and decreased libido.
◆ Other signs and symptoms include enlarged hands and feet, coarse facial features with prognathism, voice deepening, weight gain, increased blood pressure, diaphoresis, heat intolerance, hyperpigmentation, thick and oily skin, and paresthesia or sensory loss and muscle weakness in the limbs.

Renal failure, chronic
◆ Gynecomastia with decreased libido and impotence occurs.
◆ Other signs and symptoms include ammonia breath odor, oliguria, fatigue, decreased mental acuity, seizures, muscle cramps, peripheral neuropathy, anorexia, nausea, vomiting, constipation or diarrhea, bleeding tendencies, yellow-brown or bronze skin, high blood pressure, and uremic frost.

Testicular failure, secondary
◆ Gynecomastia appears after normal puberty.
◆ Other signs and symptoms include sparse facial hair, decreased libido, impotence, and testicular atrophy.

Testicular tumor
◆ Gynecomastia, nipple tenderness, and decreased libido occur.
◆ A firm mass and a heavy sensation is present in the scrotum.

Thyrotoxicosis
◆ Gynecomastia may occur with loss of libido and impotence.

◆ Other signs and symptoms include tachycardia, palpitations, weight loss despite increased appetite, diarrhea, tremors, an enlarged thyroid gland, dyspnea, nervousness, diaphoresis, heat intolerance, and exophthalmos.

OTHER
Drugs
◆ Antihypertensives, cyproterone, cimetidine, estrogens and drugs with estrogen-like effects, flutamide, ketoconazole, spironolactone, phenothiazines, and tricyclic antidepressants may cause gynecomastia.
◆ Regular use of alcohol, marijuana, or heroin reduces plasma testosterone levels, resulting in gynecomastia.

Treatments
◆ Gynecomastia may follow major surgery, testicular irradiation, or onset of hemodialysis for chronic renal failure.

NURSING CONSIDERATIONS
◆ Apply cold compresses to the breasts.
◆ Give analgesics, as prescribed.
◆ Tamoxifen, an antiestrogen, or testolactone may be helpful.
◆ If drug treatment fails, surgical removal of breast tissue may be warranted.
◆ Provide emotional support.

PEDIATRIC POINTERS
◆ In neonates, gynecomastia may be associated with galactorrhea, disappearing within a few weeks of birth.
◆ Most boys have physiologic gynecomastia at some time during adolescence, usually around age 14.

PATIENT TEACHING
◆ Explain treatments and procedures the patient needs.
◆ Teach the patient about prescribed medication administration, dosage, and possible adverse effects.
◆ Teach about the underlying diagnosis and treatment options.

Halitosis

- Unpleasant, disagreeable, or offensive breath odor

HISTORY

- Ask about the onset and characteristics of halitosis.
- Find out about associated bad taste, difficulty swallowing or chewing, reflux, regurgitation, pain, tenderness, flatus, or cough.
- Determine the pattern and characteristics of bowel movements.
- Inquire about smoking or tobacco habits.
- Obtain a description of diet and daily oral hygiene.
- Obtain a medical history, including incidence of chronic disorders and respiratory tract infection.

PHYSICAL ASSESSMENT

- Examine the mouth, throat, and nose for lesions, bleeding, drainage, foreign body obstruction, and signs of infection.
- Percuss and palpate over the sinuses for tenderness.
- Auscultate the lungs for abnormal breath sounds.
- Auscultate the abdomen for bowel sounds; percuss, noting any tympany.
- Take vital signs.

CAUSES

MEDICAL
Bowel obstruction
- Fecal halitosis is a late sign.
- Constant lower abdominal pain may occur with large-bowel obstruction.
- Other signs and symptoms (of a small-bowel obstruction) include vomiting, constipation, abdominal distention, and intermittent periumbilical cramping pain.

Bronchiectasis
- Foul or putrid halitosis is typical.
- Some patients may have a sickeningly sweet breath odor.
- Other signs and symptoms include exertional dyspnea, fatigue, malaise, weakness, weight loss, crackles, late clubbing, and a chronic productive cough with copious, foul-smelling, mucopurulent sputum.

Common cold
- A musty breath odor may be present.
- Other signs and symptoms include a dry, hacking cough with sore throat, sneezing, nasal congestion with rhinorrhea, headache, malaise, fatigue, and aching joints and muscles.

Diabetic ketoacidosis
- In this potentially life-threatening condition, the breath characteristically smells fruity.
- Other findings include blood glucose level greater than 300 mg/dl, frequent urination, increased thirst, fatigue, nausea, vomiting, tachypnea, stupor, and coma.

Esophageal cancer
- Halitosis may accompany dysphagia, hoarseness, chest pain, and weight loss.
- Nocturnal regurgitation and cachexia are late signs.

Gastric cancer
- Halitosis is a late sign.
- Other signs and symptoms include chronic dyspepsia unrelieved by antacids, a vague feeling of fullness, nausea, anorexia, fatigue, pallor,

weakness, altered bowel habits, weight loss, muscle wasting, and, if bleeding occurs, hematemesis and melena.

Gastrocolic fistula

- A fecal breath odor is preceded by intermittent diarrhea, and weight loss.

Gingivitis

- Halitosis may occur along with red, shiny, tender, edematous, bleeding gums.
- Acute necrotizing ulcerative gingivitis causes fetid breath.
- Other signs and symptoms of acute necrotizing ulcerative gingivitis include ulcers that may become covered with gray exudate, fever, cervical adenopathy, headache, and malaise.

Hepatic encephalopathy

- Fetor hepaticus (a musty, sweet, or mousy [new-mown hay] breath odor) is a late sign.
- Other signs and symptoms include coma, asterixis, and hyperactive deep tendon reflexes.

Lung abscess

- Putrid halitosis develops along with a productive cough with copious, purulent, often bloody sputum.
- Other signs and symptoms include fever with chills, dyspnea, headache, anorexia, malaise, pleuritic chest pain, asymmetrical chest movement, weight loss, and temporary clubbing.

Ozena

- This disease is characterized by atrophy of the bony ridges and mucous membranes of the nose.
- Musty or fetid breath odor occurs along with thick, green mucus and progressive loss of the sense of smell.

Periodontal disease

- Halitosis occurs with bleeding gums and pus-filled pockets around the teeth.
- Other signs and symptoms include facial pain, headache, and loose teeth covered by calculi and plaque.

Pharyngitis, gangrenous

- Halitosis occurs with an extremely sore throat.
- Other signs and symptoms include a foul taste in the mouth, choking sensation, fever, cervical lymphadenopathy, and a swollen, red, ulcerated pharynx.

Renal failure, chronic

- A urinous or ammonia breath odor occurs.
- Other signs and symptoms include signs of anemia, emotional lability, lethargy, irritability, decreased mental acuity, coarse muscular twitching, peripheral neuropathies, muscle wasting, anorexia, signs of GI bleeding, ecchymoses, yellow-brown or bronze skin, pruritus, anuria, and increased blood pressure.

Sinusitis

- Acute sinusitis causes purulent nasal discharge that leads to halitosis.
- Other signs and symptoms of acute sinusitis include a characteristic postnasal drip, nasal congestion, sore throat, cough, malaise, headache, facial pain and tenderness, and fever.
- Chronic sinusitis causes continuous mucopurulent discharge and musty breath odor.
- Other signs and symptoms of chronic sinusitis include postnasal drip, nasal congestion, and a chronic, nonproductive cough.

OTHER

Drugs

- Drugs that may cause halitosis include triamterene, inhaled anesthetics, paraldehyde, and any drugs known to cause metabolic acidosis such as nitroprusside.

NURSING CONSIDERATIONS

- To enhance appetite, provide oral hygiene before meals.

PEDIATRIC POINTERS

- In children, halitosis commonly results from physiologic causes, such as continual mouth breathing and thumb or blanket sucking.
- Phenylketonuria may produce a musty or mousy odor.

GERIATRIC POINTERS

- Dental caries, dry mouth, and poor oral hygiene can cause halitosis in elderly patients.

PATIENT TEACHING

- Teach the patient about proper oral hygiene.
- Teach the patient about causes of halitosis.

Halo vision

- Refers to seeing rainbowlike colored rings around lights or bright objects
- As light passes through tears or the cells of various anteretinal media, it breaks up into spectral colors
- Usually develops suddenly; duration dependent on the causative disorder
- Occurs in disorders associated with excessive tearing and corneal epithelial edema.

- Obtain a history, including how long the patient has been seeing halos around lights and when he usually sees them. For example, patients with glaucoma usually see halos in the morning, when intraocular pressure (IOP) is most elevated.
- Ask the patient if light bothers his eyes or if he has eye pain. Halos associated with excruciating eye pain or a severe headache may point to acute angle-closure glaucoma, an ocular emergency.
- Note a history of glaucoma, cataracts, eye surgery, and use of corrective lenses or drugs.

- Examine the patient's eyes, noting conjunctival injection, excessive tearing, and lens changes.
- Examine pupil size, shape, and response to light.
- Test visual acuity.

MEDICAL

Cataract

◆ Halo vision may be an early symptom of painless, progressive cataract formation, resulting from dispersion of light by abnormal lens opacity. The glare of headlights may blind the patient, making nighttime driving impossible.

◆ Other signs and symptoms include blurred vision, impaired visual acuity, and lens opacity, all of which develop gradually.

Corneal endothelial dystrophy

◆ Halo vision is a late symptom of this disorder, which may also cause impaired visual acuity.

Glaucoma

◆ Halo vision characterizes all types of glaucoma.

◆ Acute angle-closure glaucoma causes blurred vision, followed by a severe headache or excruciating pain in and around the affected eye. Other signs and symptoms include a moderately dilated fixed pupil that doesn't respond to light, conjunctival injection, a cloudy cornea, impaired visual acuity and, possibly, nausea and vomiting.

◆ Chronic angle-closure glaucoma usually produces no symptoms until pain and blindness occur in advanced disease. Halo vision is a late symptom (in the chronic form) that's accompanied by mild eye ache, peripheral vision loss, and impaired visual acuity.

OTHER

Drugs

◆ Digoxin (Lanoxin) can cause yellow-green halos around visual images.

Nonpathologic causes

◆ Excessive tearing associated with halo vision can be caused by poorly fitted or overworn contact lenses, emotional extremes, and exposure to intense light, as in snow blindness.

◆ To help minimize halo vision, remind the patient not to look directly at bright lights.

◆ Assess patient needs based on decreased visual acuity.

PEDIATRIC POINTERS

◆ In children, halo vision usually results from congenital cataracts or glaucoma. However, in a very young child, limited verbal ability may make halo vision difficult to assess.

◆ In preteens and teenagers, the most likely cause of halos is uncorrected nearsightedness and astigmatism.

GERIATRIC POINTERS

◆ Primary glaucoma, the most common cause of halo vision, is more common in older patients.

◆ Teach the patient the importance of follow-up care with an ophthalmologist.

◆ Teach the patient about the underlying cause of halo vision and treatment plan.

◆ Teach the patient about prescribed medications and proper technique for eyedrop administration.

◆ Teach the patient safety precautions to prevent accidents and falls.

Headache

OVERVIEW

- Most common neurologic symptom
- May be localized or generalized, producing mild to severe pain
- May be described as vascular, muscle-contraction, or a combination of both
- Benign in 90% of cases (see *Comparing benign headaches*)

HISTORY

- Ask about the onset, frequency, duration, and location of the headache.
- Obtain medical, surgical and trauma history.
- Find out about precipitating or alleviating factors.
- Obtain a drug and alcohol history.
- Ask about associated drowsiness, confusion, dizziness, seizures, fever, stiff neck, nausea, vomiting, photophobia, or vision changes.

PHYSICAL ASSESSMENT

- Evaluate level of consciousness (LOC).
- Check vital signs.
- Be alert for signs of increased intracranial pressure (ICP).
- Check pupil size and response to light.
- Note any neck stiffness.
- Palpate temporal arteries for tenderness.

Comparing benign headaches

Of the many patients who report headaches, only about 10% have an underlying medical disorder. The other 90% suffer from benign headaches, which may be classified as muscle-contraction (tension), vascular (migraine and cluster), or a combination of both.

As you review the chart below, you'll see that the two major types—muscle-contraction and vascular headaches—are quite different. In a combined headache, features of both appear; this type of headache may affect the patient with a severe muscle-contraction headache or a late-stage migraine. Treatment of a combined headache includes analgesics and sedatives.

CHARACTERISTICS	MUSCLE-CONTRACTION HEADACHES	VASCULAR HEADACHES
Incidence	◆ Most common type, accounting for 80% of all headaches	◆ More common in women and those with a family history of migraines ◆ Onset after puberty
Precipitating factors	◆ Stress, anxiety, tension, improper posture, and body alignment ◆ Prolonged muscle contraction without structural damage ◆ Eye, ear, and paranasal sinus disorders that produce reflex muscle contractions	◆ Hormone fluctuations ◆ Alcohol ◆ Emotional upset ◆ Too little or too much sleep ◆ Foods, such as chocolate, cheese, monosodium glutamate, and cured meats; caffeine withdrawal ◆ Weather changes, such as shifts in barometric pressure
Intensity and duration	◆ Produce an aching tightness or a band of pain around the head, especially in the neck and in occipital and temporal areas ◆ Occur frequently and usually last for several hours	◆ May begin with an awareness of an impending migraine or a 5- to 15-minute prodrome of neurologic deficits, such as visual disturbances, dizziness, unsteady gait, or tingling of the face, lips, or hands ◆ Produce severe, constant, throbbing pain that's typically unilateral and may be incapacitating ◆ Last for 4 to 6 hours
Associated signs and symptoms	◆ Tense neck and facial muscles	◆ Anorexia, nausea, and vomiting ◆ Occasionally, photophobia, sensitivity to loud noises, weakness, and fatigue ◆ Depending on the type (cluster headache or classic, common, or hemiplegic migraine), possibly chills, depression, eye pain, ptosis, tearing, rhinorrhea, diaphoresis, and facial flushing
Alleviating factors	◆ Mild analgesics, muscle relaxants, or other drugs during an attack ◆ Measures to reduce stress, such as biofeedback, relaxation techniques, and counseling; posture correction to prevent attacks	◆ Methysergide and propranolol to prevent vascular headache ◆ Ergot alkaloids or serotonin-receptor drugs at the first sign of a migraine ◆ Rest in a quiet, darkened room ◆ Elimination of irritating foods from diet

MEDICAL

Brain abscess
- Headache is localized to the abscess site and intensifies over a few days.
- Straining aggravates headache.
- Other signs and symptoms include nausea, vomiting, focal or generalized seizures, changes in LOC and, depending on the location of the abscess, aphasia, impaired visual acuity, hemiparesis, ataxia, tremors, and personality changes.

Brain tumor
- Headache initially is localized near the tumor site but becomes generalized as the tumor grows.
- Pain is usually intermittent, deep-seated, dull, and most intense in the morning; aggravating factors include coughing, stooping, Valsalva's maneuver, and changes in head position; and alleviating factors include sitting and rest.
- Other signs and symptoms include personality changes, altered LOC, motor and sensory dysfunction, and signs of increased ICP.

Cerebral aneurysm, ruptured
- In this life-threatening condition, headache is sudden and excruciating and usually peaks within minutes of the rupture.
- Loss of consciousness may be immediate or a variably altered LOC may occur.
- Depending on the location and severity of the bleeding, other signs and symptoms may include nausea, vomiting, nuchal rigidity, blurred vision, and hemiparesis.

Encephalitis
- A severe, generalized headache is characteristic, with mild flulike symptoms.
- Within 48 hours, the patient's LOC typically deteriorates.
- Other signs and symptoms include fever, nuchal rigidity, irritability, seizures, nausea, vomiting, photophobia, cranial nerve palsies, and focal neurologic deficits.

Epidural hemorrhage, acute
- A progressively severe headache occurs with nausea, vomiting, bladder distention, confusion, and rapid decrease in LOC.
- Other signs and symptoms include unilateral seizures, pupil dilation on affected side, hemiparesis, hemiplegia, high fever, decreased pulse rate and bounding pulse, widened pulse pressure, increased blood pressure, a positive Babinski's reflex, and decerebrate posture.

Glaucoma, acute angle-closure
- Excruciating headache as well as acute eye pain, blurred vision, halo vision, nausea, and vomiting may occur in this ophthalmic emergency.
- Other signs and symptoms include conjunctival injection, a cloudy cornea, and a moderately dilated, fixed pupil.

Hypertension
- A slightly throbbing occipital headache on awakening may occur; severity decreases during the day (if diastolic pressure remains greater than 120 mm Hg, the headache is constant).
- Other signs and symptoms include atrial gallop, restlessness, confusion, nausea, vomiting, blurred vision, seizures, and altered LOC.

Influenza
- A severe generalized or frontal headache usually begins suddenly.
- Other signs and symptoms include retro-orbital discomfort, weakness, myalgia, fever, chills, coughing, rhinorrhea, and hoarseness.

Intracerebral hemorrhage
- A severe generalized headache may develop.
- Signs and symptoms vary with the size and location of the hemorrhage and may include altered LOC, hemiplegia, hemiparesis, abnormal pupil size and response, aphasia, dizziness, nausea, vomiting, seizures, decreased sensation, irregular respirations, positive Babinski's reflex, decorticate or decerebrate posture, and increased blood pressure.

Meningitis
- Onset of a severe, constant, generalized headache is sudden and worsens with movement.
- Other signs and symptoms include altered LOC, seizures, fever, chills, nuchal rigidity, ocular palsies, facial weakness, hearing loss, positive Kernig's sign and Brudzinski's sign, hyperreflexia, opisthotonos, and signs of increased ICP.

Plague
- Pneumonic form results in sudden onset of headache, chills, fever, myalgia, productive cough, chest pain, tachypnea, dyspnea, hemoptysis, respiratory distress, and cardiopulmonary insufficiency.

Postconcussional syndrome
- A generalized or localized headache may develop 1 to 30 days after head trauma and last for 2 to 3 weeks.
- Pain may be aching, pounding, pressing, stabbing, or throbbing.
- Other signs and symptoms include giddiness or dizziness, blurred vision, fatigue, insomnia, inability to concentrate, noise and alcohol intolerance, fever, chills, malaise, chest pain, nausea, vomiting, and diarrhea.

Severe acute respiratory syndrome
- In this potentially life-threatening illness, symptoms include fever, headache, malaise, a dry nonproductive cough, and dyspnea.

(continued)

Sinusitis, acute

◆ A dull periorbital headache is usually aggravated by bending over or touching the face and is relieved by sinus drainage.
◆ Other signs and symptoms may include fever, sinus tenderness, nasal turbinate edema, sore throat, malaise, cough, and nasal discharge.

Smallpox

◆ Initial signs and symptoms include severe headache, backache, abdominal pain, high fever, malaise, prostration, and a maculopapular rash on the mucosa of the mouth, pharynx, face, and forearms, gradually developing on the trunk and legs.
◆ The rash becomes vesicular, then pustular, and finally forms a crust and scab, leaving a pitted scar.

Subarachnoid hemorrhage

◆ A sudden, violent headache occurs along with nuchal rigidity, nausea and vomiting, seizures, dizziness, ipsilateral pupil dilation, and altered LOC that may progress to coma.
◆ Other signs and symptoms include positive Kernig's sign and Brudzinski's sign, photophobia, blurred vision, fever, hemiparesis, hemiplegia, sensory disturbances, aphasia, and signs of increased ICP.

Subdural hematoma

◆ Headache develops and LOC decreases.
◆ In acute cases, early signs and symptoms include drowsiness, confusion, and agitation that may progress to coma; late signs include signs of increased ICP and focal neurologic deficits.
◆ In chronic cases, pounding headache fluctuates in severity and is located over the hematoma.
◆ Giddiness, personality changes, confusion, seizures, and progressively worsening LOC may develop weeks or months after the trauma.

Temporal arteritis

◆ A throbbing unilateral headache in the temporal or frontotemporal region may be accompanied by vision loss, hearing loss, confusion, and fever.
◆ The temporal arteries are tender, swollen, nodular and, possibly, erythematous.

Tularemia

◆ Onset of headache is abrupt in this bacterial infection.
◆ Other signs and symptoms include fever, chills, myalgia, nonproductive cough, dyspnea, pleuritic chest pain, enlarged lymph nodes, and empyema.

OTHER
Diagnostic tests

◆ Lumbar puncture or myelogram may produce a throbbing frontal headache that worsens on standing.

Drugs

◆ Indomethacin, vasodilators, and drugs with a vasodilating effect may produce headaches.
◆ Withdrawal from vasopressors may also result in headaches.

NURSING CONSIDERATIONS

◆ Monitor vital signs and LOC.
◆ Watch for a change in the headache's severity or location.
◆ Administer an analgesic, darken the room, and minimize stimuli to ease the headache.

PEDIATRIC POINTERS

◆ In children older than age 3, headache is the most common symptom of a brain tumor.
◆ Suspect a headache if a young child is banging or holding his head.

- ◆ Discuss the underlying disorder, diagnostic testing, and treatment options.
- ◆ Explain the signs of reduced LOC and seizures that the patient or his caregivers should report.
- ◆ Explain ways to maintain a safe, quiet environment and reduce environmental stress.
- ◆ Discuss the use of analgesics.

Hearing loss

OVERVIEW

- May be temporary, permanent and partial, or complete
- Classified as conductive (resulting from external or middle ear disorders), sensorineural (resulting from disorders of the inner ear or of the eighth cranial nerve), mixed (resulting from a combination of conductive and sensorineural factors), or functional (resulting from psychological factors)

HISTORY

- Ask for a description of the hearing loss.
- Obtain a medical history, including incidence of chronic ear infections, ear surgery, ear or head trauma, and recent upper respiratory tract infection.
- Obtain a drug history.
- Ask for a description of the occupational environment.
- Ask about other signs and symptoms, such as pain; discharge; ringing, buzzing, hissing, or other noises; and dizziness.

PHYSICAL ASSESSMENT

- Inspect the external ear for inflammation, boils, foreign bodies, and discharge.
- Apply pressure to the tragus and mastoid to elicit tenderness.
- During otoscopic examination, note color change, perforation, bulging, or retraction of tympanic membrane. (See *Using an otoscope.*)
- Evaluate hearing acuity.
- Perform the Weber's and Rinne tests. (See *Differentiating conductive from sensorineural hearing loss.*)

 TOP TECHNIQUE

Using an otoscope

INSERTING THE SPECULUM

Before inserting the speculum into the patient's ear, straighten the ear canal by grasping the auricle and pulling it up and back, as shown below.

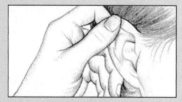

POSITIONING THE SCOPE

To examine the ear's external canal, hold the otoscope with the handle parallel to the patient's head, as shown below. Bracing your hand firmly against the patient's head keeps you from hitting the canal with the speculum.

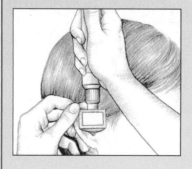

VIEWING THE STRUCTURES

When the otoscope is positioned properly, you should see the tympanic membrane structures shown here.

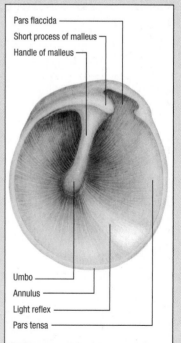

Pars flaccida

Short process of malleus

Handle of malleus

Umbo

Annulus

Light reflex

Pars tensa

CAUSES

MEDICAL

Acoustic neuroma
- Unilateral, progressive, sensorineural hearing loss occurs; tinnitus, vertigo, and facial paralysis may also develop.

Adenoid hypertrophy
- Gradual conductive hearing loss occurs.
- Other signs and symptoms include ear discharge, frequent ear infections, mouth breathing, and a sensation of ear fullness.

Allergies
- Conductive hearing loss may result.
- Other signs and symptoms include ear pain or a feeling of fullness, nasal congestion, and conjunctivitis.

Cholesteatoma
- Gradual hearing loss may be accompanied by ear ache, vertigo and facial paralysis.
- Other signs and symptoms include eardrum perforation, pearly white balls in the ear canal, and discharge.

External ear canal tumor, malignant
- Progressive conductive hearing loss occurs with deep, boring ear pain; purulent discharge; and facial paralysis.

Furuncle
- Reversible conductive hearing loss may occur.
- Other signs and symptoms include a sense of fullness in the ear, pain on palpation of the tragus or auricle and, with boil rupture, pain relief and a purulent, necrotic discharge.

Glomus jugulare tumor
- Mild, unilateral conductive hearing loss becomes progressively more severe.
- Other signs and symptoms include tinnitus that sounds like a heartbeat, gradual congestion in the affected ear, throbbing or pulsating discomfort, bloody otorrhea, facial nerve paralysis, and vertigo.

(continued)

 TOP TECHNIQUE

Differentiating conductive from sensorineural hearing loss

Weber's test and the Rinne test can help determine whether the patient's hearing loss is conductive or sensorineural. Weber's test evaluates bone conduction (BC) of sound; the Rinne test evaluates BC and air conduction (AC) of sound. Using a 512-Hz tuning fork, perform these preliminary tests as described below.

WEBER'S TEST

Place the base of a vibrating tuning fork firmly against the midline of the patient's skull at the forehead. Ask if the tone is heard equally well in both ears. If so, the test is graded midline—a normal finding. In an abnormal Weber's test (graded right or left), the sound is louder in the impaired ear, suggesting a conductive hearing loss in that ear or the sound is louder in the normal ear, suggesting sensorineural loss in the other ear.

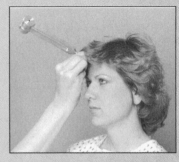

RINNE TEST

Hold the base of a vibrating tuning fork against the patient's mastoid process to test BC of the sound. Then quickly move the vibrating fork to a position in front of the ear canal to test AC of the sound. Ask the patient to tell you which location has the louder or longer sound. Repeat the procedure for the other ear. Normally, AC sound lasts longer than BC sound (a positive Rinne test). Also, AC sound is normally louder than BC sound. In conductive hearing loss, BC sound is as long as or longer than AC sound, a negative Rinne test. In sensorineural loss, AC sound is longer than BC sound, but BC sound is louder.

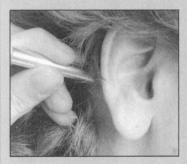

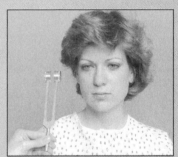

Conductive hearing loss causes:
- abnormal Weber's test result
- negative Rinne test result
- normal ability to discriminate sounds with decreased ability to detect low tones
- the patient to speak in a quiet voice.

Sensorineural hearing loss causes:
- positive Rinne test
- poor hearing in noisy areas
- difficulty hearing high-frequency sounds
- the patient to complain that others mumble or shout
- tinnitus
- the patient to speak in a loud voice.

Head trauma

◆ Conductive or sensorineural hearing loss is sudden in onset.
◆ Headache and bleeding from the ear also occur.
◆ Neurologic findings are dependent on the type of trauma that occurred.

Hypothyroidism

◆ Reversible sensorineural hearing loss may occur.
◆ Other signs and symptoms include bradycardia, weight gain despite anorexia, mental dullness, cold intolerance, facial edema, brittle hair, and dry, pale, cool and doughy skin.

Ménière's disease

◆ Intermittent, unilateral sensorineural hearing loss that involves only low tones progresses to constant hearing loss that involves other tones.
◆ Other signs and symptoms include intermittent severe vertigo, nausea, vomiting, a sensation of fullness in the ear, a roaring or hollow-seashell tinnitus, diaphoresis, and nystagmus.

Osteoma

◆ Sudden or intermittent conductive hearing loss occurs.

Otitis externa

◆ Conductive hearing loss is a characteristic symptom.
◆ Acute form produces pain, headache on the affected side, low-grade fever, lymphadenopathy, itching, and a foul-smelling sticky yellow discharge.
◆ Malignant form involves visible debris in the ear canal, pruritus, tinnitus, and severe ear pain.

Otitis media

◆ In the acute and chronic forms, hearing loss develops gradually.
◆ Other signs and symptoms of the acute form include upper respiratory tract infection with sore throat, cough, nasal discharge, headache, dizziness, a sensation of fullness in the ear, intermittent or constant ear pain, fever, nausea, and vomiting.
◆ Other signs and symptoms of the chronic form include a perforated tympanic membrane, purulent ear drainage, earache, nausea, and vertigo.
◆ In the serous form, a stuffy feeling in the ear occurs with pain that worsens at night.

Otosclerosis

◆ Unilateral conductive hearing loss usually begins in the early 20s and may gradually progress to bilateral mixed loss.
◆ Tinnitus and the ability to hear better in a noisy environment may occur.

Skull fracture

◆ Sudden, unilateral, sensorineural hearing loss may occur if the auditory nerve is damaged.
◆ Other signs and symptoms include ringing tinnitus, blood behind the tympanic membrane, and scalp wounds.

Temporal arteritis

◆ Unilateral, sensorineural hearing loss may occur along with throbbing unilateral facial pain, pain behind the eye, temporal or frontotemporal headache and, occasionally, vision loss.
◆ Other signs and symptoms include malaise, anorexia, weight loss, weakness, low-grade fever, myalgia, and a nodular, swollen artery.

Temporal bone fracture

◆ Sudden, unilateral, hearing loss is accompanied by hissing tinnitus.
◆ Other signs and symptoms may include a perforated tympanic membrane, loss of consciousness, Battle's sign, and facial paralysis.

Tuberculosis

◆ Eardrum perforation, mild conductive hearing loss, and cervical lymphadenopathy may occur if infection spreads to the ear.
◆ Other signs and symptoms include chest pain, crackles, dyspnea, fever, and tachypnea.

Tympanic membrane perforation

◆ Abrupt hearing loss occurs with ear pain, tinnitus, vertigo, and sensation of fullness in the ear.

OTHER

Drugs

◆ Chloroquine, cisplatin, vancomycin, and aminoglycosides may cause irreversible hearing loss.

◆ Loop diuretics, quinine, quinidine, and high doses of erythromycin or salicylates may cause reversible hearing loss.

Radiation therapy

◆ Radiation of the middle ear, thyroid, face, skull, or nasopharynx may cause eustachian tube dysfunction, resulting in hearing loss.

Surgery

◆ Myringotomy, myringoplasty, simple or radical mastoidectomy, or fenestrations may cause scarring that result in hearing loss.

NURSING CONSIDERATIONS

◆ When talking to the patient, face him and speak slowly and clearly.

PEDIATRIC POINTERS

◆ Hereditary disorders cause hearing loss in half of deaf infants.

◆ Congenital, sensorineural hearing loss may be caused by nonhereditary disorders, maternal use of ototoxic drugs, birth trauma, and anoxia.

◆ Unilateral, sensorineural hearing loss may be caused by mumps, meningitis, measles, influenza, and acute febrile illness.

◆ Disorders that can cause congenital, conductive hearing loss include atresia and ossicle malformation.

◆ Serous otitis media commonly causes bilateral, conductive hearing loss in children.

◆ Conductive hearing loss may occur in children who put foreign objects in their ears.

GERIATRIC POINTERS

◆ In older patients, presbyacusis (loss of ability to perceive or discriminate sounds as part of the aging process) may be aggravated by exposure to noise as well as other factors.

PATIENT TEACHING

◆ Explain the importance of ear protection and avoidance of loud noise.

◆ Stress the importance of following instructions for taking prescribed antibiotics.

◆ Teach the patient about underlying diagnosis and treatment options.

Heat intolerance

OVERVIEW

- Inability to withstand high temperatures or to maintain a comfortable body temperature
- Produces a continuous feeling of being overheated and, at times, profuse diaphoresis
- Usually develops gradually and is chronic

HISTORY

- Ask the patient when he first noticed his intolerance for heat and to describe his signs and symptoms; also ask if it occurred gradually or suddenly and if he has problems adjusting to warm weather.
- Ask about his appetite or if his weight has changed and ask about unusual nervousness or other personality changes.
- Obtain a drug history, especially noting use of amphetamines or amphetamine-like drugs and thyroid drugs.

PHYSICAL ASSESSMENT

- As you begin the examination, note how much clothing the patient is wearing.
- After taking vital signs, inspect the patient's skin for flushing and diaphoresis.
- Note tremors and lid lag.

CAUSES

MEDICAL
Hypothalamic disease
◆ In this rare disease, body temperature fluctuates dramatically, causing alternating heat and cold intolerance.
◆ Common causes of hypothalamic disease are pituitary adenoma and hypothalamic and pineal tumors.
◆ Other signs and symptoms include amenorrhea, disturbed sleep patterns, increased thirst and urination, increased appetite with weight gain, impaired visual acuity, headache, and personality changes, such as bursts of rage or laughter.

Thyrotoxicosis
◆ In thyrotoxicosis, excess thyroid hormone stimulates peripheral tissues, increasing basal metabolism and producing excess heat.
◆ Heat intolerance may be accompanied by an enlarged thyroid gland, nervousness, weight loss despite increased appetite, diaphoresis, diarrhea, tremor, and palpitations.
◆ Other signs and symptoms affect virtually every body system including irritability, difficulty concentrating, mood swings, insomnia, muscle weakness, fatigue, exophthalmos, lid lag, tachycardia, full and bounding pulse, widened pulse pressure, dyspnea, amenorrhea, and gynecomastia. Typically, the patient's skin is warm and flushed; premature graying and alopecia occur in both sexes.

OTHER
Drugs
◆ Amphetamines, amphetamine-like appetite suppressants, and excessive doses of thyroid hormone may cause heat intolerance.
◆ Anticholinergics may interfere with sweating, resulting in heat intolerance.

NURSING CONSIDERATIONS

◆ Adjust room temperature to make the patient comfortable.
◆ If the patient is diaphoretic, change his clothing and bed linens, as necessary, and encourage fluids.

PEDIATRIC POINTERS
◆ Rarely, maternal thyrotoxicosis may be passed to the neonate, resulting in heat intolerance.
◆ More commonly, acquired thyrotoxicosis appears between ages 12 and 14, although this too is infrequent.
◆ Dehydration may also make a child sensitive to heat.

PATIENT TEACHING

◆ Teach the patient about underlying disease and treatment plan.
◆ Teach about prescribed medications and the importance of maintaining proper hydration.
◆ Teach the importance of comfort measures, such as adjusting room temperature, and keeping skin dry.

Heberden's nodes

OVERVIEW

- Painless, irregular, cartilaginous or bony enlargements of the distal interphalangeal joints of the fingers
- Degeneration of articular cartilage irritates the bone and stimulates osteoblasts, causing bony enlargement
- About 2 to 3 mm in diameter, developing on one or both sides of the dorsal midline
- Larger nodes usually occur on the dominant hand, which affect one or more fingers but not the thumb (see *Recognizing Heberden's nodes*)

HISTORY

- Find out if the patient or any family members have a history of Heberden's nodes.
- Obtain a medical history, including incidence of osteoarthritis.
- Ask about joint stiffness and repeated fingertip trauma associated with his occupation or athletic activities.
- Also ask which hand is dominant.

PHYSICAL ASSESSMENT

- Carefully palpate the nodes, noting any signs of inflammation, such as redness and tenderness.
- Determine range-of-motion (ROM) in the fingers of each hand. As you do so, listen and feel for crepitation.

Recognizing Heberden's nodes

These painless bony enlargements of the distal interphalangeal finger joints appear in more than one-half of all patients with osteoarthritis.

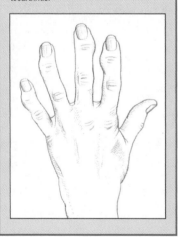

MEDICAL
Osteoarthritis
◆ This disorder commonly causes Heberden's nodes (more than one-half of all osteoarthritic patients have these nodes) and may also cause nodes in the proximal interphalangeal joints (Bouchard's nodes).
◆ Joint pain that's aggravated by movement or weight bearing is the chief symptom. Joints may also be tender and display restricted ROM.
◆ Joint stiffness is triggered by disuse and relieved by brief exercise. Stiffness may be accompanied by bony enlargement and crepitus.

OTHER
Repeated finger trauma
◆ Less commonly, repeated fingertip trauma may lead to node formation in only one joint ("baseball finger").

◆ Remind the patient to take anti-inflammatory drugs and to exercise regularly.

◆ Teach the patient the importance of avoiding joint strain by maintaining a healthy body weight.
◆ Instruct about the use of prescribed medications and their potential side effects.

Hematemesis

OVERVIEW

- Usually indicates GI bleeding above the jejunum
- May be life-threatening if massive (500 to 1,000 ml of blood)
- Bright red or blood-streaked vomitus: fresh or recent bleeding
- Dark red, brown, or black vomitus: blood retained in the stomach or partially digested (see *Rare causes of hematemesis*)

♦ **ACTION STAT!** *If the patient has massive hematemesis, check vital signs. If you detect signs of shock, place the patient in a supine position and elevate his feet. Start a large-bore I.V. line for emergency fluid replacement. Send a blood sample for typing and crossmatching, hemoglobin level, and hematocrit; administer oxygen. Emergency endoscopy may be necessary to locate the source of bleeding. Prepare to insert a nasogastric (NG) tube for suction or iced lavage. (See* **Managing hematemesis with intubation***.)*

HISTORY

- Ask about the onset, amount, color, and consistency of vomitus.
- Ask for a description of stools.
- Inquire about associated nausea, pain, flatulence, diarrhea, or weakness.
- Obtain a medical history, including incidence of ulcers or liver or coagulation disorders.
- Find out about alcohol use.
- Obtain a drug history, including aspirin and other nonsteroidal anti-inflammatory drugs (NSAIDs).

PHYSICAL ASSESSMENT

- Check for orthostatic hypotension.
- Obtain other vital signs.
- Inspect the mucous membranes, nasopharynx, and skin for signs of bleeding.
- Palpate the abdomen for tenderness, pain, or masses.
- Note lymphadenopathy.

Rare causes of hematemesis

Two rare disorders commonly cause hematemesis. *Malaria* produces this and other GI signs, but its most characteristic effects are chills, fever, headache, muscle pain, and splenomegaly. *Yellow fever* also causes hematemesis as well as sudden fever, bradycardia, jaundice, and severe prostration.

Although rare, two relatively common disorders may cause hematemesis. When acute diverticulitis affects the duodenum, GI bleeding and resultant hematemesis occur with abdominal pain and fever. With GI involvement, secondary syphilis can cause hematemesis; more characteristic signs and symptoms include a primary chancre, rash, fever, malaise, anorexia, weight loss, and headache.

Managing hematemesis with intubation

A patient with hematemesis will need to have a GI tube inserted to allow blood drainage, aspirate gastric contents, or facilitate gastric lavage, if necessary. Here are the most common tubes and their uses.

NASOGASTRIC TUBES

The Salem-Sump tube (at right), a double-lumen nasogastric (NG) tube, is used to remove stomach fluid and gas or to aspirate gastric contents. It may also be used for gastric lavage, drug administration, or feeding. Its main advantage over the Levin tube—a single-lumen NG tube—is that it allows atmospheric air to enter the patient's stomach so the tube can float freely instead of risking adhesion and damage to the gastric mucosa.

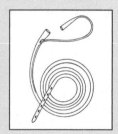

WIDE-BORE GASTRIC TUBES

The Edlich tube (at right) has one wide-bore lumen with four openings near the closed distal tip. A funnel or syringe can be connected at the proximal end. Like the other tubes, the Edlich tube can aspirate a large volume of gastric contents quickly.

The Ewald tube, a wide-bore tube that allows quick passage of a large amount of fluid and clots, is especially useful for gastric lavage in patients with profuse GI bleeding and in those who have ingested poison. Another wide-bore tube, the double-lumen Levacuator, has a large lumen for evacuation of gastric contents and a small one for lavage.

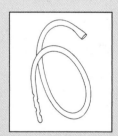

ESOPHAGEAL TUBES

The Sengstaken-Blakemore tube (at right), a triple-lumen double-balloon esophageal tube, provides a gastric aspiration port that allows drainage from below the gastric balloon. It can also be used to instill medication. A similar tube, the Linton shunt, can aspirate esophageal and gastric contents without risking necrosis because it has no esophageal balloon. The Minnesota esophagogastric tamponade tube, which has four lumina and two balloons, provides pressure-monitoring ports for both balloons without the need for Y-connectors.

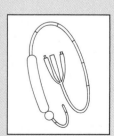

MEDICAL
Anthrax, GI
- Initial findings include loss of appetite, nausea, vomiting, and fever in this bacterial infection.
- Signs and symptoms may progress to hematemesis, abdominal pain, and severe bloody diarrhea.

Coagulation disorders
- GI bleeding and moderate to severe hematemesis may occur.
- Other signs and symptoms vary with the specific coagulation disorder and may include epistaxis and ecchymoses or petechiae.

Esophageal cancer
- Hematemesis is a late sign and occurs with steady chest pain that radiates to the back.
- Other signs and symptoms include substernal fullness, severe dysphagia, nausea, vomiting with nocturnal regurgitation and aspiration, hemoptysis, fever, hiccups, sore throat, melena, and halitosis.

Esophageal rupture
- Severity of hematemesis depends on the cause of the rupture.
- Severe retrosternal, epigastric, neck, or scapular pain accompanied by chest and neck edema may occur.
- Other signs and symptoms include subcutaneous crepitation in the chest wall, supraclavicular fossa, and neck; and signs of respiratory distress.

Esophageal varices, ruptured
- A life-threatening condition, coffee-ground or massive, bright red vomitus may occur.
- Other signs and symptoms include signs of shock, abdominal distention, and melena or painless hematochezia, ranging from slight oozing to massive rectal hemorrhage.

Gastric cancer
- Painless, bright red or dark brown vomitus is a late sign; additional late findings include fatigue, weakness, weight loss, feelings of fullness, melena, altered bowel habits, and signs of malnutrition.
- Other signs and symptoms include upper-abdominal discomfort, anorexia, mild nausea, and chronic dyspepsia unrelieved by antacids and exacerbated by food.

Gastritis, acute
- Hematemesis and melena are the most common signs.
- Other signs and symptoms include mild epigastric discomfort, nausea, fever, malaise, and, with massive blood loss, signs of shock.

GI leiomyoma
- Hematemesis occurs, possibly with dysphagia and weight loss.

Mallory-Weiss syndrome
- Hematemesis and melena may result from mucosal tear at the junction of the esophagus and the stomach, preceded by severe vomiting, retching, or straining.
- Signs of shock may accompany severe bleeding.

Peptic ulcer
- Hematemesis, possibly life-threatening, may occur.
- Other signs and symptoms include melena or hematochezia, abdominal pain, chills, fever, and signs of shock.

OTHER
Esophageal injury by caustic substances
- Hematemesis occurs with epigastric and anterior or retrosternal chest pain that's intensified by swallowing.

Treatments
- Nose or throat surgery, and traumatic NG or endotracheal intubation may cause hematemesis.

- Monitor vital signs; watch for signs of shock.
- Check stools for occult blood.
- Keep accurate intake and output records.
- Place the patient on bed rest in a low or semi-Fowler's position.
- Keep suctioning equipment nearby and use as needed.
- Provide frequent oral hygiene.
- Give a histamine-2 blocker and antacids, as prescribed.
- Prepare the patient for endoscopic evaluation, as needed.

PEDIATRIC POINTERS
- Hematemesis may be related to foreign body ingestion.
- In infants, hemorrhagic disease and esophageal erosion may cause hematemesis.

GERIATRIC POINTERS
- Hematemesis may be caused by a vascular anomaly, an aortoenteric fistula, or upper GI cancer.
- Chronic obstructive pulmonary disease, chronic liver or renal failure, and chronic NSAID use predispose elderly people to hemorrhage caused by coexisting ulcerative disorders.

- Discuss the underlying condition and treatment options.
- Explain foods or fluids the patient should avoid, as appropriate.
- Stress the importance of avoiding alcohol, if applicable.
- Teach the patient and family about all hospital procedures and testing.

Hematochezia

- Passage of bloody stools
- Usually develops abruptly and indicates bleeding below the duodenum
- May precipitate life-threatening hypovolemia

◆ **ACTION STAT!** *If the patient has severe hematochezia, check vital signs for signs of shock. Place the patient in a supine position and elevate his feet. Prepare to administer oxygen, and start a large-bore I.V. line for emergency fluid replacement. Obtain a blood sample for typing and cross-matching, hemoglobin level, and hematocrit. Insert a nasogastric tube. Iced lavage may be indicated to control bleeding. Endoscopy may be necessary to detect the source of the bleeding.*

- Ask about the onset, amount, color, and consistency of stools.
- Find out about associated signs and symptoms.
- Obtain a medical history, including incidence of GI and coagulation disorders.
- Determine the use of GI irritants, such as alcohol, aspirin, and other nonsteroidal anti-inflammatory drugs (NSAIDs).

- Check for orthostatic hypotension.
- Examine the skin for petechiae or spider angiomas.
- Palpate the abdomen for tenderness, pain, or masses.
- Note lymphadenopathy.
- Perform a digital rectal examination to detect rectal masses or hemorrhoids.

MEDICAL
Anal fissure

- Slight hematochezia occurs; blood may streak the stools or appear on toilet tissue.
- Severe rectal pain occurs, leading to reluctance to defecate and eventual constipation.

Anorectal fistula

- Blood, pus, mucus, and occasionally stools may drain from an anorectal fistula.
- Other signs and symptoms include rectal pain and pruritus.

Coagulation disorders

- GI bleeding marked by moderate to severe hematochezia may occur.
- Other signs and symptoms vary with the specific coagulation disorder but may include epistaxis and purpura.

Colitis

- Ischemic colitis commonly causes slight or massive hematochezia; severe, cramping lower abdominal pain; abdominal distention and tenderness; absent bowel sounds; and hypotension.
- Ulcerative colitis typically causes hematochezia that may also contain mucus.
- Other signs and symptoms (of ulcerative colitis) include abdominal cramps, fever, tenesmus, anorexia, nausea, vomiting, hyperactive bowel sounds, tachycardia and, later, weight loss and weakness.

Colon cancer

- Bright red rectal bleeding occurs with or without pain.
- With a left colon tumor, early signs of obstruction occur; later, obstipation, diarrhea or ribbon-shaped stools, and pain relieved by passage of stools or flatus occurs.
- With a right colon tumor, melena, abdominal aching, pressure, and dull cramps occur; later, weakness, fatigue, diarrhea, anorexia, weight loss,

anemia, vomiting, abdominal mass, and signs of obstruction develop.

Colorectal polyps
◆ Intermittent hematochezia occurs.

Crohn's disease
◆ Hematochezia isn't common unless the perineum is involved.
◆ If rectal bleeding occurs, it's likely to be massive.
◆ Other signs and symptoms include fever, abdominal distention and pain with guarding, diarrhea, hyperactive bowel sounds, anorexia, nausea, and fatigue.

Diverticulitis
◆ Mild to moderate rectal bleeding occurs after the patient feels the urge to defecate.
◆ Other signs and symptoms include left-lower-quadrant pain that's relieved by defecation, alternating episodes of constipation and diarrhea, anorexia, nausea, vomiting, rebound tenderness, and a distended, tympanic abdomen.

Dysentery
◆ Bloody diarrhea is common.
◆ Other signs and symptoms include abdominal pain or cramps, tenesmus, fever, nausea, and signs of dehydration.

Esophageal varices, ruptured
◆ A life-threatening condition, hematochezia ranges from slight rectal oozing to grossly bloody stools.
◆ Other signs and symptoms include hematemesis, melena, and signs of shock.

Food poisoning, staphylococcal
◆ Bloody diarrhea may occur 1 to 6 hours after ingesting food toxins.
◆ Other signs and symptoms include nausea, vomiting, prostration, and severe, cramping abdominal pain.

Hemorrhoids
◆ Hematochezia may accompany external hemorrhoids, causing painful defecation, possibly leading to constipation.

◆ Internal hemorrhoids usually produce chronic bleeding with bowel movements, leading to signs of anemia.

Peptic ulcer
◆ Hematochezia, hematemesis, or melena may occur.
◆ Other signs and symptoms include pain relieved by food or antacids, chills, fever, nausea, vomiting, and signs of dehydration and shock.

Small-intestine cancer
◆ Slight hematochezia or blood-streaked stools occur.
◆ Other signs and symptoms include colicky pain, postprandial vomiting, weight loss, anorexia, and fever.

Ulcerative proctitis
◆ The patient has an intense urge to defecate, but passes only bright red blood, pus, or mucus.
◆ Constipation and tenesmus (a painful spasm of the anal sphincter) may develop.

OTHER
Diagnostic tests
◆ Certain procedures, especially colonoscopy, polypectomy, and proctosigmoidoscopy may cause rectal bleeding.

Heavy metal poisoning
◆ Heavy metal poisoning may cause bloody diarrhea accompanied by cramping abdominal pain, nausea, vomiting, tachycardia, hypotension, seizures, paresthesia, depressed or absent deep tendon reflexes, and an altered level of consciousness.

NURSING CONSIDERATIONS

◆ Place the patient on bed rest.
◆ Check vital signs frequently, watching for signs of shock.
◆ Monitor intake and output hourly.
◆ Visually examine stools and test them for occult blood.
◆ If necessary, send a stool sample to the laboratory to check for parasites.

PEDIATRIC POINTERS
◆ Suspect sexual abuse in all cases of rectal bleeding in children.
◆ Hematochezia may also result from structural and inflammatory disorders.
◆ Ulcerative colitis typically produces chronic signs and symptoms in children.

GERIATRIC POINTERS
◆ Hematochezia should be evaluated (using colonoscopy) after ruling out perirectal lesions as the cause of bleeding.

PATIENT TEACHING

◆ Discuss the underlying condition, diagnostic tests, and treatment options.
◆ Explain the signs and symptoms the patient should report.
◆ Teach the patient about ostomy self-care.
◆ Discuss proper bowel elimination habits.
◆ Explain dietary recommendations and restrictions.

Hematuria

- Abnormal presence of blood in urine
- Cardinal sign of renal and urinary tract disorders
- Results from rupture or perforation of vessels in the renal system or urinary tract or from impaired glomerular filtration, which allows red blood cells (RBCs) to seep into the urine
- May be microscopic (confirmed by occult blood) or macroscopic (immediately visible)
- Classified as initial (occurring at the start of urination), terminal (occurring at the end of urination), or total (occurring throughout urination)

HISTORY

- Ask about the onset, description, and severity.
- Find out about associated pain, burning, frequency, and urgency.
- Obtain a medical history, including incidence of renal, urinary, prostatic, or coagulation disorders, and recent abdominal or flank trauma.
- Find out about recent strenuous exercise.
- Take a drug history, noting use of anticoagulants or aspirin.

PHYSICAL ASSESSMENT

- Percuss and palpate the abdomen and flanks.
- Percuss the costovertebral angle (CVA) to elicit tenderness.
- Check the urinary meatus for bleeding or other abnormalities.
- Obtain a urine specimen for testing.
- Perform a vaginal or digital rectal examination.

CAUSES

MEDICAL
Bladder cancer
- Gross hematuria occurs with pain in bladder, rectum, pelvis, flank, back, or leg.

- Other signs and symptoms include nocturia, dysuria, urinary frequency and urgency, vomiting, diarrhea, and insomnia.

Bladder trauma
- Hematuria occurs with lower abdominal pain.
- Other signs and symptoms include dysuria, anuria despite a strong urge to void; swelling of the scrotum, buttocks, or perineum; and signs of shock.

Calculi
- Bladder calculi causes gross hematuria, pain that's referred to the lower back or penile or vulvar area, and bladder distention.
- Renal calculi causes microscopic or gross hematuria, colicky pain (cardinal sign) that travels from the CVA to the flank, suprapubic region, and external genitalia when a calculus is passed; nausea; vomiting; restlessness; fever; chills; and abdominal distention.

Coagulation disorders
- Macroscopic hematuria is often the first sign of hemorrhage.
- Other signs and symptoms include epistaxis, purpura, and signs of GI bleeding.

Cystitis
- Bacterial cystitis usually produces macroscopic hematuria with urinary urgency and frequency, dysuria, perineal and lumbar pain, suprapubic discomfort, and nocturia.
- Chronic interstitial cystitis occasionally causes grossly bloody hematuria with urinary frequency, dysuria, nocturia, and tenesmus.
- Viral cystitis usually produces hematuria, urinary urgency and frequency, dysuria, nocturia, tenesmus, and fever.

Glomerulonephritis
- Acute form causes gross hematuria that tapers off to microscopic hematuria and RBC casts.
- Other acute signs and symptoms include oliguria or anuria, proteinuria,

mild fever, fatigue, flank and abdominal pain, edema, increased blood pressure, nausea, vomiting, and crackles.
- Chronic form causes hematuria that's accompanied by proteinuria, generalized edema, and increased blood pressure.

Nephritis, interstitial
- Microscopic hematuria is typical, but some patients may develop gross hematuria.
- Other signs and symptoms include fever, maculopapular rash, and oliguria or anuria.

Nephropathy, obstructive
- Microscopic or macroscopic hematuria occurs with colicky flank and abdominal pain, CVA tenderness, and anuria or oliguria that alternates with polyuria.

Polycystic kidney disease
- Microscopic or gross hematuria occurs.
- Increased blood pressure, polyuria, dull flank pain, and signs of urinary tract infection also occur.
- Late signs and symptoms include a swollen, tender abdomen and lumbar pain that's aggravated by exertion and relieved by lying down.

Prostatic hyperplasia, benign
- Macroscopic hematuria occurs with significant obstruction.
- Early signs and symptoms include diminished urinary stream, tenesmus, and a feeling of incomplete voiding.
- Late signs and symptoms include urinary hesitancy, frequency, and incontinence; nocturia; perineal pain; an enlarged prostate on rectal palpation; and constipation.

Prostatitis
- Macroscopic hematuria occurs at the end of urination.
- Urinary frequency and urgency and dysuria occurs followed by visible bladder distention.
- Acute form causes fatigue, malaise, myalgia, arthralgia, fever, chills, nau-

sea, vomiting, perineal and lower back pain, decreased libido, and a tender, swollen, firm prostate on palpation.
◆ Chronic form causes persistent urethral discharge, dull perineal pain, ejaculatory pain, and decreased libido.

Pyelonephritis, acute
◆ Microscopic or macroscopic hematuria progresses to grossly bloody hematuria.
◆ After the infection resolves, microscopic hematuria may persist for a few months.
◆ Other signs and symptoms include persistent high fever, flank pain, CVA tenderness, shaking chills, weakness, nausea, vomiting, anorexia, fatigue, dysuria, urinary frequency and urgency, nocturia, and tenesmus.

Renal cancer
◆ Grossly bloody hematuria; dull, aching flank pain; and a smooth, firm, palpable flank mass are the classic triad of signs and symptoms.
◆ Colicky pain also occurs accompanied by the passage of clots, CVA tenderness, fever, and increased blood pressure.
◆ In advanced disease, weight loss, nausea, vomiting, and leg edema with varicoceles occurs.

Renal infarction
◆ Gross hematuria occurs.
◆ Constant, severe flank and upper abdominal pain occurs with CVA tenderness, anorexia, nausea, and vomiting.
◆ Other signs and symptoms include oliguria or anuria, proteinuria, hypoactive bowel sounds, fever, and increased blood pressure.

Renal papillary necrosis, acute
◆ Grossly bloody hematuria occurs.
◆ Other signs and symptoms include intense flank pain, CVA tenderness, abdominal rigidity and colicky pain, oliguria or anuria, pyuria, fever, chills, hypertension, arthralgia, vomiting, and hypoactive bowel sounds.

Renal trauma
◆ Microscopic or gross hematuria occurs.
◆ Other signs and symptoms include flank pain, a palpable flank mass, oliguria, hematoma or ecchymoses over the upper abdomen or flank, nausea, vomiting, hypoactive bowel sounds and, in severe trauma, signs of shock.

Renal tuberculosis
◆ Gross hematuria is commonly the first sign.
◆ Other signs and symptoms include urinary frequency, dysuria, pyuria, tenesmus, colicky abdominal pain, lumbar pain, and proteinuria.

Renal vein thrombosis
◆ Grossly bloody hematuria occurs.
◆ With abrupt venous obstruction, severe flank and lumbar pain and epigastric and CVA tenderness occurs.
◆ Other signs and symptoms include fever, pallor, proteinuria, peripheral edema, and oliguria or anuria if obstruction is bilateral.

Sickle cell anemia
◆ Gross hematuria occurs.
◆ Other signs and symptoms include pallor, dehydration, chronic fatigue, tachycardia, heart murmurs, polyarthralgia, leg ulcers, dyspnea, chest pain, impaired growth and development, hepatomegaly, and jaundice.

Systemic lupus erythematosus
◆ Gross hematuria occurs along with proteinuria if the kidneys are involved.
◆ Other signs and symptoms include joint pain and stiffness, butterfly rash, photosensitivity, Raynaud's phenomenon, seizures, psychoses, recurrent fever, lymphadenopathy, oral or nasopharyngeal ulcers, anorexia, and weight loss.

Urethral trauma
◆ Initial hematuria occurs with blood at the urinary meatus, local pain, and penile or vulvar ecchymoses.

OTHER
Diagnostic tests and treatments
◆ Renal biopsy and biopsy or manipulative instrumentation of the urinary tract may result in hematuria.
◆ Kidney transplant may cause hematuria.

Drugs
◆ Drugs that may cause hematuria include anticoagulants, aspirin toxicity, analgesics, cyclophosphamide, metyrosine, phenylbutazone, penicillin, rifampin, and thiabendazole.

NURSING CONSIDERATIONS

◆ Check vital signs frequently.
◆ Monitor intake and output, including the amount and pattern of hematuria.
◆ If the patient has an indwelling urinary catheter in place, ensure its patency; irrigate if necessary.
◆ Administer analgesics, as indicated.

PEDIATRIC POINTERS
◆ Common causes of hematuria in children include congenital anomalies, birth trauma, hematologic disorders, certain neoplasms, allergies, and foreign bodies in the urinary tract.

GERIATRIC POINTERS
◆ Evaluation of hematuria should include a urine culture, excretory urography or sonography, and consultation with a urologist.

PATIENT TEACHING

◆ Discuss the underlying condition, diagnostic testing, and treatment options.
◆ Emphasize increasing fluid intake.
◆ Instruct the patient in signs and symptoms to report.

Hemianopsia

OVERVIEW

- Vision loss in one-half the visual field of one or both eyes (see *Recognizing visual field defects*)
- Caused by a lesion affecting the optic pathways

HISTORY

- Ask about associated headache, dysarthria, seizures, hallucinations, or loss of color vision.
- Determine the onset of neurologic symptoms.
- Obtain a medical history, noting eye disorders, hypertension, diabetes mellitus, and recent head trauma.

PHYSICAL ASSESSMENT

- Take vital signs.
- Evaluate level of consciousness (LOC).
- Check pupillary reaction.
- Evaluate for ptosis or facial or extremity weakness.
- Assess visual fields and plot areas of vision loss.

 TOP TECHNIQUE

Recognizing visual field defects

Lesions of the optic pathways cause visual field defects. The lesion's site determines the type of defect. For example, a lesion of the optic chiasm involving only those fibers that cross over to the opposite side causes bitemporal hemianopsia—visual loss in the temporal half of each field. However, a lesion of the optic tract or a complete lesion of the optic radiation produces visual loss in the same half of each field—either left or right homonymous hemianopsia.

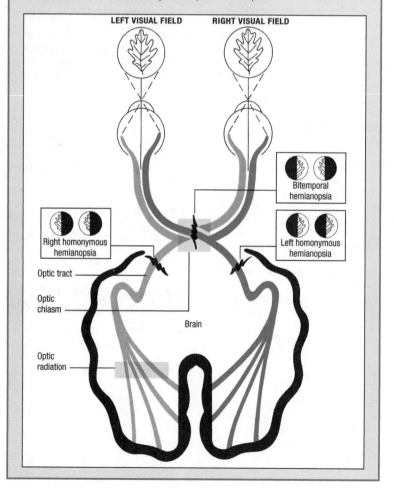

CAUSES

MEDICAL

Carotid artery aneurysm

◆ Contralateral or bilateral defects in visual fields may occur with hemiplegia, decreased LOC, headache, aphasia, behavior disturbances, and unilateral hypoesthesia.

Occipital lobe lesion

◆ Incomplete homonymous hemianopsia, scotomas, and impaired color vision are the most common symptoms.
◆ Visual hallucinations that appear in the defective field or move toward it from the intact field may also occur.

Parietal lobe lesion

◆ Homonymous hemianopsia and sensory deficits occur.
◆ Apraxia and visual or tactile agnosia may also develop.

Pituitary tumor

◆ Complete or partial bitemporal hemianopsia first occurs in the upper visual fields but later can progress to blindness.
◆ Other signs and symptoms include blurred vision, diplopia, and headache.

Stroke

◆ Hemianopsia can result when stroke affects any part of the optic pathway.
◆ Other signs and symptoms vary with the location and size of the stroke and may include decreased LOC, intellectual deficits, personality changes, emotional lability, hemiplegia, dysarthria, dysphagia, ataxia, sensory loss, apraxia, aphasia, blurred vision, urine retention or incontinence, headache, and seizures.

NURSING CONSIDERATIONS

◆ To avoid startling the patient, approach him from the unaffected side.
◆ Position the bed so that the patient's unaffected side faces the door.
◆ Remove objects that could cause falls, and alert the patient to other possible hazards.
◆ Place personal objects within field of vision; avoid putting dangerous objects where the patient can't see them.

PEDIATRIC POINTERS

◆ The most common cause of hemianopsia in children is brain tumors.

PATIENT TEACHING

◆ Discuss compensation techniques.
◆ Stress safety measures.
◆ Teach about underlying diagnosis and treatment options.

Hemoptysis

OVERVIEW

- Expectoration of blood or bloody sputum from the lungs or tracheobronchial tree (see *Identifying hemoptysis*)
- Usually results from chronic bronchitis, lung cancer, or bronchiectasis (see *What happens in hemoptysis*)

 ACTION STAT! *If the patient coughs up a copious amount of blood, endotracheal intubation may be required. Massive hemoptysis can cause airway obstruction and asphyxiation. Suction frequently to remove blood. Lavage may be necessary to loosen tenacious secretions or clots. Insert an I.V. line for fluid replacement, drug administration, and blood transfusion, if needed. Bronchoscopy may be performed to identify the bleeding site. Monitor vital signs to detect shock.*

HISTORY

- Ask about the onset and extent of hemoptysis.
- Obtain a medical history of cardiac, pulmonary, or bleeding disorders; recent infection; and exposure to tuberculosis.
- Ask about the date and results of the last tuberculin tine test.
- Obtain a drug history, including use of anticoagulants.
- Obtain a smoking history.

PHYSICAL ASSESSMENT

- Take vital signs.
- Examine the nose, mouth, and pharynx for sources of bleeding.
- Inspect the chest; look for abnormal movement during breathing and use of accessory muscles.
- Observe respiratory rate, depth, and rhythm.
- Examine skin for lesions.
- Palpate the chest for diaphragm level and for tenderness, respiratory excursion, fremitus, and abnormal pulsations.
- Percuss the chest for flatness, dullness, resonance, hyperresonance, and tympany.
- Auscultate for breath sounds.
- Auscultate for heart murmurs, bruits, and pleural rubs.
- Obtain sputum sample, and examine it for quantity, amount of blood, and color, odor, and consistency.

CAUSES

MEDICAL
Bronchial adenoma
- Recurring hemoptysis occurs along with a chronic cough and local wheezing.
- Recurrent infection, dyspnea, and wheezing may also occur.

Bronchiectasis
- Hemoptysis appearance varies from blood-tinged sputum to frank blood, depending on extent of bronchial blood vessel erosion.
- Other signs and symptoms include chronic cough, coarse crackles, late clubbing, fever, weight loss, fatigue, weakness, malaise, dyspnea on exertion, and copious, foul-smelling, and purulent sputum.

Bronchitis, chronic
- A productive cough leads to production of blood-streaked sputum.

TOP TECHNIQUE

Identifying hemoptysis

These guidelines will help you distinguish hemoptysis from epistaxis, hematemesis, and brown, red, or pink sputum.

HEMOPTYSIS

Usually frothy because it's mixed with air, blood is typically bright red with an alkaline pH (tested with Nitrazine paper). Hemoptysis is strongly suggested by the presence of respiratory signs and symptoms, including a cough, a tickling sensation in the throat, and blood produced from repeated coughing episodes. (You can rule out epistaxis because the patient's nasal passages and posterior pharynx are usually clear.)

HEMATEMESIS

The usual site of hematemesis is the GI tract; the patient vomits or regurgitates coffee-ground-like material that contains food particles, tests positive for occult blood, and has an acid pH. However, he may vomit bright red blood or swallowed blood from the oral cavity and nasopharynx. After an episode of hematemesis, the patient may have stools with traces of blood. Many patients with hematemesis also complain of dyspepsia.

BROWN, RED, OR PINK SPUTUM

Brown, red, or pink sputum can result from oxidation of inhaled bronchodilators. Sputum that looks like old blood may result from rupture of an amebic abscess into the bronchus. Red or brown sputum may occur in a patient with pneumonia caused by the enterobacterium *Serratia marcescens*. Currant-jelly–like sputum occurs with *Klebsiella* infections.

What happens in hemoptysis

Hemoptysis results when bronchial or pulmonary vessels bleed into the respiratory tract. Bleeding reflects alterations in the vascular walls and in blood-clotting mechanisms. It can result from any of the following pathophysiologic processes:

- hemorrhage and diapedesis of red blood cells from the pulmonary microvasculature into the alveoli
- necrosis of lung tissue that causes inflammation and rupture of blood vessels or hemorrhage into the alveolar spaces
- rupture of an aortic aneurysm into the tracheobronchial tree
- rupture of distended endobronchial blood vessels from pulmonary hypertension due to mitral stenosis
- rupture of a pulmonary arteriovenous fistula, of bronchial or pulmonary artery collateral channels, or of pulmonary venous collateral channels
- sloughing of a caseous lesion into the tracheobronchial tree
- ulceration and erosion of the bronchial epithelium.

- Other signs and symptoms include dyspnea, prolonged expirations, wheezing, scattered rhonchi, accessory muscle use, barrel chest, tachypnea, and late clubbing.

Coagulation disorders
- Hemoptysis occurs with multisystem hemorrhaging and purpuric lesions.

Laryngeal cancer
- Hemoptysis occurs, but hoarseness is the usual early sign.
- Other signs and symptoms include dysphagia, dyspnea, stridor, cervical lymphadenopathy, and neck pain.

Lung abscess
- Blood-streaked sputum occurs.
- Other signs and symptoms include fever, chills, diaphoresis, anorexia, dyspnea, pleuritic or dull chest pain, clubbing, and a cough with purulent, foul-smelling sputum.

Lung cancer
- Recurring hemoptysis is an early sign.
- Other signs and symptoms include a productive cough, dyspnea, fever, anorexia, weight loss, wheezing, and chest pain (a late sign).

Pneumonia
- *Klebsiella* pneumonia produces dark brown or red tenacious sputum that the patient has difficulty expelling from his mouth; it's abrupt in onset with accompanying chills, fever, dyspnea, productive cough, severe pleuritic chest pain, cyanosis, tachycardia, decreased breath sounds, and crackles.
- Pneumococcal pneumonia causes pinkish or rust-colored mucoid sputum; onset is marked by sudden shaking chills and fever, tachycardia, and tachypnea.
- Other signs and symptoms include rapid, shallow, grunting respirations with splinting; accessory muscle use; malaise; weakness; myalgia; and prostration.

Pulmonary contusion
- Cough and hemoptysis occur after blunt chest trauma.
- Other signs and symptoms include dyspnea, tachypnea, chest pain, tachycardia, hypotension, crackles, decreased or absent breath sounds over the affected area and, possibly, severe respiratory distress.

Pulmonary edema
- A life-threatening condition, frothy, blood-tinged pink sputum accompanies severe dyspnea, orthopnea, gasping, anxiety, cyanosis, diffuse crackles, a ventricular gallop, and cold, clammy skin.
- Other signs and symptoms include tachycardia, lethargy, arrhythmias, tachypnea, hypotension, and a thready pulse.

Pulmonary embolism with infarction
- Hemoptysis is a common sign of this life-threatening disorder.
- Initial symptoms typically include cough, dyspnea, anxiety, and anginal or pleuritic chest pain.

Pulmonary hypertension, primary
- Hemoptysis, exertional dyspnea, and fatigue are common, but generally develop late in the disease process.
- Other signs and symptoms include arrhythmias, syncope, cough, hoarseness, and angina-like pain that occurs with exertion and may radiate to the neck.

Pulmonary tuberculosis
- Hemoptysis is a common sign.
- Other signs and symptoms include chronic productive cough, fine crackles after coughing, dyspnea, dullness to percussion, increased tactile fremitus, amphoric breath sounds, night sweats, malaise, fatigue, fever, anorexia, weight loss, and pleuritic chest pain.

Silicosis
- A productive cough with mucopurulent sputum becomes blood-streaked, and, occasionally, massive hemoptysis may occur.

- Other signs and symptoms include exertional dyspnea, tachypnea, weight loss, fatigue, weakness, and fine, end-inspiratory crackles.

Systemic lupus erythematosus
- Pleuritis and pneumonitis may cause hemoptysis.
- Other signs and symptoms include butterfly rash, nondeforming joint pain and stiffness, photosensitivity, Raynaud's phenomenon, convulsions or psychoses, anorexia with weight loss, and lymphadenopathy.

OTHER
Diagnostic tests
- Lung or airway injury from bronchoscopy, laryngoscopy, mediastinoscopy, or lung biopsy may cause bleeding and hemoptysis.

Treatments
- Traumatic or prolonged intubation may produce hemoptysis.
- Surgery to the lungs, throat, or upper airways may cause hemoptysis.

NURSING CONSIDERATIONS

- To protect the nonbleeding lung, place the patient in the lateral decubitus position, with the suspected bleeding lung facing down.
- Monitor the patient's respiratory status, vital signs, and blood test results. especially clotting times closely.

PEDIATRIC POINTERS
- Hemoptysis in children may stem from Goodpasture's syndrome or cystic fibrosis.

PATIENT TEACHING

- Explain the importance of reporting recurrent episodes.
- Give the patient instructions for providing sputum samples
- Discuss the underlying condition, diagnostic tests, and treatment options.

Hepatomegaly

OVERVIEW

- Refers to enlargement of the liver
- Indicates potentially reversible primary or secondary liver disease
- May be confirmed by palpation, percussion, or radiologic tests

HISTORY

- Ask about alcohol use.
- Determine exposure to hepatitis.
- Obtain a drug history.
- Ask about the location and description of any associated abdominal pain.
- Ask about nausea, vomiting, fever, and weight loss.

PHYSICAL ASSESSMENT

- Inspect the skin and sclerae for jaundice, dilated veins, scars from previous surgery, and spider angiomas.
- Inspect the contour of the abdomen and measure abdominal girth.
- Percuss the liver. (See *Percussing the liver for size and position*.)
- During deep inspiration, palpate the liver's edge.
- Take vital signs.
- Assess nutritional status.
- Evaluate level of consciousness (LOC).
- Watch for personality changes, irritability, agitation, memory loss, inability to concentrate, poor mentation, and—in a severely ill patient—coma.

CAUSES

MEDICAL

Cirrhosis

- In the late stage of this disease, the liver becomes enlarged, nodular, and hard.
- Other late signs and symptoms affect all body systems and include jaundice, ascites, hypoxia, encephalopathy, bleeding disorders, and portal hypertension.

Diabetes mellitus

- Hepatomegaly, and right-upper-quadrant tenderness along with polydipsia, polyphagia, and polyuria may occur in overweight patients with poorly controlled diabetes.

Heart failure

- Hepatomegaly occurs along with jugular vein distention, cyanosis, nocturia, dependent edema of the legs and sacrum, steady weight gain, confusion and, possibly, nausea, vomiting, abdominal discomfort, and anorexia.
- Massive right-sided failure may cause anasarca, oliguria, severe weakness, and anxiety.
- If left-sided failure precedes right-sided failure, signs and symptoms include dyspnea, orthopnea, paroxysmal nocturnal dyspnea, tachypnea, arrhythmias, tachycardia, and fatigue.

Hepatitis

- Hepatomegaly occurs in the icteric phase and continues during the recovery phase.
- Early signs and symptoms include nausea, vomiting, fatigue, malaise, photophobia, sore throat, cough, and headache.
- Other signs and symptoms of the icteric phase include liver tenderness, slight weight loss, dark urine, clay-colored stools, jaundice, pruritus, right-upper-quadrant pain, and splenomegaly.

TOP TECHNIQUE

Percussing the liver for size and position

With your patient in a supine position, begin at the right iliac crest to percuss up the right midclavicular line (MCL), as shown here. The percussion note becomes dull when you reach the liver's inferior border—usually at the costal margin but sometimes at a lower point in a patient with liver disease. Mark this point and then percuss down from the right clavicle, again along the right MCL. The liver's superior border usually lies between the fifth and seventh intercostal spaces. Mark the superior border.

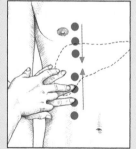

The distance between the two marked points represents the approximate span of the liver's right lobe, which normally ranges from 2¼" to 4¾" (5.5 to 12 cm).

Next, assess the liver's left lobe similarly, percussing along the sternal midline. Again, mark the points where you hear dull percussion notes. Also measure the span of the left lobe, which normally ranges from 1½" to 3⅛" (4 to 8 cm). Record your findings for use as a baseline.

Leukemia and lymphomas

◆ Moderate to massive hepatomegaly, splenomegaly, and abdominal discomfort are common.
◆ Other signs and symptoms include malaise, low-grade fever, fatigue, weakness, tachycardia, weight loss, bleeding disorders, and anorexia.

Liver cancer

◆ Primary liver tumors cause irregular, nodular, firm hepatomegaly, with pain or tenderness in the right upper quadrant and a friction rub or bruit over the liver.
◆ Metastatic liver tumors cause hepatomegaly, but accompanying signs and symptoms reflect the primary cancer.
◆ Other signs and symptoms include weight loss, anorexia, cachexia, nausea, vomiting, peripheral edema, ascites, jaundice, and a palpable right-upper-quadrant mass.

Mononucleosis, infectious

◆ Hepatomegaly may occur.
◆ Prodromal symptoms include headache, malaise, and extreme fatigue.
◆ After 3 to 5 days, signs and symptoms include sore throat, cervical lymphadenopathy, temperature fluctuations, stomatitis, palatal petechiae, periorbital edema, splenomegaly, exudative tonsillitis, pharyngitis, and a maculopapular rash.

Obesity

◆ Hepatomegaly may occur along with respiratory difficulties, cardiovascular disease, diabetes, renal disease, gallbladder disease, and psychological difficulties.

Pancreatic cancer

◆ Hepatomegaly accompanies anorexia, weight loss, abdominal or back pain, and jaundice.
◆ Other signs and symptoms include nausea, vomiting, fever, fatigue, weakness, pruritus, and skin lesions.

NURSING CONSIDERATIONS

◆ Provide bed rest, relief from stress, and adequate nutrition.
◆ Monitor and restrict dietary protein, as needed.
◆ Give hepatotoxic drugs or drugs metabolized by the liver in very small doses, if at all.

PEDIATRIC POINTERS

◆ Childhood hepatomegaly may stem from Reye's syndrome, biliary atresia, rare disorders, or poorly controlled type 1 diabetes mellitus.

PATIENT TEACHING

◆ Explain the treatment plan for underlying disorder and diagnostic tests.
◆ Stress the avoidance of alcohol and people with infections.
◆ Emphasize personal hygiene.
◆ Discuss the importance of pacing activities and rest periods.

Hiccups

OVERVIEW

- An involuntary, spasmodic contraction of the diaphragm followed by sudden closure of the glottis
- Characteristic sound reflecting the vibration of closed vocal cords as air suddenly rushes into the lungs (see *How hiccups occur*)
- Usually benign and transient and subside spontaneously

HISTORY

- Ask when the patient's hiccups began, if he's had them before, what caused them, and what makes them stop.
- Ask if the hiccups are tiring him.
- Find out if the patient has a history of abdominal or thoracic disorders.
- Ask about expsosure to fumes.

CAUSES

MEDICAL

Abdominal distention
- The most common cause of hiccups, abdominal distention also causes a feeling of fullness and, depending on the cause, abdominal pain, nausea, and vomiting.

Brain stem lesion
- Producing persistent hiccups, this type of lesion also causes decreased level of consciousness, dysphagia, dysarthria, an absent corneal reflex on the side opposite the lesion, altered respiratory pattern, abnormal pupillary response, and ocular deviation.

Gastric cancer
- Persistent hiccups can be the presenting sign of this disease.
- Other signs and symptoms include dyspepsia, abdominal pain, anorexia, early satiety, and weight loss.

Gastric dilation
- Besides hiccups, possible signs and symptoms include a sense of fullness, epigastric pain, and regurgitation or persistent vomiting.

Gastritis
- This disorder can cause hiccups along with mild epigastric discomfort (sometimes the only symptom).
- Other signs and symptoms include upper abdominal pain, eructation, fever, malaise, nausea, vomiting, hematemesis, and melena.

Increased intracranial pressure
- Early findings may include hiccups, vomiting, drowsiness, and headache.
- Classic later signs and symptoms include changes in pupillary reactions and respiratory pattern, increased systolic pressure, and bradycardia.

Pancreatitis
- Hiccups, vomiting, and sudden and steady epigastric pain (often radiating to the back) may occur in this disorder.

How hiccups occur

Hiccups may result from irritations in the chest or abdomen that trigger transmission of impulses through the vagus (afferent) and phrenic (efferent) nerves to the diaphragm. Upon completion of this reflex arc, the diaphragm contracts, and the resulting abrupt intake of air is promptly cut off as the glottis snaps shut.

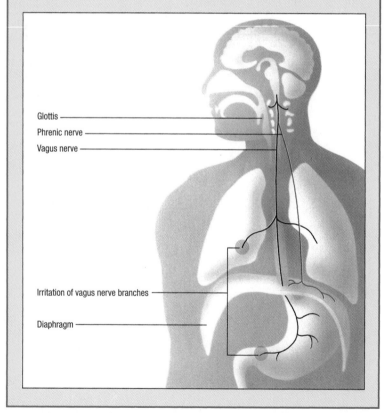

Glottis
Phrenic nerve
Vagus nerve

Irritation of vagus nerve branches

Diaphragm

- A severe attack may cause persistent vomiting, extreme restlessness, fever, and abdominal tenderness and rigidity.

Pleural irritation
- Besides hiccups, this condition may cause cough, dyspnea, or chest pain.

Renal failure
- Hiccups may occur in the late stages of both chronic and acute renal failure.
- Other signs and symptoms affect every body system and include fatigue, oliguria or anuria, nausea, vomiting, confusion, flank pain, yellow-brown or bronze skin, uremic frost, ammonia breath odor, bleeding tendencies, gum ulcerations, asterixis, and Kussmaul's respirations.

OTHER
Surgery
- Mild and transient attacks of hiccups occasionally follow abdominal surgery.

NURSING CONSIDERATIONS

- Treatment for hiccups includes gastric lavage or applying finger pressure on the eyeballs (through closed lids).
- Hiccups may also be relieved by briefly applying ice cubes to both sides of the neck at the level of the larynx.
- If hiccups persist, a phenothiazine (especially chlorpromazine), metoclopramide (Reglan), or nasogastric intubation may provide relief. (*Caution*: The tube may cause vomiting.)
- If simpler methods fail, treatment may include a phrenic nerve block.

PEDIATRIC POINTERS
- In an infant, hiccups usually result from rapid ingestion of liquids without adequate burping. Tell parents to hold the infant upright during feedings.

PATIENT TEACHING

- Teach the patient simple methods of relieving hiccups, such as holding his breath repeatedly or rebreathing into a paper bag (both of which increase his serum carbon dioxide level, which inhibits hiccups).
- If abdominal distention is the probable cause of hiccups, teach the patient lifestyle changes, such as eating smaller, more frequent meals and avoiding large meals before bedtime.
- Advise the patient to increase fiber and fluid intake to avoid constipation.
- Warn the patient with chronic renal failure that persistent hiccups, usually accompanied by nausea and vomiting, can indicate worsening or acute decompensation of renal function.

Hirsutism

OVERVIEW

- Refers to excessive growth of coarse body and facial hair, especially in females
- Involves excessive androgen production or an increased sensitivity of the skin to androgens
- May be mild, moderate, or severe
- Further virilization caused by extremely high androgen levels (see *Recognizing signs of virilization*)

HISTORY

- Ask about the onset of hirsutism.
- Inquire about the use of hair removal techniques.
- Obtain a menstrual history.
- Obtain a drug history, including drugs containing an androgen or progestin compound.

PHYSICAL ASSESSMENT

- Examine the hirsute areas, noting the distribution pattern of the hair.
- Observe the patient for obesity.
- Observe for other signs of virilization.

TOP TECHNIQUE

Recognizing signs of virilization

Excessive androgen levels produce severe hirsutism and other marked signs of virilization. As you examine your patient, look for the signs of virilization shown below.

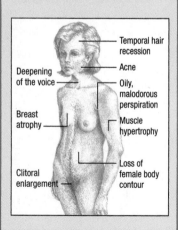

- Temporal hair recession
- Acne
- Deepening of the voice
- Oily, malodorous perspiration
- Breast atrophy
- Muscle hypertrophy
- Clitoral enlargement
- Loss of female body contour

CAUSES

MEDICAL

Acromegaly
- Hirsutism may be accompanied by enlarged hands and feet, coarsened facial features, prognathism, increased diaphoresis, oily skin, fatigue, weight gain, heat intolerance, and lethargy.

Adrenocortical carcinoma
- Hirsutism progresses rapidly.
- Truncal obesity, buffalo hump, moon face, oligomenorrhea, amenorrhea, muscle wasting, and thin skin with purple striae develop.
- Other signs and symptoms include muscle weakness, excessive diaphoresis, poor wound healing, acne, deepened voice, weakness, fatigue, hypertension, hyperpigmentation, and personality changes.

Androgen overproduction by ovaries
- Hirsutism and anovulation occur with other signs of virilization.

Cushing's syndrome (hypercortisolism)
- Hair growth increases on the face, abdomen, breasts, chest, or upper thighs.
- Other signs and symptoms include truncal obesity, buffalo hump, moon face, thin skin, purple striae, ecchymoses, petechiae, muscle wasting and weakness, poor wound healing, hypertension, weakness, fatigue, excessive diaphoresis, hyperpigmentation, menstrual irregularities, and personality changes.

Hyperprolactinemia
- Hirsutism, hypogonadism, galactorrhea, amenorrhea, and acne develop.
- Infertility may be present.
- Visual field defects may occur if a pituitary tumor is the cause.

Idiopathic hirsutism
- Excess hair growth occurs at puberty, increasing in early adulthood.
- Other signs and symptoms include acne, obesity, infrequent menses or anovulation, and thick, oily skin.

Ovarian tumor
◆ If tumor produces androgens, rapidly progressing hirsutism may occur with amenorrhea and rapidly developing virilization.

Polycystic ovary disease
◆ Hirsutism occurs after onset of menstrual irregularities.
◆ Other signs and symptoms include obesity, amenorrhea, oligomenorrhea, menometrorrhagia, infertility, insulin-reistant diabetes, and acne.

OTHER
Drugs
◆ Aminoglutethimide, cyclosporine, drugs containing androgens or progestins, glucocorticoids, metoclopramide, and minoxidil can result in hirsutism.

NURSING CONSIDERATIONS

◆ Prepare the patient for tests to determine blood levels of luteinizing hormone, follicle-stimulating hormone, prolactin, and other hormones.
◆ Encourage verbalization of concerns about self-image.

PEDIATRIC POINTERS
◆ Hirsutism can stem from congenital adrenal hyperplasia.
◆ Hirsutism that occurs at or after puberty commonly results from polycystic ovary disease.

GERIATRIC POINTERS
◆ Hirsutism can occur after menopause if peripheral conversion of estrogen is poor.

PATIENT TEACHING

◆ Explain the cause of the patient's hirsutism.
◆ Explain the treatment.
◆ Discuss hair removal techniques.

Hoarseness

OVERVIEW

- Characterized as a rough or harsh sound to the voice
- May be acute or chronic

HISTORY

- Ask about the onset and quality of hoarseness and aggravating factors.
- Inquire about associated shortness of breath, sore throat, dry mouth, cough, or difficulty swallowing dry food.
- Find out about exposure to fire or noxious fume inhalation within the past 48 hours or overuse of voice.
- Obtain a medical history, including incidence of cancer, rheumatoid arthritis, or aortic aneurysm.
- Find out about alcohol and smoking habits.

PHYSICAL ASSESSMENT

- Inspect the oral cavity and pharynx for redness or exudate.
- Palpate the neck for masses and the cervical lymph nodes and the thyroid gland for enlargement.
- Palpate the trachea.
- Ask the patient to stick out his tongue; if he can't, he may have paralysis from cranial nerve involvement.
- Examine the eyes for corneal ulcers and enlarged lacrimal ducts.
- Examine for dilated jugular and chest veins.
- Take vital signs.
- Inspect for asymmetrical chest expansion or signs of respiratory distress.
- Auscultate for crackles, rhonchi, wheezing, and tubular sounds.
- Percuss the chest for dullness.

CAUSES

MEDICAL

Gastroesophageal reflux
- Hoarseness, sore throat, cough, heartburn, throat clearing, and feeling of a lump in the throat may occur.
- The laryngeal tissue and vocal cords may appear red and swollen.

Hypothyroidism
- Hoarseness may occur early.
- Other signs and symptoms include fatigue, cold intolerance, coarse hair, alopecia, weight gain despite anorexia, menorrhagia, thinning nails, and dry, flaky skin.

Laryngeal cancer
- Hoarseness is an early sign but may not occur until later in disease process.
- Other signs and symptoms include a long history of smoking, persistent minor throat discomfort, dysphagia, otalgia, hemoptysis, and a mild, dry cough.

Laryngeal leukoplakia
- Hoarseness is common, especially in smokers.
- Mild, moderate, or severe dysphagia may also occur.

Laryngitis
- Persistent hoarseness may be the only sign in the chronic form.
- Hoarseness or complete loss of voice develops suddenly in the acute form.
- Other signs and symptoms include pain (especially during swallowing or speaking), cough, fever, profuse diaphoresis, sore throat, and rhinorrhea.

Thoracic aortic aneurysm
- Hoarseness may occur with thoracic aortic aneurysm.
- The most common symptom is penetrating pain that's especially severe when the patient is supine.

- Other signs and symptoms include brassy cough, dyspnea, and a substernal aching in the shoulders, lower back, or abdomen.

Tracheal trauma
- Hoarseness occurs with hemoptysis, dysphagia, neck pain, airway occlusion, and respiratory distress.
- Cervical spine injuries may also be present.

Vocal cord paralysis
- Hoarseness and vocal weakness occurs with vocal cord paralysis.
- Other signs and symptoms include signs of head or neck trauma, dyspnea, and dysphagia.

Vocal cord polyps or nodules
- Raspy hoarseness accompanies chronic cough and crackling voice.

OTHER
Inhalation injury
- Inhalation injury from a fire or explosion produces hoarseness, coughing, singed nasal hairs, orofacial burns, soot-stained sputum and, possibly, respiratory distress.

Treatments
- Prolonged intubation may cause temporary hoarseness.
- Surgical trauma to the laryngeal nerve may cause temporary or permanent vocal cord paralysis.

NURSING CONSIDERATIONS
- Observe the patient for stridor.
- When hoarseness lasts for longer than 2 weeks, indirect or fiberoptic laryngoscopy is indicated.

PEDIATRIC POINTERS
- In infants and young children, hoarseness may result from congenital anomalies, but may also result from croup.
- In prepubescent boys, hoarseness can stem from juvenile papillomatosis of the upper respiratory tract.

PATIENT TEACHING
- Discuss the underlying condition, diagnostic tests, and treatment options.
- Explain the importance of resting the voice.
- Teach the patient alternative ways to communicate.
- Stress the avoidance of alcohol, smoking, and second-hand smoke.

Homans' sign

OVERVIEW

- ◆ Reflects deep calf pain that results from strong and abrupt dorsiflexion of ankle (see *Eliciting Homans' sign*)
- ◆ Results from venous thrombosis or inflammation of calf muscles
- ◆ Unreliable indicator of venous disorders
- ◆ If deep vein thrombosis is suspected, should be elicited very carefully to avoid dislodging a clot and, possibly, causing pulmonary embolism

HISTORY

- ◆ Ask about signs and symptoms of deep vein thrombosis or thrombophlebitis, such as calf and leg pain.
- ◆ Ask about associated shortness of breath or chest pain.
- ◆ Inquire about predisposing events, such as leg injury, recent surgery, childbirth, use of hormonal contraceptives, associated diseases, and prolonged inactivity.

PHYSICAL ASSESSMENT

- ◆ Inspect and palpate the calf for warmth, tenderness, redness, swelling, and a palpable vein.
- ◆ Measure circumferences of both calves.

TOP TECHNIQUE

Eliciting Homans' sign

To elicit Homans' sign, first support the patient's thigh with one hand and his foot with the other. Bend his leg slightly at the knee; then firmly and abruptly dorsiflex the ankle as shown. Resulting deep calf pain indicates a positive Homans' sign. (The patient may also resist ankle dorsiflexion or flex the knee involuntarily if Homans' sign is positive.)

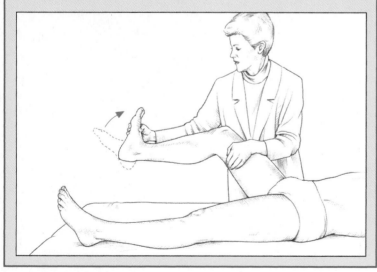

CAUSES

MEDICAL

Deep vein thrombophlebitis

◆ Positive Homans' sign and calf tenderness may be the only signs.
◆ Other signs and symptoms include severe pain, heaviness, warmth, and swelling of the affected leg; visible, engorged superficial veins or palpable, cordlike veins; and fever, chills, and malaise.

Deep vein thrombosis

◆ Positive Homans' sign occurs with tenderness over the deep calf veins, slight edema of the calves and thighs, a low-grade fever, and tachycardia.
◆ Cyanosis and cool skin in the affected leg may occur with venous obstruction.

Popliteal cyst, ruptured

◆ Positive Homans' sign and sudden onset of calf tenderness, swelling, and redness occur.
◆ Bruising may be observed on the popliteal space and calf.

NURSING CONSIDERATIONS

◆ Place the patient on bed rest with the affected leg elevated above heart evel.
◆ Apply warm, moist compresses to the affected area.
◆ Administer analgesics, as needed.
◆ Have the patient keep the affected leg elevated while sitting and avoid crossing his legs at the knees.
◆ Administer anticoagulants and thrombolytic therapy, as ordered, for thrombophlebitis.

PATIENT TEACHING

◆ Explain the signs of prolonged clotting time the patient should report, if anticoagulant is ordered.
◆ Emphasize the avoidance of alcohol, dietary recommendations, and drug interactions related to anticoagulation therapy.
◆ Stress the importance of follow-up appointments.
◆ Explain drugs the patient will need.
◆ Explain the use of elastic support stockings.
◆ Discuss the importance of checking with the physician before taking any new drugs.

Hyperpigmentation

OVERVIEW

- Excessive skin coloring that reflects overproduction, abnormal location, or maldistribution of melanin—the dominant brown or black pigment found in skin, hair, mucous membranes, nails, brain tissue, cardiac muscle, and parts of the eye
- May also reflect abnormalities of other skin pigments: carotenoids (yellow), oxyhemoglobin (red), and hemoglobin (blue)
- Typically asymptomatic and chronic but a common problem that can have distressing psychological and social implications

HISTORY

- Obtain a detailed patient and family history about hyperpigmentation, including if it was present at birth and other signs or symptoms that accompany it.
- Obtain a history of medical disorders (especially endocrine) as well as contact with or ingestion of chemicals, metals, plants, vegetables, citrus fruits, sunlight, or perfumes.
- Find out if the patient is pregnant or taking prescription or over-the-counter drugs.
- Ask about other signs and symptoms such as fatigue; weakness; muscle aches; chills; irritability; fainting; pruritus; cardiopulmonary signs or symptoms, such as cough, shortness of breath, or swelling of the ankles, hands, or other areas; and GI complaints, such as anorexia, nausea, vomiting, weight loss, abdominal pain, diarrhea, constipation, or epigastric fullness.
- Also ask about genitourinary signs and symptoms, such as dark or pink urine, increased or decreased urination, menstrual irregularities, and loss of libido.

PHYSICAL ASSESSMENT

- Examine the patient's skin. Note the color of hyperpigmented areas: brown suggests excess melanin in the epidermis; slate gray or a bluish tone suggests excess pigment in the dermis.
- Inspect for other skin changes—thickening and leatherlike texture as well as changes in hair distribution.
- Check the patient's skin and sclerae for jaundice, and note any spider angiomas, palmar erythema, or purpura.
- Take the patient's vital signs, noting fever, hypotension, or pulse irregularities.
- Evaluate his general appearance looking for exophthalmos and an enlarged jaw, nose, or hands.
- Palpate for an enlarged thyroid gland, and auscultate for a bruit over the gland.
- Palpate the muscles for atrophy and the joints for swelling and tenderness.
- Assess the abdomen for ascites and edema, and palpate and percuss the liver and spleen to evaluate their size and position.
- Check the male patient for testicular atrophy and gynecomastia.

CAUSES

MEDICAL
Acanthosis nigricans

- This soft velvety-brown pigmentation with wart-like elevations is found most commonly in the skin folds and may have associated skin tags.
- It typically occurs in individuals younger than age 40, may be genetically inherited, and is associated with obesity or endocrinopathies, such as hypothyroidism or hyperthyroidism, acromegaly, polycystic ovary disease, insulin-resistant diabetes, or Cushing's syndrome.
- When seen in individuals older than age 40, this disorder is commonly associated with an internal malignancy, usually adenocarcinoma, and most commonly of the GI tract or uterus; less commonly of the lung, prostate, breast, or ovary.
- Acanthosis nigricans of the oral mucosa or tongue is highly suggestive of a neoplasm, especially of the GI tract.

Acromegaly

- This disorder results from a pituitary tumor that secretes excessive amounts of growth hormone after puberty.
- Hyperpigmentation (possibly acanthosis nigricans) may affect the face, neck, genitalia, axillae, palmar creases, and new scars. The skin appears oily, sweaty, thick, and leathery, with furrows and ridges formed over the face, neck, and scalp.
- The tongue is enlarged and furrowed; lips are thick; hands are broad and spadelike; body hair is markedly increased; and the nose is large.
- Marked prognathism interferes with chewing.

Adrenocortical insufficiency (Addison's disease)

- This disorder produces diffuse tan, brown, or bronze-to-black hyperpigmentation of both exposed and unexposed areas of the face, knees, knuckles, elbows, antecubital areas, beltline, palmar creases, lips, gums, tongue, and buccal mucosa (where hyperpigmentation may be bluish black).
- Normally pigmented areas, moles, and scars become darker.
- Early in the disorder, hyperpigmentation occurs as persistent tanning after exposure to the sun.
- Some patients (usually female) lose axillary and pubic hair; about 15% have vitiligo.
- Other signs and symptoms include slowly progressive fatigue, weakness, anorexia, nausea, vomiting, weight loss, orthostatic hypotension, abdominal pain, irritability, weak and irregular pulse, diarrhea or constipation, decreased libido, amenorrhea, syncope and, sometimes, an enhanced sense of taste, smell, and hearing.

Cirrhosis, biliary

- Hyperpigmentation is a classic feature of this disorder, which primarily affects women between ages 40 and 60.
- A widespread and accentuated brown hyperpigmentation appears on areas exposed to sunlight, but not on the mucosa.
- Pruritus that worsens at bedtime may be the earliest symptom.
- Fatigue, weight loss, and vague abdominal pain may appear years before the onset of jaundice.
- Malabsorption may cause nocturnal diarrhea, frothy and bulky stools, weight loss, purpura, and osteomalacia with bone and back pain.
- Other signs and symptoms include hematemesis from esophageal varices, xanthomas and xanthelasmas, hepatosplenomegaly, ascites, edema, spider angiomas, and palmar erythema.

Cirrhosis, Laënnec's

- After about 10 years of excessive alcohol ingestion, progressive liver dysfunction causes diffuse, generalized hyperpigmentation on sun-exposed areas.
- Early in the disorder, the patient may complain of increasing weakness, fatigue, anorexia, slight weight loss, nausea and vomiting, indigestion, constipation or diarrhea, and a dull abdominal ache.
- As the disorder progresses, the patient may display major signs and symptoms in every body system resulting from hepatic insufficiency and portal hypertension.

Cushing's syndrome, hypercortisolism

- Most common in females, this syndrome is caused by excessive levels of adrenocortical hormones or related corticosteroids.
- In addition to hyperpigmentation, other signs and symptoms include diabetes mellitus, hypertension, left ventricular hypertrophy, capillary fragility, increased susceptibility to infection, decreased resistance to stress, suppressed inflammatory response, muscle weakness, pathologic changes from bone demineralization, gynecomastia in males, and mild virilism and amenorrhea or oligomenorrhea in females.

Hemochromatosis

- In this inherited disorder (also called *bronzed diabetes*), most common in men between ages 40 and 60, early and progressive hyperpigmentation results from melanin (and possibly iron) deposits in the skin.
- Hyperpigmentation develops as generalized bronzing and metallic gray areas accentuated over sun-exposed areas, genitalia, and scars.
- Early signs and symptoms include weakness, lassitude, weight loss, abdominal and joint pain, loss of libido, and signs of diabetes, such as polydipsia and polyuria.
- Later, signs of liver and cardiac involvement become prominent.

Malignant melanoma

- This form of cancer causes malignant lesions of pigmented skin, commonly moles.
- Common sites include the head and neck in men, the legs in women, and the back in both men and women exposed to excessive sunlight.
- Up to 70% of these lesions arise from a preexisting nevus.
- Metastatic melanoma may produce generalized hyperpigmentation.
- The cardinal sign of malignant melanoma is a skin lesion or nevus that enlarges, changes color, becomes inflamed, itches, ulcerates, bleeds, changes texture, or develops an associated halo nevus or vitiligo.

Melasma

- This light or dark brown hyperpigmentation occurs on areas exposed to sunlight, most notably on the face, and is associated with use of hormonal contraceptives or pregnancy.
- Some cases are idiopathic.
- Lesions are symmetrical and usually involve the cheeks, forehead, and upper lip.
- When related to pregnancy, the pigmentation may decrease after delivery.

Porphyria cutanea tarda

- Primarily affecting men between ages 40 and 60, this disorder produces generalized brownish hyperpigmentation on sun-exposed areas and extreme skin fragility (particularly on a bald scalp and on the face and hands).
- It also causes pink or brownish urine (from porphyrin excretion), anorexia, jaundice, hepatomegaly, abdominal pain or cramping, muscle weakness, and personality changes.

Scleroderma, progressive systemic sclerosis

- Both localized and systemic scleroderma produce generalized dark brown hyperpigmentation that's unrelated to sun exposure; other findings include areas of depigmentation and spider angiomas.

(continued)

- Early signs and symptoms include those of Raynaud's phenomenon— blanching, cyanosis, and erythema of the fingers and toes when exposed to cold or stress, and possible finger shortening, fingertip ulcerations, and gangrene of the fingers and toes.
- Later signs and symptoms include pain, stiffness, and swelling of the fingers and joints; skin thickening that progresses to taut, shiny, leathery skin over the entire hands and forearms and then over the upper arms, chest, abdomen, and back; masklike facial skin and a pinched mouth; and, possibly, contractures.

Thyrotoxicosis
- This disorder can cause hyperpigmentation on the face, neck, genitalia, axillae, and palmar creases as well as in new scars.
- Classic signs and symptoms of Graves' disease, the most common form of thyrotoxicosis, include an enlarged thyroid gland, nervousness, heat intolerance, weight loss despite increased appetite, profuse diaphoresis, diarrhea, tremor, and palpitations.
- Other signs and symptoms include vitiligo; warm, moist skin; erythematous palms; fine scalp hair with premature graying; and Plummer's nails.
- Exophthalmos, although characteristic, is absent in many patients.

Tinea versicolor
- This benign fungal skin infection produces raised or macular, scaly lesions, usually on the upper trunk, neck, and arms, which range from hyperpigmented patches in fair-skinned patients to hypopigmented patches in dark-skinned patients.

OTHER
Arsenic poisoning
- Chronic arsenic poisoning can cause diffuse hyperpigmentation with scattered freckle-size areas of normal or depigmented skin.
- Other signs and symptoms may include weakness, muscle aches, peripheral neuropathy, headache, drowsiness, confusion, seizures, and mucous membrane involvement (conjunctivitis, photophobia, pharyngitis, or an irritating cough).

Drugs
- Hyperpigmentation can stem from use of barbiturates; salicylates; chemotherapeutic drugs, such as busulfan, cyclophosphamide, procarbazine, and nitrogen mustard; chlorpromazine; antimalarial drugs, such as hydroxychloroquine; hydantoin; minocycline; metals, such as silver (in argyria) and gold (in chrysiasis); corticotropin; and phenothiazines.

NURSING CONSIDERATIONS

- Wood's lamp, a special ultraviolet light, helps enhance the contrast between normal and hyperpigmented epidermis.
- A skin biopsy can help confirm the cause of hyperpigmentation.
- Hyperpigmentation may persist even after treatment of the underlying disorder or withdrawal of the causative drug.
- Bleaching creams may not be effective if most of the excess melanin lies in subepidermal skin layers. In addition, over-the-counter bleaching creams tend to be ineffective because they contain less than 2% hydroquinone.

PEDIATRIC POINTERS

- Most moles that are found in children are junctional nevi—flat, well demarcated, brown to bluish-black—that can appear anywhere on the skin.
- Although these lesions are considered benign, recent evidence suggests that some of them may become malignant in later life.
- Some physicians recommend removal of junctional nevi; others advise regular inspection.
- Congenital melanocytic nevi present at birth should be removed, especially if large (greater than 20 cm), because they become malignant in about 20% of cases. Some of these lesions may have an increased amount of hair.
- Bizarre arrangements of linear or streaky hyperpigmented lesions on a child's sun-exposed lower legs suggest phytophotodermatitis. Advise parents to protect the child's skin with long pants and socks.
- Congenital hyperpigmented lesions include benign mongolian spots and sharply defined or diffuse lesions occurring in such disorders as neurofibromatosis, xeroderma pigmentosum, Albright's syndrome, Fanconi's syndrome, Gaucher's disease, Niemann-Pick disease, Peutz-Jeghers syndrome, phenylketonuria, and Wilson's disease.

PATIENT TEACHING

- Advise the patient to use corrective cosmetics, to avoid excessive sun exposure, and to apply a sunscreen or sun blocker such as zinc oxide cream.
- Advise patients who stop using bleaching agents to continue using sun blockers because rebound hyperpigmentation can occur.
- Warn every patient with a benign hyperpigmented area to consult his physician if the lesion's size, shape, or color changes; this may signal a developing skin cancer.

Hyperpnea

- Refers to breathing at normal or increased rate with marked chest expansion during inhalation in response to oxygen demand
- May result in hyperventilation
- May be a sign of a life-threatening condition (see *Managing hyperpnea*)
- Known as Kussmaul's respirations when it's a compensatory mechanism in metabolic acidosis (see *Kussmaul's respirations: A compensatory mechanism*)

HISTORY

- Ask about recent illnesses or infections.
- Find out about the ingestion of aspirin or other drugs or inhalation of drugs or chemicals.
- Obtain a medical history, including incidence of diabetes mellitus, renal disease, or pulmonary conditions.
- Ask about associated signs and symptoms, such as thirst, hunger, nausea, vomiting, severe diarrhea, or upper respiratory tract infection.

PHYSICAL ASSESSMENT

- Assess level of consciousness (LOC).
- Observe for clues to abnormal breathing pattern.
- Examine for cyanosis, restlessness, and anxiety.
- Observe for intercostal and abdominal retractions, accessory muscle use, and diaphoresis.
- Inspect for draining wounds or signs of infection.
- Take vital signs, including oxygen saturation.

 ACTION STAT!

Managing hyperpnea

Carefully examine the patient with hyperpnea for related signs of life-threatening conditions, such as increased intracranial pressure (ICP), metabolic acidosis, diabetic ketoacidosis, and uremia. Be prepared for rapid interventions.

INCREASED ICP

If you observe hyperpnea in a patient who has signs of head trauma (soft-tissue injury, edema, or ecchymoses on the face or head) from a recent accident and has lost consciousness, act quickly to prevent further brain stem injury and irreversible deterioration. Take the patient's vital signs, noting bradycardia, increased systolic blood pressure, and widening pulse pressure—signs of increased ICP.

Examine his pupillary reaction. Elevate the head of the bed 30 degrees (unless you suspect spinal cord injury), insert an artificial airway, and administer oxygen. Connect the patient to a cardiac monitor and continuously observe his respiratory pattern. (Irregular respirations signal deterioration.) Start an I.V. line at a slow infusion rate and prepare to administer an osmotic diuretic, such as mannitol, to decrease cerebral edema. Obtain a blood sample for arterial blood gas analysis to help guide treatments.

METABOLIC ACIDOSIS

If the patient with hyperpnea doesn't have a head injury, his increased respiratory rate probably indicates metabolic acidosis. Suspect shock if the patient has cold, clammy skin. Palpate for a rapid, thready pulse and take his blood pressure, noting hypotension. Elevate the patient's legs 30 degrees, apply pressure dressings to any obvious hemorrhage, start several large-bore I.V. lines, and prepare to administer fluids, vasopressors, and blood transfusions.

A patient with hyperpnea who has a history of alcohol abuse, is vomiting profusely, has diarrhea or profuse abdominal drainage, has ingested an overdose of aspirin, or is cachectic and has a history of starvation may also have metabolic acidosis. Inspect his skin for dryness and poor turgor, indicating dehydration. Take his vital signs, looking for low-grade fever and hypotension. Start an I.V. line for fluid replacement. Draw blood for electrolyte studies, and prepare to administer sodium bicarbonate.

DIABETIC KETOACIDOSIS

If the patient has a history of diabetes mellitus, is vomiting, and has a fruity breath odor (acetone breath), suspect diabetic ketoacidosis. Catheterize him to monitor increased urine output, and infuse normal saline solution. Perform a fingerstick to estimate blood glucose levels with a reagent strip. Obtain a urine specimen to test for glucose and acetone, and draw blood for glucose and ketone tests. Also, administer fluids, insulin, potassium, and sodium bicarbonate I.V., as ordered.

UREMIA

If the patient has a history of renal disease, an ammonia breath odor (uremic fetor), and a fine, white powder on his skin (uremic frost), suspect uremia. Start an I.V. line at a slow rate, and prepare to administer sodium bicarbonate. Monitor his electrocardiogram for arrhythmias due to hyperkalemia. Monitor his serum electrolyte, blood urea nitrogen, and creatinine levels as well until hemodialysis or peritoneal dialysis begins.

Kussmaul's respirations: A compensatory mechanism

Kussmaul's respirations—fast, deep breathing without pauses—characteristically sound labored, with deep breaths that resemble sighs. This breathing pattern develops when respiratory centers in the medulla detect decreased blood pH, thereby triggering compensatory fast and deep breathing to remove excess carbon dioxide and restore pH balance.

Disorders (such as diabetes mellitus and renal failure), drug effects, and other conditions cause metabolic acidosis (loss of bicarbonate ions and retention of acid).

↓

Blood pH decreases.

↓

Kussmaul's respirations develop to blow off excess carbon dioxide

↓

Blood pH rises.

↓

Respiratory rate and depth decrease (corrected pH) in effective compensation.

- Auscultate the heart and lungs.
- Assess for dehydration.

CAUSES

MEDICAL
Head injury
- Hyperpnea occurs along with signs of increased intracranial pressure; loss of consciousness; soft-tissue injury or bony deformity of the face, head, or neck; facial edema; cloudy or bloody drainage from the mouth, nose, or ears; raccoon eyes; Battle's sign; an absent doll's eye sign; and motor and sensory disturbances.

Hyperventilation syndrome
- Acute anxiety triggers episodic hyperpnea.
- Other signs and symptoms include agitation, vertigo, syncope, pallor, circumoral and peripheral cyanosis, muscle twitching, carpopedal spasm, weakness, and arrhythmias.

Hypoxemia
- Many pulmonary disorders that cause hypoxemia may cause hyperpnea and episodes of hyperventilation with chest pain, dizziness, and paresthesia.
- Other signs and symptoms include dyspnea, cough, crackles, rhonchi, wheezing, and decreased breath sounds.

Ketoacidosis
- In alcoholic ketoacidosis, Kussmaul's respirations begin abruptly and are accompanied by vomiting for several days, fruity breath odor, dehydration, abdominal pain and distention, and absent bowel sounds.
- In diabetic ketoacidosis, a potentially life-threatening disorder, Kussmaul's respirations occur with polydipsia, polyphagia, and polyuria.
- Other signs and symptoms of diabetic ketoacidosis include fruity breath odor, orthostatic hypotension, weakness, decreased LOC, nausea, vomiting, anorexia, abdominal pain, and a rapid, thready pulse.

- In starvation ketoacidosis, also a life-threatening disorder, Kussmaul's respirations occur gradually and may be accompanied by cachexia, dehydration, decreased LOC, bradycardia, and a history of severely limited food intake.

Renal failure
- Life-threatening acidosis and Kussmaul's respirations can occur.
- Other signs and symptoms include oliguria or anuria, uremic fetor, severe pruritus, uremic frost, purpura, ecchymoses, nausea, vomiting, weakness, burning in the legs and feet, diarrhea or constipation, altered LOC, seizures, and yellow, dry, scaly skin.

Sepsis
- Severe infection may cause acidosis, resulting in Kussmaul's respirations.
- Other signs and symptoms include tachycardia, hypotension, oliguria, fever or a low temperature, chills, headache, lethargy, profuse diaphoresis, anorexia, cough, change in mental status, and signs of infection.

Shock
- A life-threatening condition, Kussmaul's respirations, hypotension, tachycardia, narrowed pulse pressure, weak pulse, dyspnea, oliguria, anxiety, restlessness, stupor that can progress to coma, and cool, clammy skin occurs.
- Other signs and symptoms include external or internal bleeding, in hypovolemic shock; chest pain, arrhythmias, and signs of heart failure, in cardiogenic shock; high fever and chills, in septic shock; or stridor, in anaphylactic shock.

OTHER
Drugs
- Toxic levels of salicylates, ammonium chloride, acetazolamide, and other carbonic anhydrase inhibitors can cause Kussmaul's respirations.
- Ingestion of methanol and ethylene glycol can also cause Kussmaul's respirations.

NURSING CONSIDERATIONS

- Monitor vital signs, including oxygen saturation.
- Observe for increasing respiratory distress or an irregular respiratory pattern.
- Start an I.V. line for administration of fluids, blood transfusions, and vasopressor drugs, as ordered.
- Prepare to give ventilatory support.

PEDIATRIC POINTERS
- Hyperpnea in a child indicates the same metabolic or neurologic causes as in an adult.
- The most common cause of metabolic acidosis in a child is diarrhea.

PATIENT TEACHING

- Discuss the underlying condition, diagnostic tests, and treatment options.
- Teach the diabetic patient how to monitor his blood glucose level, and stress the importance of compliance with diabetes therapy.
- Explain fluids and foods the patient should avoid.
- Discuss pulmonary hygiene.
- Teach the patient ways to avoid respiratory infections.
- Emphasize the importance of alcohol cessation and provide information about groups or other resources that can help, as appropriate.

Hypopigmentation

OVERVIEW

- Refers to a decrease in normal skin, hair, mucous membrane, or nail color resulting from deficiency, absence, or abnormal degradation of the pigment melanin
- May be congenital or acquired, asymptomatic, or associated with other findings
- Typically chronic and can be difficult to identify if the patient is light-skinned or has only slightly decreased coloring

HISTORY

- Obtain a detailed patient history including family history of hypopigmentation.
- Find out if it developed after skin lesions or a rash, or if it has been present since birth and if the lesions are painful.
- Obtain a medical history, including incidence of burns, physical injury, or physical contact with chemicals.
- Ask about prescription or over-the-counter drugs.
- Find out if he has noticed other skin changes—such as erythema, scaling, ulceration, or hyperpigmentation—or if sun exposure causes unusually severe burning.

PHYSICAL ASSESSMENT

- Examine the patient's skin, noting erythema, scaling, ulceration, areas of hyperpigmentation, and other findings.

CAUSES

MEDICAL
Albinism
- This genetically inherited disease involves alterations of the melanin pigment system that affects skin, hair, and eyes.
- There are various forms of albinism, all of which are present at birth.
- Skin and hair color vary from snow white to brown, but the universal finding of iris translucency confirms the diagnosis.
- Other optic signs and symptoms include nystagmus, decreased visual acuity, decreased pigmentation of the retina, and strabismus.

Burns
- Thermal and radiation burns can cause transient or permanent hypopigmentation.

Discoid lupus erythematosus
- This form of lupus erythematosus may produce hypopigmentation after inflammatory skin eruptions.
- Lesions are sharply defined, separate or fused macules, papules, or plaques; they vary from pink to purple, with a yellowish or brown crust and scaly, enlarged hair follicles.
- Although they may occur on other parts of the body, the lesions are typically distributed in a butterfly pattern over the cheeks and bridge of the nose. Telangiectasia may occur.
- After the inflammatory eruptive stage, noncontractile scarring and atrophy commonly affect the face and may also involve sun-exposed areas of the neck, ears, scalp (with possible alopecia), lips, and oral mucosa.

Hypomelanosis, idiopathic guttate
- Common in lightly pigmented people older than age 30, this skin disorder produces sharply marginated, angular white spots on sun-exposed extremities.
- In blacks, hypopigmentation occurs mainly on the upper arms.

Inflammatory and infectious disorders
- Skin disorders, such as psoriasis, and infectious disorders, such as viral exanthemas or syphilis, can cause transient or permanent hypopigmentation.

Tinea versicolor
- This benign fungal skin infection produces scaly, sharply defined lesions that usually appear on the upper trunk, neck, and arms.
- The lesions range from hypopigmented patches in dark-skinned patients to hyperpigmented patches in fair-skinned patients.

Tuberculoid leprosy
- This chronic disorder affects the skin and peripheral nervous system. Erythematous or hypopigmented macules have decreased or absent sensation for light, touch, and warmth.
- Because the lesions don't sweat, the skin feels dry and rough and may be scaly.
- Other signs and symptoms may include very painful, palpable peripheral nerves; muscle atrophy and contractures; and ulcers of the fingers and toes.

Vitiligo
- This common skin disorder produces sharply defined, flat white macules and patches ranging in diameter from 1 to over 20 cm.
- The hypopigmented areas commonly have hyperpigmented borders.
- Usually bilaterally symmetrical, lesions appear on sun-exposed areas; in body folds; around the eyes, nose, mouth, and rectum; and over bony prominences.

- Patches of vitiligo may coalesce to form universal lack of pigment and may involve the hair, eyebrows, and eyelashes.
- Spontaneous repigmentation can occur.
- Hypopigmented patches (halo nevi) may surround pigmented moles.

OTHER
Chemicals
- Most phenolic compounds—for example, amylphenol (a dye) and paratertiary butylphenol (PTBP), which are used in plastics and glues, and germicides, which are used in many household and industrial products—can cause hypopigmentation.

Drugs
- Topical or intralesional administration of corticosteroids causes hypopigmentation at the treatment site. Chloroquine, an antimalarial drug, may cause depigmentation of hair (including eyebrows and lashes) and poor tanning 2 to 5 months after therapy begins.

NURSING CONSIDERATIONS

- In fair-skinned patients, a special ultraviolet (UV) light (Wood's lamp) can help differentiate hypopigmented lesions, which appear pale, from depigmented lesions, which appear white.
- Repigmentation therapy may be prescribed, combining a photosensitizing drug (psoralen) and UVA light.
- Refer patients for counseling, as appropriate.
- Suggest referral to a support group, such as the National Organization for Albinism and Hypomelanosis (NOAH).

PEDIATRIC POINTERS
- In children, hypopigmentation results from genetic or acquired disorders, including albinism, phenylketonuria, and tuberous sclerosis.
- In neonates, hypopigmentation may indicate a metabolic or nervous system disorder.

GERIATRIC POINTERS
- In elderly people, hypopigmentation is usually the result of cumulative exposure to UV light, which may also cause hyperpigmentation, telangiectasia, and purpura. These changes are known as *dermatoheliosis*.

PATIENT TEACHING

- Teach patients with albinism that lifelong diligence is needed to protect the skin from sun exposure, including using sunblock with an SPF greater than 30; wearing protective clothing, hats, and sunglasses (even for infants); and avoiding the sun during high solar intensity.
- Encourage regular examinations for early detection and treatment of lesions that may become premalignant or malignant.
- Advise patients to use corrective cosmetics to help hide skin lesions.

Impotence

- Refers to the inability to achieve and maintain penile erection sufficient to complete satisfactory sexual intercourse; ejaculation may or may not be affected
- Varies from occasional and minimal to permanent and complete.
- Occasional impotence: occurs in about one-half of adult American men; chronic impotence: affects about 10 million American men
- May be classified as primary or secondary

- Obtain a psychosocial history including patient's marital or relationship status, how long he has been in the relationship, the age and health status of his sexual partner, past relationships, sexual activity outside marriage or his primary sexual relationship, occupational history, his typical daily activities, and his living situation.
- Obtain a medical history, including incidence of cancer and its treatment, diabetes mellitus, hypertension, heart disease, neurologic disorders such as multiple sclerosis, or stroke, and psychological history.
- Obtain a surgical history, emphasizing neurologic, vascular, and urologic surgery.
- Ask about recent trauma and the date of the injury as well as its severity, associated effects, and treatment.
- Ask about intake of alcohol, drug use or abuse, smoking, diet, and exercise.
- Obtain a urologic history, including voiding problems, especially incontinence and past injury.
- Ask the patient when his impotence began, how it progressed, and its current status. Make your questions specific, but be sensitive to the fact that many patients have difficulty discussing sexual problems.
- Ask the patient to rate the quality of a typical erection on a scale of 0 to 10, with 0 being completely flaccid and 10 being completely erect. Using the same scale, also ask him to rate his ability to ejaculate during sexual activity, with 0 being never and 10 being always.

- Perform a brief physical examination; inspect and palpate the genitalia and prostate for structural abnormalities.
- Assess the patient's sensory function, concentrating on the perineal area.
- Test motor strength and deep tendon reflexes in all extremities, and note other neurologic deficits.
- Take the patient's vital signs and palpate his pulses for quality. Note any signs of peripheral vascular disease, such as cyanosis and cool extremities. Auscultate for abdominal aortic, femoral, carotid, or iliac bruits, and palpate for thyroid gland enlargement.

MEDICAL
Central nervous system disorders
- Spinal cord lesions from trauma produce sudden impotence.
- A complete lesion above S2 (upper-motor-neuron lesion) disrupts descending motor tracts to the genital area, causing loss of voluntary erectile control but not of reflex erection and reflex ejaculation.
- A complete lesion in the lumbosacral spinal cord (lower-motor-neuron lesion) causes loss of reflex ejaculation and reflex erection.
- Spinal cord tumors and degenerative diseases of the brain and spinal cord (such as multiple sclerosis and amyotrophic lateral sclerosis) cause progressive impotence.

Endocrine disorders
- Hypogonadism from testicular or pituitary dysfunction may lead to impotence from deficient secretion of androgens (primarily testosterone).
- Adrenocortical and thyroid dysfunction and chronic hepatic disease may also cause impotence because these organs play a role (although minor) in sex hormone regulation.

Penile disorders

◆ With Peyronie's disease, the penis is bent, making erection painful and penetration difficult and eventually impossible.
◆ Phimosis prevents erection until circumcision releases constricted foreskin.
◆ Other inflammatory, infectious, or destructive diseases of the penis, such as sexually transmitted diseases, may also cause impotence.

Peripheral neuropathy

◆ Systemic diseases, such as chronic renal failure and diabetes mellitus, can cause progressive impotence if the patient develops peripheral neuropathy. This condition affects about 50% of males with diabetes.
◆ Other signs and symptoms of diabetic neuropathy include bladder distention with overflow incontinence, orthostatic hypotension, syncope, paresthesia and other sensory disturbances, muscle weakness, and leg atrophy.

Psychological distress

◆ Impotence can result from diverse psychological causes, including depression, performance anxiety, memories of previous traumatic sexual experiences, moral or religious conflicts, and troubled emotional or sexual relationships.

Trauma

◆ Traumatic injury involving the penis, urethra, prostate, perineum, or pelvis may cause sudden impotence due to structural alteration, nerve damage, or interrupted blood supply.

Vascular disorders

◆ Various vascular disorders can cause impotence and include advanced arteriosclerosis affecting both major and peripheral blood vessels, Leriche's syndrome (slowly developing occlusion of the terminal abdominal aorta), and arteriosclerosis, thrombosis, or embolization of smaller vessels supplying the penis.

OTHER
Alcohol and drugs

◆ Alcoholism and drug abuse are associated with impotence as are many prescription drugs, especially antihypertensives and psychotropics. (See *Drugs that may cause impotence.*)

Surgery

◆ Surgical injury to the penis, bladder neck, urinary sphincter, rectum, or perineum can cause impotence as can injury to local nerves or blood vessels.

NURSING CONSIDERATIONS

◆ Care begins by ensuring privacy, confirming confidentiality, and establishing a rapport with the patient. No other medical condition affecting males is as potentially frustrating, humiliating, and devastating to self-esteem and significant relationships as impotence. Help the patient feel comfortable about discussing his sexuality. This begins with feeling comfortable about your own sexuality and adopting an accepting attitude about the sexual experiences and preferences of others.
◆ Prepare the patient for screening tests for hormonal irregularities and for Doppler studies of penile blood pressure to rule out vascular insufficiency. Other tests include voiding studies, nerve conduction tests, evaluation of nocturnal penile tumescence, and psychological screening.
◆ Treatment of psychogenic impotence may involve counseling for the patient and his sexual partner; treatment of organic impotence focuses on reversing the cause, if possible.
◆ Other forms of treatment include surgical revascularization, drug-induced erection, surgical repair of a venous leak, and penile prostheses.

GERIATRIC POINTERS

◆ Impotence isn't a normal finding in elderly men and should be addressed appropriately regardless of age.

PATIENT TEACHING

◆ Encourage your patient to talk openly about his needs and desires, fears and anxieties, or misconceptions. Urge him to discuss these issues with his partner as well as what role both of them want sexual activity to play in their lives.
◆ Teach the patient about impotence and it's causes and treatment options.
◆ Teach the patient about all tests and procedures he will be undergoing to help with diagnosis.
◆ Advise the patient to maintain follow-up appointments and therapy for underlying medical disorders.

Drugs that may cause impotence

Many commonly used drugs—especially antihypertensives—can cause impotence, which may be reversible if the drug is discontinued or the dosage reduced. Here are some examples:

amitriptyline	imipramine
atenolol	methyldopa
bicalutamide	nortriptyline
carbamazepine	perphenazine
cimetidine	prazosin
clonidine	propranolol
desipramine	telmisartan
digoxin	thiazide diuretics
escitalopram	thioridazine
finasteride	tranylcypromine
hydralazine	valsartan

Insomnia

- Inability to fall asleep, remain asleep, or feel refreshed by sleep
- May have a physiologic or pathophysiologic cause

HISTORY

- Obtain a sleep history.
- Determine when the onset of insomnia occurred.
- Obtain a drug history, noting the use of central nervous system stimulants and over-the-counter medications.
- Ask about the use of caffeine and caffeinated beverages.
- Obtain a medical history of chronic or acute conditions, including painful or pruritic conditions.
- Ask about alcohol use.
- Determine emotional status and stress factors.
- Obtain a psychosocial history, noting factors such as frequent travel, exercise, and personal or job-related problems.

PHYSICAL ASSESSMENT

- Perform a complete physical examination.
- Pay close attention to findings that suggest a neurologic, cardiac, respiratory, or endocrine disorder.

CAUSES

MEDICAL
Alcohol withdrawal syndrome
- Insomnia may persist for up to 2 years.
- Other early effects include excessive diaphoresis, tachycardia, hypertension, tremors, restlessness, irritability, headache, nausea, flushing, and nightmares.
- Progression to alcohol withdrawal delirium as soon as 48 hours after cessation produces confusion, disorientation, paranoia, delusions, hallucinations, and seizures.

Depression
- Chronic insomnia occurs with difficulty falling asleep, waking and being unable to fall back to sleep, or waking early in the morning.
- The patient also experiences loss of interest in usual activities, feelings of worthlessness and guilt, fatigue, difficulty concentrating, indecisiveness, and recurrent thoughts of death.
- Other signs and symptoms include dysphoria, decreased appetite with weight loss or increased appetite with weight gain, and psychomotor agitation or retardation.

Generalized anxiety disorder
- Chronic insomnia occurs with fatigue, restlessness, diaphoresis, dyspepsia, high resting pulse and respiratory rates, and signs of apprehension.

Nocturnal myoclonus
- Involuntary and fleeting muscle jerks of the legs occur every 5 to 90 seconds, disturbing sleep.
- The patient reports poor sleep and daytime somnolence.
- The condition can occur in patients with diabetes or restless leg syndrome.

Pain
- Conditions that cause pain can also cause insomnia.
- Behavioral responses include altered body position, moaning, grimacing, withdrawal, crying, restlessness, muscle twitching, and immobility.
- With mild or moderate pain, signs and symptoms include pallor, elevated blood pressure, dilated pupils, skeletal muscle tension, dyspnea, tachycardia, and diaphoresis.
- With severe and deep pain, signs and symptoms include pallor, decreased blood pressure, bradycardia, nausea, vomiting, weakness, dizziness, and loss of consciousness.

Pruritus
- Insomnia results because of itching.

Sleep apnea syndrome
- Sleep is disturbed by apneic periods that end with a series of gasps and eventual wakefulness.
- With central sleep apnea, respiratory movement ceases for the apneic period.
- With obstructive sleep apnea, upper airway obstruction blocks incoming air, but breathing movements continue.
- Other signs and symptoms include morning headache, daytime fatigue, hypertension, ankle edema, and personality changes.

Thyrotoxicosis
- Difficulty falling asleep and then sleeping for only a brief period is a characteristic symptom.
- Other signs and symptoms include dyspnea, tachycardia, palpitations, atrial or ventricular gallop, weight loss despite increased appetite, diarrhea, tremors, nervousness, diaphoresis, hypersensitivity to heat, an enlarged thyroid gland, and exophthalmos.

OTHER
Drugs
- Use of, abuse of, or withdrawal from sedatives or hypnotics may produce insomnia.
- Central nervous system stimulants may also produce insomnia.

◆ Prepare the patient for tests to evaluate his insomnia.
◆ Institute measures to help relieve insomnia. (See *Tips for relieving insomnia.*)

PEDIATRIC POINTERS

◆ Insomnia in early childhood may develop along with separation anxiety (ages 2 to 3), after a stressful or tiring day, or during illness or teething.
◆ In children ages 6 to 11, insomnia usually reflects residual excitement from the day's activities.
◆ Caffeine intake should be avoided, especially 2 to 4 hours before bedtime.

GERIATRIC POINTERS

◆ Sleep patterns of older people are marked by frequent awakenings, diminished stage III and stage IV nonrapid eye movement time, increased time spent awake at night, and more frequent daytime naps.

PATIENT TEACHING

◆ Teach the patient techniques to increase comfort and relaxation, and address underlying cause.
◆ Discuss the appropriate use of tranquilizers or sedatives.
◆ Refer the patient to counseling or sleep disorder clinic, as needed.

Tips for relieving insomnia

COMMON PROBLEMS	CAUSES	INTERVENTIONS
Acroparesthesia	Improper positioning may compress superficial (ulnar, radial, and peroneal) nerves, disrupting circulation to the compressed nerve. This causes numbness, tingling, and stiffness in an arm or leg.	Teach the patient to assume a comfortable position in bed with his limbs unrestricted. If he tends to awaken with a numb arm or leg, tell him to massage and move it until sensation returns completely and then to assume an unrestricted position.
Anxiety	Physical and emotional stress produces anxiety, which causes autonomic stimulation.	Encourage the patient to discuss his fears and concerns and teach him relaxation techniques, such as guided imagery and deep breathing. Give a mild sedative, such as temazepam or another sedative hypnotic, before bedtime. Emphasize that these drugs are to be used for the short-term only.
Dyspnea	With many cardiac and pulmonary disorders, a recumbent position and inactivity cause restricted chest expansion, secretion pooling, and pulmonary vascular congestion, leading to coughing and shortness of breath.	Elevate the head of the bed or provide at least two pillows or a reclining chair to help the patient sleep. Suction him when he awakens and encourage deep breathing and incentive spirometry every 2 to 4 hours. Also, provide supplementary oxygen by nasal cannula. If the patient is pregnant, encourage her to sleep on her left side at a comfortable elevation.
Pain	Chronic or acute pain can prevent or disrupt sleep.	Give drugs for pain 20 minutes before bedtime, and teach deep, even, slow breathing to promote relaxation. If the patient has back pain, help him lie on his side with his legs flexed. If he has epigastric pain, encourage him to take an antacid before bedtime and to sleep with the head of the bed elevated. If he has incisions, instruct him to splint during coughing or movement.
Pruritus	A localized skin infection or a systemic disorder, such as liver failure, may produce intensely annoying itching, even during the night.	Wash the patient's skin with a mild soap and water and dry the skin thoroughly. Apply moisturizing lotion on dry, unbroken skin and an antipruritic such as calamine lotion on pruritic areas. Administer diphenhydramine or hydroxyzine, as ordered, to help minimize itching.
Restless leg syndrome	Irresistible urge to move legs starts or becomes worse at rest, especially when lying down, and requires movement for relief.	Help the patient exercise his legs gently by slowly walking with him around the room and down the hall. If ordered, administer a muscle relaxant such as diazepam.

Intermittent claudication

OVERVIEW

◆ Cramping limb pain
◆ Brought on by exercise; relieved by 1 to 2 minutes of rest
◆ May be acute or chronic

ACTION STAT! *If the patient has sudden intermittent claudication with severe or aching leg pain at rest, check the temperature and color of his leg and palpate femoral, popliteal, posterior tibial, and dorsalis pedis pulses. Suspect acute arterial occlusion if pulses are absent; if the leg feels cold and looks pale, cyanotic, or mottled; and if paresthesia and pain are present.*

Mark areas of pallor, cyanosis, or mottling, and reassess frequently. Don't elevate the leg. Protect it, allowing nothing to press on it. Start an I.V. line, and administer an anticoagulant and analgesic, as prescribed. Anticipate diagnostic tests and, possibly, surgery.

HISTORY

◆ Ask the patient how far he can walk before pain occurs, how long it takes for pain to subside, and recent changes in the pain's pattern and characteristics.
◆ Explore risk factors, such as smoking, diabetes, hypertension, and hyperlipidemia.
◆ Ask about associated signs and symptoms, such as paresthesia in the affected limb and visible changes in the color of the fingers.

PHYSICAL ASSESSMENT

◆ Palpate lower extremity pulses; note character, strength, and bilateral equality.
◆ Note color and temperature differences between the legs and compare with the arms.
◆ Auscultate for bruits over major arteries.
◆ Elevate the affected leg for 2 minutes and assess color changes; note how long it takes for color to return when legs are dependent.
◆ Examine the feet, toes, and fingers for ulceration.
◆ Inspect the hands and lower legs for small, tender nodules and erythema along blood vessels.
◆ If the patient has arm pain, inspect the arms for a change in color (to white) on elevation.
◆ Palpate and compare upper extremity pulses.

CAUSES

MEDICAL
Aortic arteriosclerotic occlusive disease
◆ Intermittent claudication occurs in the buttock, hip, thigh, and calf, along with absent or diminished femoral pulses.
◆ Other signs and symptoms include bruits over the femoral and iliac arteries, pallor and coolness of the affected limb on elevation, and profound limb weakness.

Arterial occlusion, acute
◆ Intense intermittent claudication occurs.
◆ The limb is cool, pale, and cyanotic with absent pulses below the occlusion.
◆ Other signs and symptoms include paresthesia, paresis, increased capillary refill time, and a sensation of cold in the affected limb.

Arteriosclerosis obliterans
◆ Intermittent claudication appears in the calf along with diminished or absent popliteal and pedal pulses, coolness in the affected limb, pallor on elevation, and profound limb weakness with continuing exercise.
◆ Other signs and symptoms include numbness; paresthesia; and, in more severe disease, pain in the toes or foot while at rest; ulceration; and gangrene.

Buerger's disease
◆ Intermittent claudication of the instep is typical in this inflammatory vascular disorder.
◆ Early signs include migratory superficial nodules and erythema along extremity blood vessels and migratory venous phlebitis.
◆ With exposure to cold, feet initially become cold, cyanotic, and numb; later, they redden, become hot, and tingle.
◆ Other signs and symptoms include impaired peripheral pulses, paresthesia of the hands and feet, and migratory superficial thrombophlebitis.

Leriche's syndrome

◆ Arterial occlusion causes intermittent claudication of the hip, thigh, buttocks, and calf and also causes impotence in men.
◆ Other signs and symptoms include bruits, global atrophy, absent or diminished pulses, gangrene of the toes, and legs that become cool and pale with elevation.

Neurogenic claudication

◆ Pain from intermittent claudication requires a longer rest time than pain from vascular claudication.
◆ Other signs and symptoms include paresthesia, weakness and clumsiness when walking, and hypoactive deep tendon reflexes after walking.

NURSING CONSIDERATIONS

◆ Encourage the patient to exercise.
◆ Advise the patient to avoid prolonged sitting or standing as well as crossing his legs at the knees.

PEDIATRIC POINTERS

◆ Intermittent claudication rarely occurs in children.
◆ Intermittent claudication may develop in children with coarctation of the aorta; however, extensive compensatory collateral circulation typically prevents manifestation of this sign.

PATIENT TEACHING

◆ Discuss with the patient the risk factors, diagnostic tests, and treatment options, including medications, for intermittent claudication.
◆ Stress the importance of inspecting his legs and feet for ulcers.
◆ Explain ways the patient can protect his extremities from injury and elements.
◆ Teach the patient the signs and symptoms he should report.
◆ Teach the patient exercises to improve circulation in his legs. (See *Improving leg circulation*.)

Improving leg circulation

To help stimulate circulation in the legs, instruct the patient to do the following:

Perform these exercises (called Berger's exercises) as part of your regular exercise program. Do them four times each day or as often as your physician specifies.

Begin by lying flat on your back; then raise your legs straight up at a 90-degree angle, and hold this position for 2 minutes.

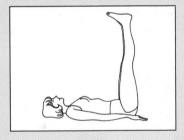

Now sit on the edge of a table or any flat surface that's high enough so that your legs don't touch the floor. Dangle your legs and swirl them in circles for 2 minutes.

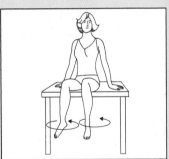

Finally, lie flat for 2 minutes; then repeat the sequence twice.

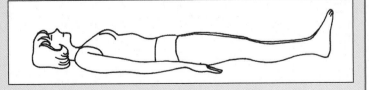

Janeway's lesions

- Slightly raised but usually flat, irregular, nontender, small (1 to 4 mm in diameter), erythematous lesions on the palms and soles that disappear spontaneously
- Blanch with pressure or elevation of the affected extremity
- Occasionally form a diffuse rash over the trunk and extremities

- Obtain a medical history from the patient, especially noting valvular or rheumatic heart disease; prosthetic valve replacement; meningitis; recent dental procedures or invasive diagnostic tests; any skin, bone, or respiratory infections; renal disease requiring an arteriovenous shunt; or long-term I.V. therapy, such as total parenteral nutrition.
- Find out if the patient has weakness, fatigue, chills, anorexia, or night sweats, possibly indicating an infection.
- Obtain a drug history including use of prophylactic antibiotics for rheumatic heart disease, I.V. drug use, or any immunosuppressant.

- Perform a physical examination, carefully inspecting the skin for other lesions, such as petechiae on his trunk or mucous membranes, and Osler's nodes on his palms, soles, or finger or toe pads.
- Inspect fingers for clubbing and splinter hemorrhages.
- Take vital signs, noting fever and tachycardia (which may indicate heart failure if it persists after fever disappears).
- Inspect and palpate his extremities for edema.
- Auscultate for gallops and murmurs.
- Assess other body systems for embolic complications of infective endocarditis, such as acute abdominal pain and hematuria.

MEDICAL

Infective endocarditis, acute

- Janeway's lesions are a late sign of this infectious disorder. They were once a common finding, possibly reflecting an immunologic reaction to the infecting organisms (usually bacteria), but these lesions are rarely seen today as the disease is detected and managed at an earlier stage.
- Early signs and symptoms include a sudden onset of shaking chills and fever, peripheral edema, dyspnea, petechiae, Osler's nodes, Roth's spots, and hematuria.

Infective endocarditis, subacute

- Janeway's lesions may appear late in this disorder, which has an insidious onset.
- Embolization may produce acute signs and symptoms, such as chest, abdominal, and extremity pain; paralysis; hematuria; and blindness.
- Early signs and symptoms include weakness, fatigue, weight loss, fever, night sweats, anorexia, and arthralgia.
- Other signs and symptoms include an elevated pulse, pale skin, Osler's nodes, splinter hemorrhages under the fingernails, petechiae, Roth's spots, clubbing of the fingers (in long-standing disease), splenomegaly, and murmurs.

- Treatment of infective endocarditis includes an antibiotic and—with complications such as heart failure—a diuretic and cardiac glycoside.
- Monitor the patient's intake, output, and cardiac status, and be alert for embolic complications, such as acute chest pain, abdominal pain, and paralysis.

PEDIATRIC POINTERS

- In children, Janeway's lesions result from infective endocarditis, which commonly stems from congenital heart defects or rheumatic fever.

- Explain to the patient that Janeway's lesions will disappear without damaging his skin.
- Teach the patient about diagnostic tests, such as blood cultures and an echocardiogram.
- Teach the patient about the importance of prescribed medications, how to take them, and possible side effects.

Jaundice

- Yellow discoloration of skin, mucous membranes, or sclerae of the eyes
- Indicates excessive levels of bilirubin in the blood (see *Impaired bilirubin metabolism in jaundice*)
- Easier to detect in natural light
- Also known as *icterus*

- Ask about the onset of jaundice.
- Inquire about associated pruritus, clay-colored stools, dark urine, fatigue, fever, chills, GI signs or symptoms, and cardiopulmonary symptoms.
- Obtain a medical history, including incidence of cancer; liver, pancreatic or gallbladder disease; hepatitis; or gallstones.
- Ask about drug and alcohol use.
- Find out about recent weight loss.

- Perform the physical examination in a room with natural light.
- Rule out hypercarotenemia, which is more prominent on the palms and soles and doesn't affect the sclera.
- Inspect the skin for texture, dryness, hyperpigmentation, spider angiomas, petechiae, and xanthomas.
- Note clubbed fingers and gynecomastia.
- Palpate the abdomen for tenderness, pain, and swelling.
- Palpate and percuss the liver and spleen for enlargement.
- Test for ascites.
- Auscultate for arrhythmias, murmurs, or gallops.
- Palpate lymph nodes for swelling.
- Obtain baseline data on mental status.

Impaired bilirubin metabolism in jaundice

Jaundice occurs in three forms: prehepatic, hepatic, and posthepatic. In all three, bilirubin levels in the blood increase because of impaired metabolism.

With *prehepatic jaundice*, certain conditions and disorders, such as transfusion reactions and sickle cell anemia, cause massive hemolysis. Red blood cells rupture faster than the liver can conjugate bilirubin, so large amounts of unconjugated bilirubin pass into the blood, causing increased intestinal conversion of this bilirubin to water-soluble urobilinogen for excretion in urine and stools. (Unconjugated bilirubin is insoluble in water, so it can't be directly excreted in urine.)

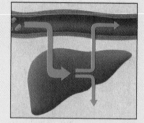

With *hepatic jaundice*, the liver's inability to conjugate or excrete bilirubin leads to increased blood levels of conjugated and unconjugated bilirubin. This occurs with such disorders as hepatitis, cirrhosis, and metastatic cancer and during the prolonged use of drugs metabolized by the liver.

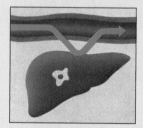

With *posthepatic jaundice*, which occurs in patients with a biliary or pancreatic disorder, bilirubin forms at its normal rate, but inflammation, scar tissue, a tumor, or gallstones block the flow of bile into the intestine. This causes an accumulation of conjugated bilirubin in the blood. Water-soluble, conjugated bilirubin is excreted in the urine.

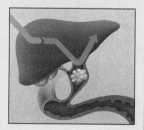

MEDICAL
Carcinoma

◆ Cancer of the hepatopancreatic ampulla produces fluctuating jaundice, occult bleeding, mild abdominal pain, recurrent fever, weight loss, pruritus, back pain, and chills.
◆ Hepatic cancer produces jaundice, right-upper-quadrant discomfort and tenderness, nausea, weight loss, slight fever, ascites, edema, and an irregular, nodular, firm, enlarged liver.
◆ With pancreatic cancer, progressive jaundice may be the only sign; other signs and symptoms include weight loss, back or abdominal pain, anorexia, nausea, vomiting, fever, steatorrhea, fatigue, weakness, diarrhea, pruritus, and skin lesions.

Cholangitis

◆ Jaundice along with right-upper-quadrant pain and high fever with chills make up Charcot's triad.
◆ Other signs and symptoms include pruritus and clay-colored stools.

Cholecystitis

◆ Nonobstructive jaundice occurs.
◆ Biliary colic typically peaks abruptly, persisting for 2 to 4 hours, then localizes to the right upper quadrant and becomes constant.
◆ Other signs and symptoms include nausea, vomiting, fever, profuse diaphoresis, chills, tenderness on palpation, a positive Murphy's sign, and abdominal distention and rigidity.

Cholelithiasis

◆ Jaundice and biliary colic are common.
◆ Pain is severe and steady in the right upper quadrant or epigastrium, radiates to the right scapula or shoulder, and intensifies over several hours.
◆ Other signs and symptoms include nausea, vomiting, tachycardia, restlessness and, if the common bile duct is occluded, fever, chills, jaundice, clay-colored stools, and abdominal tenderness.

Cholestasis

◆ Prolonged attacks of jaundice (sometimes spaced several years apart) are accompanied by pruritus.
◆ Other signs and symptoms include fatigue, nausea, weight loss, anorexia, pale stools, and right-upper-quadrant pain.

Cirrhosis

◆ With Laënnec's cirrhosis, mild to moderate jaundice occurs with pruritus; common early signs and symptoms include ascites, weakness, leg edema, nausea, vomiting, diarrhea or constipation, anorexia, massive hematemesis, weight loss, and right-upper-quadrant pain.
◆ With primary biliary cirrhosis, fluctuating jaundice may appear years after the onset of other signs and symptoms, such as pruritus that worsens at bedtime (commonly the first sign), weakness, fatigue, weight loss, and vague abdominal pain.

Glucose-6-phosphate dehydrogenase deficiency

◆ Jaundice occurs along with pallor, dyspnea, tachycardia, malaise, and hepatosplenomegaly in this congenital abnormality.

Heart failure

◆ Jaundice occurs with severe right-sided heart failure due to liver dysfunction.
◆ Other signs and symptoms include jugular vein distention, cyanosis, dependent edema, weight gain, weakness, confusion, hepatomegaly, nausea, vomiting, abdominal discomfort, anorexia, and ascites (a late sign).

Hemolytic anemia, acquired

◆ Prominent jaundice appears with dyspnea, fatigue, pallor, tachycardia, and palpitations.
◆ With rapid hemolysis, chills, fever, irritability, headache, abdominal pain, and signs of shock may appear.

(continued)

Hepatitis

◆ Jaundice occurs late and is preceded by dark urine and clay-colored stools.
◆ Signs and symptoms during the icteric phase include weight loss, anorexia, right-upper-quadrant pain and tenderness, and an enlarged liver.
◆ Other signs and symptoms include fatigue, nausea, vomiting, malaise, arthralgias, myalgias, headache, anorexia, photophobia, pharyngitis, cough, diarrhea or constipation, and low-grade fever.

Pancreatitis, acute

◆ Jaundice may occur.
◆ The primary symptom is usually severe epigastric pain that may radiate to the back and is relieved by lying with the knees flexed on the chest or sitting up and leaning forward.
◆ Other signs and symptoms include nausea, persistent vomiting, Turner's or Cullen's sign, fever, and abdominal distention, rigidity, and tenderness.

Sickle cell anemia

◆ Jaundice occurs with impaired growth and development, increased susceptibility to infection, thrombotic complications, leg ulcers, swollen and painful joints, fever, chills, bone aches, and chest pain.

OTHER
Drugs

◆ Jaundice may occur with drugs that cause hepatic injury, such as acetaminophen, isoniazid, hormonal contraceptives, sulfonamides, mercaptopurine, erythromycin estolate, niacin, troleandomycin, androgenic steroids, 3-hydroxy-3-methylglutaryl coenzyme A (HMG-CoA) reductase inhibitors, phenothiazines, ethanol, methyldopa, rifampin, dilantin, phenylbutazone, and I.V. tetracycline.

Treatments

◆ Upper abdominal surgery may result in jaundice due to organ manipulation leading to edema and obstructed bile flow.
◆ Surgical shunts used to reduce portal hypertension may also produce jaundice.
◆ Prolonged surgery resulting in shock, blood loss, or blood transfusion can cause jaundice.

NURSING CONSIDERATIONS

◆ To decrease pruritus:
- Frequently bathe the patient.
- Apply an antipruritic lotion such as calamine.
- Administer diphenhydramine or hydroxyzine.
◆ Provide emotional support.

PEDIATRIC POINTERS

◆ Physiologic jaundice is common in neonates, developing 3 to 5 days after birth.
◆ In infants, obstructive jaundice usually results from congenital biliary atresia.

GERIATRIC POINTERS

◆ In patients older than age 60, jaundice is usually caused by cholestasis resulting from extrahepatic obstruction.

PATIENT TEACHING

◆ Discuss the underlying condition, diagnostic tests, and treatment options.
◆ Teach the patient appropriate dietary changes he can make.
◆ Discuss ways to reduce pruritus.

Jaw pain

- May arise from the maxilla, mandible, or temporomandibular joint (TMJ)
- Usually results from disorders of the teeth, soft tissue, or glands of the mouth or throat or from local trauma or infection
- May develop gradually or abruptly
- May signal a life-threatening disorder

  ◆ **ACTION STAT!** *Sudden severe jaw pain, especially when associated with chest pain, shortness of breath, or arm pain, may signal an acute coronary syndrome or a myocardial infarction. Perform an electrocardiogram and obtain blood samples for cardiac enzyme levels. Administer oxygen, morphine sulfate, and a vasodilator, as indicated.*

HISTORY

- Determine the onset, character, intensity, and frequency of jaw pain.
- Ask whether the jaw pain radiates to other areas.
- Ask about recent trauma, surgery, or procedures.
- Inquire about associated signs and symptoms, such as joint or chest pain, dyspnea, palpitations, fatigue, headache, malaise, anorexia, weight loss, intermittent claudication, diplopia, and hearing loss.
- Ask about aggravating or alleviating factors.

PHYSICAL ASSESSMENT

- Inspect the painful area for redness; palpate for edema or warmth.
- Look for facial asymmetry.
- Check the TMJs, noting crepitus and ability to open the mouth.
- Palpate the parotid area for pain and swelling.
- Inspect and palpate the oral cavity for lesions, elevation of the tongue, or masses.

CAUSES

MEDICAL
Angina pectoris
- Jaw and left arm pain may radiate from the substernal area.
- It may be triggered by exertion, emotional stress, or ingestion of a heavy meal and subsides with rest or administration of nitroglycerin.
- Other signs and symptoms include shortness of breath, nausea, vomiting, tachycardia, dizziness, diaphoresis, and palpitations.

Arthritis
- Osteoarthritis causes aching jaw pain that increases with activity and may be accompanied by crepitus, enlarged joints with restricted range of motion, and stiffness on awakening that improves with activity.
- Rheumatoid arthritis causes symmetrical pain in all joints, including the jaw.
- Other signs and symptoms of rheumatoid arthritis include tender, swollen joints with limited range of motion that are stiff after inactivity; myalgia; fatigue; weight loss; malaise; anorexia; lymphadenopathy; mild fever; painless, movable nodules on the elbows, knees, and knuckles; joint deformities and crepitus; and multiple systemic complications.

Head and neck cancer
- Jaw pain has an insidious onset.
- Other signs and symptoms include a history of leukoplakia ulcers on the mucous membranes; palpable masses in the jaw, mouth, and neck; dysphagia; bloody discharge; drooling; lymphadenopathy; and trismus.

Hypocalcemic tetany
- Painful muscle contractions of the jaw and mouth occur with paresthesia and carpopedal spasms.
- Other signs and symptoms include weakness, fatigue, palpitations, hyperreflexia, positive Chvostek's and Trousseau's signs, muscle twitching, choreiform movements, muscle cramps and, with severe hypocalcemia, laryngospasm with stridor, cyanosis, seizures, and arrhythmias.

Ludwig's angina
- Severe jaw pain in the mandibular area occurs with tongue elevation, sublingual edema, fever, and drooling caused by cellulitis.
- Progressive disease produces dysphagia, dysphonia, stridor, and dyspnea.

Myocardial infarction
- A life-threatening disorder, crushing substernal pain may radiate to the lower jaw, left arm, neck, back, or shoulder blades.
- Other signs and symptoms include pallor, clammy skin, dyspnea, excessive diaphoresis, nausea, vomiting, anxiety, restlessness, a feeling of impending doom, low-grade fever, decreased or increased blood pressure, arrhythmias, an atrial gallop, new murmurs, and crackles.

Osteomyelitis
- Aching jaw pain may occur along with warmth, swelling, tenderness, erythema, and restricted jaw movement.
- Tachycardia, sudden fever, nausea, and malaise may occur with acute osteomyelitis.

Sinusitis
- Maxillary sinusitis produces intense boring pain in the maxilla and cheek that may radiate to the eye along with a feeling of fullness, increased pain on percussion of the first and second molars and, in those with

nasal obstruction, the loss of the sense of smell.
- Sphenoid sinusitis produces chronic pain at the mandibular ramus and vertex of the head and in the temporal area.
- Other signs and symptoms of both types of sinusitis include fever, halitosis, headache, malaise, cough, sore throat, and fever.

Suppurative parotitis
- Onset of jaw pain, high fever, and chills is abrupt.
- Other signs and symptoms include erythema and edema of the overlying skin; a tender, swollen gland; and pus at the second molar.

Temporal arteritis
- Sharp jaw pain occurs after chewing or talking.
- Other signs and symptoms include low-grade fever; generalized muscle pain; malaise; fatigue; anorexia; weight loss; throbbing, unilateral headache in the frontotemporal regions; swollen, nodular, tender and, possibly, pulseless temporal arteries; and erythema of the overlying skin.

Temporomandibular joint disorders
- Jaw pain at the TMJ; spasm and pain of the masticating muscle; clicking, popping, or crepitus of the TMJ; and restricted jaw movement may occur.
- Other signs and symptoms include localized pain that may radiate to other head and neck areas, teeth clenching, bruxism, ear pain, headache, deviation of the jaw to the affected side upon opening the mouth, and jaw subluxation or dislocation, especially after yawning.

Trauma
- Jaw pain may occur with swelling and decreased jaw mobility.
- Other signs and symptoms include hypotension, tachycardia, lacerations, ecchymoses, hematomas, blurred vision, and rhinorrhea or otorrhea.

Trigeminal neuralgia
- Paroxysmal attacks of intense unilateral jaw pain (stopping at the facial midline) or rapid-fire shooting sensations in one division of the trigeminal nerve (usually the mandibular or maxillary division) occur.
- Pain is felt mainly over the lips and chin and in the teeth; mouth and nose areas may be hypersensitive; and corneal reflexes are diminished or absent (if the ophthalmic branch is involved).

OTHER
Drugs
- Some drugs, such as phenothiazines, affect the extrapyramidal tract, causing dyskinesias; others cause tetany of the jaw from hypocalcemia.

Jugular vein distention

OVERVIEW

- Abnormal fullness and height of pulse waves in internal or external jugular veins
- Involves a pulse wave height greater than 1¼″ to 1½″ (3 to 4 cm) above the angle of Louis with the patient in a supine position and his head elevated 45 degrees (see *Evaluating jugular vein distention*)
- Reflects increased venous pressure in the right side of the heart, which in turn, indicates increased central venous pressure
- Occurs in cardiovascular disorders

 ACTION STAT! *If you detect jugular vein distention in a patient with pale, clammy skin who suddenly appears anxious and dyspneic, take his blood pressure. If you note hypotension and paradoxical pulse, suspect cardiac tamponade. Elevate the foot of the bed 20 to 30 degrees, give supplemental oxygen, and monitor cardiac status and rhythm, oxygen saturation, and mental status. Start an I.V. line for medication administration and keep cardiopulmonary resuscitation equipment readily available. Assemble equipment for emergency pericardiocentesis.*

HISTORY

- Find out about recent weight gain or swelling.
- Inquire about associated chest pain, shortness of breath, paroxysmal nocturnal dyspnea, anorexia, nausea, or vomiting.
- Obtain a medical history, including incidence of cancer or cardiac, pulmonary, hepatic, or renal disease, recent trauma or surgery.
- Obtain a drug history, noting use of diuretics.
- Inquire about diet history, especially sodium intake.

PHYSICAL ASSESSMENT

- Check vital signs.
- Inspect and palpate for edema.
- Weigh the patient and compare weight to his baseline.
- Auscultate lungs for crackles and heart for gallops, pericardial friction rub, and muffled heart sounds.
- Inspect abdomen for distention.
- Palpate and percuss for an enlarged liver.

TOP TECHNIQUE

Evaluating jugular vein distention

With the patient in a supine position, elevate the head of the bed 45 to 90 degrees. (In the normal patient, veins distend only when the patient lies flat.)

Next, locate the angle of Louis (sternal notch)—the reference point for measuring various pressure. To do so, palpate the clavicles where they join the sternum (the suprasternal notch). Place your first two fingers on the suprasternal notch. Then, without lifting them from the skin, slide them down the sternum until you feel a bony protuberance—this is the angle of Louis.

Find the internal jugular vein (which indicates venous pressure more reliably than the external jugular vein). Shine a flashlight across the patient's neck to create shadows that highlight his venous pulse. Be sure to distinguish jugular vein pulsations from carotid artery pulsations. One way to do this is to palpate the vessel: Arterial pulsations continue, whereas venous pulsations disappear with light finger pressure. Also, venous pulsations increase or decrease with changes in body position; arterial pulsations remain constant.

Next, locate the highest point along the vein where you can see pulsations. Using a centimeter ruler, measure the distance between the high point and the sternal notch. Record this finding as well as the angle at which the patient was lying. A finding greater than 1¼″ to 1½″ (3 to 4 cm) above the sternal notch, with the head of the bed at a 45-degree angle, indicates jugular vein distention.

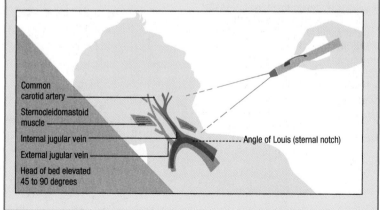

Common carotid artery

Sternocleidomastoid muscle

Internal jugular vein

External jugular vein

Head of bed elevated 45 to 90 degrees

Angle of Louis (sternal notch)

MEDICAL
Cardiac tamponade
◆ A life-threatening condition, jugular vein distention occurs along with anxiety, restlessness, cyanosis, chest pain, dyspnea, hypotension, and clammy skin.
◆ Other signs and symptoms include tachycardia, tachypnea, muffled heart sounds, a pericardial friction rub, weak or absent peripheral pulses that decrease during inspiration (pulsus paradoxus), and hepatomegaly.

Heart failure
◆ Right-sided heart failure commonly causes jugular vein distention, weakness, cyanosis, dependent edema, steady weight gain, confusion, and hepatomegaly.
◆ Other signs and symptoms of right-sided failure include nausea, vomiting, abdominal discomfort, anorexia, and ascites (a late sign).
◆ Jugular vein distention is a late sign in left-sided heart failure.
◆ Other signs and symptoms of left-sided failure include fatigue, dyspnea, orthopnea, paroxysmal nocturnal dyspnea, tachypnea, tachycardia, crackles, a ventricular gallop, and arrhythmias.

Hypervolemia
◆ Jugular vein distention occurs along with rapid weight gain, elevated blood pressure, bounding pulse, peripheral edema, dyspnea, and crackles.

Pericarditis, chronic constrictive
◆ Jugular vein distention is a progressive sign and more prominent on inspiration (known as Kussmaul's sign).
◆ Other signs and symptoms include chest pain, dependent edema, hepatomegaly, ascites, and pericardial friction rub.

Superior vena cava obstruction
◆ Jugular vein distention may occur along with facial, neck, and upper arm edema.

NURSING CONSIDERATIONS

◆ If the patient has cardiac tamponade, prepare him for pericardiocentesis.
◆ Restrict fluids and monitor intake and output.
◆ Insert an indwelling urinary catheter, if necessary.
◆ If the patient has heart failure, administer a diuretic, as ordered.
◆ Routinely change the patient's position to avoid skin breakdown from peripheral edema.
◆ Prepare the patient for central venous or pulmonary artery catheter insertion.

PEDIATRIC POINTERS
◆ Jugular vein distention is difficult to evaluate in infants, toddlers, and children because of their short, thick necks.

PATIENT TEACHING

◆ Discuss the underlying condition, diagnostic tests, and treatment options.
◆ Explain foods or fluids the patient should avoid.
◆ Teach the patient to perform daily weight monitoring.
◆ Explain what signs and symptoms he should report.
◆ Explain the importance of scheduled rest periods and help him plan for them.

Kehr's sign

OVERVIEW

- Referred left shoulder pain due to diaphragmatic irritation by intraperitoneal blood
- Cardinal sign of hemorrhage within the peritoneal cavity
- Pain usually arising when the patient assumes the supine position or lowers his head, which increases contact of free blood or clots with the left diaphragm, involving the phrenic nerve

ACTION STAT! *After you detect Kehr's sign, quickly take the patient's vital signs. If the patient shows signs of hypovolemia, elevate his feet 30 degrees. In addition, insert a large-bore I.V. line for fluid and blood replacement and an indwelling urinary catheter. Begin monitoring intake and output. Draw blood to determine hematocrit, and provide supplemental oxygen.*

HISTORY

- Ask patient about abdominal or shoulder pain
- Ask female patient whether she might be pregnant
- Obtain history of trauma
- Obtain complete drug history

PHYSICAL ASSESSMENT

- Inspect the patient's abdomen for bruises and distention, and palpate for tenderness.
- Percuss for Ballance's sign—an indicator of massive perisplenic clotting and free blood in the peritoneal cavity from a ruptured spleen.

CAUSES

MEDICAL
Intra-abdominal hemorrhage
♦ Kehr's sign usually accompanies intense abdominal pain, abdominal rigidity, and muscle spasm and usually develops right after the hemorrhage; however, its onset is sometimes delayed up to 48 hours.
♦ Other signs and symptoms vary with the cause of bleeding, including ruptured spleen, ruptured ectopic pregnancy, or a history of blunt or penetrating abdominal injuries.

NURSING CONSIDERATIONS

♦ In anticipation of surgery, withhold oral intake, and prepare the patient for abdominal X-rays, a computed tomography scan, an ultrasound and, possibly, paracentesis, peritoneal lavage, and culdocentesis.
♦ Give an analgesic, if needed.

PEDIATRIC POINTERS
♦ Because a child may have difficulty describing pain, watch for nonverbal clues such as rubbing the shoulder.

PATIENT TEACHING

♦ Teach the patient and family about all hospital procedures, including surgery and tests.
♦ Discuss the diagnosis and treatment plan.
♦ Teach the patient and family about prescribed medications, dietary modifications, and appropriate postoperative activities, as indicated.

Kernig's sign

- Indicates meningeal irritation, herniated disk, or spinal tumor
- Elicits resistance and hamstring muscle pain when the knee attempts to extend while the hip and knee are flexed 90 degrees (see *Eliciting Kernig's sign*)

- Obtain medical and drug history, including use of illegal drugs.
- Ask about back pain that radiates to the legs, numbness, tingling, or weakness.
- Inquire about a history of cancer, infection, or back injury.

- Assess motor function by inspecting the muscles and testing muscle tone and strength.
- Perform cerebellar testing.
- Assess sensory function by checking the patient's sensitivity to pain, light touch, vibration, position, and discrimination.

TOP TECHNIQUE

Eliciting Kernig's sign

To elicit Kernig's sign, place the patient in a supine position. Flex the leg at the hip and knee, as shown below. Then try to extend the leg while you keep the hip flexed. If the patient has pain and, possibly, a spasm in the hamstring muscle and resists further extension, you can assume that meningeal irritation is present.

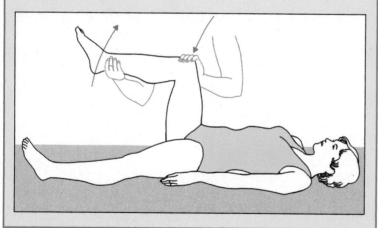

CAUSES

MEDICAL
Lumbosacral herniated disk
◆ Positive Kernig's sign may be elicited.
◆ Sciatic pain on the affected side or both sides is an early symptom.

Meningitis
◆ Positive Kernig's sign usually occurs early, along with fever and, possibly, chills.

Spinal cord tumor
◆ Kernig's sign can be occasionally elicited.
◆ The earliest symptom of spinal cord tumor is pain felt locally or along the spinal nerve, commonly in the leg.

Subarachnoid hemorrhage
◆ Kernig's sign and Brudzinski's sign can be elicited within minutes after the initial bleeding. (See *When Kernig's sign signals CNS crisis.*)

NURSING CONSIDERATIONS

◆ Closely monitor vital signs, intracranial pressure (ICP), and cardiopulmonary and neurologic status.
◆ Ensure bed rest, quiet, and minimal stress.
◆ For those with subarachnoid hemorrhage, darken the room and elevate the head of the bed at least 30 degrees to reduce ICP.
◆ If the patient has a herniated disk or spinal tumor, he may require pelvic traction.

PEDIATRIC POINTERS
◆ Kernig's sign is considered ominous in children because of the greater potential for rapid deterioration.

PATIENT TEACHING

◆ Discuss the underlying disorder, diagnostic tests, and treatment options.
◆ Teach the patient the signs and symptoms of meningitis.
◆ Discuss ways to prevent meningitis.
◆ Teach the patient with a herniated disk about activities he should avoid.
◆ Teach the patient how to apply his back brace or cervical collar, as needed.

 ACTION STAT!

When Kernig's sign signals CNS crisis

Because Kernig's sign may signal meningitis or subarachnoid hemorrhage—both life-threatening central nervous system (CNS) disorders—take the patient's vital signs immediately to obtain baseline information. Then test for Brudzinski's sign to obtain further evidence of meningeal irritation. Next, ask the patient or his family to describe the onset of illness. Typically, the progressive onset of headache, fever, nuchal rigidity, and confusion suggests meningitis. The sudden onset of a severe headache, nuchal rigidity, photophobia and, possibly, loss of consciousness usually indicates subarachnoid hemorrhage.

MENINGITIS

If meningitis is suspected, ask about recent infections, especially tooth abscesses. Ask about exposure to infected people or to places where meningitis is endemic. Meningitis is usually a complication of another bacterial infection;

draw blood for culture studies to determine the causative organism. If a tumor or abscess can be ruled out, prepare the patient for a lumbar puncture. Find out if the patient has a history of I.V. drug abuse, an open-head injury, or endocarditis. Insert an I.V. line and immediately begin giving an antibiotic, as ordered.

SUBARACHNOID HEMORRHAGE

If subarachnoid hemorrhage is suspected, ask about a history of hypertension, cerebral aneurysm, head trauma, or arteriovenous malformation. Also ask about sudden withdrawal of an antihypertensive.

Check the patient's pupils for dilation, and assess him for signs of increasing intracranial pressure, such as bradycardia, increased systolic blood pressure, and widened pulse pressure. Insert an I.V. line and administer supplemental oxygen.

Leg pain

OVERVIEW

- May be gradual or sudden, localized or diffuse
- May feel dull, burning, sharp, shooting, or tingling

ACTION STAT! *If the patient has acute leg pain and a history of trauma, quickly take his vital signs and determine the leg's neurovascular status. Observe the leg's position and check for swelling, gross deformities, or abnormal rotation. Check distal pulses and note skin color and temperature. A pale, cool, and pulseless leg may indicate impaired circulation, which may require emergency surgery. (See* Highlighting causes of local leg pain.*)*

HISTORY

- Ask about the onset and description of pain.
- Obtain a medical history, including incidence of cancer, injury, surgery, or joint, vascular, or back problems.
- Inquire about the use of assistive devices.
- Obtain a drug history.
- Ask about recent airplane travel.

PHYSICAL ASSESSMENT

- Observe the leg while the patient walks (if possible), stands, and sits.
- If the leg isn't fractured, test hip and knee range-of-motion (ROM).
- Check reflexes in the legs.
- Compare both legs for symmetry, movement, and active ROM.
- Assess sensation and strength.
- If the leg is immobilized, check distal circulation, sensation, and mobility; stretch the toes to elicit associated pain.

Highlighting causes of local leg pain

Various disorders cause hip, knee, ankle, or foot pain, which may radiate to surrounding tissues and be reported as leg pain. Local pain is commonly accompanied by tenderness, swelling, and deformity in the affected area.

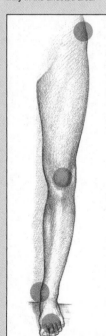

HIP PAIN
Arthritis
Avascular necrosis
Bursitis
Dislocation
Fracture
Sepsis
Tumor

KNEE PAIN
Arthritis
Bursitis
Chondromalacia
Contusion
Cruciate ligament injury
Dislocation
Fracture
Meniscal injury
Osteochondritis dissecans
Phlebitis
Popliteal cyst
Radiculopathy
Ruptured extensor mechanism
Sprain

ANKLE PAIN
Achilles tendon contracture
Arthritis
Dislocation
Fracture
Sprain
Tenosynovitis

FOOT PAIN
Arthritis
Bunion
Callus or corn
Dislocation
Flatfoot
Fracture
Gout
Hallux rigidus
Hammer toe
Ingrown toenail
Köhler's disease
Morton's neuroma
Occlusive vascular disease
Plantar fasciitis
Plantar wart
Radiculopathy
Tabes dorsalis
Tarsal tunnel syndrome

MEDICAL
Bone cancer
◆ The initial symptom is continuous, deep or boring pain that worsens at night
◆ Later signs and symptoms include skin breakdown, impaired circulation, cachexia, fever, and impaired mobility

Compartment syndrome
◆ Swelling or bleeding within a muscle compartment can interfere with circulation.
◆ Progressive, intense lower leg pain that increases with passive muscle stretching is a major sign of this limb-threatening disorder.
◆ Pain typically worsens despite analgesia.
◆ Other symptoms include muscle weakness and paresthesia, but normal distal circulation.

Fracture
◆ Severe, acute leg pain accompanies swelling and ecchymosis.
◆ Other signs and symptoms include deformity, muscle spasms, bony crepitation, paresthesia, absent pulse, mottled cyanosis, cool skin, and pain with movement.

Infection
◆ Local leg pain occurs with erythema, swelling, streaking, and warmth.
◆ Other signs and symptoms include fever, tachycardia, and loss of function of the affected limb.

Occlusive vascular disease
◆ Continuous cramping pain may worsen with walking.
◆ Other signs and symptoms include pain at night, cold feet, cold intolerance, numbness, tingling, ankle and lower leg edema, decreased or absent pulses, and increased capillary refill time.

Sciatica
◆ Shooting, aching, or tingling pain radiates down the back of the leg.

◆ Typically, activity exacerbates the pain and rest relieves it.

Strain or sprain
◆ Acute strain causes sharp, transient pain and rapid swelling, followed by leg tenderness and ecchymosis.
◆ Chronic strain produces stiffness, soreness, generalized leg tenderness, and pain on passive or active motion.
◆ Sprain causes local pain, especially during joint movement; ecchymosis; local swelling; and loss of mobility.

Thrombophlebitis
◆ Discomfort ranges from calf tenderness to severe pain and swelling, warmth, and heaviness.
◆ Other signs and symptoms include fever, chills, malaise, muscle cramps, a positive Homans' sign, and superficial veins that are engorged, sensitive to pressure, and hard, thready, and cordlike.

Varicose veins
◆ Nocturnal cramping; heaviness; diffuse, dull aching after prolonged standing or walking; and aching during menses occur.
◆ Other signs and symptoms include palpable nodules, orthostatic edema, and stasis pigmentation of the calves and ankles.

Venous stasis ulcers
◆ Localized pain and bleeding occur.
◆ Mottled, bluish pigmentation is characteristic, and local edema may occur.

◆ Check distal pulses and evaluate the legs for temperature, color, and sensation.
◆ Monitor thigh and calf circumference.
◆ Give an anticoagulant, analgesic, and antibiotic, as ordered.
◆ Use sandbags to immobilize the leg; apply ice and, if needed, implement skeletal traction.
◆ Maintain adequate hydration and nutrition.

PEDIATRIC POINTERS
◆ Common causes of leg pain in children include fracture, osteomyelitis, and bone cancer.
◆ If parents fail to give adequate explanation for a leg fracture, consider child abuse.

◆ Discuss the underlying condition, diagnostic tests, and treatment options.
◆ Explain the use of anti-inflammatory drugs, ROM exercises, and assistive devices.
◆ Discuss lifestyle changes the patient should make.
◆ Teach appropriate positioning to enhance blood flow and venous return.
◆ Discuss the need for physical therapy, as appropriate.
◆ Teach cast care.
◆ Discuss signs and symptoms to report.

Level of consciousness, decreased

OVERVIEW

- Ranges from lethargy to stupor to coma
- Involves cerebral disturbance to any part of the communication within the reticular activating system
- May signal a life-threatening disorder
- May deteriorate suddenly or gradually and can remain altered temporarily or permanently
- Changes in mental status the most sensitive indicators of decreased level of consciousness (LOC)

 ACTION STAT! After evaluating the patient's airway, breathing, and circulation, use the Glasgow Coma Scale to determine LOC and to obtain baseline data. (See Using the Glasgow Coma Scale.*)*

Insert an artificial airway, elevate the head of the bed 30 degrees and, if spinal cord injury has been ruled out, turn the patient's head to the side. Prepare to suction the patient, if needed. He may require hyperventilation to reduce carbon dioxide levels and decrease intracranial pressure (ICP). Then determine the rate, rhythm, and depth of spontaneous respirations. Support breathing with a handheld resuscitation bag, if needed.

If Glasgow Coma Scale score is 7 or lower, intubation and resuscitation may be needed. Continue to monitor vital signs, looking for signs of increasing ICP, such as bradycardia and widening pulse pressure. When airway, breathing, and circulation are stabilized, perform a neurologic examination.

HISTORY

- Ask family about headaches, dizziness, nausea, vision or hearing disturbances, weakness, and fatigue.
- Determine whether the family has noticed any changes in behavior, personality, memory, or temperament.
- Obtain a medical history, including incidence of neurologic disease or cancer and recent trauma or infection.
- Obtain a history of drug and alcohol use.

PHYSICAL ASSESSMENT

- Perform a complete neurologic examination.
- Perform a physical assessment.

TOP TECHNIQUE

Using the Glasgow Coma Scale

To use the Glasgow Coma Scale, test the patient's ability to respond to verbal, motor, and sensory stimulation and grade the reaction according to the chart. The scoring system doesn't determine exact level of consciousness, but it does provide an easy way to describe the patient's mental status and helps to detect and interpret changes from baseline findings. A decreased reaction score in one or more categories may signal an impending neurologic crisis. A score of 7 or lower indicates severe neurologic damage.

TEST	REACTION	SCORE
Eye opening response	Open spontaneously	4
	Open to verbal command	3
	Open to pain	2
	No response	1
Best motor response	Obeys verbal command	6
	Localizes painful stimulus	5
	Flexion—withdrawal	4
	Flexion—abnormal (decorticate rigidity)	3
	Extension (decerebrate rigidity)	2
	No response	1
Best verbal response	Oriented and converses	5
	Disoriented and converses	4
	Inappropriate words	3
	Incomprehensible sounds	2
	No response	1
Total		3 to 15

MEDICAL

Adrenal crisis

- Decreased LOC, ranging from lethargy to coma, may develop within 12 hours of onset.
- Early signs and symptoms include progressive weakness, irritability, anorexia, headache, nausea, vomiting, diarrhea, abdominal pain, and fever.
- Later signs and symptoms include hypotension; rapid, thready pulse; oliguria; cool, clammy skin; and flaccid extremities.

Brain abscess

- Decreased LOC varies from drowsiness to deep stupor.
- Early signs and symptoms include constant intractable headache, nausea, vomiting, and seizures.
- Later signs and symptoms include ocular disturbances and signs of infection.
- Other signs and symptoms include personality changes, confusion, abnormal behavior, dizziness, facial weakness, aphasia, ataxia, tremor, and hemiparesis.

Brain tumor

- LOC decreases slowly, from lethargy to coma.
- Apathy, behavior changes, memory loss, decreased attention span, morning headache, dizziness, aphasia, seizures, vision loss, ataxia, and sensorimotor disturbances may occur.
- In later stages, signs and symptoms include, papilledema, vomiting, bradycardia, and widening pulse pressure.
- In the final stages, signs include decorticate or decerebrate posture.

Cerebral aneurysm, ruptured

- Somnolence, confusion and, at times, stupor characterize moderate bleeding.
- Deep coma occurs with severe bleeding, which can be fatal.

- Onset is usually abrupt with sudden, severe headache, nausea, and vomiting.
- Nuchal rigidity, back and leg pain, fever, restlessness, irritability, seizures, and blurred vision point to meningeal irritation.
- Other signs and symptoms include hemiparesis, hemisensory defects, dysphagia, and visual defects.

Cerebral contusion

- Unconscious patients may have dilated, nonreactive pupils and decorticate or decerebrate posture.
- Conscious patients may be drowsy, confused, disoriented, agitated, or violent.
- Other signs and symptoms include blurred or double vision, fever, headache, pallor, diaphoresis, seizures, impaired mental status, slight hemiparesis, tachycardia, altered respirations, aphasia, and hemiparesis.

Diabetic ketoacidosis

- Decrease in LOC is rapid and ranges from lethargy to coma.
- Polydipsia, polyphagia, and polyuria precede decreased LOC secondary to fluid shift from elevated glucose level.
- Other signs and symptoms include weakness, anorexia, abdominal pain, nausea, vomiting, orthostatic hypotension, fruity breath odor, Kussmaul's respirations, warm and dry skin, and a rapid, thready pulse.

Encephalitis

- Decreased LOC may range from lethargy to coma within 48 hours of onset.
- Other signs and symptoms may include abrupt onset of fever, headache, nuchal rigidity, nausea, vomiting, irritability, personality changes, seizures, aphasia, ataxia, hemiparesis, nystagmus, photophobia, myoclonus, and cranial nerve palsies.

Encephalopathy

- Hepatic encephalopathy produces decreased LOC that ranges from

slight personality changes to coma depending on the stage.

- Hypertensive encephalopathy produces LOC that progressively decreases from lethargy to stupor to coma.
- Hypoglycemic encephalopathy produces LOC that rapidly deteriorates from lethargy to coma.
- Hypoxic encephalopathy produces a sudden or gradual decrease in LOC, leading to coma and brain death.
- Uremic encephalopathy produces LOC that decreases gradually from lethargy to coma.

Epidural hemorrhage, acute

- Momentary loss of consciousness is sometimes followed by a lucid interval.
- While the patient is lucid, signs and symptoms include severe headache, nausea, vomiting, and bladder distention.
- Rapid deterioration in consciousness follows, possibly leading to coma.
- Other signs and symptoms include irregular respirations, seizures, decreased and bounding pulse, increased pulse pressure, hypertension, fixed and dilated pupils, unilateral hemiparesis or hemiplegia, decerebrate posture, and positive Babinski's reflex.

Heatstroke

- As body temperature increases, LOC gradually decreases from lethargy to coma.
- At the onset, skin is hot, flushed, and diaphoretic with blotchy cyanosis; when body temperature exceeds 105° F (40.5° C), skin is no longer diaphoretic.
- Other early signs and symptoms include irritability, anxiety, severe headache, malaise, tachycardia, tachypnea, orthostatic hypotension, muscle cramps, rigidity, and syncope.

(continued)

Hypernatremia

◆ LOC deteriorates from lethargy to coma.
◆ The patient is irritable and exhibits twitches that progress to seizures.
◆ Other signs and symptoms include nausea, malaise, fever, thirst, flushed skin, dry mucous membranes, and a weak, thready pulse.

Hyperosmolar hyperglycemic nonketotic syndrome

◆ LOC decreases rapidly from lethargy to coma.
◆ Early signs and symptoms include polyuria, polydipsia, weight loss, and weakness.
◆ Later signs and symptoms include hypotension, poor skin turgor, dry skin and mucous membranes, tachycardia, tachypnea, oliguria, and seizures.

Hypokalemia

◆ LOC gradually decreases to lethargy.
◆ Other signs and symptoms include confusion, nausea, vomiting, diarrhea, polyuria, weakness, decreased reflexes, malaise, dizziness, hypotension, arrhythmias, and abnormal electrocardiogram results.

Hyponatremia

◆ Decreased LOC occurs in late stages.
◆ Early nausea and malaise may progress to behavior changes, confusion, lethargy, incoordination and, eventually, seizures and coma.

Hypothermia

◆ When severe, LOC decreases from lethargy to coma.
◆ Mild to moderate cases produce memory loss, slurred speech, shivering, weakness, fatigue, and apathy.
◆ Other early signs and symptoms include ataxia, muscle stiffness, hyperactive deep tendon reflexes (DTRs), diuresis, tachycardia, bradypnea, decreased blood pressure, and cold, pale skin.
◆ Later signs and symptoms include muscle rigidity, decreased reflexes, peripheral cyanosis, bradycardia, arrhythmias, severe hypotension, shal-

low respirations, oliguria and, possibly, cardiopulmonary arrest.

Intracerebral hemorrhage

◆ In this life-threatening disorder, rapid, steady loss of consciousness occurs within hours and is accompanied by severe headache, dizziness, nausea, and vomiting.
◆ Other signs and symptoms include increased blood pressure, irregular respirations, Babinski's reflex, seizures, aphasia, decreased sensations, hemiplegia, decorticate or decerebrate posture, and dilated pupils.

Meningitis

◆ Confusion and irritability occur; stupor, coma, and seizures may occur in severe cases.
◆ Other signs and symptoms include fever, chills, severe headache, nuchal rigidity, hyperreflexia, Kernig's and Brudzinski's signs, ocular palsies, photophobia, facial weakness, hearing loss, and opisthotonos.

Myxedema crisis

◆ Decline in LOC may be swift due to hypothyroidism.
◆ Other signs and symptoms include severe hypothermia, hypoventilation, hypotension, bradycardia, hypoactive reflexes, periorbital and peripheral edema, impaired hearing and balance, and seizures.

Pontine hemorrhage

◆ A sudden, rapid decrease in LOC to the point of coma occurs within minutes.
◆ Death occurs within hours.
◆ Other signs and symptoms include total paralysis, decerebrate posture, Babinski's reflex, absent doll's eye sign, and bilateral miosis.

Seizure disorders

◆ A complex partial seizure causes decreased LOC, manifested as a blank stare, purposeless behavior, and unintelligible speech; an aura may precede the seizure; several minutes of mental confusion may follow the seizure.

◆ An absence seizure involves a brief change in LOC, indicated by blinking or eye rolling, blank stare, and slight mouth movements.
◆ A generalized tonic-clonic seizure typically begins with a loud cry and sudden loss of consciousness; consciousness returns after the seizure, but the patient remains confused and may fall into deep sleep.
◆ An atonic seizure produces sudden unconsciousness for a few seconds.
◆ Status epilepticus, a life-threatening condition, involves rapidly recurring seizures.

Shock

◆ Decreased LOC occurs late.
◆ Other signs and symptoms include confusion, anxiety, restlessness, hypotension, tachycardia, weak pulse with narrowing pulse pressure, dyspnea, oliguria, and cool, clammy skin.

Stroke

◆ In thrombotic stroke, LOC changes may be abrupt or take several minutes, hours, or days to evolve.
◆ In embolic stroke, LOC changes occur suddenly and peak immediately.
◆ In hemorrhagic stroke, LOC changes develop over minutes or hours, depending on the extent of the bleeding.
◆ Other signs and symptoms of stroke include disorientation, intellectual deficits, personality changes, emotional lability, dysarthria, dysphagia, ataxia, aphasia, agnosia, unilateral sensorimotor loss, vision disturbances, incontinence, and seizures.

Subdural hematoma, chronic

◆ LOC deteriorates slowly.
◆ Other signs and symptoms include confusion, decreased ability to concentrate, personality changes, headache, light-headedness, seizures, and a dilated ipsilateral pupil with ptosis.

Subdural hemorrhage, acute

◆ In this life-threatening condition, agitation and confusion are followed by LOC progressively decreasing from somnolence to coma.

- Other signs and symptoms include headache, fever, unilateral pupil dilation, decreased pulse and respiratory rates, widening pulse pressure, seizures, hemiparesis, and Babinski's reflex.

Thyroid storm
- LOC decreases suddenly and can progress to coma.
- Irritability, restlessness, confusion, and psychotic behavior precede the deterioration.
- Other signs and symptoms include tremors, weakness, vision disturbances, tachycardia, arrhythmias, angina, acute respiratory distress, vomiting, diarrhea, and fever.

Transient ischemic attack
- LOC decreases abruptly (with varying severity) and gradually returns to normal within 24 hours.
- Other signs and symptoms include transient vision loss, nystagmus, aphasia, dizziness, dysarthria, unilateral hemiparesis or hemiplegia, tinnitus, paresthesia, dysphagia, and uncoordinated gait.

West Nile encephalitis
- Stupor, disorientation, and coma occur with severe infection.
- Skin rash and lymphadenopathy may also develop.
- Other signs and symptoms of severe infection include high fever, headache, neck stiffness, tremors, occasional seizures, and paralysis; rarely, death can occur.

OTHER
Alcohol
- Alcohol causes varying degrees of sedation, irritability, and incoordination; intoxication causes stupor.

Drugs
- Overdose of barbiturates, other central nervous system depressants, or aspirin can cause sedation and other degrees of decreased LOC.

Poisoning
- Toxins, such as lead, carbon monoxide, and snake venom, can cause varying degrees of decreased LOC.

NURSING CONSIDERATIONS

- Reassess LOC and neurologic status at least hourly.
- Monitor ICP and intake and output.
- Ensure airway patency and proper nutrition.
- Keep the patient on bed rest with the side rails up.
- Keep the head of the bed elevated to at least 30 degrees.
- Maintain seizure precautions.
- Don't give an opioid or a sedative.

PEDIATRIC POINTERS
- The primary cause of decreased LOC in children is head trauma.
- Other causes include poisoning, hydrocephalus, meningitis, or brain abscess following an ear or a respiratory infection.

PATIENT TEACHING

- Discuss the underlying condition, diagnostic tests, and treatment options with the patient and his family, as appropriate for the patient's mental status or LOC.
- Teach safety and seizure precautions.
- Provide referrals to sources of support.
- Discuss quality-of-life issues.

Light flashes

OVERVIEW

◆ Occur locally or throughout the visual field
◆ Complaints of seeing spots, stars, or lightning-type streaks
◆ May occur suddenly or gradually and can indicate temporary or permanent vision impairment
◆ Usually signal the splitting of the posterior vitreous membrane into two layers, with the inner layer detaching from the retina, and the outer layer remaining fixed to it

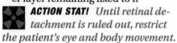 **ACTION STAT!** *Until retinal detachment is ruled out, restrict the patient's eye and body movement.*

HISTORY

◆ Obtain a history of when the light flashes began and their location.
◆ Ask about eye pain or headache and if the patient wears or has ever worn corrective lenses and if he or a family member has a history of eye or vision problems.
◆ Obtain a medical history, including incidence of hypertension, diabetes mellitus, or trauma.
◆ Obtain an occupational history because light flashes may be related to job stress or eye strain.

PHYSICAL ASSESSMENT

◆ Perform a complete eye and vision examination, including visual acuity and visual fields, especially if trauma is apparent or suspected.
◆ Inspect the external eye, lids, lashes, and tear puncta for abnormalities and the iris and sclera for signs of bleeding.
◆ Observe pupillary size and shape; check for reaction to light, accommodation, and consensual light response.

CAUSES

MEDICAL
Head trauma
- A patient who has sustained minor head trauma may report "seeing stars" when the injury occurs.
- Later, he may develop nausea, vomiting, and decreased level of consciousness.
- Other signs and symptoms include localized pain at the injury site, generalized headache, and dizziness.

Migraine headache
- Light flashes—possibly accompanied by an aura—may herald a classic migraine headache.
- As these symptoms subside, the patient typically experiences a severe, throbbing, unilateral headache that usually lasts 1 to 12 hours and may be accompanied by paresthesia of the lips, face, or hands; slight confusion; dizziness; photophobia; nausea; and vomiting.

Retinal detachment
- Light flashes described as floaters or spots are localized in the portion of the visual field where the retina is detaching.
- With macular involvement, the patient may experience painless visual impairment resembling a curtain covering the visual field.

Vitreous detachment
- Visual floaters may accompany a sudden onset of light flashes.
- Usually, one eye is affected at a time.

NURSING CONSIDERATIONS

- If the patient has retinal detachment, prepare him for reattachment surgery.
- If the patient doesn't have retinal detachment, reassure him that his light flashes are temporary and don't indicate eye damage.

PEDIATRIC POINTERS
- Children may experience light flashes after minor head trauma.

PATIENT TEACHING

- If the patient had surgery, teach postoperative care, including the need to wear bilateral eye patches and limit activity, lifting, and positions until the retina heals completely.
- Teach the patient about the underlying diagnosis.
- Teach about prescribed medications.
- For the patient with a migraine headache, teach him about maintaining a quiet, dark environment; importance of getting enough sleep; and taking an analgesic, as appropriate.

Low birth weight

- Normal minimum birth weight less than 5½ lb (2,500 g)
- Associated with higher neonate morbidity and mortality
- Classified as two groups: preterm infants (before the 37th week of gestation); and small for gestational age (SGA)
- Preterm neonate: usually results from a disorder that prevents the uterus from retaining the fetus, interferes with the normal course of pregnancy, causes premature separation of the placenta, or stimulates uterine contractions before term
- SGA neonate: intrauterine growth possibly retarded by a disorder that interferes with placental circulation, fetal development, or maternal health (see *Maternal causes of low birth weight*)
- SGA nenates who demonstrate catch-up growth, do so by 8 to 12 months
- Some remaining below the 10th percentile

Maternal causes of low birth weight

If the neonate is small for gestational age, consider these possible maternal causes:

- acquired immunodeficiency syndrome
- alcohol or opioid abuse
- chronic maternal illness
- cigarette smoking
- hypertension
- hypoxemia
- malnutrition
- toxemia.

If the neonate is born prematurely, consider these common maternal causes:

- abruptio placentae
- amnionitis
- cocaine or crack use
- incompetent cervix
- placenta previa
- polyhydramnios
- preeclampsia
- premature rupture of membranes
- severe maternal illness
- urinary tract infection.

ACTION STAT! *Because low birth weight may be associated with poorly developed body systems, particularly the respiratory system, your priority is to monitor the neonate's respiratory status. Be alert for signs of distress, such as apnea, grunting respirations, intercostal or xiphoid retractions, or a respiratory rate exceeding 60 breaths/minute after the first hour of life. If you detect any of these signs, prepare to provide respiratory support. Endotracheal intubation or supplemental oxygen with an oxygen hood may be needed.*

Monitor the neonate's axillary temperature. Decreased fat reserves may keep him from maintaining normal body temperature, and a drop below 97.8° F (36.5° C) exacerbates respiratory distress by increasing oxygen consumption. To maintain normal body temperature, use an overbed warmer or an Isolette. (If these are unavailable, use a wrapped rubber bottle filled with warm water, but be careful to avoid hyperthermia.) Cover the neonate's head to prevent heat loss.

- Obtain prenatal history from parents
- Obtain maternal drug and alcohol history
- Ask about maternal medical history.

- As soon as possible, evaluate the neonate's neuromuscular and physical maturity to determine gestational age. (See *Ballard Scale for calculating gestational age.*)
- Follow with a routine neonatal examination.

MEDICAL
Chromosomal aberrations

- Abnormalities in the number, size, or configuration of chromosomes can cause low birth weight and possibly multiple congenital anomalies in a preterm or SGA neonate. For example, a neonate with trisomy 21 (Down syndrome) may be SGA and have prominent epicanthal folds, a flat-bridged nose, a protruding tongue, palmar simian creases, muscular hypotonia, and an umbilical hernia.

Cytomegalovirus infection

- Although low birth weight in this disorder is usually associated with preterm birth, some neonates may be SGA.
- Assessment at birth may reveal these classic signs: petechiae and ecchymoses, jaundice, and hepatosplenomegaly, which increases for several days.
- Other signs and symptoms include high fever, lymphadenopathy, tachypnea, and dyspnea, along with prolonged bleeding at puncture sites.

Placental dysfunction

- Low birth weight and a wasted appearance occur in an SGA neonate.
- The neonate may be symmetrically short or may appear relatively long for his low weight.
- Additional signs and symptoms reflect the underlying cause. For example, if maternal hyperparathyroidism caused placental dysfunction, the neonate may exhibit muscle jerking and twitching, carpopedal spasm, ankle clonus, vomiting, tachycardia, and tachypnea.

Ballard Scale for calculating gestational age

GESTATIONAL MATURITY

NEUROMUSCULAR MATURITY SIGN	SCORE							RECORD SCORE HERE
	-1	0	1	2	3	4	5	
POSTURE	—						—	
SQUARE WINDOW (Wrist)	>90°	90°	60°	45°	30°	0°	—	
ARM RECOIL	—	180°	140° to 180°	110° to 140°	90° to 110°	<90°	—	
POPLITEAL ANGLE	180°	160°	140°	120°	100°	90°	<90°	
SCARF SIGN							—	
HEEL TO EAR							—	

TOTAL NEUROMUSCULAR MATURITY SCORE

PHYSICAL MATURITY

PHYSICAL MATURITY SIGN	SCORE							RECORD SCORE HERE
	-1	0	1	2	3	4	5	
SKIN	Sticky, friable, transparent	Gelatinous, red, translucent	Smooth, pink; visible vessels	Superficial peeling or rash; few visible vessels	Cracking; pale areas; rare visible vessels	Parchment-like; deep cracking; no visible vessels	Leathery, cracked, wrinkled	
LANUGO	None	Sparse	Abundant	Thinning	Bald areas	Mostly bald	—	
PLANTAR SURFACE	Heel-toe 40 to 50 mm: −1; <40 mm: −2	>50 mm; no crease	Faint red marks	Anterior transverse crease only	Creases over anterior two-thirds	Creases over entire sole	—	
BREAST	Imperceptible	Barely perceptible	Flat areola, no bud	Stippled areola; 1- to 2-mm bud	Raised areola; 3- to 4-mm bud	Full areola; 5- to 10-mm bud	—	
EYE AND EAR	Lids fused, loosely: −1; tightly: −2	Lids open; pinna flat, stays folded	Slightly curved pinna; soft, slow recoil	Well-curved pinna; soft but ready recoil	Formed and firm; instant recoil	Thick cartilage; ear stiff	—	
GENITALIA, (Male)	Scrotum flat, smooth	Scrotum empty; faint rugae	Testes in upper canal; rare rugae	Testes descending; few rugae	Testes down; good rugae	Testes pendulous; deep rugae	—	
GENITALIA, (Female)	Clitoris prominent; labia flat	Prominent clitoris; small labia minora	Prominent clitoris; enlarging minora	Majora and minora equally prominent	Majora large; minora small	Majora cover clitoris and minora	—	

TOTAL PHYSICAL MATURITY SCORE

SCORE

Neuromuscular _____
Physical_____
Total _____

MATURITY RATINGS

TOTAL MATURITY SCORE	GESTATIONAL AGE (WEEKS)
-10	20
-5	22
0	24
5	26
10	28
15	30
20	32
25	34
30	36
35	38
40	40
45	42
50	44

GESTESTIONAL AGE (WEEKS)

By dates _____
By ultrasound_____
By score _____

Adapted with permission from Ballard, J.L. "New Ballard Scale Expanded To Include Extremely Premature Infants," *Journal of Pediatrics* 119:417-23, 1991.

(continued)

Rubella, congenital

♦ The low-birth-weight neonate with this disease is born at term but is usually SGA.
♦ A characteristic "blueberry muffin" rash accompanies cataracts, purpuric lesions, hepatosplenomegaly, and a large anterior fontanel.
♦ Abnormal heart sounds, if present, vary with the type of associated congenital heart defect.

Toxoplasmosis, congenital

♦ The low-birth-weight neonate may be either preterm or SGA and may have hydrocephalus or microcephalus.
♦ Associated signs and symptoms include fever, seizures, lymphadenopathy, hepatosplenomegaly, jaundice, and rash.
♦ Other defects, which may occur months or years later, include strabismus, blindness, epilepsy, and mental retardation.

Varicella, congenital

♦ Low birth weight is accompanied by cataracts and skin vesicles.

NURSING CONSIDERATIONS

♦ To make up for low fat and glycogen stores in the low-birth-weight neonate, initiate feedings as soon as possible and continue to feed every 2 to 3 hours.
♦ Provide gavage or I.V. feeding for sick or very premature neonates.
♦ Check abdominal girth daily or more frequently if indicated, and check stools for blood because increasing girth and bloody stools may indicate necrotizing enterocolitis.
♦ A sepsis workup may be necessary if signs of infection are associated with low birth weight.
♦ Check the neonate's vital signs every 15 minutes for the first hour and at least once every hour thereafter until his condition stabilizes.
♦ Be alert for changes in temperature or behavior, feeding problems, respiratory distress, or periods of apnea—possible indications of infection.

♦ Monitor blood glucose levels and watch for signs and symptoms of hypoglycemia, such as irritability, jitteriness, tremors, seizures, irregular respirations, lethargy, and a high-pitched or weak cry.
♦ If the neonate is receiving supplemental oxygen, carefully monitor arterial blood gas values and the oxygen concentration of inspired air to prevent retinopathy.
♦ Monitor the neonate's urine output by weighing diapers before and after voiding. Check urine color, measure specific gravity, and test for the presence of glucose, blood, or protein.
♦ Watch for changes in the neonate's skin color because increasing jaundice may indicate hyperbilirubinemia.

- Teach the parents how to participate in their neonate's care to strengthen bonding, and allow ample time for their questions.
- Teach the parents about the underlying medical diagnosis and treatment plan.
- At discharge, teach the parents how to care for the neonate at home.
- Stress the importance of follow-up visits.

Lymphadenopathy

OVERVIEW

- Refers to enlargement of one or more lymph nodes
- May be generalized or localized (see *Areas of localized lymphadenopathy* and *Causes of localized lymphadenophathy*)
- Cause for concern if node is more than ⅜″ (1 cm) in diameter

HISTORY

- Ask about the onset, location, and description of swelling.
- Find out about recent infections or health problems.
- Ask about previous biopsies and personal or family history of cancer.

PHYSICAL ASSESSMENT

- Note the size of any palpable lymph nodes and whether they're fixed or mobile, tender or nontender, and erythematous.
- Note the texture of palpable nodes.
- If lymph nodes are erythematous, check the area drained by that part of the lymph system for signs of infection.
- Palpate and percuss the spleen.

CAUSES

MEDICAL
Acquired immunodeficiency syndrome
- Lymphadenopathy occurs with fatigue, night sweats, afternoon fevers, diarrhea, weight loss, and cough with several concurrent infections.

Anthrax, cutaneous
- Lymphadenopathy, malaise, headache, and fever may develop.
- A small, elevated itchy lesion resembling an insect bite may progress into a painless, necrotic-centered ulcer.

Chronic fatigue syndrome
- Lymphadenopathy may occur with incapacitating fatigue, sore throat, low-grade fevers, myalgia, cognitive dysfunction, and sleep disturbances.

Areas of localized lymphadenopathy

When you detect an enlarged lymph node, palpate the entire lymph node system to determine the extent of lymphadenopathy. Include the lymph nodes indicated below in your assessment.

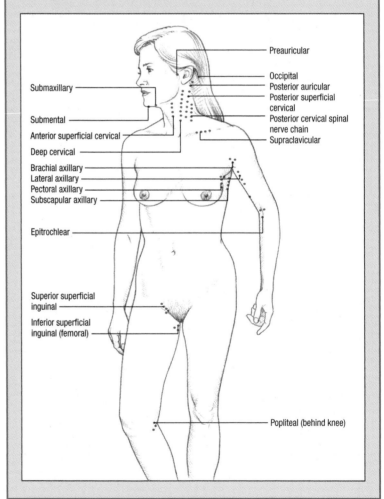

Labels: Preauricular, Occipital, Posterior auricular, Posterior superficial cervical, Posterior cervical spinal nerve chain, Supraclavicular, Submaxillary, Submental, Anterior superficial cervical, Deep cervical, Brachial axillary, Lateral axillary, Pectoral axillary, Subscapular axillary, Epitrochlear, Superior superficial inguinal, Inferior superficial inguinal (femoral), Popliteal (behind knee)

- Other signs and symptoms include arthralgia with arthritis, headache, and memory deficits.

Cytomegalovirus infection
- Generalized lymphadenopathy is accompanied by fever, malaise, and hepatosplenomegaly.
- Other signs and symptoms include a pruritic rash of small, erythematous macules that progresses to papules and then to vesicles.

Hodgkin's disease
- Extent of lymphadenopathy reflects stage of malignancy.
- Early signs and symptoms include pruritus, fatigue, weakness, night sweats, malaise, weight loss, and fever.

Leukemia
- In acute lymphocytic leukemia, generalized lymphadenopathy is accompanied by fatigue, malaise, pallor, prolonged bleeding time, swollen gums, weight loss, bone or joint pain, hepatosplenomegaly, and low fever.

- In chronic lymphocytic leukemia, generalized lymphadenopathy appears early along with fatigue, malaise, and fever.
- Late signs and symptoms of the chronic form include hepatosplenomegaly, severe fatigue, weight loss, bone tenderness, edema, pallor, dyspnea, tachycardia, palpitations, bleeding, anemia, and macular or nodular lesions.

Lyme disease
- As disease progresses, lymphadenopathy, constant malaise and fatigue, and intermittent headache, fever, chills, and aches develop.
- Arthralgia and, eventually, neurologic and cardiac abnormalities may develop.

Mononucleosis, infectious
- Painful lymphadenopathy involves cervical, axillary, and inguinal nodes.
- Prodromal symptoms of headache, malaise, and fatigue appear 3 to 5 days before the appearance of the classic triad of lymphadenopathy,

sore throat, and temperature fluctuations with an evening peak.
- Other signs and symptoms include hepatosplenomegaly, stomatitis, exudative tonsillitis, or pharyngitis.

Non-Hodgkin's lymphoma
- Painless enlargement of one or more peripheral lymph nodes is the most common sign.
- Generalized lymphadenopathy characterizes stage IV.
- Other signs and symptoms include dyspnea, cough, hepatosplenomegaly, fever, night sweats, fatigue, malaise, and weight loss.

Rheumatoid arthritis
- Lymphadenopathy is an early, nonspecific finding.
- Later signs and symptoms include joint tenderness, swelling, and warmth; joint stiffness after inactivity; subcutaneous nodules on the elbows; joint deformity; muscle weakness; and muscle atrophy.
- Other signs and symptoms include fatigue, malaise, low fever, weight loss, and vague arthralgia and myalgia.

Sarcoidosis
- Generalized hilar and right paratracheal forms of lymphadenopathy with splenomegaly are common.
- Initial signs and symptoms include arthralgia, fatigue, malaise, weight loss, and pulmonary symptoms.
- Other signs and symptoms vary and may include breathlessness, cough, substernal chest pain, arrhythmias, muscle weakness and pain, phalangeal and nasal mucosal lesions, subcutaneous skin nodules, eye pain, photophobia, nonreactive pupils, seizures, and cranial or peripheral nerve palsies.

Causes of localized lymphadenopathy

Various disorders can cause localized lymphadenopathy, but this sign usually results from infection or trauma affecting the specific area. Here are some common causes of lymphadenopathy, listed according to the area affected.

OCCIPITAL
- Infection
- Roseola
- Scalp infection
- Seborrheic dermatitis
- Tick bite
- Tinea capitis

AURICULAR
- Erysipelas
- Herpes zoster ophthalmicus
- Infection
- Rubella
- Squamous cell carcinoma
- Styes or chalazion
- Tularemia

CERVICAL
- Cat-scratch fever
- Facial or oral cancer
- Infection
- Mononucleosis
- Monocutaneous lymph node syndrome
- Rubella
- Rubeola
- Thyrotoxicosis
- Tonsillitis
- Tuberculosis
- Varicella

SUBMAXILLARY AND SUBMENTAL
- Cystic fibrosis
- Dental infection
- Gingivitis
- Glossitis
- Infection

SUPRACLAVICULAR
- Infection
- Neoplastic disease

AXILLARY
- Breast cancer
- Infection
- Lymphoma
- Mastitis

INGUINAL AND FEMORAL
- Carcinoma
- Chancroid
- Infection
- Lymphogranuloma venereum
- Syphilis

POPLITEAL
- Infection

(continued)

Syphilis
◆ Localized lymphadenopathy occurs with a painless canker that develops at site of sexual exposure.
◆ In the second stage, generalized lymphadenopathy occurs along with a macular, papular, pustular, or nodular rash on the arms, trunk, palms (a diagnostic sign), soles, face, and scalp.
◆ Other signs and symptoms include headache, malaise, anorexia, weight loss, nausea, vomiting, sore throat, and low fever.

Systemic lupus erythematosus
◆ Generalized lymphadenopathy accompanies butterfly rash (hallmark sign), photosensitivity, Raynaud's phenomenon, and joint pain and stiffness.
◆ Other signs and symptoms include pleuritic chest pain, cough, fever, anorexia, and weight loss.

Tuberculous lymphadenitis
◆ Lymphadenopathy may be generalized or restricted to superficial lymph nodes.
◆ Lymph nodes may become fluctuant and drain to surrounding tissue.
◆ Other signs and symptoms include fever, chills, weakness, and fatigue.

OTHER
Drugs
◆ Phenytoin may cause generalized lymphadenopathy.

Immunizations
◆ Typhoid vaccination may cause generalized lymphadenopathy.

NURSING CONSIDERATIONS

◆ If the patient is uncomfortable, provide an antipyretic, a tepid sponge bath, or a hypothermia blanket.
◆ If diagnostic tests reveal infection, check your facility's policy regarding infection control.

PEDIATRIC POINTERS
◆ Infection is the most common cause of lymphadenopathy in children.
◆ If the child has a history of febrile seizures, provide an antipyretic.

◆ Teach the patient about the underlying condition, diagnostic tests, and treatment options.
◆ Teach the patient ways to prevent infection.
◆ Explain the signs and symptoms of infection the patient should report.
◆ Explain the reasons for isolation, as needed.
◆ Stress the importance of a healthy diet and rest.

Masklike facies

- Total loss of facial expression
- Results from bradykinesia usually due to extrapyramidal damage
- Rate of eye blinking reduced to 1 to 4 blinks per minute, producing a characteristic "reptilian" stare
- Commonly develops insidiously; may initially be mistaken by the observer for depression or apathy

- Ask the patient and his family or friends when they first noticed the masklike facial expression and any other signs or symptoms.
- Obtain a medication history.

- Determine the degree of facial muscle weakness by asking the patient to smile and to wrinkle his forehead. Typically, the patient's responses are slowed.
- Assess the patient's neurologic status.

MEDICAL

Dermatomyositis

- Masklike facies reflects muscle soreness, weakness, and destruction extending from the face and neck to the shoulder and pelvic girdle.
- Dysphagia and dysphonia develop.
- Other characteristic cutaneous signs involve edema and dusky lilac suffusion of the eyelid margin or periorbital tissue; an erythematous rash on the face, neck, upper back, chest, arms, and nail beds; and violet (Gottron's) papules dorsal to the interphalangeal joint.

Facial palsy

- Masklike facies is a hallmark of bilateral Bell's palsy and is characterized by periaural pain, hyperacusis, and disturbance of taste.

Guillain-Barré syndrome

- Bilateral facial weakness may occur and is accompanied by hypoactive reflexes, paresthesia in the extremities, and limb weakness in this inflammatory neurologic disorder.
- Respiratory insufficiency may also occur, which requires pulmonary function testing and respiratory support.

Myasthenia gravis

- Ptosis and generalized facial muscle weakness are common and may be accompanied by diplopia, dysarthria, dysphagia, and limb weakness due to nerve transmission disturbance.
- Weakness typically worsens with repetitive use of muscles and also later in the day.
- Pulmonary function tests may be needed to rule out impending respiratory crisis.

Parkinson's disease

- Masklike facies occurs early but is commonly overlooked because the signs are subtle and include raised eyebrows and smooth facial muscles.
- More noticeable signs of central nervous system decline include muscle rigidity, which may be uniform (lead-pipe rigidity) or jerky (cogwheel rigidity), and an insidious tremor, which usually begins in the fingers (pill-roll tremor), increases during stress or anxiety, and decreases during purposeful movement or sleep.
- Other typical signs and symptoms include stooped posture and propulsive gait, monotone voice and, possibly, drooling, dysphagia, and dysarthria.

Scleroderma

- A late sign of this connective tissue disorder, masklike facies develops along with a smooth, wrinkle-free appearance, "pinching" of the mouth and, possibly, contractures as facial skin becomes tight and inelastic.
- Other late signs and symptoms include pain, stiffness, and swelling of joints and foreshortened fingers.
- Skin on the fingers and then on the hands and forearms thickens and becomes taut and shiny.
- GI dysfunction produces frequent reflux and heartburn, weight loss, diarrhea or constipation, and malodorous floating stools.

OTHER

Carbon monoxide poisoning

◆ Masklike facies usually develops several weeks after acute carbon monoxide poisoning.
◆ Other signs and symptoms include rigidity, dementia, impaired sensory function, choreoathetosis, generalized seizures, and myoclonus.

Drugs

◆ Phenothiazines (particularly piperazine derivatives) and other antipsychotic drugs commonly cause masklike facies as well as other extrapyramidal effects.
◆ In addition, metoclopramide (Reglan) and metyrosine (Demser) can sometimes cause masklike facies. This sign usually improves when the drug dosage is reduced or the drug therapy discontinued.

Manganese poisoning, chronic

◆ Masklike facies develops gradually, along with a resting tremor and personality changes.
◆ The patient may also experience Huntington's disease, propulsive gait, dystonia, and rigidity.
◆ Later, extreme muscle weakness and fatigue occur.

NURSING CONSIDERATIONS

◆ If the patient's facial weakness results from Guillain-Barré syndrome or myasthenia gravis, be prepared to initiate emergency respiratory support.
◆ If the patient's masklike facies results from Parkinson's disease, explain to his family that the sign may hide facial clues to depression—a common symptom of Parkinson's disease.

PEDIATRIC POINTERS

◆ Masklike facies occurs in the juvenile form of Parkinson's disease.

PATIENT TEACHING

◆ Teach the patient about underlying diagnosis and treatment plan.
◆ Teach about prescribed medications.

McBURNEY'S sign

- Tenderness elicited by palpating the right-lower-quadrant over McBurney's point (see *Eliciting McBurney's sign*)
- Indicator of localized peritoneal inflammation in acute appendicitis

- Ask about the onset, location, and description of abdominal pain.
- Determine what aggravates and alleviates the tenderness.
- Find out about last bowel movement and other signs and symptoms, such as vomiting and a low-grade fever.

- Before eliciting McBurney's sign, inspect the abdomen for distention, auscultate for hypoactive or absent bowel sounds, and test for tympany.
- Lightly palpate the abdomen to detect tenderness, rigidity, guarding, or pain.
- Observe the patient's facial expression for signs of pain.
- Obtain vital signs.

TOP TECHNIQUE

Eliciting McBurney's sign

To elicit McBurney's sign, help the patient into a supine position with his knees slightly flexed and his abdominal muscles relaxed. Palpate deeply and slowly in the right lower quadrant over McBurney's point—located about 2″ (5 cm) from the right anterior superior spine of the ilium, on a line between the spine and the umbilicus. Point pain and tenderness, a positive McBurney's sign, indicates appendicitis.

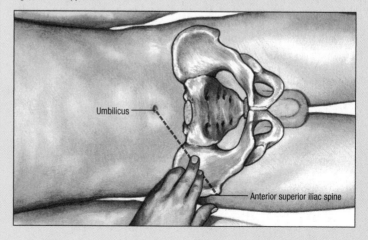

Umbilicus

Anterior superior iliac spine

MEDICAL

Appendicitis

◆ McBurney's sign appears within the first 2 to 12 hours after the onset of appendicitis, after initial pain in the epigastric and periumbilical area shifts to the right lower quadrant.
◆ Persistent pain increases with walking or coughing.
◆ Nausea and vomiting occur at onset.
◆ Boardlike abdominal rigidity and rebound tenderness—that worsen as the condition progresses—accompany cutaneous hyperalgia, fever, constipation or diarrhea, tachycardia, retractive respirations, anorexia, and moderate malaise.
◆ Rupture causes sudden end to pain and the development of signs and symptoms of peritonitis.

◆ Make sure the patient receives nothing by mouth.
◆ Prepare the patient for appendectomy.
◆ Avoid administration of a cathartic or enema, which may cause the appendix to rupture.

PEDIATRIC POINTERS

◆ McBurney's sign is also elicited in children with appendicitis.

GERIATRIC POINTERS

◆ In elderly patients, McBurney's sign may be decreased or absent.

◆ Explain which postoperative signs and symptoms the patient should report.
◆ Instruct the patient on wound care.
◆ Explain the needed activity restrictions.
◆ Instruct the patient about prescribed medications.

McMurray's sign

OVERVIEW

- Palpable, audible click or pop elicited by rotating the tibia on the femur (see *Eliciting McMurray's sign*)
- Indicator of medial meniscal injury
- Shouldn't be elicited in patient with suspected fractures of the tibial plateau or femoral condyles

HISTORY

- Ask about the onset and description of acute knee pain.
- Find out what aggravates and alleviates the pain.
- Obtain a medical history, including previous knee surgery, prosthetic replacement, and joint problems such as arthritis.

PHYSICAL ASSESSMENT

- Assess the leg's range-of-motion (ROM), both passive and with resistance.
- Check for cruciate ligament stability by noting anterior or posterior movement of the tibia on the femur (drawer sign).
- Measure the quadriceps muscles in both legs for symmetry.

 TOP TECHNIQUE

Eliciting McMurray's sign

Eliciting McMurray's sign requires special training and gentle manipulation of the patient's leg to avoid extending a meniscal tear or locking the knee. If you've been trained to elicit McMurray's sign, place the patient in a supine position and flex his affected knee until his heel nearly touches his buttock. Place your thumb and index finger on either side of the knee joint space and grasp his heel with your other hand. Then rotate the foot and lower leg laterally to test the posterior aspect of the medial meniscus.

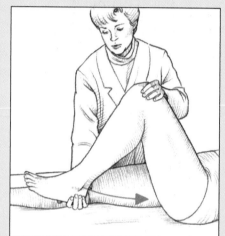

Keeping his foot in this position, extend the knee to a 90-degree angle to test the front side of the medial meniscus. A palpable or audible click—a positive McMurray's sign—indicates injury to meniscal structures.

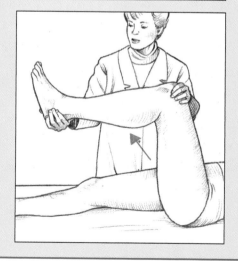

CAUSES

MEDICAL
Meniscal tear
◆ McMurray's sign is usually elicited.
◆ Other signs and symptoms include acute knee pain at the medial or lateral joint line, quadriceps weakening and atrophy, and decreased ROM or locking of the knee joint.

NURSING CONSIDERATIONS

◆ If trauma is the cause of the knee pain and the presence of McMurray's sign, prepare the patient for aspiration of the joint.
◆ Immobilize and apply ice to the knee.
◆ Apply a knee immobilizer or assist with casting, as appropriate.

PEDIATRIC POINTERS
◆ McMurray's sign in adolescents is usually elicited in meniscal tears caused by sports injury.
◆ It may also be elicited in children with congenital discoid meniscus.

PATIENT TEACHING

◆ Explain to the patient the purpose of elevating the affected leg.
◆ Teach about appropriate knee exercises; provide referral to physical therapy, as needed.
◆ Explain the proper use of assistive devices the patient needs.
◆ Explain the proper use of analgesics and anti-inflammatories.

Melena

OVERVIEW

- Passage of black, tarry stools containing digested blood (see *Comparing melena to hematochezia*)
- Commonly indicates upper GI bleeding
- When severe, can signal acute bleeding and life-threatening hypovolemic shock

 ACTION STAT! *If the patient has severe melena, take orthostatic vital signs and look for other signs of hypovolemic shock. Insert a large-bore I.V. line to administer replacement fluids and allow blood transfusion. Obtain hematocrit, prothrombin time, International Normalized Ratio, and partial thromboplastin time. Place the patient flat with his head turned to the side and his feet elevated. Administer supplemental oxygen, as needed.*

HISTORY

- Ask about the onset of melena.
- Determine the frequency and quantity of bowel movements.
- Ask about hematemesis or hematochezia.
- Find out about the use of anti-inflammatory drugs, alcohol, other GI irritants, or iron supplements.
- Obtain a drug history, noting the use of warfarin and other anticoagulants.

PHYSICAL ASSESSMENT

- Inspect the mouth and nasopharynx for bleeding.
- Auscultate, percuss, and palpate the abdomen.
- Perform a cardiovascular assessment to detect signs and symptoms of shock.

CAUSES

MEDICAL
Colon cancer
- Early right-sided tumor growth may cause melena and abdominal aching, pressure, or cramps.
- As the right-sided tumor progresses, signs and symptoms include weakness, fatigue, anemia, diarrhea or obstipation, anorexia, weight loss, vomiting, and signs and symptoms of obstruction.
- Early left-sided tumor growth may cause rectal bleeding with intermittent abdominal fullness or cramping and rectal pressure.
- As the left-sided tumor progresses, signs and symptoms include melena (usually develops late in the disease), obstipation, diarrhea, and pencil-shaped stools.

Esophageal cancer
- Melena is a late sign along with painful dysphagia, anorexia, and regurgitation.
- Earlier signs and symptoms include painless dysphagia, rapid weight loss, steady chest pain with substernal fullness, nausea, vomiting, and hematemesis.

Esophageal varices, ruptured
- A life-threatening disorder; melena, hematochezia, and hematemesis may occur.
- Melena is preceded by signs of shock.
- Agitation or confusion signal developing hepatic encephalopathy.

Gastric cancer
- Melena and altered bowel habits may occur late.
- Common signs and symptoms include insidious onset of upper abdominal or retrosternal discomfort and chronic dyspepsia unrelieved by antacids and exacerbated by food.
- Other signs and symptoms include anorexia, nausea, hematemesis, pallor, fatigue, weight loss, and a feeling of abdominal fullness.

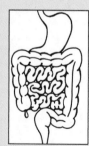

TOP TECHNIQUE

Comparing melena to hematochezia

With GI bleeding, the site, amount, and rate of blood flow through the GI tract determine if a patient will develop melena (black, tarry stools) or hematochezia (bright red, bloody stools). Usually, melena indicates upper GI bleeding, and hematochezia indicates lower GI bleeding. However, with some disorders, melena may alternate with hematochezia. This chart helps differentiate these two commonly related signs.

SIGN	SITES	CHARACTERISTICS
Melena	Esophagus, stomach, duodenum; rarely, jejunum, ileum, ascending colon	Black, loose, tarry stools; delayed or minimal passage of blood through GI tract
Hematochezia	Usually affects the colon or lower; rapid hemorrhage of 1 L or more associated with esophageal, stomach, or duodenal bleeding	Bright red or dark, mahogany-colored stools; pure blood; blood mixed with formed stool; or bloody diarrhea; reflects lower GI bleeding or rapid blood loss and passage of undigested blood through GI tract

---

Gastritis

◆ Melena and hematemesis are common signs.
◆ Other signs and symptoms include mild epigastric or abdominal discomfort that's made worse by eating, belching, nausea, vomiting, and malaise.

Mallory-Weiss syndrome

◆ Massive bleeding from the upper GI tract is characteristic following a tear to the mucous membrane of the esophagus or esophageal gastric junction.
◆ Melena and hematemesis follow vomiting.
◆ Epigastric or back pain, and signs and symptoms of shock may occur.

Mesenteric vascular occlusion

◆ Slight melena occurs along with 2 to 3 days of persistent, mild abdominal pain.
◆ Later, abdominal pain becomes severe and may be accompanied by tenderness, distention, guarding, and rigidity.
◆ Anorexia, vomiting, fever, and profound shock may also develop.

Peptic ulcer

◆ Melena may signal life-threatening hemorrhage.
◆ Other signs and symptoms include decreased appetite; nausea; vomiting; hematemesis; hematochezia; left epigastric pain that's gnawing, burning, or sharp; and signs and symptoms of shock.

Small-bowel tumors

◆ Tumors may bleed and produce melena.
◆ Other signs and symptoms include abdominal pain, distention, and increasing frequency and rising pitch of bowel sounds.

Thrombocytopenia

◆ Melena or hematochezia may accompany other manifestations of bleeding tendency.
◆ Malaise, fatigue, weakness, and lethargy are typical.

OTHER
Drugs

◆ Aspirin, other nonsteroidal antiinflammatory drugs (NSAIDs), or alcohol can cause melena.

NURSING CONSIDERATIONS

◆ Monitor vital signs, and look closely for signs of hypovolemic shock.
◆ Encourage bed rest.
◆ Keep the perianal area clean and dry to prevent skin irritation and breakdown.
◆ A nasogastric tube may be needed to drain gastric contents and for decompression.
◆ Give blood transfusions, as ordered.

PEDIATRIC POINTERS

◆ Neonates may experience melena neonatorum from extravasation of blood into the alimentary canal.
◆ In older children, melena usually results from peptic ulcer, gastritis, or Meckel's diverticulum.

GERIATRIC POINTERS

◆ Patients with recurrent intermittent GI bleeding without a clear cause should be considered for angiography or an exploratory laparotomy.

PATIENT TEACHING

◆ Explain the changes in bowel elimination that the patient needs to report.
◆ Stress the importance of undergoing colorectal cancer screening.
◆ Explain the need to avoid aspirin, other NSAIDs, and alcohol.

Menorrhagia

OVERVIEW

- Abnormally heavy or long menstrual bleeding, 80 ml or more per monthly period
- Occurs as a single episode or a chronic sign

✦ *ACTION STAT! Evaluate hemodynamic status by taking orthostatic vital signs. Insert a large-gauge I.V. line to begin fluid replacement if the patient shows an increase of 10 beats/minute in pulse rate, a decrease of 10 mm Hg in systolic blood pressure, or other signs of hypovolemic shock, such as pallor, tachycardia, tachypnea, and cool, clammy skin. Place the patient in a supine position with her feet elevated, and administer supplemental oxygen, as needed.*

Use menstrual pads to examine the quality and quantity of bleeding. Then prepare the patient for a pelvic examination to help determine the cause of bleeding.

HISTORY

- Obtain a menstural history including age at menarche, average duration of menstrual periods, interval between them, date of the last menses, and recent changes in her normal menstrual pattern. Have the patient describe the character and amount of bleeding.
- Obtain information about method of birth control, the number of pregnancies and outcome of each, dates of her most recent pelvic examination and Papanicolaou smear, and the details of any previous gynecologic infections or neoplasms.
- If possible, obtain a pregnancy history of the patient's mother, and determine if the patient was exposed in utero to diethylstilbestrol. (This drug has been linked to vaginal and cervical diseases.)
- Ask about general health and medical history including a history of thyroid, adrenal, or hepatic disease; blood dyscrasias; or tuberculosis, because these may predispose the patient to menorrhagia; and about past surgical procedures; and any recent emotional stress.
- Find out if the patient has undergone X-ray or other radiation therapy because this may indicate prior treatment for menorrhagia.
- Obtain a thorough drug and alcohol history, noting the use of anticoagulants or aspirin.

PHYSICAL ASSESSMENT

- Perform a pelvic examination.
- Obtain blood and urine samples for pregnancy testing.

CAUSES

MEDICAL
Blood dyscrasias
- Menorrhagia is one of several possible signs of a bleeding disorder.
- Other associated signs and symptoms include epistaxis, bleeding gums, purpura, hematemesis, hematuria, and melena.

Endometriosis
- Menorrhagia may be a sign of this disorder, in which endometrial tissue is found outside the lining of the uterine cavity. However, the classic symptom is dysmenorrhea.
- Often a tender fixed adnexal mass is palpable on bimanual examination.
- Other signs and symptoms depend on the location of the ectopic tissue outside the uterus but may include dyspareunia, suprapubic pain, dysuria, nausea, vomiting, abdominal cramps, cyclic pelvic pain, and infertility.

Hypothyroidism
- Menorrhagia is a common early sign and is accompanied by such nonspecific findings as fatigue, cold intolerance, constipation, and weight gain despite anorexia.
- As hypothyroidism progresses, intellectual and motor activity decrease; the skin becomes dry, pale, cool, and doughy; the hair becomes dry and sparse; and the nails become thick and brittle.
- Myalgia, hoarseness, decreased libido, and infertility also commonly occur.
- Eventually, the patient develops a characteristic dull, expressionless face and edema of the face, hands, and feet.
- Deep tendon reflexes are delayed, and bradycardia and abdominal distention may occur.

Uterine fibroids
◆ Menorrhagia is the most common sign, but other forms of abnormal uterine bleeding as well as dysmenorrhea or leukorrhea, can also occur.
◆ Other related signs and symptoms include abdominal pain, a feeling of abdominal heaviness, backache, constipation, urinary urgency or frequency, and an enlarged uterus, which is usually nontender.

OTHER
Drugs
◆ Use of hormonal contraceptives may cause sudden onset of profuse, prolonged menorrhagia.
◆ Anticoagulants also have been associated with excessive menstrual flow.

Intrauterine devices
◆ Menorrhagia can result from the use of intrauterine contraceptive devices.

NURSING CONSIDERATIONS

◆ Monitor the patient closely for signs of hypovolemia.
◆ Encourage the patient to maintain adequate fluid intake.
◆ Monitor intake and output, and estimate uterine blood loss by recording the number of sanitary napkins or tampons used during an abnormal period and comparing this with usage during a normal period.
◆ To help decrease blood flow, encourage the patient to rest and to avoid strenuous activities.
◆ Obtain blood samples for hematocrit, prothrombin time, partial thromboplastin time, and International Normalized Ratio levels.

PEDIATRIC POINTERS
◆ Irregular menstrual function in young girls may be accompanied by hemorrhage and resulting anemia.

GERIATRIC POINTERS
◆ In postmenopausal women, menorrhagia can't occur. In such patients, vaginal bleeding is usually caused by endometrial atrophy; however, malignancy must be ruled out.

PATIENT TEACHING

◆ Teach the patient about the cause of menorrhagia and treatment options.
◆ Teach her how to monitor blood loss and maintain fluid volume by adequate fluid intake.

Metrorrhagia

- Uterine bleeding that occurs irregularly between menstrual periods
- Usually light, but may range from staining to hemorrhage
- Usually indicative of slight physiologic bleeding from the endometrium during ovulation

- Obtain a menstrual history including age at menarche, average duration of menstrual periods, interval between them, date of the last menses, and recent changes in her normal menstrual pattern. Have the patient describe the character and amount of bleeding.
- Ask when metrorrhagia usually occurs in relation to her period and if she experiences other signs or symptoms.
- Ask about previous gynecologic problems.
- Obtain a contraceptive and obstetric history, the dates of her last Papanicolaou smear and pelvic examination, and when she last had sexual intercourse and whether or not it was with protection.
- Ask about her general health, any recent changes, and if she's been under emotional stress.
- If possible, obtain a pregnancy history of the patient's mother, and determine if the patient was exposed in utero to diethylstilbestrol. (This drug has been linked to vaginal and cervical diseases.)

- Perform a pelvic examination, if indicated.
- Obtain blood samples and urine specimen for pregnancy testing.

MEDICAL

Cervicitis

- Cervicitis is a nonspecific infection that may cause spontaneous bleeding, spotting, or posttraumatic bleeding.
- Assessment reveals red, granular, irregular lesions on the external cervix.
- Purulent vaginal discharge (with or without odor), lower abdominal pain, and a fever may occur.

Dysfunctional uterine bleeding

- Abnormal uterine bleeding not caused by pregnancy or major gynecologic disorders usually occurs as metrorrhagia, although menorrhagia is possible.
- Bleeding may be profuse or scant, intermittent or constant.

Endometrial polyps

- In most patients, endometrial polyps cause abnormal bleeding, usually intermenstrual or postmenopausal; however, some patients remain asymptomatic.

Endometriosis

◆ Metrorrhagia (usually premenstrual) may be the only indication of endometriosis or it may accompany cyclical pelvic discomfort, infertility, and dyspareunia.
◆ A tender, fixed adnexal mass may be palpable on bimanual examination.

Endometritis

◆ Endometritis causes metrorrhagia, purulent vaginal discharge, and enlargement of the uterus.
◆ Other signs and symptoms include fever, lower abdominal pain, and abdominal muscle spasm.

Gynecologic cancer

◆ Metrorrhagia is commonly an early sign of cervical or uterine cancer.
◆ Later signs and symptoms include weight loss, pelvic pain, fatigue and, possibly, an abdominal mass.

Uterine leiomyomas

◆ Besides metrorrhagia, uterine leiomyomas may cause increasing abdominal girth and heaviness in the abdomen, constipation, and urinary frequency or urgency.
◆ The patient may report pain if the uterus attempts to expel the tumor through contractions and if the tumors twist or necrose after circulatory occlusion or infection; however, the patient with leiomyomas is usually asymptomatic.

Vaginal adenosis

◆ Vaginal adenosis commonly produces metrorrhagia.
◆ Palpation reveals roughening or nodules in affected vaginal areas.

OTHER
Contraceptives

◆ Oral, injectable, or implanted contraceptives may cause metrorrhagia.

Drugs

◆ Anticoagulants may cause metrorrhagia.

Herbal remedies

◆ Herbal remedies, such as ginseng, can cause postmenopausal bleeding.

Surgery and procedures

◆ Cervical conization and cauterization may cause metrorrhagia.

NURSING CONSIDERATIONS

◆ Encourage bed rest to reduce bleeding.
◆ Give an analgesic for discomfort.

PATIENT TEACHING

◆ Teach the patient about the cause of metrorrhagia and treatment options.
◆ Teach her how to monitor blood loss.

Miosis

- Pupillary constriction caused by contraction of the sphincter muscle in the iris
- Occurs normally as a response to fatigue, increased light, or administration of a miotic; as part of the eye's accommodation reflex; and as part of the aging process (pupil size steadily decreases from adolescence to about age 60)

HISTORY

- Obtain a history of ocular symptoms including onset, duration, and intensity.
- Ask about trauma, serious systemic disease, use of topical and systemic drugs, and contact lens use.

PHYSICAL ASSESSMENT

- Perform a thorough eye examination including visual acuity in each eye, with and without correction, paying particular attention to blurred or decreased vision in the miotic eye.
- Compare both pupils for size (many people have a normal discrepancy), color, shape, reaction to light, accommodation, and consensual light response.
- Evaluate extraocular muscle function by assessing the six cardinal fields of gaze.

CAUSES

MEDICAL
Cerebrovascular arteriosclerosis
- Miosis is usually unilateral, depending on the site and extent of vascular damage.
- Other signs and symptoms include visual blurring; slurred speech or, possibly, aphasia; loss of muscle tone; memory loss; vertigo; and headache.

Cluster headache
- Ipsilateral miosis, tearing, conjunctival injection, and ptosis commonly accompany a severe cluster headache, along with facial flushing and sweating, bradycardia, restlessness, and nasal stuffiness or rhinorrhea.

Corneal foreign body
- Miosis in the affected eye occurs with pain, a foreign-body sensation, slight vision loss, conjunctival injection, photophobia, and profuse tearing.

Corneal ulcer
- Miosis in the affected eye appears with moderate pain; visual blurring and, possibly, some vision loss; and diffuse, conjunctival injection.

Horner's syndrome
- Moderate miosis is common in this neurologic syndrome and occurs ipsilaterally to the spinal cord lesion.
- Related ipsilateral signs and symptoms include a sluggish pupillary reflex, slight enophthalmos, moderate ptosis, facial anhidrosis, transient conjunctival injection, and vascular headache.
- When the syndrome is congenital, the iris on the affected side may appear lighter.

Hyphema
- Usually the result of blunt trauma, hyphema can cause miosis with moderate pain, visual blurring, diffuse conjunctival injection, and slight eyelid swelling.
- The eyeball may feel harder than normal.

Iritis, acute
- Miosis typically occurs in the affected eye along with decreased pupillary reflex, severe eye pain, photophobia, visual blurring, conjunctival injection and, possibly, pus accumulation in the anterior chamber.
- The eye appears cloudy, the iris bulges, and the pupil is constricted.

Neuropathy
- Two forms of neuropathy occasionally produce Argyll Robertson pupils, which are bilateral miotic (often pinpoint), unequal, and irregularly shaped pupils that don't dilate properly with mydriatic use and fail to react to light, although they do constrict on accommodation.
- With diabetic neuropathy, related signs and symptoms include paresthesia and other sensory disturbances, extremity pain, orthostatic hypotension, impotence, incontinence, and leg muscle weakness and atrophy.
- With alcoholic neuropathy, related signs and symptoms include progressive, variable muscle weakness and wasting, various sensory disturbances, and hypoactive deep tendon reflexes.

Parry-Romberg syndrome
- This facial hemiatrophy typically produces miosis, sluggish pupillary reflexes, enophthalmos, nystagmus, ptosis, and different-colored irises.

Pontine hemorrhage
- Bilateral miosis is characteristic, along with rapid onset of coma, total paralysis, decerebrate posture, absent doll's eye sign, and a positive Babinski's reflex.

Tabes dorsalis
- This tertiary form of syphilis is marked by Argyll Robertson pupils, a wide base ataxic gait, paresthesia, loss of proprioception, analgesia, thermanesthesia, Charcot's joints, incontinence and, possibly, impotence.

Uveitis
- With anterior uveitis, miosis is accompanied by moderate to severe eye pain, severe conjunctival injection, photophobia, and pus in the anterior chamber.
- With posterior uveitis, miosis is accompanied by gradual onset of eye pain, photophobia, visual floaters, visual blurring, conjunctival injection and, commonly, distorted pupil shape.

OTHER
Chemical burns
- An opaque cornea may make miosis hard to detect; however, signs and symptoms may include moderate to severe pain, diffuse conjunctival injection, inability to keep the eye open, visual blurring, and blistering.

Drugs
- Such topical drugs as acetylcholine, carbachol, echothiophate iodide, and pilocarpine are used to treat eye disorders specifically for their miotic effect.
- Systemic drugs such as barbiturates, cholinergics, anticholinesterases, clonidine hydrochloride (overdose), opiates, and reserpine also cause miosis, as does deep anesthesia.

NURSING CONSIDERATIONS
- Because any ocular abnormality can be a source of fear and anxiety, reassure and support the patient.
- Administer medications, as ordered, including pain control as needed.

PEDIATRIC POINTERS
- Miosis is common in neonates, simply because they're asleep or sleepy most of the time.
- Bilateral miosis occurs with congenital microcoria, an uncommon bilateral disease transmitted as an autosomal dominant trait and marked by the absence of the dilator muscle of the pupil. At birth, these infants have pupils less than 2 mm and seem to gaze far away.

PATIENT TEACHING
- Teach the patient about underlying diagnosis and treatment plan.
- Clearly explain any diagnostic tests ordered, which may include a complete ophthalmologic examination or a neurologic workup.

Moon facies

- Distinctive facial adiposity, characterized by marked facial roundness and puffiness, a double chin, a prominent upper lip, and full supraclavicular fossae
- Usually caused by ectopic or excessive pituitary production of corticotropin, adrenal adenoma or carcinoma, or long-term glucocorticoid therapy

- Find out about the onset of facial adiposity.
- Ask about recent weight gain and any personal or family history of endocrine disorders, obesity, or cancer.
- Ask about fatigue, irritability, depression, or confusion
- If the patient is a female of childbearing age, determine the date of her last menses and whether she's experienced any menstrual irregularities.
- If the patient is receiving a glucocorticoid, ask the name of the drug, dosage, schedule, route of administration, and reason for therapy.

- Take the patient's vital signs, weight, and height.
- Assess the patient's overall appearance.
- Perform a complete physical examination, specifically focusing on the musculoskeletal and integumentary systems.
- Obtain blood samples for testing, as ordered.

MEDICAL

Hypercortisolism

◆ Moon face varies in severity, depending on the degree of cortisol excess and weight gain.
◆ The patient typically exhibits buffalo hump, truncal obesity with slender arms and legs, and thin, transparent skin with purple striae and ecchymoses.
◆ Other cushingoid signs and symptoms include acne, diaphoresis, fatigue, muscle wasting and weakness, poor wound healing, elevated blood pressure, personality changes, and skeletal growth retardation (in children).
◆ Related signs and symptoms include hirsutism and amenorrhea or oligomenorrhea (in a female) and gynecomastia and impotence (in a male).

OTHER

Drugs

◆ Most cases of moon face result from prolonged use of a glucocorticoid, such as cortisone, dexamethasone (Mymethasone), hydrocortisone, or prednisone.

◆ Relieve the patient's concern about his body image by explaining that moon face and other disconcerting cushingoid effects can usually be corrected by treating the underlying disorder or by discontinuing or modifying glucocorticoid therapy.

PEDIATRIC POINTERS

◆ Moon face is rare in children.
◆ In an infant or a young child, it usually indicates adrenal adenoma or carcinoma or, rarely, cri du chat syndrome.
◆ After age 7, it usually indicates abnormal pituitary secretion of corticotropin in bilateral adrenal hyperplasia.

◆ Teach the patient about the underlying diagnosis and treatment plan.
◆ Teach about prescribed medications and how to take them.
◆ Explain to the patient that he should only discontinue or modify glucocorticoid therapy as directed by a physician.
◆ Clearly explain any diagnostic tests ordered. These may include serum and urine 17-hydroxycorticosteroid studies; a 2-day, low-dose dexamethasone test followed by a 2-day, high-dose dexamethasone test; plasma corticotropin studies; and a corticotropin-releasing hormone test.

Mouth lesions

OVERVIEW

- Include ulcers (most common), cysts, firm nodules, hemorrhagic lesions, papules, vesicles, bullae, and erythematous lesions
- May occur anywhere on the lips, cheeks, hard and soft palate, salivary glands, tongue, gingivae, or mucous membranes (see *Common mouth lesions*)

HISTORY

- Ask about the onset of lesions.
- Find out about pain, odor, drainage, or skin lesions.
- Obtain a drug history, including drug allergies and antibiotic use.
- Obtain a medical history, including incidence of malignancies, sexually transmitted diseases, I.V. drug use, recent infection, or trauma.
- Ask about dental history and oral hygiene habits.

PHYSICAL ASSESSMENT

- Note lesion sites and character.
- Examine the lips for color and texture.
- Inspect and palpate the buccal mucosa and tongue for color, texture, contour, and lesions.
- Examine the oropharynx.
- Inspect the teeth and gums.
- Palpate the neck for adenopathy.

CAUSES

MEDICAL

Acquired immunodeficiency syndrome
- Oral lesions may be an early sign of immunosuppression.
- Kaposi's sarcoma may appear on the hard palate as a flat or raised lesion, ranging in color from red to blue to purple; lesion may ulcerate and become painful.

Candidiasis
- Soft elevated plaques usually develop on the buccal mucosa and tongue.

- In acute atrophic form, lesions are red and painful.
- In chronic hyperplastic form, lesions are white and firm.

Discoid lupus erythematosus
- Erythematous areas with white spots and radiating white striae appear on the tongue, buccal mucosa, and palate.
- Other signs and symptoms include skin lesions on the face, enlarged hair follicles filled with scale, and alopecia.

Erythema multiforme
- Onset of vesicles and bullae on the lips and buccal mucosa is sudden.
- Erythematous macules and papules may form symmetrically on the hands, arms, feet, face, and neck and, possibly, in the eyes and on genitalia.
- Other signs and symptoms include lymphadenopathy, fever, malaise, cough, throat and chest pain, vomiting, diarrhea, myalgia, arthralgia, fingernail loss, blindness, hematuria, and signs of renal failure.

Gingivitis, acute necrotizing ulcerative
- Gingival ulcers occur suddenly and are covered with a grayish-white pseudomembrane.
- Other signs and symptoms include tender or painful gingivae, intermittent gingival bleeding, halitosis, enlarged cervical lymph nodes, and fever.

Gonorrhea
- Painful lip ulcerations may occur, along with rough, reddened, bleeding gingivae and a swollen, ulcerated tongue.
- Female patients may be asymptomatic or develop inflammation and a greenish-yellow vaginal discharge.
- Male patients may develop dysuria, purulent urethral discharge, and a reddened, edematous urinary meatus.

Herpes simplex 1
- Small, irritating vesicles develop on the oral mucosa following a brief pe-

---

Common mouth lesions

SQUAMOUS CELL CARCINOMA

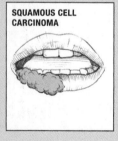

LICHEN PLANUS

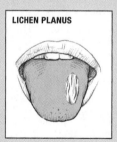

ULCERATION FROM TONGUE BITING

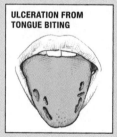

GINGIVAL HYPERPLASIA

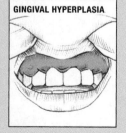

APHTHOUS STOMATITIS

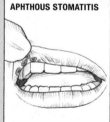

SYPHILITIC CHANCRE (RARE)

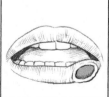

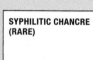

riod of prodromal tingling, itching, fever, and pharyngitis.
- Vesicles form on an erythematous base and then rupture, leaving a painful ulcer, followed by a yellowish crust.
- Other signs and symptoms include submaxillary lymphadenopathy, increased salivation, halitosis, anorexia, and keratoconjunctivitis.

Herpes zoster
- Painful vesicles develop on the buccal mucosa, tongue, uvula, pharynx, and larynx.
- Small red nodules erupt on one side of the thorax or up and down the arms and legs and rapidly become vesicles filled with clear fluid or pus; vesicles dry and form scabs about 10 days after the eruption.
- Other signs and symptoms include fever, malaise, pruritus, paresthesia or hyperesthesia, and tenderness along the course of the involved sensory nerve.

Leukoplakia, erythroplakia
- Leukoplakia is a white lesion that can't be removed by rubbing the mucosal surface.
- Erythroplakia is red and edematous and has a velvety surface.

Lichen planus
- White or gray, velvety, threadlike papules develop on the buccal mucosa or the tongue.
- Violet papules with white lines or spots then erupt on the genitalia, lower back, ankles, and anterior lower legs along with pruritus, nails with longitudinal ridges, and alopecia.

Squamous cell carcinoma
- A painless ulcer with an elevated, indurated border most commonly appears on the lower lip.

Stomatitis, aphthous
- In the minor form, one or more erosions covered by a gray membrane and surrounded by a red halo appear on the mucosa.

- In the major form, large, painful ulcers occur on the lips, cheek, tongue, and soft palate.

Syphilis
- In the primary stage, a solitary painless, red ulcer (chancre) appears on the lip or in the mouth; the ulcer appears as a crater with undulated, raised edges and a shiny center and may develop a crust.
- In the secondary stage, multiple painless ulcers covered by grayish plaque erupt in the mouth; a macular, papular, pustular, or nodular rash appears on the arms, trunk, palms, soles, face, and scalp.
- Other signs and symptoms in the secondary stage include lymphadenopathy, headache, malaise, anorexia, weight loss, nausea, vomiting, sore throat, low fever, metrorrhagia, and postcoital bleeding.
- At the tertiary stage, chronic, painless, superficial nodules or deep granulomatous lesions develop on skin and mucous membranes, especially the tongue and palate.

Systemic lupus erythematosus
- Oral lesions appear as erythematous areas from edema, petechiae, and superficial ulcers with a red halo and tendency to bleed.
- Other signs and symptoms include nondeforming arthritis, butterfly rash across the nose and cheeks, and photosensitivity.

OTHER
Drugs
- Chemotherapeutic drugs produce stomatitis, which can lead to oral lesions.
- Allergic reactions to penicillin, sulfonamides, gold, quinine, streptomycin, phenytoin, aspirin, and barbiturates can also cause oral lesions.
- Inhaled steroids used for pulmonary disorders can also lead to oral lesions.

Treatments
- Radiation therapy may cause oral lesions.

NURSING CONSIDERATIONS
- Provide a topical anesthetic such as lidocaine.
- Provide oral hygiene.

PEDIATRIC POINTERS
- Causes of mouth ulcers in children include chickenpox, measles, scarlet fever, diphtheria, and hand-foot-and-mouth disease.
- In neonates, mouth ulcers can result from candidiasis or congenital syphilis.

GERIATRIC POINTERS
- Ill-fitting dentures can cause irritation, leading to inflammation and ulcers.

PATIENT TEACHING

- Explain to the patient which irritants to avoid.
- Teach the patient proper mouth care and oral hygiene.
- Explain the signs and symptoms the patient should report.

Murmurs

- Auscultatory sounds heard within the heart chambers or major arteries
- Classified by their timing and duration in the cardiac cycle, auscultatory location, loudness, configuration, pitch, and quality (see *Classifying murmurs*)
- Reflect accelerated, forward, or backward blood flow or decreased blood viscosity

 ACTION STAT! *In patients with bacterial endocarditis, new murmurs with crackles, distended jugular veins, orthopnea, and dyspnea may signal heart failure. In patients with acute myocardial infarction, a loud decrescendo holosystolic murmur at the apex that radiates to the axilla and left sternal border or throughout the chest is significant, particularly with a widely split S_2 and an atrial gallop. This murmur, with signs of acute pulmonary edema, usually indicates acute mitral insufficiency from the rupture of the chordae tendineae—a medical emergency.*

- Ask whether the murmur is new or existing.
- Find out about other symptoms, including palpitations, dizziness, syncope, chest pain, dyspnea, and fatigue.
- Obtain a medical history, including incidence of rheumatic fever, recent dental work, heart disease, or heart surgery.

- Auscultate the heart and determine the type of murmur. (See *Identifying common murmurs*. Also see *Positioning the patient for auscultation*, page 370.)
- Note the presence of cardiac arrhythmias, jugular vein distention, dyspnea, orthopnea, and crackles.
- Palpate the liver for enlargement or tenderness.

 TOP TECHNIQUE

Classifying murmurs

After you've auscultated a murmur, determine its timing in the cardiac cycle, location, loudness, configuration, pitch, and quality. Identifying these qualities will help you establish the type of murmur your patient has.

Timing can be characterized as systolic (between S_1 and S_2), holosystolic (continuous throughout systole), diastolic (between S_2 and S_1), or continuous throughout systole and diastole; systolic and diastolic murmurs can be further characterized as early, middle, or late.

Location refers to the area of maximum loudness, such as the apex, the lower left sternal border, or an intercostal space.

Loudness is graded on a scale of 1 to 6. A grade 1 murmur is very faint, detected only after careful auscultation. A grade 2 murmur is a soft, evident murmur. A grade 3 murmur is moderately loud. A grade 4 murmur is loud with a possible intermittent thrill. A grade 5 murmur is loud and associated with a palpable precordial thrill. A grade 6 murmur is loud and, like grade 5 murmurs, is associated with a thrill. Further, a grade 6 murmur is audible even when the stethoscope is lifted from the thoracic wall.

Configuration, or shape, refers to the nature of loudness—crescendo (grows louder), decrescendo (grows softer), crescendo-decrescendo (first rises, then falls), decrescendo-crescendo (first falls, then rises), plateau (even intensity), or variable (uneven intensity).

Pitch may be high or low.

Quality may be described as harsh, rumbling, blowing, scratching, buzzing, musical, or squeaking.

MEDICAL

Aortic insufficiency

♦ In acute form, a soft, short diastolic murmur is heard over the left sternal border that's best heard with the patient leaning forward and at the end of a forced held expiration.

♦ Other acute signs and symptoms include tachycardia, dyspnea, jugular vein distention, crackles, increased fatigue, and pale, cool extremities.

♦ In chronic form, a high-pitched, blowing, decrescendo diastolic murmur is heard over the second or third right intercostal space or the left sternal border; an Austin Flint murmur—a rumbling, mid-to-late diastolic murmur best heard at the apex—may also occur.

♦ Other chronic signs and symptoms include palpitations, tachycardia, angina, increased fatigue, dyspnea, orthopnea, and crackles.

Aortic stenosis

♦ Murmur is systolic, harsh and grating, medium-pitched, crescendo-decrescendo, and heard loudest over the second right intercostal space with the patient leaning forward.

♦ Other signs and symptoms include dizziness, syncope, dyspnea on exertion, paroxysmal nocturnal dyspnea, fatigue, and angina.

Cardiomyopathy, hypertrophic

♦ A harsh, late systolic murmur commonly accompanies an audible S_3 or S_4.

♦ Murmur decreases with squatting and increases with sitting down.

♦ Other signs and symptoms include dyspnea, chest pain, palpitations, dizziness, and syncope.

Mitral insufficiency

♦ Acute form produces medium-pitched blowing, early systolic or holosystolic decrescendo murmur at apex, along with a widely split S_2 and, commonly, S_4.

♦ Other acute signs and symptoms include tachycardia and signs of acute pulmonary edema.

♦ Chronic form produces high-pitched, blowing, holosystolic plateau murmur that's loudest at apex and may radiate to axilla or back.

♦ Other chronic signs and symptoms include fatigue, dyspnea, and palpitations.

Mitral prolapse

♦ Midsystolic to late-systolic click with high-pitched late-systolic crescendo murmur occurs, best heard at the apex.

♦ Other signs and symptoms include cardiac awareness, migraine headaches, dizziness, weakness, syncope, palpitations, chest pain, dyspnea, severe episodic fatigue, mood swings, and anxiety.

Mitral stenosis

♦ Murmur is soft, low-pitched, rumbling, crescendo-decrescendo, and diastolic; is accompanied by a loud S_1 or opening snap; and is best heard with the patient lying on his left side.

♦ With severe stenosis, murmur of mitral insufficiency may also be heard.

♦ Other signs and symptoms include hemoptysis, exertional dyspnea, fatigue, and signs of acute pulmonary edema.

TOP TECHNIQUE

Identifying common murmurs

The timing and configuration of a murmur can help you identify its underlying cause. Learn to recognize the characteristics of these common murmurs.

AORTIC INSUFFICIENCY (CHRONIC)

Thickened valve leaflets fail to close correctly, permitting backflow of blood into the left ventricle.

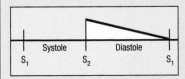

AORTIC STENOSIS

Thickened, scarred, or calcified valve leaflets impede ventricular systolic ejection.

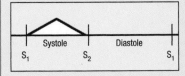

MITRAL PROLAPSE

Incompetent mitral valve bulges into the left atrium because of an enlarged posterior leaflet and elongated chordae tendineae.

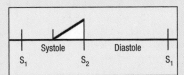

MITRAL INSUFFICIENCY (CHRONIC)

Incomplete mitral valve closure permits backflow of blood into the left atrium.

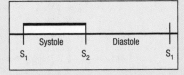

MITRAL STENOSIS

Thickened or scarred valve leaflets cause valve stenosis and restrict blood flow.

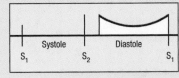

(continued)

Papillary muscle rupture

- A life-threatening disorder, a loud holosystolic murmur can be auscultated at the apex.
- Other signs and symptoms include severe dyspnea, chest pain, syncope, hemoptysis, tachycardia, and hypotension.

Rheumatic fever with pericarditis

- A systolic murmur of mitral insufficiency, midsystolic murmur from swelling of the leaflet of the mitral valve, and a diastolic murmur of aortic insufficiency are common.
- A pericardial friction rub, along with murmurs and gallops, is best heard with the patient leaning forward during forced expiration.
- Other signs and symptoms include fever, joint and sternal pain, edema, and tachypnea.

Tricuspid insufficiency

- Soft, high-pitched, holosystolic blowing murmur increases with inspiration and decreases with exhalation and Valsalva's maneuver; it's best heard over the lower left sternal border and the xiphoid area.
- Late signs and symptoms include exertional dyspnea, orthopnea, jugular vein distention, ascites, peripheral cyanosis and edema, muscle wasting, fatigue, weakness, and syncope.

Tricuspid stenosis

- A diastolic murmur similar to that of mitral stenosis, but louder with inspiration and decreased with exhalation and Valsalva's maneuver, is produced.
- Other signs and symptoms include fatigue, syncope, peripheral edema, jugular vein distention, ascites, hepatomegaly, and dyspnea.

OTHER
Treatments

- Prosthetic valve replacement may cause variable murmurs.

 TOP TECHNIQUE

Positioning the patient for auscultation

If heart sounds are faint or undetectable, try listening to them with the patient seated and leaning forward or lying on his left side, which brings the heart closer to the surface of the chest. These illustrations show how to position the patient for high- and low-pitched sounds.

FORWARD LEANING

The forward-leaning position is best suited for hearing high-pitched sounds related to semilunar valve problems, such as aortic and pulmonic valve murmurs. To auscultate for these sounds, place the diaphragm of the stethoscope over the aortic and pulmonic areas in the right and left second intercostal spaces, as shown below.

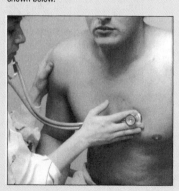

LEFT LATERAL RECUMBENT

The left lateral recumbent position is best suited for hearing low-pitched sounds, such as mitral valve murmurs and extra heart sounds. To hear these sounds, place the bell of the stethoscope over the apical area, as shown below.

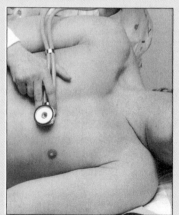

- Monitor cardiovascular status with acute conditions.
- Give an antibiotic and an anticoagulant, if needed.

PEDIATRIC POINTERS

- Innocent murmurs are commonly heard in young children.
- Pathognomonic heart murmurs in infants and young children usually result from congenital heart disease.
- Other murmurs can be acquired, as with rheumatic heart disease.

- Discuss underyling condition, diagnostic tests, and treatment options.
- Explain the need for prophylactic antibiotics prior to certain procedures, such as dental work.
- Explain the signs and symptoms the patient should report.

Muscle atrophy

OVERVIEW

- Results from denervation or prolonged muscle disuse
- Causes loss of motion or power

HISTORY

- Ask about the onset and progression of muscle atrophy.
- Inquire about other signs and symptoms, such as weakness, pain, loss of sensation, and recent weight loss.
- Obtain a medical history, including incidence of musculoskeletal, endocrine, metabolic, or neurologic disorders, and trauma.
- Ask about the use of drugs, particularly steroids.
- Find out about alcohol use.

PHYSICAL ASSESSMENT

- Check all muscle groups for size, tonicity, and strength.
- Measure the circumference of all limbs. (See *Measuring limb circumference.*)
- Check for muscle contractures in all limbs by fully extending joints, noting any pain resistance.
- Palpate peripheral pulses for quality and rate.
- Assess sensory function in and around the atrophied area.
- Test deep tendon reflexes (DTRs).

CAUSES

MEDICAL

Amyotrophic lateral sclerosis
- Muscle weakness and atrophy that begins in one hand, spreads to the arm, and then develops in the other hand and arm are initial symptoms.
- Eventually, weakness and atrophy spread to the trunk, neck, tongue, larynx, pharynx, and legs; progressive respiratory muscle weakness leads to respiratory insufficiency.
- Other signs and symptoms include muscle flaccidity, fasciculations, hyperactive DTRs, slight leg muscle spasticity, dysphagia, impaired speech, excessive drooling, and depression.

Burns
- Limited muscle movements from fibrous scar tissue, pain, and loss of serum proteins lead to atrophy.

Compartment syndrome and Volkmann's ischemic contracture
- Muscle atrophy is a late sign along with contractures, paralysis, and loss of pulses.
- Earlier signs and symptoms include severe pain that increases with passive muscle movement, weakness, and paresthesia.

Herniated disk
- Muscle weakness, disuse and, ultimately, atrophy develop.
- Severe lower back pain, possibly radiating to the buttocks, legs, and feet is the primary symptom.
- Other signs and symptoms include muscle spasm, diminished reflexes, and sensory changes.

Hypercortisolism
- Limb weakness and eventually atrophy occur.
- Other cushingoid signs and symptoms include buffalo hump, moon face, truncal obesity, purple striae, thin skin, acne, easy bruising, poor wound healing, elevated blood pressure, fatigue, hyperpigmentation, and diaphoresis.
- Related signs and symptoms include hirsutism and menstrual irregularities (in females) and impotence (in males).

Measuring limb circumference

Measure the limb at the place of largest muscle circumference. To ensure accurate and consistent limb circumference measurements, mark and use the same reference point each time and measure with the limb in full extension. The illustration shows the correct reference points for arm and leg measurements.

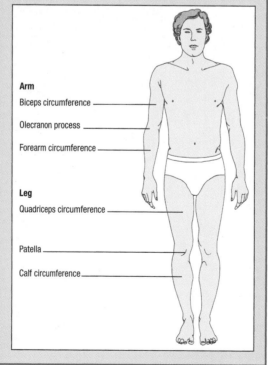

Arm
Biceps circumference
Olecranon process
Forearm circumference

Leg
Quadriceps circumference
Patella
Calf circumference

Hypothyroidism

- Reversible weakness and atrophy of proximal limb muscles may occur.
- Other signs and symptoms include muscle cramps and stiffness, cold intolerance; weight gain despite anorexia; mental dullness; dry, pale, cool, doughy skin; puffy face, hands, and feet; and bradycardia.

Meniscal tear

- Quadriceps muscle atrophy is a classic sign.

Multiple sclerosis

- Arm and leg atrophy, spasticity, and contractures result from progressive demyelination.
- Other signs and symptoms include diplopia, blurred vision, nystagmus, hyperactive DTRs, sensory loss or paresthesia, dysarthria, dysphagia, incoordination, ataxic gait, intention tremors, emotional lability, impotence, and urinary dysfunction.

Osteoarthritis

- Atrophy proximal to involved joints eventually occurs.
- Other late signs and symptoms include Heberden's nodes, Bouchard's nodes, crepitus and fluid accumulation, and contractures.

Parkinson's disease

- Muscle rigidity, weakness, and disuse produces muscle atrophy.
- Other signs and symptoms include resting tremors, bradykinesia, a propulsive gait, a high-pitched and monotone voice, masklike facies, drooling, dysphagia, dysarthria, and oculogyric crisis or blepharospasm.

Peripheral nerve trauma

- Muscle weakness and atrophy develop.
- Other signs and symptoms include paresthesia or sensory loss, pain, loss of reflexes supplied by the damaged nerve and, possibly, paralysis.

Peripheral neuropathy

- Muscle weakness progresses slowly to flaccid paralysis and eventually to atrophy.

- Other signs and symptoms include loss of vibration sense; paresthesia, hyperesthesia, or anesthesia in the hands and feet; mild to sharp, burning pain; anhidrosis; glossy red skin; and diminished or absent DTRs.

Protein deficiency

- Muscle weakness and atrophy develop if the deficiency is chronic.
- Other signs and symptoms include chronic fatigue, apathy, anorexia, dry skin, peripheral edema, and dull, sparse, dry hair.

Radiculopathy

- Muscle atrophy and weakness develop along with paralysis, severe pain and, at times, loss of feeling in the areas supplied by the affected nerve.

Rheumatoid arthritis

- Muscle atrophy occurs in the late stages.
- Other late signs and symptoms include deformities, crepitation with joint rotation, and multiple systemic complications.

Spinal cord injury

- Muscle weakness and flaccid, then spastic, paralysis eventually lead to atrophy.
- Other signs and symptoms depend on the level of injury but may include respiratory insufficiency or paralysis, sensory loss, bowel and bladder dysfunction, hyperactive DTRs, positive Babinski's reflex, sexual dysfunction, and anhidrosis.

Stroke

- Muscle weakness and, eventually, atrophy of the arms, legs, face, and tongue occurs.
- Other signs and symptoms vary but may include dysarthria, aphasia, ataxia, apraxia, agnosia, visual disturbances, altered level of consciousness, personality changes, bowel and bladder dysfunction, seizures, and ipsilateral paresthesia or sensory loss.

Thyrotoxicosis

- Insidious, generalized muscle weakness and atrophy occur.
- Other signs and symptoms include extreme anxiety, fatigue, heat intolerance, diaphoresis, tremors, tachycardia, palpitations, ventricular or atrial gallop, dyspnea, weight loss, an enlarged thyroid gland, and exophthalmos.

OTHER

Drugs

- Prolonged steroid therapy interferes with muscle metabolism and leads to atrophy.

Treatments

- Prolonged immobilization from bed rest, casts, splints, or traction may cause muscle weakness and atrophy.

NURSING CONSIDERATIONS

- Encourage frequent active or passive range-of-motion exercises.
- Apply splints or braces, if needed.
- If you find resistance to full extension during exercise, consult the physical therapist.
- Use heat, drugs, or relaxation techniques to relax resistant muscles.

PEDIATRIC POINTERS

- In young children, profound muscle weakness and atrophy can result from muscular dystrophy.
- Muscle atrophy may also result from cerebral palsy and poliomyelitis, and from paralysis from meningocele and myelomeningocele.

PATIENT TEACHING

- Discuss underlying condition, diagnostic tests, and treatment options.
- Show the patient how to use assistive devices, as needed.
- Emphasize safety measures the patient should adopt.
- Teach the patient an exercise regimen to follow.

Muscle flaccidity

- Weak, soft muscles with decreased resistance to movement, increased mobility, and greater than normal range-of-motion (ROM)
- Result of disrupted muscle innervation
- May be localized to a limb or muscle group or generalized over the entire body
- Onset may be acute, as in trauma, or chronic, as in neurologic disease

◼ *ACTION STAT! If the patient's muscle flaccidity results from trauma, make sure his cervical spine has been stabilized. Quickly determine his respiratory status. If you note signs and symptoms of respiratory insufficiency—dyspnea, shallow respirations, nasal flaring, cyanosis, and decreased oxygen saturation—administer oxygen by nasal cannula or mask. Intubation and mechanical ventilation may be necessary.*

HISTORY

- Ask about the onset and duration of muscle flaccidity and any precipitating factors.
- Ask about associated signs and symptoms, notably weakness, other muscle changes, and sensory loss or paresthesia.

PHYSICAL ASSESSMENT

- Examine the affected muscles for atrophy, which indicates a chronic problem.
- Test muscle strength, and check deep tendon reflexes in all limbs.

CAUSES

MEDICAL
Amyotrophic lateral sclerosis
- Progressive muscle weakness and paralysis are accompanied by generalized flaccidity.
- Effects typically begin in one hand, spread to the arm, and then develop in the other hand and arm. Eventually, they spread to the trunk, neck, tongue, larynx, pharynx, and legs; progressive respiratory muscle weakness leads to respiratory insufficiency.
- Other signs and symptoms include muscle cramps and coarse fasciculations, hyperactive deep tendon reflexes (DTRs), slight leg muscle spasticity, dysphagia, dysarthria, excessive drooling, and depression.

Brain lesions
- Frontal and parietal lobe lesions may cause contralateral flaccidity, weakness or paralysis, and eventually, spasticity and, possibly, contractures.
- Other signs and symptoms include hyperactive DTRs, positive Babinski's reflex, loss of proprioception, stereognosis, graphesthesia, anesthesia, and thermanesthesia.

Cerebellar disease
- Generalized muscle flaccidity or hypotonia is accompanied by ataxia, dysmetria, intention tremor, slight muscle weakness, fatigue, and dysarthria.

Guillain-Barré syndrome
- Progression of muscle flaccidity is typically symmetrical and ascending, moving from the feet to the arms and facial nerves within 24 to 72 hours of onset of this inflammatory disorder.
- Associated signs and symptoms include sensory loss or paresthesia, absent DTRs, tachycardia (or, less often, bradycardia), fluctuating hypertension and orthostatic hypotension, diaphoresis, incontinence, dysphagia, dysarthria, hypernasality, and facial diplegia.
- Weakness may progress to total motor paralysis and respiratory failure.

Huntington's disease
- Besides flaccidity, progressive mental status changes up to and including dementia and choreiform movements are major symptoms of this hereditary disease.
- Other signs and symptoms include poor balance, hesitant or explosive speech, dysphagia, impaired respirations, and incontinence.

Muscle disease
- Muscle weakness and flaccidity are features of myopathies and muscular dystrophies.

Peripheral nerve trauma
- Flaccidity, paralysis, and loss of sensation and reflexes in the innervated area can occur.

Peripheral neuropathy

◆ Flaccidity usually occurs in the legs as a result of chronic progressive muscle weakness and paralysis, which may also cause mild to sharp burning pain, glossy red skin, anhidrosis, and loss of vibration sensation.
◆ Paresthesia, hyperesthesia, or anesthesia may affect the hands and feet.
◆ DTRs may be hypoactive or absent.

Poliomyelitis

◆ Damage to the anterior horn cells in the spinal cord and brain stem causes flaccid weakness and loss of reflexes.
◆ The large proximal muscles of the limbs are most commonly affected.

Seizure disorder

◆ Brief periods of syncope and generalized flaccidity commonly follow a generalized tonic-clonic seizure.

Spinal cord injury

◆ Spinal shock can result in acute muscle flaccidity or spasticity below the level of injury.
◆ Other signs and symptoms that occur below the level of injury may include paralysis; absent deep tendon reflexes; analgesia; thermanesthesia; loss of proprioception and vibration, touch, and pressure sensation; anhidrosis (usually unilateral); hypotension; bowel and bladder dysfunction; and impotence or priapism.
◆ Injury in the C1 to C5 region can produce respiratory paralysis and bradycardia.

◆ Provide regular, systematic, passive ROM exercises to preserve joint mobility and to increase circulation.
◆ Reposition and assess a patient with generalized flaccidity every 2 hours to protect him from skin breakdown.
◆ Pad bony prominences and other pressure points, and prevent thermal injury by testing bath water yourself before the patient bathes.
◆ Treat isolated flaccidity by supporting the affected limb in a sling or with a splint.
◆ Ensure patient safety and reduce the risk of falls by introducing assistive devices and their proper use.
◆ Consult physical and occupational therapist to formulate a personalized therapy regimen and foster independence.
◆ Prepare the patient for diagnostic tests, such as cranial and spinal X-rays, computed tomography scans, and electromyography.

PEDIATRIC POINTERS

◆ Pediatric causes of muscle flaccidity include myelomeningocele, Lowe's disease, Werdnig-Hoffmann disease, and muscular dystrophy.
◆ An infant or young child with generalized flaccidity may lie in a froglike position, with his hips and knees abducted.

◆ Teach the patient and family how to do ROM exercises at home.
◆ Teach the patient and family the importance of doing ROM exercises at home.
◆ Teach the patient and family the importance of frequent position changes and other pressure ulcer prevention techniques.
◆ Teach the patient and family about the underlying diagnosis and treatment plan.
◆ Teach the patient and family about any prescribed medications and their use.
◆ Encourage the patient to use assistive devices, as instructed.

Muscle spasms

OVERVIEW

- Strong, painful muscle contractions
- Most commonly occur in the calf and foot

◆ **ACTION STAT!** *If the patient complains of frequent or unrelieved spasms in many muscles with paresthesia in his hands and feet, quickly attempt to elicit Chvostek's and Trousseau's signs. If these signs are present, suspect hypocalcemia. Evaluate respiratory function, watching for the development of laryngospasm. Provide supplemental oxygen, as needed, and anticipate intubation and mechanical ventilation. Insert an I.V. line for administration of a calcium supplement. Monitor cardiac status and begin resuscitation, if needed.*

HISTORY

- Ask about the onset and description of spasms.
- Find out what causes, aggravates, or alleviates the spasms.
- Inquire about weakness, sensory loss, or paresthesia.
- Obtain a drug and diet history.
- Ask about recent vomiting or diarrhea.

PHYSICAL ASSESSMENT

- Check muscle strength and tone.
- Check all major muscle groups and note whether movements precipitate spasms.
- Palpate peripheral pulses for presence and quality.
- Examine limbs for color, capillary refill, edema, and temperature changes.
- Test reflexes and sensory function in all limbs.

CAUSES

MEDICAL

Amyotrophic lateral sclerosis
- Muscle spasms may accompany progressive muscle weakness and atrophy that typically begin in one hand, spread to the arm, and then spread to the other hand and arm.
- Eventually, muscle weakness and atrophy affect the trunk, neck, tongue, larynx, pharynx, and legs.
- Other signs and symptoms include respiratory insufficiency, muscle spasticity, coarse fasciculations, hyperactive deep tendon reflexes (DTRs), dysphagia, impaired speech, excessive drooling, and depression.

Arterial occlusive disease
- Spasms and intermittent claudication occur in the leg.
- Other signs and symptoms include loss of peripheral pulses, pallor or cyanosis, decreased sensation, hair loss, dry or scaling skin, edema, and ulcerations.

Cholera
- Muscle spasms, severe water and electrolyte loss, thirst, weakness, decreased skin turgor, tachycardia, and hypotension occur along with abrupt watery diarrhea and vomiting.

Dehydration
- Limb and abdominal cramps, and muscle twitching may occur.
- Other signs and symptoms include a slight fever, decreased skin turgor, dry mucous membranes, tachycardia, orthostatic hypotension, muscle twitching, seizures, nausea, vomiting, and oliguria.

Fracture
- Localized spasms and pain are mild if fracture is nondisplaced; intense, if severely displaced.
- Other signs and symptoms include swelling, limited mobility, and bony crepitation.

Hypocalcemia
◆ Tetany is the classic feature.
◆ Other signs and symptoms include Chvostek's and Trousseau's signs; paresthesia of the lips, fingers, and toes; choreiform movements; hyperactive DTRs; fatigue; palpitations; and arrhythmias.

Hypomagnesemia
◆ Tetany, leg and foot cramps may occur.
◆ Other signs and symptoms include Chvostek's sign, hyperneuromuscular irritability, cardiac arrhythmias, vasodilation, hypotension, confusion, and seizures.

Hypothyroidism
◆ Spasms and stiffness occur with leg muscle hypertrophy or proximal limb weakness and atrophy.
◆ Other signs and symptoms include forgetfulness and mental instability; fatigue; cold intolerance; dry, pale, cool, doughy skin; puffy face, hands, and feet; periorbital edema; dry, sparse, brittle hair; bradycardia; and weight gain despite anorexia.

Muscle trauma
◆ Excessive muscle strain may cause mild to severe spasms.
◆ The injured area may be painful, swollen, reddened, and warm.

Respiratory alkalosis
◆ Acute onset of muscle spasms may be accompanied by twitching and weakness, carpopedal spasms, circumoral and peripheral paresthesia, vertigo, syncope, pallor, and anxiety.
◆ Cardiac arrhythmias may occur with severe alkalosis.

Spinal injury or disease
◆ Resulting muscle spasms worsen with movement.

OTHER
Drugs
◆ Corticosteroids, diuretics, and estrogens may result in spasms.

NURSING CONSIDERATIONS
◆ Help alleviate spasms by slowly stretching the affected muscle in the direction opposite the contraction.
◆ Give a mild analgesic, as needed.

PEDIATRIC POINTERS
◆ Muscle spasms may indicate hypoparathyroidism, osteomalacia, rickets or, rarely, congenital torticollis.

PATIENT TEACHING
◆ Discuss underlying condition, diagnostic tests, and treatment options.
◆ Explain immobilization and wrapping the injured area.
◆ Discuss pain relief measures.
◆ Help the patient learn to use assistive devices, as needed.

Muscle spasticity

OVERVIEW

- State of excessive muscle tone manifested by increased resistance to stretching and heightened reflexes
- Caused by an upper-motor-neuron lesion; usually occurs in the arm and leg muscles (see *How spasticity develops*)
- Also known as *muscle hypertonicity*

  ▲ *ACTION STAT! In a patient with a recent skin puncture or laceration, generalized spasticity and trismus may indicate tetanus; if you suspect tetanus, look for signs of respiratory distress. Provide ventilatory support, if needed, and monitor the patient closely.*

HISTORY

- Ask about the onset, duration, and progression of spasticity.
- Ask about how the spasticity started and what aggravates it.
- Find out about other muscular changes or other symptoms, such as pain.
- Obtain a medical history, including incidence of trauma or degenerative or vascular disease.

PHYSICAL ASSESSMENT

- Take vital signs.
- Perform a neurologic assessment.
- Test reflexes and evaluate motor and sensory function in all limbs.
- Evaluate muscles for wasting and contractures.

CAUSES

MEDICAL
Amyotrophic lateral sclerosis

- Early signs and symptoms include progressive muscle weakness and flaccidity that typically begin in the hands and arms, and eventually spread to the trunk, neck, larynx, pharynx, and legs.
- Spasticity, spasms, coarse fasciculations, hyperactive deep tendon reflexes (DTRs), and a positive Babinski's reflex also occur.
- Other signs and symptoms include respiratory insufficiency, dysphagia, dysarthria, excessive drooling, and depression.

Epidural hemorrhage

- Limb spasticity is a late and ominous sign and may be preceded by momentary loss of consciousness after

---

How spasticity develops

Motor activity is controlled by pyramidal and extrapyramidal tracts that originate in the motor cortex, basal ganglia, brain stem, and spinal cord. Nerve fibers from the various tracts converge and synapse at the anterior horn in the spinal cord. Together, they maintain segmental muscle tone by modulating the stretch reflex arc. This arc, shown in simplified form below, is basically a negative feedback loop in which muscle stretch (stimulation) causes reflexive contraction (inhibition), thus maintaining muscle length and tone.

Damage to certain tracts results in loss of inhibition and disruption of the stretch reflex arc. Uninhibited muscle stretch produces exaggerated, uncontrolled muscle activity, accentuating the reflex arc and eventually resulting in spasticity.

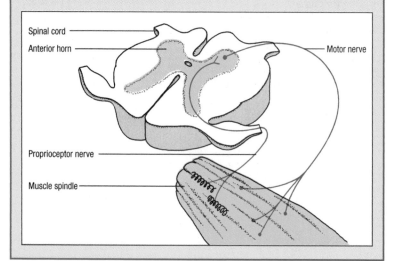

Spinal cord

Anterior horn

Motor nerve

Proprioceptor nerve

Muscle spindle

---

head trauma, followed by a lucid interval, and then a rapid deterioration in level of consciousness (LOC).
- Other signs and symptoms include hemiparesis or hemiplegia; seizures; fixed, dilated pupils; high fever; decreased and bounding pulse; widened pulse pressure; elevated blood pressure; irregular respiratory pattern; a positive Babinski's reflex; and decerebrate posture.

Multiple sclerosis
- Muscle spasticity, hyperreflexia, and contractures may eventually develop as demyelination advances.
- Progressive weakness and atrophy occur early.
- Other signs and symptoms include diplopia, blurring or loss of vision, nystagmus, sensory loss or paresthesia, dysarthria, dysphagia, incoordination, ataxic gait, intention tremors, emotional lability, impotence, and urinary dysfunction.

Spinal cord injury
- Spastic paralysis in the affected limbs follows initial flaccid paralysis.
- Spasticity and muscle atrophy increase for up to 2 years after the injury, then gradually regress to flaccidity.
- Other signs and symptoms vary with the level of the injury and may include respiratory insufficiency or paralysis, sensory losses, bowel and bladder dysfunction, hyperactive DTRs, positive Babinski's reflex, anhidrosis, and bradycardia.

Stroke
- Spastic paralysis may develop on the affected side following the acute stage.
- Other signs and symptoms vary and may include dysarthria, aphasia, ataxia, apraxia, agnosia, ipsilateral paresthesia or sensory loss, visual disturbance, altered LOC, personality changes, emotional lability, bowel and bladder dysfunction, and seizures.

NURSING CONSIDERATIONS

- Give drugs for pain and an antispasmodic.
- Passive range-of-motion exercises, splinting, traction, and application of heat may help relieve spasms and prevent contractures.
- Maintain a calm, quiet environment, and encourage bed rest.
- In cases of prolonged, uncontrollable spasticity, nerve blocks or surgical transection may be needed.

PEDIATRIC POINTERS
- In children, muscle spasticity may be a sign of cerebral palsy.

PATIENT TEACHING

- Discuss underlying condition, diagnostic tests, and treatment options.
- Teach the patient to use assistive devices, as needed.
- Discuss ways of maintaining independence.
- Teach about prescribed medications.

Muscle weakness

OVERVIEW

- Detected by observing and measuring the strength of an individual muscle or muscle group

HISTORY

- Determine the onset and location of weakness.
- Ask what aggravates the weakness.
- Find out about other symptoms, including muscle or joint pain, altered sensory function, and fatigue.
- Obtain a medical history, including incidence of hyperthyroidism, musculoskeletal or neurologic problems, recent trauma, and family history of chronic muscle weakness.
- Obtain an alcohol and drug history.

PHYSICAL ASSESSMENT

- Test major muscles on both sides. (See *Testing muscle strength*.)
- Test for range-of-motion (ROM) at all major joints.
- Test sensory function in the involved areas.
- Test deep tendon reflexes (DTRs) on both sides.

CAUSES

MEDICAL
Amyotrophic lateral sclerosis
- Muscle weakness and atrophy in one hand rapidly spread to the arm and then to the other hand and arm.
- Eventually, weakness and atrophy spread to the trunk, neck, tongue, larynx, pharynx, and legs; respiratory insufficiency results from progressive respiratory muscle weakness.

Brain tumor
- Weakness varies with the tumor's location and size.
- Other signs and symptoms include headache, vomiting, diplopia, decreased visual acuity, decreased level of consciousness (LOC), pupillary changes, decreased motor strength, hemiparesis, hemiplegia, diminished sensations, ataxia, seizures, and behavioral changes.

Guillain-Barré syndrome
- Rapidly progressive, symmetrical weakness and pain ascend from the feet to the arms and facial nerves, and may progress to motor paralysis and respiratory failure.
- Other signs and symptoms include sensory loss or paresthesia, muscle flaccidity, absent DTRs, tachycardia or bradycardia, fluctuating hypertension and orthostatic hypotension, diaphoresis, bowel and bladder incontinence, facial diplegia, dysphagia, dysarthria, and hypernasality.

Head trauma
- Varying degrees of muscle weakness occur.
- Other signs and symptoms include decreased LOC, otorrhea or rhinorrhea, raccoon eyes and Battle's sign, sensory disturbances, and signs of increased intracranial pressure.

Herniated disk
- Muscle weakness, disuse and, ultimately, atrophy occurs.

(Text continues on page 382.)

TOP TECHNIQUE

Testing muscle strength

Obtain an overall picture of your patient's motor function by testing strength in 10 selected muscle groups. Ask the patient to attempt normal range-of-motion movements against your resistance. If the muscle group is weak, vary the amount of resistance, as necessary, to permit accurate assessment. If necessary, position the patient so his limbs don't have to resist gravity, and repeat the test.

Rate muscle strength on a scale from 0 to 5:
0 = No evidence of muscle contraction; no movement
1 = Visible or palpable contraction, but no movement
2 = Full muscle movement with force of gravity eliminated
3 = Full muscle movement against gravity, but no movement against resistance
4 = Full muscle movement against gravity; partial movement against resistance
5 = Full muscle movement against both gravity and resistance—normal strength

ARM MUSCLES

Biceps. With your hand on the patient's hand, have him flex his forearm against your resistance. Watch for biceps contraction.

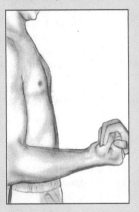

Deltoid. With the patient's arm fully extended, place one hand over his deltoid muscle and the other on his wrist. Ask him to abduct his arm to a horizontal position against your resistance; as he does so, palpate for deltoid contraction.

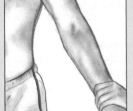

Triceps. Have the patient abduct and hold his arm midway between flexion and extension. Hold and support his arm at the wrist, and ask him to extend it against your resistance. Watch for triceps contraction.

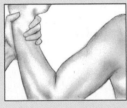

Dorsal interossei. Have the patient extend and spread his fingers, and tell him to try to resist your attempt to squeeze them together.

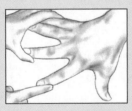

Forearm and hand (grip). Have the patient grasp your middle and index fingers and squeeze as hard as he can. To prevent pain or injury to the examiner, the examiner should cross his fingers.

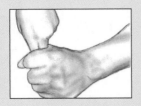

LEG MUSCLES

Anterior tibial. With the patient's leg extended, place your hand on his foot and ask him to dorsiflex his ankle against your resistance. Palpate for anterior tibial contraction.

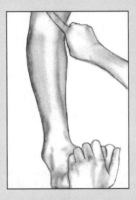

Psoas. While you support his leg, have the patient raise his knee and then flex his hip against your resistance. Watch for psoas contraction.

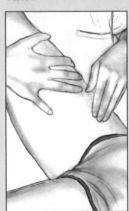

Extensor hallucis longus. With your finger on the patient's great toe, have him dorsiflex the toe against your resistance. Palpate for extensor hallucis contraction.

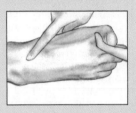

Quadriceps. Have the patient bend his knee slightly while you support his lower leg. Then ask him to extend the knee against your resistance; as he's doing so, palpate for quadriceps contraction.

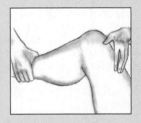

Gastrocnemius. With the patient on his side, support his foot and ask him to plantarflex his ankle against your resistance. Palpate for gastrocnemius contraction.

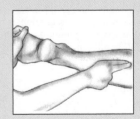

- Severe lower back pain, possibly radiating to the buttocks, legs, and feet—usually on one side—is the primary symptom.
- Diminished reflexes and sensory changes may occur.

Hodgkin's disease
- Muscle weakness may accompany painless, progressive lymphadenopathy.
- Other signs and symptoms include paresthesia, fatigue, persistent fever, night sweats, and weight loss.

Hypercortisolism
- Limb weakness and atrophy occur.
- Related cushingoid features include buffalo hump, moon face, truncal obesity, purple striae, thin skin, acne, elevated blood pressure, fatigue, hyperpigmentation, easy bruising, poor wound healing, and diaphoresis.
- Other signs and symptoms may include impotence (in males) and hirsutism and menstrual irregularities (in females).

Hypothyroidism
- Reversible weakness and atrophy of proximal limb muscles may occur.
- Other signs and symptoms include muscle cramps; cold intolerance; weight gain despite anorexia; mental dullness; dry, pale, doughy skin; puffy face, hands, and feet; impaired hearing and balance; and bradycardia.

Multiple sclerosis
- Muscle weakness in one or more limbs may progress to atrophy, spasticity, and contractures.
- Other signs and symptoms include diplopia, blurred vision, vision loss, nystagmus, hyperactive DTRs, sensory loss or paresthesia, dysarthria, dysphagia, incoordination, ataxic gait, intention tremors, emotional lability, and urinary dysfunction.

Myasthenia gravis
- Gradually progressive skeletal muscle weakness and fatigue are the principal symptoms.
- Other early signs include weak eye closure, ptosis, diplopia, a masklike facies, difficulty chewing and swallowing, nasal regurgitation of fluid with hypernasality, and a hanging jaw and bobbing head.
- Respiratory failure may eventually occur.

Osteoarthritis
- Progressive muscle disuse and weakness lead to atrophy.
- Other signs and symptoms include crepitation; enlarged edematous joints; Heberden's nodes; increased pain in damp, cold weather; joint stiffness; limited ROM; pain relieved by resting joints; and smooth, taut, shiny skin.

Paget's disease
- Muscle weakness, paralysis, paresthesia, and pain may develop.
- Other signs and symptoms may include bowed tibias, frequent fractures, and kyphosis.

Parkinson's disease
- Muscle weakness accompanies rigidity.
- Other signs and symptoms include a pill-rolling tremor in one hand, propulsive gait, dysarthria, bradykinesia, drooling, dysphagia, a masklike facies, and a high-pitched, monotonous voice.

Peripheral nerve trauma
- Muscle weakness and atrophy are accompanied by paresthesia, pain, and loss of reflexes supplied by damaged nerve.

Peripheral neuropathy
- Muscle weakness progresses slowly to flaccid paralysis.
- Other signs and symptoms include loss of vibration sense; paresthesia, hyperesthesia, or anesthesia in the hands and feet; hypoactive or absent DTRs; mild to sharp burning pain; anhidrosis; and glossy, red skin.

Potassium imbalance
- With hypokalemia, temporary muscle weakness occurs and may be accompanied by nausea, vomiting, diarrhea, decreased mentation, leg cramps, diminished reflexes, malaise, polyuria, dizziness, hypotension, and arrhythmias.
- With hyperkalemia, weakness progresses to flaccid paralysis and may be accompanied by irritability, confusion, hyperreflexia, paresthesia or anesthesia, oliguria, anorexia, nausea, diarrhea, abdominal cramps, tachycardia or bradycardia, and arrhythmias.

Rhabdomyolysis
- Muscle weakness or pain occurs with fever, nausea, vomiting, malaise, dark urine, and signs of acute renal failure.

Rheumatoid arthritis
- Symmetric muscle weakness may accompany increased warmth, swelling, and tenderness in involved joints; pain; and stiffness.

Seizure disorder
- Temporary generalized muscle weakness may occur after generalized tonic-clonic seizure; aura may precede the seizure.
- Other postictal signs and symptoms include headache, muscle soreness, and profound fatigue.

Spinal trauma and disease
- Severe muscle weakness, leading to flaccidity or spasticity and, eventually, paralysis, occurs.

Stroke

◆ Weakness may progress to hemiplegia and atrophy.
◆ Other signs and symptoms include dysarthria, aphasia, ataxia, apraxia, agnosia, ipsilateral paresthesia or sensory loss, visual disturbance, altered LOC, personality changes, bowel and bladder dysfunction, headache, and seizures.

Thyrotoxicosis

◆ Insidious, generalized muscle weakness and atrophy may occur.
◆ Other signs and symptoms include anxiety, fatigue, heat intolerance, diaphoresis, tremors, tachycardia, palpitations, ventricular or atrial gallop, dyspnea, weight loss, enlarged thyroid gland, exophthalmos, and warm, flushed skin.

OTHER

Drugs

◆ Aminoglycoside antibiotics may worsen weakness in patients with myasthenia gravis.
◆ Generalized muscle weakness can result from prolonged corticosteroid use, digoxin, and excessive doses of dantrolene.

Immobility

◆ Immobilization, prolonged bed rest, or inactivity can lead to muscle weakness in the involved extremity.

NURSING CONSIDERATIONS

◆ Provide assistive devices, as needed.
◆ Protect the patient from injury.
◆ If sensory loss occurs, guard against pressure ulcer formation and thermal injury.
◆ With chronic weakness, provide ROM exercises or splint the limbs, as needed.
◆ Allow for adequate rest periods.
◆ Give medications for pain, as needed.

PEDIATRIC POINTERS

◆ Muscular dystrophy is a major cause of muscle weakness in children.

PATIENT TEACHING

◆ Teach the patient how to use assistive devices, as needed.
◆ Explain the importance of frequent position changes and rest periods.
◆ Teach patient about prescribed medications.

Mydriasis

OVERVIEW

- Pupillary dilation caused by contraction of the dilator of the iris
- May be a normal response to stimuli or drugs

HISTORY

- Ask about other eye problems, such as pain, blurring, diplopia, or visual field defects.
- Obtain a health history, focusing on incidence of eye or head trauma, glaucoma and other ocular problems, and neurologic and vascular disorders.
- Obtain a complete drug history.

PHYSICAL ASSESSMENT

- Inspect and compare the pupils' size, color, and shape. (See *Grading pupil size*.)
- Test each pupil for light reflex, consensual response, and accommodation.
- Perform a swinging flashlight test to evaluate a decreased response to direct light coupled with a normal consensual response.
- Check eyes for ptosis, swelling, and ecchymosis.
- Test visual acuity in both eyes with and without correction.
- Evaluate extraocular muscle function by checking the six cardinal fields of gaze.

CAUSES

MEDICAL
Aortic arch syndrome
- Mydriasis in both eyes occurs late due to decreased circulation.
- Related ocular signs and symptoms include visual blurring, transient vision loss, and diplopia.
- Other signs and symptoms include dizziness and syncope; neck, shoulder, and chest pain; bruits; loss of radial and carotid pulses; paresthesia; intermittent claudication; and, possibly, decreased blood pressure in the arms.

Carotid artery aneurysm
- Mydriasis in one eye may be accompanied by bitemporal hemianopsia, decreased visual acuity, hemiplegia, decreased level of consciousness, headache, aphasia, behavioral changes, and hypoesthesia.

Glaucoma, acute angle-closure
- Moderate mydriasis and loss of pupillary reflex occur with excruciating pain, redness, decreased visual acuity, visual blurring, halo vision, conjunctival injection, a cloudy

 TOP TECHNIQUE

Grading pupil size

To ensure accurate evaluation of pupillary size, compare your patient's pupils to the scale below. Keep in mind that maximum constriction may be less than 1 mm and maximum dilation greater than 9 mm.

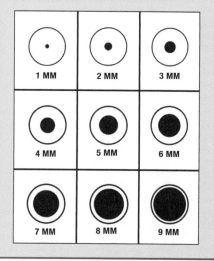

cornea and, in 2 to 5 days without treatment, permanent blindness.

Oculomotor nerve palsy
◆ Mydriasis in one eye is commonly the first sign.
◆ Other signs and symptoms include ptosis, diplopia, decreased pupillary reflexes, exotropia, and complete loss of accommodation.

Traumatic iridoplegia
◆ Mydriasis and loss of pupillary reflex (caused by paralysis of sphincter of iris) are usually transient.
◆ Other signs and symptoms include a quivering iris, ecchymosis, pain, and swelling.

OTHER
Drugs
◆ Mydriasis can be caused by anesthesia induction, anticholinergics, antihistamines, sympathomimetics, barbiturates (overdose), estrogens, and tricyclic antidepressants.
◆ Topical mydriatic drugs and cycloplegics are given for their mydriatic effect.

Surgery
◆ Traumatic mydriasis commonly results from ocular surgery.

NURSING CONSIDERATIONS
◆ If the patient is experiencing photophobia, darken the room, and encourage the patient to close or shade his eyes or wear sunglasses.
◆ Administer eye drops or ointments, as prescribed.

PEDIATRIC POINTERS
◆ Mydriasis occurs in children as a result of ocular trauma, drugs, Adie's syndrome and, most commonly, increased intracranial pressure.

PATIENT TEACHING
◆ Discuss the effects of mydriatic drugs and reducing their adverse effects.
◆ Teach about the underlying diagnosis and treatment plan.

Myoclonus

- Involves sudden, shock-like contractions of the muscles
- May be isolated or repetitive, rhythmic or arrhythmic, symmetrical or asymmetrical, synchronous or asynchronous, generalized or focal
- May be triggered by certain stimuli

✦ **ACTION STAT!** *Check for seizure activity. Take vital signs to rule out arrhythmias or a blocked airway. If the patient has a seizure, gently help him lie down. Place a pillow or a rolled-up towel under the head to prevent concussion. Loosen any constrictive clothing, especially around the neck, and turn the head to one side to prevent airway occlusion or aspiration of secretions.*

HISTORY

- Ask about the frequency, severity, location, and circumstances of myoclonus.
- Determine whether the patient has had previous seizures.
- Find out what causes the patient's myoclonus.

PHYSICAL ASSESSMENT

- Evaluate level of consciousness (LOC) and mental condition.
- Check for muscle rigidity and wasting.
- Test for deep tendon reflexes.
- Complete neurologic and musculoskeletal assessments.

CAUSES

MEDICAL
Alzheimer's disease
- Generalized myoclonus may occur in advanced stages.
- Other late signs and symptoms include mild choreoathetoid movements, muscle rigidity, bowel and bladder incontinence, delusions, and hallucinations.

Creutzfeldt-Jakob disease
- Diffuse myoclonic jerks are initially random; they gradually become rhythmic and symmetrical in response to sensory stimuli in this progressive neurologic disease.
- Other signs and symptoms include ataxia, aphasia, hearing loss, muscle rigidity and wasting, fasciculations, hemiplegia, vision disturbances and, possibly, blindness.

Encephalitis, viral
- Myoclonus is intermittent.
- Other signs and symptoms vary but may include rapidly decreasing LOC, fever, headache, irritability, nuchal rigidity, vomiting, seizures, aphasia, ataxia, hemiparesis, facial muscle weakness, nystagmus, ocular palsies, and dysphagia.

Encephalopathy
- In hepatic encephalopathy, myoclonic jerks are produced in association with asterixis and focal or generalized seizures.
- In hypoxic encephalopathy, generalized myoclonus or seizures occur almost immediately after restoration of cardiopulmonary function.
- In uremic encephalopathy, myoclonic jerks and seizures are common.

Epilepsy

◆ With idiopathic epilepsy, localized myoclonus usually occurs singly or in short bursts in an arm or leg upon awakening.
◆ With myoclonic epilepsy, myoclonus is initially infrequent and localized but becomes more frequent and generalized over a period of months.

OTHER
Drug withdrawal

◆ Myoclonus may be seen in patients with alcohol, opioid, or sedative withdrawal or alcohol withdrawal delirium.

Poisoning

◆ Acute intoxication with methylbromide, bismuth, or strychnine may produce an acute onset of myoclonus and confusion.

NURSING CONSIDERATIONS

◆ If myoclonus is progressive, take seizure precautions.
◆ Keep an oral airway and suction equipment at the bedside.
◆ Pad the bed's side rails and remove potentially harmful objects.
◆ Remain with the patient while he walks.
◆ Give drugs that suppress myoclonus, as ordered.

PEDIATRIC POINTERS

◆ Myoclonus may result from subacute sclerosing panencephalitis, severe meningitis, progressive poliodystrophy, childhood myoclonic epilepsy, and encephalopathies.

PATIENT TEACHING

◆ Disuss underlying condition, diagnostic tests, and treatment options.
◆ Talk with the patient about taking safety measures and seizure precautions.
◆ Refer the patient to social service or community resources, as needed.
◆ Teach the patient about prescribed medications.

Nasal flaring

◆ Abnormal dilation of the nostrils

ACTION STAT! *If you note nasal flaring in the patient, quickly evaluate his respiratory status. Absent breath sounds, cyanosis, diaphoresis, and tachycardia point to complete airway obstruction. As necessary, deliver back blows or abdominal thrusts (Heimlich maneuver) to relieve the obstruction. If these don't clear the airway, emergency intubation or tracheostomy and mechanical ventilation may be necessary.*

If the patient's airway isn't obstructed but he displays breathing difficulty, give oxygen by nasal cannula or face mask. Intubation and mechanical ventilation may be necessary. Insert an I.V. line for fluid and drug administration. Begin cardiac monitoring. Obtain a chest X-ray and samples for arterial blood gas (ABG) analysis and electrolyte studies.

HISTORY

◆ Obtain a pertinent history, including incidence of cardiac and pulmonary disorders such as asthma, allergies, respiratory tract infection, or trauma.
◆ Obtain a smoking and drug history.

PHYSICAL ASSESSMENT

◆ Take vital signs.
◆ Auscultate breath sounds.

CAUSES

MEDICAL

Acute respiratory distress syndrome (ARDS)

◆ ARDS causes increased respiratory difficulty and hypoxemia, with nasal flaring, dyspnea, tachypnea, diaphoresis, cyanosis, scattered crackles, rhonchi, wheezing, and use of accessory muscles. It also produces tachycardia, anxiety, and a decreased level of consciousness (LOC).

Airway obstruction

◆ Complete obstruction above the tracheal bifurcation causes sudden nasal flaring; absent breath sounds, despite intercostal retractions and marked accessory muscle use; tachycardia; diaphoresis; cyanosis; a decreasing LOC; and, eventually, respiratory arrest.
◆ Partial obstruction causes nasal flaring with inspiratory stridor, gagging, wheezing, a violent cough, marked accessory muscle use, agitation, cyanosis, and hoarseness.

Anaphylaxis

◆ Severe reactions can produce respiratory distress with nasal flaring, stridor, wheezing, accessory muscle use, intercostal retractions, and chest tightness.
◆ Associated signs and symptoms include nasal congestion, sneezing, pruritus, urticaria, erythema, diaphoresis, angioedema, weakness, hoarseness, dysphagia and, rarely, vomiting, nausea, diarrhea, urinary urgency, and incontinence.
◆ Cardiac arrhythmias, hypotension, and signs of shock may occur late.

Asthma, acute

◆ An asthma attack can cause nasal flaring, dyspnea, tachypnea, prolonged expiratory wheezing, accessory muscle use, cyanosis, and a dry or productive cough.
◆ Auscultation may reveal rhonchi, crackles, wheezing, and decreased or absent breath sounds.
◆ Other signs and symptoms include anxiety, tachycardia, and increased blood pressure.

Chronic obstructive pulmonary disease (COPD)

◆ Nasal flaring is accompanied by prolonged pursed-lip expiration; accessory muscle use; a loose, rattling, productive cough; cyanosis; reduced chest expansion; crackles; rhonchi; wheezing; and dyspnea.
◆ COPD can lead to acute respiratory failure secondary to pulmonary infection or edema.

Pneumothorax

◆ Pneumothorax is an acute disorder that can result in respiratory distress with nasal flaring, dyspnea, tachypnea, shallow respirations, hyperresonance or tympany on percussion, agitation, jugular vein distention, tracheal deviation, and cyanosis.

- Breath sounds may be decreased or absent on the affected side; similarly, chest wall motion may be decreased on the affected side and mediastinal or tracheal shift may occur.
- Other signs and symptoms typically include sharp chest pain, tachycardia, hypotension, cold and clammy skin, diaphoresis, subcutaneous crepitation, and anxiety.

Pulmonary edema
- Pulmonary edema typically produces nasal flaring, severe dyspnea, wheezing, and a cough that produces frothy, pink sputum. Increased accessory muscle use may occur with tachycardia, cyanosis, hypotension, crackles, jugular vein distention, peripheral edema, and a decreased LOC.

Pulmonary embolus
- A potentially life-threatening disorder, nasal flaring may be accompanied by dyspnea, tachypnea, wheezing, cyanosis, a pleural friction rub, and a productive cough (possibly hemoptysis).
- Other signs and symptoms include sudden chest tightness or pleuritic pain, tachycardia, atrial arrhythmias, hypotension, a low-grade fever, syncope, marked anxiety, and restlessness.

OTHER
Diagnostic tests
- Pulmonary function tests, such as vital capacity testing, can produce nasal flaring with forced inspiration or expiration.

Treatments
- Certain respiratory treatments, such as deep breathing, can cause nasal flaring.

NURSING CONSIDERATIONS

- To help ease breathing, place the patient in high Fowler's position.
- If he's at risk for aspirating secretions, place him in a modified Trendelenburg's or side-lying position.
- Suction frequently to remove oropharyngeal secretions, if necessary.
- Administer humidified oxygen to thin secretions and decrease airway drying and irritation. Provide adequate hydration to liquefy secretions.
- Reposition the patient every hour, and encourage coughing and deep breathing.
- Avoid administering sedatives or opiates, which can depress the cough reflex or respirations.
- Continually assess the patient's respiratory status, and check his vital signs and oxygen saturation every 30 minutes, or as necessary.

PEDIATRIC POINTERS
- Nasal flaring is an important sign of respiratory distress in infants and very young children, who can't verbalize their discomfort.
- Common causes include airway obstruction, hyaline membrane disease, croup, and acute epiglottiditis.
- The use of a croup tent may improve oxygenation and humidification for such patients.

PATIENT TEACHING

- Teach the patient about underlying diagnosis and treatment plan.
- Prepare the patient for diagnostic tests, such as chest X-rays, a lung scan, pulmonary arteriography, sputum culture, complete blood count, ABG analysis, and 12-lead electrocardiogram.
- Teach about prescribed medications.
- Teach about the importance of proper positioning.
- Teach the patient how to do coughing and deep breathing exercises.

Nasal obstruction

OVERVIEW

- Typically benign, but may cause discomfort or voice changes or alter sense of taste and smell
- May result from an allergic, inflammatory, neoplastic, endocrine, or metabolic disorder; a structural abnormality; a traumatic injury; or a foreign object

HISTORY

- Ask about the onset, duration, frequency, and description of obstruction.
- Inquire about associated drainage, sinus pain, or headaches.
- Take a drug and alcohol history.
- Find out about previous trauma or surgery.
- Ask about recent travel.

PHYSICAL ASSESSMENT

- Assess airflow and the condition of the turbinates and nasal septum.
- Evaluate the orbits for any evidence of decreased vision, excess tearing, or abnormal appearance of the eye.
- Palpate over the frontal and maxillary sinuses for tenderness.
- Examine the ears for effusions.
- Inspect the oral cavity, pharynx, nasopharynx, and larynx.
- Palpate the neck for adenopathy.

CAUSES

MEDICAL

Basilar skull fracture
- Cerebrospinal fluid rhinorrhea may develop.
- Related signs and symptoms include epistaxis, otorrhea, and a bulging tympanic membrane from blood or fluid.
- Other signs and symptoms include headache, facial paralysis, nausea, vomiting, impaired eye movement, ocular deviation, vision and hearing loss, depressed level of consciousness, Battle's sign, and raccoon eyes.

Common cold
- Watery discharge, sneezing, and nasal obstruction occur.
- Other signs and symptoms include sinus pain, reduced sense of taste and smell, sore throat, malaise, myalgia, arthralgia, and mild headache.

Hypothyroidism
- Nasal obstruction may occur due to vasodilation in the nasal mucosa.
- Other signs and symptoms include fatigue, weight gain despite anorexia, cold intolerance, pallor, facial edema, impaired memory, brittle hair, thick skin and tongue, bradycardia, and a hoarse voice.

Nasal deformities
- A deviated nasal septum may cause nasal obstruction.
- A perforated nasal septum may cause a sensation of nasal congestion due to altered airflow.

Nasal fracture
- Mucosal swelling, epistaxis, abscess, or a septal deviation caused by trauma results in nasal obstruction.
- Other signs and symptoms include periorbital ecchymoses and edema, nasal deformity and pain, and crepitation of the nasal bones.

Nasal polyps
- Nasal obstruction, anosmia, and clear, watery drainage develop.
- Translucent, pear-shaped polyps occur.

Nasal tumors
- Nasal obstruction, rhinorrhea, epistaxis, pain, foul discharge, and cheek swelling may occur.

Nasopharyngeal tumors
- Nasal obstruction, rhinorrhea, epistaxis, otitis media, and nasal speech may occur.
- Neck mass or conductive hearing loss may be the first sign of cancer.

Pregnancy

◆ Vascular engorgement of the mucosa results in obstruction.
◆ Other signs and symptoms include clear or blood-tinged drainage, sneezing, and edematous and bluish turbinates.

Rhinitis

◆ Allergic rhinitis produces watery discharge and nasal obstruction as well as sneezing, increased lacrimation, decreased sense of smell, postnasal drip, and itching of the eyes, nose, and ears.
◆ Vasomotor rhinitis produces a profuse, watery nasal discharge and nasal obstruction as well as sneezing, postnasal drip, and swollen turbinates.
◆ Atrophic rhinitis produces chronic and continuous nasal obstruction along with intermittent, foul-smelling, purulent drainage.

Sinusitis

◆ Acute sinusitis produces marked nasal obstruction along with fever, severe pain over the involved sinuses, and thick, purulent drainage.
◆ Chronic sinusitis produces persistent or recurrent nasal obstruction as well as thick, intermittently purulent rhinorrhea and discomfort over the involved sinuses.

Wegener's granulomatosis

◆ Besides nasal obstruction, other nasal signs and symptoms include paranasal sinus pain, crusting, epistaxis, mucopurulent discharge, and cartilaginous necrosis of the septum and bridge of the nose.

OTHER

Drugs

◆ Topical nasal vasoconstrictors may cause rebound rhinorrhea and nasal obstruction.
◆ Antihypertensives may cause nasal congestion.

Surgery

◆ Nasal obstruction may occur after sinus or cranial surgery or rhinoplasty.

NURSING CONSIDERATIONS

◆ Promote fluid intake to thin secretions, as needed.
◆ Give an antihistamine, a decongestant, an analgesic, or an antipyretic, as prescribed.

PEDIATRIC POINTERS

◆ Acute nasal obstruction in children commonly results from the common cold; chronic obstruction typically results from large adenoids.
◆ In neonates, choanal atresia is the most common congenital cause of nasal obstruction.
◆ Cystic fibrosis may cause nasal polyps, resulting in obstruction.

PATIENT TEACHING

◆ Disuss underlying condition, diagnostic tests, and treatment options.
◆ Teach the patient proper use of nasal vasoconstrictor sprays.
◆ Explain activity restrictions to a patient requiring surgery.

Nausea

- Sensation of profound revulsion to food or of impending vomiting

HISTORY

- Ask about the onset and description of nausea.
- Determine aggravating or alleviating factors.
- Obtain a medical history, including incidence of GI, endocrine, and metabolic disorders; cancer; and infections.
- Ask about vomiting, abdominal pain, and changes in bowel habits.
- Ask about the possibility of pregnancy.

PHYSICAL ASSESSMENT

- Inspect the skin for jaundice, bruises, and spider angiomas; assess skin turgor.
- Inspect for abdominal distention.
- Auscultate for bowel sounds and bruits.
- Palpate for abdominal rigidity and tenderness and test for rebound tenderness.
- Palpate and percuss the liver.

CAUSES

MEDICAL

Anthrax, GI
- Initial signs and symptoms include nausea, vomiting, loss of appetite, and fever which may progress to abdominal pain, severe bloody diarrhea, and hematemesis.

Appendicitis
- A brief period of nausea may accompany onset of abdominal pain.
- Other signs and symptoms include abdominal rigidity and tenderness, cutaneous hyperalgesia, fever, constipation or diarrhea, tachycardia, anorexia, and malaise.

Cholecystitis, acute
- Nausea typically follows severe right-upper-quadrant pain that may radiate to the back or shoulders, commonly after meals.
- Other signs and symptoms include vomiting, flatulence, abdominal tenderness, rigidity and distention, fever with chills, diaphoresis, and a positive Murphy's sign.

Cholelithiasis
- Nausea accompanies severe right-upper-quadrant or epigastric pain.
- Other signs and symptoms include vomiting, abdominal tenderness and guarding, flatulence, belching, epigastric burning, tachycardia, restlessness and, with occlusion of the common bile duct, jaundice, clay-colored stools, fever, and chills.

Cirrhosis
- Nausea, vomiting, anorexia, abdominal pain, and constipation or diarrhea occur.
- As the disease progresses, jaundice and hepatomegaly may occur with abdominal distention, spider angiomas, fetor hepaticus, enlarged superficial abdominal veins, and mental changes.

Diverticulitis
- Nausea, intermittent crampy abdominal pain, constipation or diarrhea, low-grade fever and, in many cases, a palpable, fixed mass occur.
- Other signs and symptoms include anorexia, bloody stools, and flatulence.

Electrolyte imbalances
- Nausea and vomiting occur with cardiac arrhythmias, tremors or seizures, anorexia, malaise, and weakness.

Escherichia coli 0157:H7
- Nausea, watery or bloody diarrhea, vomiting, fever, and abdominal cramps occur.

Gastritis
- Nausea is common, especially after ingestion of alcohol, aspirin, spicy foods, or caffeine.
- Vomiting, epigastric pain, belching, and malaise may also occur.

Gastroenteritis
- Nausea, vomiting, diarrhea, and abdominal cramping occur.
- Other signs and symptoms include fever, malaise, hyperactive bowel sounds, abdominal pain and tenderness, and signs of dehydration and electrolyte imbalance.

Hepatitis
- Nausea is an early symptom.
- Vomiting, fatigue, myalgia, arthralgia, headache, anorexia, photophobia, pharyngitis, cough, and fever also occur early in the preicteric phase.

Hyperemesis gravidarum
- Unremitting nausea and vomiting persist beyond the first trimester of pregnancy.
- Other signs and symptoms include weight loss, signs of dehydration, headache, and delirium.

Inflammatory bowel disease
- Nausea, vomiting, abdominal pain, and anorexia may occur, but the most common sign is recurrent diarrhea with blood, pus, and mucus.

Intestinal obstruction

◆ Nausea, vomiting, constipation, and abdominal pain occur.
◆ Other signs and symptoms include abdominal distention and tenderness, visible peristaltic waves, and hyperactive (in partial obstruction) or hypoactive or absent bowel sounds (in complete obstruction).

Irritable bowel syndrome

◆ Nausea, dyspepsia, and abdominal distention may occur.
◆ Other signs and symptoms include lower abdominal pain and tenderness relieved by defecation, diurnal diarrhea alternating with constipation or normal bowel function, small stools with visible mucus, and a feeling of incomplete evacuation.

Labyrinthitis

◆ Nausea and vomiting occur with vertigo, progressive hearing loss, nystagmus, and tinnitus.

Lactose intolerance

◆ Nausea, diarrhea, cramps, bloating, and gas occur after eating dairy products.

Ménière's disease

◆ Sudden, brief, recurrent attacks of nausea, vomiting, vertigo, tinnitus, nystagmus and, eventually, hearing loss occur.

Metabolic acidosis

◆ Nausea, vomiting, anorexia, diarrhea, Kussmaul's respirations, and decreased level of consciousness may develop.

Migraine headache

◆ Nausea and vomiting may occur along with photophobia, light flashes, increased sensitivity to noise, light-headedness, partial vision loss, and paresthesia of the lips, face, and hands.

Motion sickness

◆ Nausea and vomiting occur along with possible headache, dizziness, fatigue, diaphoresis, hypersalivation, and dyspnea.

Myocardial infarction

◆ Nausea and vomiting may occur, but the cardinal symptom is severe substernal chest pain that may radiate to the left arm, jaw, or neck.
◆ Other signs and symptoms include dyspnea, pallor, clammy skin, diaphoresis, altered blood pressure, and arrhythmias.

Pancreatitis, acute

◆ Nausea, usually followed by vomiting, is an early symptom.
◆ Other signs and symptoms include severe upper abdominal pain that may radiate to the back; abdominal tenderness and rigidity; anorexia; diminished bowel sounds; and fever.

Peptic ulcer

◆ Nausea and vomiting follow attacks of sharp or gnawing, burning epigastric pain when the stomach is empty or after ingesting alcohol, caffeine, or aspirin.

Peritonitis

◆ Nausea and vomiting accompany acute abdominal pain.
◆ Other signs and symptoms include fever, chills, tachycardia, hypoactive or absent bowel sounds, abdominal rigidity and tenderness, diaphoresis, hypotension, and shallow respirations.

Rhabdomyolysis

◆ Nausea, vomiting, fever, malaise, and dark urine are common due to renal damage.
◆ Tenderness, swelling, and muscle weakness or pain may also develop.

Thyrotoxicosis

◆ Nausea and vomiting may accompany severe anxiety, heat intolerance, diaphoresis, diarrhea, tremor, tachycardia, palpitations, fatigue and weakness.
◆ Other signs and symptoms include exophthalmos, ventricular or atrial gallop, and an enlarged thyroid gland.

OTHER
Drugs

◆ Antineoplastics, opiates, ferrous sulfate, levodopa, oral potassium chloride replacements, estrogens, sulfasalazine, antibiotics, quinidine, anesthetics, digoxin, theophylline overdose, and nonsteroidal anti-inflammatory drugs can cause nausea.

Radiation and surgery

◆ Radiation therapy can cause nausea and vomiting.
◆ Postoperative nausea and vomiting is common.

NURSING CONSIDERATIONS

◆ Provide measures to ease the patient's nausea.
◆ Evaluate fluid, electrolyte, and acid-base balance.
◆ Elevate the patient's head or position him on his side.
◆ Be prepared to insert a nasogastric tube, if needed.

PATIENT TEACHING

◆ Discuss what aggravates nausea and how to avoid it.
◆ Teach the patient about underlying diagnosis and treatment plan.

Neck pain

OVERVIEW

- May originate from any neck structure
- May be referred from other areas of the body

 ACTION STAT! *If the patient's neck pain results from trauma, first immobilize the cervical spine, preferably with a long backboard and Philadelphia collar. Take vital signs and perform a quick neurologic examination. Give oxygen, as needed. Intubation or tracheostomy and mechanical ventilation may be necessary. Ask how the injury occurred. Examine the neck for abrasions, swelling, lacerations, erythema, and ecchymoses.*

HISTORY

- Find out about the onset and description of pain.
- Ask about alleviating, aggravating, or precipitating factors.
- Find out about associated symptoms such as headache.
- Obtain a medical and drug history.

PHYSICAL ASSESSMENT

- Inspect the neck, shoulders, and cervical spine for swelling, masses, erythema, and ecchymoses.
- Assess active range-of-motion (ROM) in the neck and note any pain.
- Examine posture.
- Test and compare bilateral muscle strength and sensation.
- Assess hand grasp and arm reflexes.
- If the patient's condition permits, test for Brudzinski's and Kernig's signs.
- Palpate the cervical lymph nodes for enlargement.

CAUSES

MEDICAL

Cervical extension injury
- Anterior pain usually diminishes within several days after injury.
- Posterior pain persists and may even intensify.
- Other signs and symptoms include tenderness, swelling and nuchal rigidity, arm or back pain, occipital headache, muscle spasms, visual blurring, and unilateral miosis on the affected side.

Cervical spine fracture
- Severe neck pain may occur with intense occipital headache, quadriplegia, deformity, and respiratory paralysis.

Cervical spine tumor
- Metastatic tumors typically produce persistent neck pain; primary tumors cause mild to severe pain along a specific nerve root.
- Other signs and symptoms may include paresthesia, arm and leg weakness that progresses to atrophy and paralysis, and bowel and bladder incontinence.

Cervical spondylosis
- Posterior neck pain that may radiate is aggravated by and restricts movement.
- Other signs and symptoms include paresthesia, weakness, and stiffness.

Cervical stenosis
- Neck and arm pain, paresthesia, muscle weakness or paralysis, gait and balance problems, and decreased ROM may occur.

Herniated cervical disk
- Variable neck pain that's referred along a specific dermatome is aggravated by and restricts movement.
- Paresthesia and other sensory disturbances and arm weakness may also occur.

Hodgkin's disease
- Generalized pain may eventually affect the neck.
- Lymphadenopathy, the classic sign, may accompany paresthesia, muscle weakness, fever, fatigue, weight loss, malaise, and hepatomegaly.

Laryngeal cancer
- Neck pain radiating to the ear is a late sign.
- Other signs and symptoms include dysphagia, dyspnea, hemoptysis, stridor, hoarseness, and cervical lymphadenopathy.

Lymphadenitis
- Enlarged and inflamed cervical lymph nodes cause acute pain.
- Fever, chills, and malaise may also occur.

Meningitis
- Neck pain may accompany nuchal rigidity.
- Other signs and symptoms include fever, headache, photophobia, positive Brudzinski's and Kernig's signs, and decreased level of consciousness (LOC).

Neck sprain
- Pain, slight swelling, stiffness, and restricted ROM result.

◆ Ligament rupture causes severe pain, marked swelling, ecchymosis, muscle spasms, and nuchal rigidity with head tilt.

Paget's disease
◆ Cervical vertebrae deformity may produce severe neck pain, paresthesia, and arm weakness as the disease progresses.

Rheumatoid arthritis
◆ Moderate to severe pain may radiate along a specific nerve root.
◆ Other signs and symptoms include increasingly stiff joints; paresthesia; muscle weakness; low-grade fever; anorexia; malaise; fatigue; neck deformity; and warmth, swelling, and tenderness in involved joints.

Spinous process fracture
◆ Fracture near the cervicothoracic junction produces acute pain that radiates to shoulders.
◆ Other signs and symptoms include swelling, tenderness, restricted ROM, muscle spasm, and deformity.

Subarachnoid hemorrhage
◆ A life-threatening condition, moderate to severe neck pain and rigidity, headache, and decreased LOC may occur.
◆ Kernig's and Brudzinski's signs are present.

Torticollis
◆ Severe neck pain accompanies recurrent, unilateral muscle stiffness and spasms, followed by a momentary twitching or contraction that pulls the head to the affected side.

Tracheal trauma
◆ Torn tracheal mucosa produces mild to moderate pain and may result in airway occlusion, hemoptysis, hoarseness, and dysphagia.

NURSING CONSIDERATIONS

◆ Give an anti-inflammatory and an analgesic, as needed.
◆ Apply a cervical collar, as appropriate. (See *Applying a Philadelphia collar*.)
◆ Neck trauma may not initially produce a lot of pain; however, immobilization is necessary until significant injury is ruled out.

PEDIATRIC POINTERS
◆ The most common causes of neck pain in children are meningitis and trauma.

PATIENT TEACHING

◆ Explain any activities the patient needs to limit.
◆ Teach the patient to apply the cervical collar, if needed.
◆ Provide reinforcement for exercises the patient needs to perform.
◆ Discuss underlying diagnosis, diagnostic tests, and treatment options.

Applying a Philadelphia collar

A lightweight, molded polyethylene collar designed to hold the neck straight with the chin slightly elevated and tucked in, the Philadelphia cervical collar immobilizes the cervical spine, decreases muscle spasms, and relieves some pain. It also prevents further injury and promotes healing. When applying the collar, fit it snugly around the patient's neck and attach the Velcro fasteners or buckles at the back. Check the patient's airway and his neurovascular status to ensure that the collar isn't too tight. Also, make sure that the collar isn't placed too high in front, which can hyperextend the neck. In a patient with a neck sprain, hyperextension may cause the ligaments to heal in a shortened position; in a patient with a cervical spine fracture, it could cause serious neurologic damage.

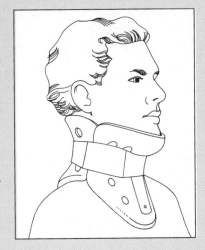

Nipple discharge

OVERVIEW

- Characterized as intermittent or constant, unilateral or bilateral, and by color, consistency, and composition
- Relatively common and often normal in parous women
- Galactorrhea: abnormal flow of milk from the breast other than normal lactation

HISTORY

- Ask about the onset, duration, and description of discharge.
- Inquire about associated pain, tenderness, itching, warmth, and changes in breast or nipple contour.
- Ask about use of herbs; some have estrogenic effects and cause nipple discharge as an adverse effect.
- Determine the onset and growth of any breast lumps.
- Find out about the use of hormones.
- Obtain a complete gynecologic and obstetric history.
- Determine the patient's normal menstrual cycle and date of last menses.
- Ask about breast swelling and tenderness, bloating, irritability, headaches, abdominal cramping, nausea, or diarrhea related to menses.
- Assess her risk factors for breast cancer.

PHYSICAL ASSESSMENT

- Characterize the discharge. (See *Eliciting nipple discharge*.)
- Inspect the nipples for deviation, flattening, retraction, redness, asymmetry, thickening, excoriation, erosion, or cracking.
- Inspect the breasts for asymmetry, irregular contours, dimpling, erythema, and peau d'orange.
- With the patient in a supine position, palpate breasts and axillae for lumps.
- Note the size, location, delineation, consistency, and mobility of any lumps.

CAUSES

MEDICAL
Breast abscess
- A thick, purulent discharge may be produced from a cracked nipple or an infected duct.
- Other signs and symptoms include abrupt onset of high fever with chills; breast pain, tenderness, and erythema; a palpable soft nodule or generalized induration; and nipple retraction.

Breast cancer
- Bloody, watery, or purulent discharge may emit from a normal-appearing nipple.
- Characteristic signs and symptoms include a hard, irregular, fixed lump; erythema; dimpling; peau d'orange; changes in contour; nipple deviation, flattening, or retraction; axillary lymphadenopathy; and breast pain.

Choriocarcinoma
- A white or grayish milky discharge may occur with persistent uterine bleeding and bogginess, and vaginal masses.

 TOP TECHNIQUE

Eliciting nipple discharge

If your patient has a history or evidence of nipple discharge, you can attempt to elicit it during your examination. Help the patient into a supine position, and gently squeeze the nipple between your thumb and index finger (as shown below left); note any discharge through the nipple. Then place your fingers on the areola, as shown below right, and palpate the entire areolar surface, watching for any discharge through areolar ducts.

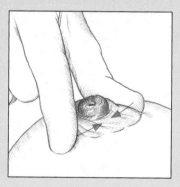 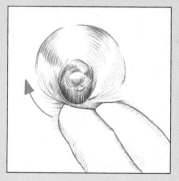

Herpes zoster
- Bilateral, spontaneous, intermittent galactorrhea may occur.
- Other characteristic signs and symptoms include shooting or burning pain; eruption of small red nodules or vesicles on the thorax and, possibly, the arms and legs; headache; fever; malaise; and pruritus, paresthesia, or hyperesthesia in affected areas.

Intraductal papilloma
- Discharge is unilateral, serous, serosanguineous, or bloody from only one duct.
- Subareolar nodules, breast pain, and tenderness may occur.

Mammary duct ectasia
- A thick, sticky, grayish discharge from multiple ducts may be the first sign; discharge may be bilateral and is usually spontaneous.
- Other signs and symptoms include a rubbery, poorly delineated lump beneath the areola, with a blue-green discoloration of the overlying skin; nipple retraction; and redness, swelling, tenderness, and burning pain in the areola and nipple.

Paget's disease
- Serous or bloody unilateral discharge emits from denuded skin on the nipple, which is red, intensely itchy and, possibly, eroded or excoriated.

Prolactin-secreting pituitary tumor
- Bilateral galactorrhea may occur.
- Other signs and symptoms include amenorrhea, infertility, decreased libido, vaginal secretions, headaches, and blindness.

Proliferative (fibrocystic) breast disease
- Bilateral clear, milky, or straw-colored discharge occurs.
- Multiple round, soft, tender, mobile nodules are palpable on both breasts in the upper outer quadrants.
- Nodule size, tenderness, and discharge increase during the luteal phase of the menstrual cycle.

Trauma
- Bilateral galactorrhea can result from trauma to the breasts.
- Other signs and symptoms vary with the cause and severity of trauma but may include chest pain; dyspnea; bruising; flail chest; cardiac tamponade; pulmonary artery tears; ventricular rupture; shock; and bronchial, tracheal, or esophageal tears.

OTHER
Drugs
- Antihypertensives, cimetidine, hormonal contraceptives, metoclopramide, psychotropic agents, or verapamil may cause galactorrhea.

Surgery
- Chest wall surgery may stimulate thoracic nerves, causing intermittent bilateral galactorrhea.

NURSING CONSIDERATIONS
- Clearly explain the nature and origin of the discharge.
- Apply a breast binder.

PEDIATRIC POINTERS
- Nipple discharge in children and adolescents is rare.
- Infants may produce a milky discharge between 3 days and 2 weeks after birth due to maternal hormonal influences.

GERIATRIC POINTERS
- In postmenopausal women, breast changes are considered malignant until proven otherwise.

PATIENT TEACHING
- Discuss underlying condition, diagnostic tests, and treatment options.
- Explain the importance of being aware of discharge characteristics.
- Explain when to seek medical attention.
- Discuss the importance of breast self-examinations, medical appointments, and mammograms.

Nipple retraction

OVERVIEW

- Inward displacement of the nipple below the level of surrounding breast tissue
- Results from scar tissue formation within a lesion or large mammary duct

HISTORY

- Ask the patient when she first noticed the nipple retraction and if she has experienced other nipple changes, such as itching, discoloration, discharge, or excoriation.
- Ask about breast pain, lumps, redness, swelling, or warmth.
- Obtain a history, noting risk factors for breast cancer, such as a family history or previous malignancy.

PHYSICAL ASSESSMENT

- Examine both nipples and breasts with the patient sitting upright with her arms at her sides, with her hands pressing on her hips, with her arms overhead, and leaning forward so her breasts hang. Look for redness, excoriation, and discharge; nipple flattening and deviation; and breast asymmetry, dimpling, or contour differences. (See *Differentiating nipple retraction from inversion.*)
- Try to evert the nipple by gently squeezing the areola.
- With the patient in a supine position, palpate both breasts for lumps, especially beneath the areola.
- Mold breast skin over the lump or gently pull it up toward the clavicle, looking for accentuated nipple retraction.
- Palpate axillary lymph nodes.

Differentiating nipple retraction from inversion

Nipple retraction is sometimes confused with nipple inversion, a common abnormality that's congenital in many patients and doesn't usually signal underlying disease. A retracted nipple (left) appears flat and broad, whereas an inverted nipple (right) can be pulled out from the sulcus where it hides.

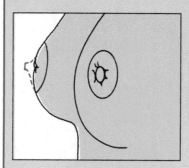 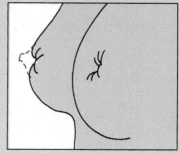

CAUSES

MEDICAL
Breast abscess
◆ Breast abscess, most common in breast-feeding women, occasionally produces unilateral nipple retraction.
◆ Other signs and symptoms include a high fever with chills; breast pain, erythema, and tenderness; breast induration or a soft mass; and cracked, sore nipples, possibly with a purulent discharge.

Breast cancer
◆ Unilateral nipple retraction is commonly accompanied by a hard, fixed, nontender nodule beneath the areola as well as other breast nodules.
◆ Other nipple changes include itching, burning, erosion, and watery or bloody discharge.
◆ Breast changes commonly include dimpling, altered contour, peau d'orange, ulceration, tenderness (possibly pain), redness, and warmth. Axillary lymph nodes may be enlarged.

Mammary duct ectasia
◆ Nipple retraction commonly occurs along with a poorly defined, rubbery nodule beneath the areola, with a blue-green skin discoloration; areolar burning, itching, swelling, tenderness, and erythema; and nipple pain with a thick, sticky, grayish, multiductal discharge.

Mastitis
◆ Nipple retraction, deviation, cracking, or flattening may occur with a firm and indurated or tender, flocculent, discrete breast nodule; warmth; erythema; tenderness; and edema.
◆ Fatigue, high fevers, and chills also may be present.

OTHER
Surgery
◆ Previous breast surgery may cause underlying scarring and retraction.

NURSING CONSIDERATIONS

◆ Prepare the patient for diagnostic tests, including mammography, cytology of nipple discharge, and biopsy.

PEDIATRIC POINTERS
◆ Nipple retraction doesn't occur in prepubescent females.

PATIENT TEACHING

◆ Teach your patient breast self-examination.
◆ Teach her to seek medical evaluation when breast changes occur.
◆ Teach about underlying diagnosis and treatment plan.

Nocturia

- Excessive urination of 500 ml or more at night
- Urination may occur one or more times during the night

HISTORY

- Ask about the onset, frequency, and pattern of nocturia.
- Inquire about precipitating factors.
- Determine the volume voided.
- Find out about associated color, odor, or consistency changes of urine.
- Note the pattern of fluid intake, including use of caffeinated and alcoholic beverages.
- Review associated pain, burning, difficulty urinating, and costovertebral angle (CVA) tenderness.
- Obtain a medical history, including a personal or family history of renal or urinary tract disorders, or endocrine and metabolic diseases.
- Obtain a drug history, noting use and timing of diuretics, a cardiac glycoside, or an antihypertensive.

PHYSICAL ASSESSMENT

- Palpate and percuss the kidneys, CVA, and bladder.
- Inspect the urinary meatus.
- Inspect urine specimen for color, odor, and presence of sediment.

CAUSES

MEDICAL
Benign prostatic hyperplasia
- Nocturia occurs along with possible frequency, hesitation, urgency, incontinence, reduced force and caliber of the urine stream, terminal dribbling, hematuria, lower abdominal fullness, perineal pain, and constipation.
- Palpation reveals an enlarged prostate.

Bladder neoplasm
- Nocturia, a late sign, is marked by frequent voiding of small to moderate amounts of urine.
- Characteristic signs and symptoms include hematuria, bladder distention, urinary frequency and urgency; dysuria; pyuria; vomiting; diarrhea; insomnia; and bladder, rectal, flank, back, or leg pain.

Cystitis
- Nocturia is marked by frequent, small voidings and accompanied by dysuria and tenesmus in all forms of cystitis.
- In bacterial cystitis, findings include urinary urgency; hematuria; fatigue; suprapubic, perineal, flank, and lower back pain; and, occasionally, low-grade fever.
- In chronic interstitial cystitis, Hunner's ulcers and gross hematuria may occur.
- In viral cystitis, urinary urgency, hematuria, and fever may develop.

Diabetes insipidus
- Nocturia occurs early and involves periodic voiding of moderate to large amounts of urine.
- Polydipsia and dehydration may also develop.

Diabetes mellitus
- Nocturia, an early sign, is marked by frequent, large voidings.
- Other signs and symptoms include daytime polyuria, polydipsia, polyphagia, frequent urinary tract infections, recurrent yeast infections, vaginitis, weakness, fatigue, weight loss, and signs of dehydration.

Hypercalcemic nephropathy
- Nocturia is marked by periodic voiding of moderate to large amounts of urine.
- Other signs and symptoms include daytime polyuria, polydipsia and, occasionally, hematuria and pyuria.

Hypokalemic nephropathy
- Nocturia is marked by periodic voiding of moderate to large amounts of urine.
- Other signs and symptoms include polydipsia, daytime polyuria, muscle weakness or paralysis, hypoactive bowel sounds, and increased susceptibility to pyelonephritis.

Prostate cancer
- Nocturia occurs late and is characterized by infrequent voidings of moderate amounts of urine.
- Other signs and symptoms include dysuria; difficulty initiating a urine stream; interrupted urine stream; bladder distention; urinary frequency; weight loss; pallor; weakness; perineal pain; constipation; and a hard, irregularly shaped nodular prostate on palpation.

Pyelonephritis, acute

◆ Nocturia is common and is characterized by infrequent voiding of moderate amounts of urine; urine may appear cloudy.
◆ Related signs and symptoms include a high, sustained fever with chills, fatigue, flank pain, CVA tenderness, weakness, dysuria, hematuria, urinary frequency and urgency, and tenesmus.
◆ Occasionally, anorexia, nausea, vomiting, diarrhea, and hypoactive bowel sounds occur.

Renal failure, chronic

◆ Nocturia is characterized by infrequent voiding of moderate amounts of urine and occurs relatively early; oliguria or anuria may also develop.
◆ Other signs and symptoms include fatigue, ammonia breath odor, Kussmaul's respirations, peripheral edema, elevated blood pressure, decreased level of consciousness, confusion, emotional lability, muscle twitching, anorexia, metallic mouth taste, constipation or diarrhea, petechiae, ecchymoses, pruritus, yellow- or bronze-tinged skin, nausea, and vomiting.

OTHER
Drugs

◆ Drugs that mobilize edematous fluid or produce diuresis may cause nocturia.

NURSING CONSIDERATIONS

◆ Maintain fluid balance.
◆ Monitor vital signs, intake and output, and daily weight.
◆ Document frequency of nocturia, amount, and specific gravity.
◆ Plan administration of a diuretic for daytime hours, if possible.
◆ Plan rest periods to compensate for sleep lost.

PEDIATRIC POINTERS

◆ With the exception of prostate disorders, causes of nocturia are generally the same for children and adults.

GERIATRIC POINTERS

◆ Postmenopausal women have decreased bladder elasticity, but urine output remains constant, resulting in nocturia.

PATIENT TEACHING

◆ Explain the importance of reducing fluid intake and voiding before bedtime.
◆ Teach patient about underlying diagnosis and treatment plan.

Nuchal rigidity

◆ Neck stiffness that prevents flexion

■ ***ACTION STAT!*** *After eliciting nuchal rigidity, attempt to elicit Kernig's and Brudzinski's signs. Quickly evaluate the patient's level of consciousness (LOC). Take his vital signs. If you note signs of increased intracranial pressure (ICP), such as increased systolic pressure, bradycardia, and a widened pulse pressure, start an I.V. line for drug administration and deliver oxygen, as necessary. Keep the head of the bed elevated at least 30 degrees. Draw a specimen for blood studies, such as a complete blood count and electrolytes.*

HISTORY

◆ Obtain a patient history, relying on family members if an altered LOC prevents the patient from responding. Ask about the onset and duration of neck stiffness; precipitating factors; associated signs and symptoms, such as a headache, fever, nausea and vomiting; and motor and sensory changes.
◆ Check for a history of hypertension, head trauma, cerebral aneurysm or arteriovenous malformation, endocarditis, recent infection (such as sinusitis or pneumonia), or recent dental work.
◆ Obtain a complete drug history.
◆ If the patient has no other signs of meningeal irritation, ask about a history of arthritis or neck trauma

PHYSICAL ASSESSMENT

◆ Attempt to passively flex the patient's neck and touch his chin to his chest. If nuchal rigidity is present, this maneuver triggers pain and muscle spasms. Make sure that there's no cervical spine misalignment, such as a fracture or dislocation, before testing for nuchal rigidity. Severe spinal cord damage could result.
◆ Inspect the patient's hands for swollen, tender joints, and palpate the neck for pain or tenderness.
◆ Assess neurologic system.

CAUSES

MEDICAL
Cervical arthritis

◆ With cervical arthritis, nuchal rigidity develops gradually. Initially, the patient may complain of neck stiffness in the early morning or after a period of inactivity. Stiffness then becomes increasingly severe and frequent, and may even affect other joints, especially those in the hands.
◆ Pain on movement, especially with lateral motion or head turning, is common.

Encephalitis

◆ Encephalitis is a viral infection that may cause nuchal rigidity accompanied by other signs of meningeal irritation, such as positive Kernig's and Brudzinski's signs.
◆ Usually, nuchal rigidity appears abruptly and is preceded by a headache, vomiting, and fever.
◆ Other signs and symptoms include a rapidly decreasing LOC, progressing from lethargy to coma within 24 to 48 hours of onset, seizures, ataxia, hemiparesis, nystagmus, and cranial nerve palsies, such as dysphagia and ptosis.

Listeriosis

◆ Nuchal rigidity occurs with fever, headache, and a change in the LOC.
◆ Initial signs and symptoms include myalgia, abdominal pain, nausea, vomiting, and diarrhea.
◆ If listeriosis spreads to the nervous system, meningitis may develop.
◆ Listeriosis infection during pregnancy may lead to premature delivery, infection of the neonate, or still birth.

Meningitis

◆ Nuchal rigidity is an early sign of meningitis and is accompanied by other signs of meningeal irritation—positive Kernig's and Brudzinski's signs, hyperreflexia and, possibly, opisthotonos.

◆ Other early signs and symptoms include a fever with chills, confusion, headache, photophobia, irritability, and vomiting; later signs and symptoms include stupor, seizures, and coma.

◆ Cranial nerve involvement may cause ocular palsies, facial weakness, and hearing loss.

◆ An erythematous papular rash occurs in some forms of viral meningitis; a purpuric rash may occur in meningococcal meningitis.

Subarachnoid hemorrhage

◆ Nuchal rigidity develops immediately after bleeding into the subarachnoid space.

◆ Related signs and symptoms include positive Kernig's and Brudzinski's signs; an abrupt onset of a severe headache; photophobia; fever; nausea and vomiting; dizziness; cranial nerve palsies; focal neurologic signs, such as hemiparesis or hemiplegia; and signs of increased ICP, such as bradycardia and altered respirations.

◆ LOC may deteriorate rapidly, possibly progressing to coma.

NURSING CONSIDERATIONS

◆ Prepare the patient for diagnostic tests, such as computed tomography scans, magnetic resonance imaging, and cervical spinal X-rays.

◆ Monitor the patient's vital signs, intake and output, and neurologic status closely.

◆ Avoid routine administration of opioid analgesics because these may mask signs of increasing ICP.

◆ Enforce strict bed rest; keep the head of the bed elevated at least 30 degrees to help minimize ICP.

◆ Assist the patient in finding a comfortable position to obtain adequate rest.

PEDIATRIC POINTERS

◆ Tests for nuchal rigidity are generally less reliable in children, especially in infants.

◆ In younger children, move the head gently in all directions, observing for resistance.

◆ In older children, ask the child to sit upright and touch his chin to his chest. Resistance to this movement may indicate meningeal irritation.

PATIENT TEACHING

◆ Teach the patient about underlying diagnosis and treatment plan.

◆ Teach family members how they can participate in the care of the patient.

Nystagmus

OVERVIEW

- Involuntary oscillations of one or both eyeballs
- May be pendular (equal in rate in both directions) or jerk (fast and then slow) (see *Assessing nystagmus*)
- May be rhythmic and may be horizontal, vertical, rotary, or mixed
- May be transient or sustained and occur spontaneously or on deviation or fixation of the eyes
- Results from pathology in the visual perceptual area, vestibular system, cerebellum, or brain stem

HISTORY

- Ask about the onset, duration, and description of nystagmus.
- Inquire about recent infection of the ear or respiratory tract.
- Note a history of head trauma or cancer.
- Find out about associated vertigo, dizziness, tinnitus, nausea or vomiting, numbness, weakness, bladder dysfunction, and fever.

PHYSICAL ASSESSMENT

- Evaluate level of consciousness (LOC) and vital signs.
- Be alert for signs of increased intracranial pressure (ICP), such as pupillary changes, drowsiness, elevated systolic pressure, and altered respirations.
- Test extraocular muscle function.
- Note when nystagmus occurs as well as its velocity and direction.
- Test reflexes and cranial nerves.
- Evaluate motor and sensory function.

 TOP TECHNIQUE

Assessing nystagmus

The various types of jerk and pendular nystagmus are illustrated here.

Jerk nystagmus
Convergence-retraction nystagmus refers to the irregular jerking of the eyes back into the orbit during upward gaze. It can indicate midbrain tegmental damage.

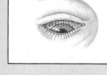

Downbeat nystagmus refers to the irregular downward jerking of the eyes during downward gaze. It can signal lower medullary damage.

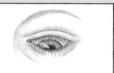

Vestibular nystagmus, the horizontal or rotary movement of the eyes, suggests vestibular disease or cochlear dysfunction.

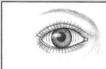

Pendular nystagmus
Horizontal, or pendular, nystagmus refers to oscillations of equal velocity around a center point. It can indicate congenital loss of visual acuity or multiple sclerosis.

Vertical, or seesaw, nystagmus is the rapid, seesaw movement of the eyes: One eye appears to rise while the other appears to fall. It suggests an optic chiasm lesion.

CAUSES

MEDICAL
Encephalitis
◆ Jerk nystagmus is typically accompanied by altered LOC ranging from lethargy to coma.
◆ It may be preceded by sudden onset of fever, headache, and vomiting.
◆ Other signs and symptoms include nuchal rigidity, seizures, aphasia, ataxia, photophobia, and cranial nerve palsies.

Head trauma
◆ Brain stem injury may cause horizontal jerk nystagmus.
◆ Other signs and symptoms include pupillary changes, altered respiratory pattern, coma, and decerebrate posture.

Labyrinthitis, acute
◆ Sudden onset of jerk nystagmus is accompanied by dizziness, vertigo, tinnitus, nausea, and vomiting.
◆ Fast component of the fluctuating nystagmus rate is toward the unaffected ear.
◆ Gradual sensorineural hearing loss may occur.

Ménière's disease
◆ Acute attacks of jerk nystagmus, severe nausea, dizziness, vertigo, progressive hearing loss, and tinnitus occur.
◆ Direction of jerk nystagmus varies from one attack to the next.

Multiple sclerosis
◆ Jerk or pendular nystagmus may occur intermittently.
◆ It may be preceded by diplopia, blurred vision, and paresthesia.
◆ Other signs and symptoms include muscle weakness or paralysis; spasticity; hyperreflexia; intention tremor; gait ataxia; dysphagia; dysarthria; impotence; constipation; emotional instability; and urinary frequency, urgency, and incontinence.

Stroke
◆ A stroke involving the posterior inferior cerebellar artery may cause sudden horizontal or vertical jerk nystagmus that may be gaze dependent.
◆ Other signs and symptoms include dysphagia, dysarthria, loss of pain and temperature sensation in the ipsilateral face and contralateral trunk and limbs, ipsilateral Horner's syndrome, cerebellar signs, and signs of increased ICP.

OTHER
Drugs
◆ Jerk nystagmus may result from barbiturate, phenytoin, or carbamazepine toxicity and alcohol intoxication.

NURSING CONSIDERATIONS

◆ Monitor the patient for changes in neurologic status.
◆ Provide for the patient's safety.

PEDIATRIC POINTERS
◆ In children, pendular nystagmus may be idiopathic, or it may result from early impaired vision associated with certain disorders.

PATIENT TEACHING

◆ Instruct the patient about safety measures.
◆ Caution the patient about the importance of avoiding sudden position changes.
◆ Discuss the underlying diagnosis, diagnostic tests and treatment options.

Ocular deviation

OVERVIEW

- Abnormal eye movement
- May be conjugate (both eyes move together) or disconjugate (one eye moves separately from the other)

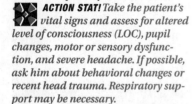 **ACTION STAT!** *Take the patient's vital signs and assess for altered level of consciousness (LOC), pupil changes, motor or sensory dysfunction, and severe headache. If possible, ask him about behavioral changes or recent head trauma. Respiratory support may be necessary.*

HISTORY

- Find out the duration of ocular deviation.
- Ask about associated signs and symptoms, such as double vision, eye pain, headache, motor or sensory changes, or fever.
- Obtain an ocular history, noting recent eye or head trauma or surgery.
- Obtain a medical history, including incidence of hypertension; diabetes; allergies; and thyroid, neurologic, and muscular disorders.

PHYSICAL ASSESSMENT

- Perform a complete neurologic assessment, including a complete eye assessment.
- Observe for partial or complete ptosis.
- Observe for spontaneous head tilts or turns that compensate for ocular deviation.
- Check for eye redness or periorbital edema.
- Assess visual acuity.
- Evaluate extraocular muscle function by testing the six cardinal positions of gaze. (See *Testing the six cardinal positions of gaze.*)

CAUSES

MEDICAL
Brain tumor
- Ocular deviation depends on the site and extent of the tumor.
- Related signs and symptoms include headaches that are most severe in the morning, behavioral changes, memory loss, dizziness, confusion, vision loss, motor and sensory dysfunction, aphasia, signs of hormonal imbalance, and slowly deteriorating LOC from lethargy to coma.
- Other late signs and symptoms include papilledema, vomiting, increased systolic pressure, widening pulse pressure, and decorticate posture.

Cerebral aneurysm
- Typically, ocular deviation and diplopia are the first signs.

- Ptosis and a severe headache (on one side, usually in the front) are other major signs and symptoms.
- With aneurysm rupture, abrupt intensification of pain, nausea, and vomiting occur.
- With bleeding from the site, meningeal irritation, back and leg pain, fever, irritability, seizures, blurred vision, hemiparesis, dysphagia, and visual defects may develop.

Diabetes mellitus
- Ocular deviation, ptosis, and the sudden onset of diplopia and pain occur due to nerve damage, especially in long-standing diabetics.

Encephalitis
- Ocular deviation and diplopia may occur.
- Fever, headache, and vomiting are followed by signs of meningeal irritation and neuronal damage.
- Rapid deterioration of LOC may occur within 24 to 48 hours.

 TOP TECHNIQUE

Testing the six cardinal positions of gaze

To perform an assessment of extraocular muscle function, sit directly in front of the patient and ask her to remain still while you hold a cylindrical object, such as a penlight, directly in front of and about 18″ (46 cm) away from her nose. Ask the patient to hold her head still and to watch the object as you move it clockwise through each of the six cardinal positions, returning the object to midpoint after each movement. (Three positions are shown here: left superior, left lateral, and left inferior.)

The ocular muscles must work with the muscles producing the opposite movement. Normally, when one muscle contracts, its opposite relaxes to produce a smooth motion.

Throughout the test, the patient's eyes should remain parallel as they move. Note any abnormal findings, such as nystagmus or the deviation of one eye away from the object.

LEFT SUPERIOR

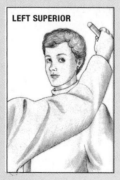

LEFT LATERAL

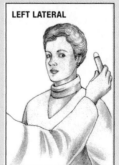

LEFT INFERIOR

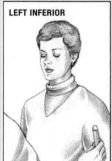

Head trauma

- The nature of ocular deviation depends on the site and extent of head trauma.
- Visible soft-tissue injury, bony deformity, facial edema, and clear or bloody otorrhea or rhinorrhea may be present.
- Other signs and symptoms include blurred vision, diplopia, nystagmus, behavioral changes, headache, motor and sensory dysfunction, signs of increased intracranial pressure, and a decreased LOC that may progress to coma.

Multiple sclerosis

- Ocular deviation may be an early sign.
- Diplopia, blurred vision, and sensory dysfunction occur.
- Other signs and symptoms include nystagmus; constipation; muscle weakness; paralysis; spasticity; hyperreflexia; intention tremor; gait ataxia; dysphagia; dysarthria; impotence; emotional lability; and urinary frequency, urgency, and incontinence.

Myasthenia gravis

- Ocular deviation may accompany the more common initial signs of diplopia and ptosis.
- It may affect only the eye muscles or progress to other muscle groups, causing altered facial expression, difficulty chewing, dysphagia, weakened voice, impaired fine hand movements, and respiratory distress.

Ophthalmoplegic migraine

- Ocular deviation and diplopia persist for days after the pain subsides.
- Other signs and symptoms include headache on one side with possible ptosis on the same side; temporary hemiplegia; irritability, depression, or slight confusion; and sensory deficits.

Orbital blowout fracture

- Limited extraocular movement and ocular deviation may occur.
- Typically, upward gaze is absent.

- Other signs and symptoms include pain, diplopia, nausea, periorbital edema, ecchymosis, and a globe that may be displaced downward and inward.

Orbital tumor

- Ocular deviation occurs as the tumor gradually enlarges.
- Other signs and symptoms include an edematous eyelid, proptosis, diplopia, and blurred vision.

Stroke

- Ocular deviation depends on the site and extent of the stroke.
- Related signs and symptoms vary and may include altered LOC, contralateral hemiplegia and sensory loss, dysarthria, dysphagia, homonymous hemianopsia, blurred vision, and diplopia.
- Other signs and symptoms include urine retention or incontinence or both, constipation, behavioral changes, headache, vomiting, and seizures.

Thyrotoxicosis

- Exophthalmos occurs, which causes limited extraocular movement and ocular deviation.
- Usually, the upward gaze weakens first, followed by diplopia.
- Related signs and symptoms include lid retraction, a wide-eyed staring gaze, excessive tearing, edematous eyelids and, sometimes, inability to close the eyes.
- Other signs and symptoms include tachycardia, palpitations, weight loss despite increased appetite, diarrhea, tremors, an enlarged thyroid gland, dyspnea, nervousness, diaphoresis, heat intolerance, and an atrial or ventricular gallop.

NURSING CONSIDERATIONS

- If you suspect an acute neurologic disorder, assess vital signs and neurologic status and report abnormal finding to the physician.
- Evaluate patient areas for safety concerns, and anticipate needs due to visual deficit.

PEDIATRIC POINTERS

- In children, the most common cause of ocular deviation is nonparalytic strabismus.

PATIENT TEACHING

- Explain the disorder and its treatment.
- Explain changes in LOC that need to be reported.
- Provide information about maintaining a safe environment.
- Teach ways of reducing environmental stress.

Oligomenorrhea

- Abnormally infrequent menstrual bleeding (three to six menstrual cycles per year)
- Common in infertile, early postmenarchal, and perimenopausal women
- May develop gradually or may follow a period of gradually lengthening cycles
- May alternate with normal menses or progress to secondary amenorrhea

HISTORY

- Ask the patient's age.
- Obtain a menstrual history, including age at menarche, and characteristics and duration of bleeding.
- Note hormonal contraceptive use.
- Note previous gynecologic disorders.
- Ask about problems with breast-feeding.
- Determine weight gain or loss and exercise patterns.
- Find out about excessive thirst, frequent urination, fatigue, jitteriness, palpitations, headache, dizziness, and impaired peripheral vision.
- Obtain a drug history.

PHYSICAL ASSESSMENT

- Take vital signs and weigh the patient.
- Inspect for increased facial hair growth, sparse body hair, male distribution of fat and muscle, acne, and clitoral enlargement.
- Note if the skin is abnormally dry or moist; check hair texture.
- Look for signs of psychological or physical stress.
- Rule out pregnancy.

CAUSES

MEDICAL
Adrenal hyperplasia

- Oligomenorrhea may occur with signs of androgen excess, such as clitoral enlargement, deepening voice, acne, and male distribution of hair, fat, and muscle mass.

Anorexia nervosa

- Sporadic oligomenorrhea or amenorrhea may occur along with a morbid fear of being fat and a weight loss of more than 20% of the patient's ideal body weight.
- Other signs and symptoms include dramatic skeletal muscle atrophy and loss of fatty tissue; dry or sparse scalp hair; lanugo on the face and body; constipation; decreased libido; and blotchy or sallow, dry skin.

Diabetes mellitus

- Oligomenorrhea may be an early sign; in juvenile-onset diabetes, the patient may never have had normal menses.
- Other signs and symptoms include excessive hunger, polydipsia, polyuria, polyphagia, weakness, fatigue, dry mucous membranes, poor skin turgor, irritability, emotional lability, and weight loss.

Hypothyroidism

- Oligomenorrhea may occur.
- Other signs and symptoms include fatigue; cold intolerance; dry, flaky, inelastic skin; constipation; puffy face, hands, and feet; bradycardia; decreased mental acuity; hoarseness; periorbital edema; ptosis; dry, sparse hair; thick, brittle nails; and unexplained weight gain.

Polycystic ovary disease

- Oligomenorrhea, amenorrhea, menometrorrhagia, or irregular menses may occur.
- Infertility, anovulation, and enlarged, palpable ovaries are common.
- Other signs and symptoms include male distribution of body hair and muscle mass, facial hair growth, acne, and obesity.

Prolactin-secreting pituitary tumor

- Oligomenorrhea or amenorrhea may be the first sign.
- Headache and visual field disturbances signal tumor expansion.
- Other signs and symptoms include galactorrhea, infertility, loss of libido, and sparse pubic hair.

Thyrotoxicosis

- Oligomenorrhea may occur with reduced fertility.
- Other signs and symptoms include irritability; weight loss despite increased appetite; dyspnea; tachycardia; palpitations; diarrhea; tremors; diaphoresis; heat intolerance; an enlarged thyroid and possibly, exophthalmos.

OTHER
Drugs

- Drugs that increase androgen level—such as corticosteroids, corticotropin, anabolic steroids, danazol, and injectable and implantable contraceptives—may cause oligomenorrhea.
- Other drugs that may cause oligomenorrhea include phenothiazine derivatives, amphetamines, and antihypertensives.

NURSING CONSIDERATIONS

- Prepare the patient for diagnostic tests.
- Provide emotional support related to altered body or self-image.

PEDIATRIC POINTERS

- Oligomenorrhea in adolescents is associated with immature hormonal function.
- Prolonged oligomenorrhea may signal congenital adrenal hyperplasia or Turner's syndrome.

GERIATRIC POINTERS

- Oligomenorrhea in perimenopausal women usually indicates impending onset of menopause.

PATIENT TEACHING

- Discuss underlying condition, diagnostic tests, and treatment options.
- Teach the patient techniques of recording basal body temperature to determine ovulation cycles.
- Explain the use of a home ovulation test.
- Provide information about the use of contraceptives.

Oliguria

OVERVIEW

- Defined as urine output of less than 400 ml/24 hours
- Major sign of renal and urinary tract disorders (see *How oliguria develops*)
- Typically occurs abruptly and may herald serious, possibly life-threatening hemodynamic instability

HISTORY

- Ask about usual voiding patterns and the onset and description of oliguria.
- Find out about pain or burning on urination, fever, loss of appetite, thirst, dyspnea, chest pain, or recent weight gain or loss.
- Record the patient's daily fluid intake.
- Obtain a medical history, including incidence of renal, urinary tract, or cardiovascular disorders; recent traumatic injury or surgery with significant blood loss; and recent transfusions.
- Ask about use of alcohol.
- Obtain a drug history.
- Note exposure to nephrotoxic agents, such as heavy metals, organic solvents, anesthetics, or radiographic contrast media.

PHYSICAL ASSESSMENT

- Take vital signs and weigh the patient.
- Palpate the kidneys for tenderness and enlargement.
- Percuss for costovertebral angle (CVA) tenderness.
- Inspect the flanks for edema or erythema.
- Auscultate the heart and lungs for abnormal sounds and the flank area for bruits.
- Assess for edema or signs of dehydration.
- Obtain a urine specimen, and inspect it for abnormal color, odor, or sediment; measure its specific gravity.

(Text continues on page 412.)

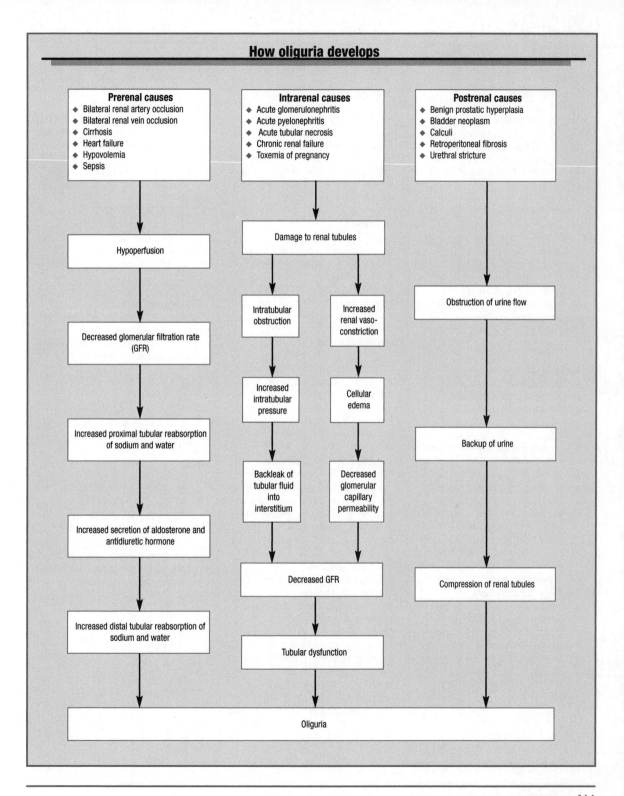

How oliguria develops

Prerenal causes
- Bilateral renal artery occlusion
- Bilateral renal vein occlusion
- Cirrhosis
- Heart failure
- Hypovolemia
- Sepsis

Intrarenal causes
- Acute glomerulonephritis
- Acute pyelonephritis
- Acute tubular necrosis
- Chronic renal failure
- Toxemia of pregnancy

Postrenal causes
- Benign prostatic hyperplasia
- Bladder neoplasm
- Calculi
- Retroperitoneal fibrosis
- Urethral stricture

Hypoperfusion

Damage to renal tubules

Decreased glomerular filtration rate (GFR)

Intratubular obstruction

Increased renal vaso-constriction

Obstruction of urine flow

Increased proximal tubular reabsorption of sodium and water

Increased intratubular pressure

Cellular edema

Increased secretion of aldosterone and antidiuretic hormone

Backleak of tubular fluid into interstitium

Decreased glomerular capillary permeability

Backup of urine

Increased distal tubular reabsorption of sodium and water

Decreased GFR

Compression of renal tubules

Tubular dysfunction

Oliguria

MEDICAL

Acute tubular necrosis

- Oliguria, an early sign, may occur abruptly (in shock) or gradually (in nephrotoxicity) and persist for about 2 weeks, followed by polyuria.
- Other signs and symptoms include signs of hyperkalemia, uremia, and heart failure.

Calculi

- Oliguria or anuria may occur.
- Excruciating pain radiates from the CVA to the flank, the suprapubic region, and the external genitalia.
- Other signs and symptoms include urinary frequency and urgency, dysuria, hematuria or pyuria, nausea, vomiting, hypoactive bowel sounds, abdominal distention and, possibly, fever and chills.

Gestational hypertension

- Oliguria may be accompanied by elevated blood pressure, dizziness, diplopia, blurred vision, nausea and vomiting, irritability, and frontal headache.
- Oliguria is preceded by generalized edema and sudden weight gain of more than 3 lb (1.4 kg) per week during the second trimester or more than 1 lb (0.5 kg) per week during the third trimester.
- If the condition progresses to eclampsia, seizures and coma may occur.

Glomerulonephritis, acute

- Oliguria or anuria occurs.
- Other signs and symptoms include mild fever, fatigue, gross hematuria, proteinuria, generalized edema, elevated blood pressure, headache, nausea, vomiting, flank and abdominal pain, and signs of pulmonary congestion.

Heart failure

- In left-sided heart failure, oliguria occurs due to decreased renal perfusion.
- In advanced failure, orthopnea, cyanosis, clubbing, ventricular gallop, diastolic hypertension, cardiomegaly, and hemoptysis occur.
- Other signs and symptoms include dyspnea, fatigue, weakness, peripheral edema, distended neck veins, tachycardia, tachypnea, crackles, and a dry or productive cough.

Hypovolemia

- Oliguria may occur.
- Other signs and symptoms include orthostatic hypotension, apathy, lethargy, fatigue, muscle weakness, anorexia, nausea, thirst, dizziness, sunken eyeballs, poor skin turgor, and dry mucous membranes.

Pyelonephritis, acute

- Oliguria, high fever with chills, fatigue, flank pain, CVA tenderness, weakness, nocturia, dysuria, hematuria, urinary frequency and urgency, and tenesmus occur.
- Anorexia, nausea, diarrhea, and vomiting may also develop.

Renal artery occlusion, bilateral

- Oliguria or, more commonly, anuria may accompany severe, constant upper abdominal and flank pain, nausea and vomiting, hypoactive bowel sounds, fever, and diastolic hypertension.

Renal failure, chronic

- Oliguria is a major sign of end-stage chronic renal failure.
- Eventually, seizures, coma, and uremic frost develop.
- Other signs and symptoms include fatigue, weakness, irritability, uremic fetor, ecchymoses, petechiae, peripheral edema, elevated blood pressure, confusion, emotional lability, drowsiness, coarse muscle twitching, muscle cramps, peripheral neuropathies, anorexia, metallic taste in the mouth, nausea, vomiting, constipation or diarrhea, stomatitis, pruritus, pallor, and yellow- or bronze-tinged skin.

Renal vein occlusion, bilateral

- Occasionally, oliguria occurs with acute low back and flank pain, CVA tenderness, fever, pallor, hematuria, enlarged and palpable kidneys, edema and, possibly, signs of uremia.

Sepsis

- Oliguria, fever, chills, restlessness, confusion, diaphoresis, anorexia, vomiting, diarrhea, pallor, hypotension, and tachycardia occur.
- Signs of local infection may also develop.

Urethral stricture

- Oliguria is accompanied by chronic urethral discharge, urinary frequency and urgency, dysuria, pyuria, and diminished urine stream.

OTHER

Diagnostic tests

- Radiographic studies that use contract media may cause nephrotoxicity and oliguria.

Drugs

- Oliguria may result from drugs that cause decreased renal perfusion (diuretics), nephrotoxicity (most notably aminoglycosides and chemotherapeutics), urine retention (adrenergics and anticholinergics), or urinary obstruction associated with precipitation of urinary crystals (sulfonamides and acyclovir).

- Monitor vital signs, intake and output, and daily weight.
- Restrict fluids to 600 ml to 1 L more than the urinary output for the previous day, if indicated.
- Provide diet low in sodium, potassium, and protein.

PEDIATRIC POINTERS

- In a neonate, oliguria may result from edema or dehydration, congenital heart disease, respiratory distress syndrome, sepsis, congenital hydronephrosis, acute tubular necrosis, and renal vein thrombosis.
- Causes of oliguria in children ages 1 to 5 include hemolytic-uremic syndrome and acute poststreptococcal glomerulonephritis.

GERIATRIC POINTERS

- In elderly patients, oliguria may result from an underlying disorder, overall poor muscle tone because of inactivity, poor fluid intake, and infrequent voiding attempts.

- Explain fluid and dietary restrictions the patient needs.
- Teach patient about prescribed medications.
- Teach about underlying diagnosis and treatment plan.

Opisthotonos

OVERVIEW

◆ Severe, prolonged spasm characterized by a strongly arched, rigid back; hyperextended neck; the heels bent back; and the arms and hands flexed at the joints
◆ Sign of severe meningeal irritation
◆ Occurs spontaneously and continuously, but may be aggravated by movement
◆ May be a protective reflex because it immobilizes the spine, alleviating the pain associated with meningeal irritation

ACTION STAT! *If the patient is stuporous or comatose, immediately evaluate his vital signs. Employ resuscitative measures, as appropriate. Place the patient in a bed, with rails raised and padded, or in a crib.*

HISTORY

◆ Obtain a history noting incidence of cerebral aneurysm, arteriovenous malformation, hypertension, or recent infection that may have spread to the nervous system.
◆ Explore associated signs and symptoms, such as headache, chills, and vomiting.

PHYSICAL ASSESSMENT

◆ Evaluate level of consciousness (LOC) and test sensorimotor and cranial nerve function.
◆ Check for Brudzinski's and Kernig's signs and for nuchal rigidity.
◆ Obtain vital signs.

CAUSES

MEDICAL
Arnold-Chiari syndrome
◆ Opisthotonos typically occurs with hydrocephalus, with its characteristic enlarged head; thin, shiny scalp with distended veins; and underdeveloped neck muscles.
◆ Other signs and symptoms include a high-pitched cry, abnormal leg muscle tone, anorexia, vomiting, nuchal rigidity, irritability, noisy respirations, and a weak sucking reflex.

Meningitis
◆ Opisthotonos accompanies other signs of meningeal irritation, including nuchal rigidity, positive Brudzinski's and Kernig's signs, and hyperreflexia.
◆ Related cardinal signs and symptoms include moderate to high fever with chills and malaise, headache, vomiting and, eventually, papilledema.
◆ Other signs and symptoms include irritability; photophobia; diplopia, deafness, and other cranial nerve palsies; and decreased LOC that may progress to seizures and coma.

Subarachnoid hemorrhage
◆ Opisthotonos may occur along with other signs of meningeal irritation, such as nuchal rigidity and positive Kernig's and Brudzinski's signs.
◆ Focal signs of hemorrhage, such as severe headache, hemiplegia or hemiparesis, aphasia, and photophobia, along with other vision problems, may also occur.
◆ With increasing intracranial pressure, the patient may develop bradycardia, elevated blood pressure, altered respiratory pattern, seizures, and vomiting.
◆ LOC may rapidly deteriorate, resulting in coma; then, decerebrate posture may alternate with opisthotonos.

Tetanus

- A life-threatening infection, opisthotonos may occur.
- Initially, trismus occurs.
- Eventually, muscle spasms may affect the abdomen, producing board-like rigidity; the back, resulting in opisthotonos; or the face, producing risus sardonicus. Spasms may also affect the respiratory muscles, causing distress.
- Other signs and symptoms include tachycardia, diaphoresis, hyperactive deep tendon reflexes, and seizures.

OTHER
Drugs

- Phenothiazines and other antipsychotics may cause opisthotonos, usually as part of an acute dystonic reaction.

NURSING CONSIDERATIONS

- Assess neurologic status and check vital signs frequently.
- Make the patient as comfortable as possible; place him in a side-lying position with pillows for support.
- If meningitis is suspected, institute respiratory isolation. Lumbar puncture may be ordered to identify pathogens and analyze cerebrospinal fluid.
- If subarachnoid hemorrhage is suspected, prepare the patient for a computed tomography scan or magnetic resonance imaging.

PEDIATRIC POINTERS

- Opisthotonos is far more common in children—especially infants—than in adults.
- It's also more exaggerated in children because of nervous system immaturity. (See *Opisthotonos: Sign of meningeal irritation.*)

PATIENT TEACHING

- Teach the patient and family about underlying diagnosis and treatment plan.
- Teach the patient and family about all tests and hospital procedures.
- Teach the patient and family about prescribed medications.

Opisthotonos: Sign of meningeal irritation

In the characteristic posture, the back is severely arched with the neck hyperextended. The heels bend back on the legs, and the arms and hands flex rigidly at the joints, as shown.

Orthopnea

OVERVIEW

- Characterized by difficulty breathing in a supine position
- Common symptom of cardiopulmonary disorders that produce dyspnea
- Results from increased hydrostatic pressure in the pulmonary vasculature related to being in the supine position
- May be reported that patient can't catch his breath when lying down or that he sleeps in a reclining chair or propped up by pillows
- May be classified as two- or three-pillow orthopnea

HISTORY

- Ask about the onset and description of orthopnea.
- Note how many pillows are used for sleeping.
- Obtain a medical history, including incidence of cardiopulmonary disorders, such as myocardial infarction, rheumatic heart disease, heart failure, valvular disease, asthma, emphysema, or chronic bronchitis.
- Find out about smoking and alcohol habits.
- Inquire about associated cough, dyspnea, fatigue, weakness, loss of appetite, or chest pain.
- Obtain a drug history.

PHYSICAL ASSESSMENT

- Take vital signs.
- Check for other signs of increased respiratory effort, such as accessory muscle use, shallow respirations, and tachypnea.
- Note barrel chest.
- Inspect skin for pallor or cyanosis, and inspect the fingers for clubbing.
- Observe and palpate for edema.
- Check jugular vein distention.
- Auscultate the lungs and heart.
- Monitor oxygen saturation.

CAUSES

MEDICAL
Chronic obstructive pulmonary disease

- Orthopnea and other dyspneic complaints are accompanied by accessory muscle use, tachypnea, tachycardia, and paradoxical pulse.
- Related signs and symptoms include diminished breath sounds, rhonchi, crackles, and wheezing on auscultation; dry or productive cough with copious sputum; anorexia; weight loss; and edema.
- Barrel chest, cyanosis, and clubbing are late signs.

Left-sided heart failure

- If heart failure is acute, orthopnea may begin suddenly; if chronic, it may be constant.
- Early signs and symptoms include progressively severe dyspnea, Cheyne-Stokes respirations, paroxysmal nocturnal dyspnea, fatigue, weakness, a cough that may occasionally produce clear or blood-tinged sputum, tachycardia, tachypnea, and crackles.
- Late signs and symptoms include cyanosis, clubbing, ventricular gallop, and hemoptysis.

Mediastinal tumor

- Orthopnea is an early sign.
- As the tumor enlarges, signs and symptoms include retrosternal chest pain; dry cough; hoarseness; dysphagia; stertorous respirations; palpitations; cyanosis; suprasternal retractions on inspiration; tracheal deviation; dilated jugular and superficial chest veins; and edema of the face, neck, and arms.

Valvular heart disease

◆ Orthopnea may occur.
◆ Signs and symptoms may vary according to valve involved.
◆ Signs and symptoms of aortic insufficiency include fatigue, dyspnea, palpitations, dizziness, and angina. With heart failure, orthopnea, paroxysmal nocturnal dyspnea, and cough may also occur.
◆ Signs and symptoms of aortic stenosis include syncope, angina, and dyspnea on exertion. With left-sided heart failure, orthopnea may also occur.
◆ Signs and symptoms of mitral insufficiency include fatigue, dyspnea, palpitations, angina, and orthopnea.
◆ Signs and symptoms of mitral stenosis include fatigue, weakness, dyspnea on exertion, nocturnal dyspnea, palpitations, and orthopnea.

NURSING CONSIDERATIONS

◆ Place the patient in semi-Fowler's or high Fowler's position.
◆ Alternatively, have the patient lean over a bedside table with his chest forward.
◆ If needed, administer oxygen via nasal cannula.
◆ To reduce lung fluid, give a diuretic, as ordered.
◆ Monitor intake and output.
◆ For the patient with left-sided heart failure, give angiotensin-converting enzyme inhibitors, as ordered.
◆ Assist with insertion of a central venous line or pulmonary artery catheter, as needed.

PEDIATRIC POINTERS

◆ Common causes of orthopnea in children include heart failure, croup syndrome, cystic fibrosis, and asthma.
◆ Sleeping in an infant seat may improve symptoms for a young child.

GERIATRIC POINTERS

◆ If the patient is using more than one pillow in bed, consider a noncardiogenic pulmonary cause.

PATIENT TEACHING

◆ Discuss underlying condition, diagnostic tests, and treatment options.
◆ Explain the signs and symptoms the patient should report.
◆ Explain dietary and fluid restrictions the patient needs.
◆ Discuss daily weight measurement.
◆ Explain energy conservation measures, as appropriate.

Orthostatic hypotension

OVERVIEW

- Characterized by a blood pressure drop of 15 to 20 mm Hg or more (with or without an increase in the heart rate of at least 20 beats/minute) upon rising from a supine to a sitting or standing position
- Failure of compensatory vasomotor responses to adjust to position changes
- Produces light-headedness, syncope, or blurred vision
- Also called *postural hypotension*

  ACTION STAT! *Check for tachycardia, altered level of consciousness (LOC), and pale, clammy skin. If present, suspect hypovolemic shock. Insert a large-bore I.V. line for fluid or blood replacement. Take vital signs frequently, and monitor the patient's intake and output.*

HISTORY

- Ask about dizziness, weakness, or fainting when standing.
- Inquire about fatigue, orthopnea, nausea, headache, abdominal or chest discomfort, and GI bleeding.
- Obtain a drug history.

PHYSICAL ASSESSMENT

- Obtain vital signs and weight.
- Check skin turgor.
- Palpate peripheral pulses.
- Auscultate the heart and lungs.
- Test muscle strength and observe gait for unsteadiness.
- Obtain blood samples for laboratory studies.

CAUSES

MEDICAL
Adrenal insufficiency
- Orthostatic hypotension may be accompanied by fatigue, muscle weakness, poor coordination, anorexia, nausea, vomiting, fasting hypoglycemia, weight loss, irritability, abdominal pain, hyperpigmentation, and a weak, irregular pulse.
- Other signs and symptoms include diarrhea; constipation; decreased libido; amenorrhea; syncope; and enhanced taste, smell, and hearing.

Amyloidosis
- Orthostatic hypotension is common.
- Other signs and symptoms include angina, tachycardia, dyspnea, orthopnea, fatigue, and cough.

Diabetic autonomic neuropathy
- Orthostatic hypotension is accompanied by syncope, dysphagia, constipation or diarrhea, painless bladder distention with overflow incontinence, impotence, and retrograde ejaculation.

Hyperaldosteronism
- Orthostatic hypotension with sustained elevated blood pressure occurs.
- Other signs and symptoms include muscle weakness, intermittent flaccid paralysis, fatigue, headache, paresthesia, vision disturbance, nocturia, polydipsia, personality changes and, possibly, tetany.

Hyponatremia
- Orthostatic hypotension occurs with headache, profound thirst, nausea, vomiting, muscle twitching and weakness, fatigue, oliguria or anuria, tachycardia, abdominal cramps, irritability, seizures, decreased LOC, and cold clammy skin.
- If severe, cyanosis, thready pulse and, eventually, vasomotor collapse occurs.

Hypovolemia
- Orthostatic hypotension occurs with apathy, fatigue, muscle weakness, anorexia, nausea, and profound thirst.
- Other signs and symptoms include dizziness, oliguria, sunken eyeballs, poor skin turgor, and dry mucous membranes.

OTHER
Drugs
- Antihypertensives, diuretics in large doses, levodopa, monoamine oxidase inhibitors, morphine, nitrates, phenothiazines, spinal anesthesia, and tricyclic antidepressants may cause orthostatic hypotension.

Treatments
- Orthostatic hypotension is common with prolonged bed rest.
- Sympathectomy may cause orthostatic hypotension by disrupting normal vasoconstrictive mechanisms.

NURSING CONSIDERATIONS

◆ Elevate the head of the bed, and help the patient to a sitting position with his feet dangling over the side of the bed; if tolerated, have him sit in a chair briefly.
◆ Monitor intake and output and weigh the patient daily.
◆ Evaluate the need for assistive devices.
◆ Help the patient with walking.

PEDIATRIC POINTERS
◆ Causes of orthostatic hypotension in children may be the same as those in adults.

GERIATRIC POINTERS
◆ Elderly patients commonly experience autonomic dysfunction, which can present as orthostatic hypotension.
◆ Postprandial hypotension may occur 45 to 60 minutes after a meal.

PATIENT TEACHING

◆ Discuss the underlying condition, diagnostic tests, and treatment options.
◆ Explain the importance of avoiding volume depletion.
◆ Explain how to change position gradually.
◆ Teach the patient preambulation exercises to do before getting out of bed. (See *Performing preambulation exercises*.)

Performing preambulation exercises

To help minimize the effects of orthostatic hypotension, such as dizziness and blurred vision, teach the patient to perform these leg exercises before getting out of bed.

Lying flat on her back, the patient should flex one knee slightly, keeping her heel on the bed.

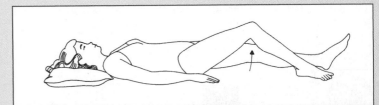

The patient should then extend her leg and raise her heel off the bed.

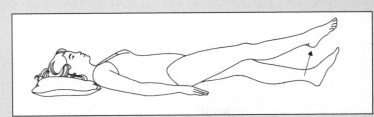

Next, the patient should flex her knee again, and lower her heel to the bed.

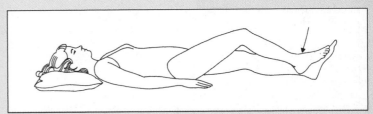

The patient should then straighten her leg.

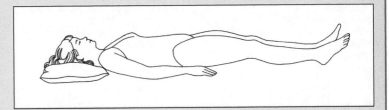

Instruct the patient to repeat the procedure for the other leg. She should alternate sides, performing the exercises six times for each leg.

Ortolani's sign

- Click, clunk, or popping sensation that's felt and commonly heard when a neonate's hip is flexed 90 degrees and abducted
- Results when the femoral head enters or exits the acetabulum

- Find out if the infant has been screened for Ortolani's sign in the past. Screening for this sign is an important part of neonatal care because early detection and treatment of developmental dysplasia of the hip (DDH) improves the neonate's chances of growing with a correctly formed, functional joint.
- Ask parents about a family history of DDH.
- Ask if infant was breech delivery, one of twins, or large for gestational age at birth.

- During assessment for Ortolani's sign, the neonate should be relaxed and lying supine. (See *Detecting developmental dysplasia of the hip*.)
- After eliciting Ortolani's sign, evaluate the neonate for asymmetrical gluteal folds, limited hip abduction, and unequal leg length.

TOP TECHNIQUE

Detecting developmental dysplasia of the hip

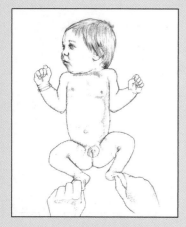

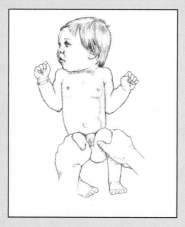

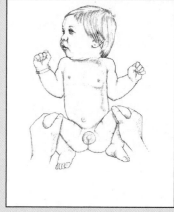

When assessing the neonate, attempt to elicit Ortolani's sign to detect developmental dysplasia of the hip (DDH). Begin by placing the infant in a supine position with his knees and hips flexed. Observe for symmetry.

Place your hands on the infant's knees, with your index fingers along his lateral thighs on the greater trochanter. Then raise his knees to a 90-degree angle with his back.

Abduct the infant's thighs so that the lateral aspect of his knees lies almost flat on the table. If the infant has a dislocated hip, you'll feel and often hear a click, clunk, or popping sensation (Ortolani's sign) as the head of the femur moves out of the acetabulum. The infant may also give a sudden cry of pain. Be sure to distinguish a positive Ortolani's sign from the normal clicks due to rotation of the hip, which don't elicit the sensation of instability, or simultaneous movement of the knee.

CAUSES

MEDICAL
DDH
- With complete dysplasia, the affected leg may appear shorter, or the affected hip may appear more prominent.
- Most common in the female, DDH produces Ortolani's sign, which may be accompanied by limited hip abduction and unequal gluteal folds. Usually, the neonate with DDH has no gross deformity or pain.

NURSING CONSIDERATIONS

- Ortolani's sign can be elicited only during the first 4 to 6 weeks of life; this is also the optimum time for effective corrective treatment.
- If treatment is delayed, DDH may cause degenerative hip changes, lordosis, joint malformation, and soft-tissue damage.
- Various methods of abduction can be used to produce a stable joint. These methods include using soft splinting devices and a plaster hip spica cast.

PEDIATRIC POINTERS
- A strong relationship between hip dysplasia and methods of handling neonates has been demonstrated. For instance, Inuit and Navajo Indians have a high incidence of DDH, which may be related to their practice of wrapping neonates in blankets or strapping them to cradleboards. In cultures where mothers carry neonates on their backs or hips, such as in the Far East and Africa, hip dysplasia is rarely seen.

PATIENT TEACHING

- Teach parents the importance of early screening and treatment.
- Teach parents about the treatment plan.

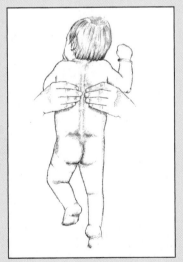

If you elicit a positive Ortolani's sign, observe for asymmetrical gluteal folds and unequal leg length.

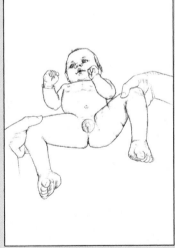

Flex the infant's hips to detect limited abduction.

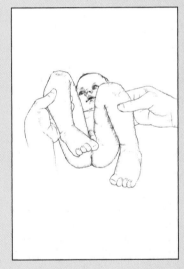

Flex the infant's knees, and observe for apparent shortening of the femur.

Osler's nodes

OVERVIEW

- Tender, raised, pea-sized, red or purple lesions that erupt on the palms and soles, especially the pads of the fingers and toes
- Usually develop after other telling signs and symptoms of endocarditis and disappear spontaneously within several days
- May result from bacterial emboli caught in peripheral capillaries or may reflect an immunologic reaction to the causative organism
- Must be distinguished from the even less common Janeway's lesions—small, painless, erythematous lesions that also erupt on the palms and soles

HISTORY

- If you discover Osler's nodes, obtain a history for clues to the cause of infective endocarditis, such as recent surgery or dental work; invasive procedures of the urinary or gynecologic tract; a prosthetic valve or an arteriovenous fistula for hemodialysis; cardiac disorders and murmurs; or recent upper respiratory, skin, or urinary tract infection.
- Find out if the patient has been using I.V. drugs and explore associated complaints, such as chills, fatigue, anorexia, and night sweats.

PHYSICAL ASSESSMENT

- Take vital signs and auscultate the heart for murmurs and gallops and the lungs for crackles.
- Inspect the skin and mucous membranes for petechiae and other lesions.
- If you suspect I.V. drug abuse, inspect the patient's arms and other areas for needle tracks.

MEDICAL

Acute infective endocarditis

◆ Osler's nodes may occur.
◆ Classic signs and symptoms include acute onset of high, intermittent fever with chills and signs of heart failure, such as dyspnea, peripheral edema, and distended jugular veins.
◆ Janeway's lesions and Roth's spots are more common in this form than in the subacute form; petechiae may also occur.
◆ Embolization may abruptly occur, causing organ infarction or peripheral vascular occlusion with hematuria, chest or limb pain, paralysis, blindness, and other diverse effects.

Subacute infective endocarditis

◆ Osler's nodes are characteristic of this form of endocarditis.
◆ A suddenly changing murmur or the discovery of a new murmur is another cardinal sign.
◆ Related signs and symptoms include intermittent fever, pallor, weakness, fatigue, arthralgia, night sweats, tachycardia, anorexia and weight loss, splenomegaly, clubbing, and petechiae.
◆ Occasionally, Janeway's lesions, subungual splinter hemorrhages, and Roth's spots also appear. Signs of heart failure may occur with extensive valvular damage.
◆ Embolization may also develop, producing signs and symptoms that vary depending on the location of the emboli.

◆ Monitor the patient's vital signs to evaluate the effectiveness of antibiotic therapy against infective endocarditis.
◆ Prepare the patient for blood studies, such as a complete blood count, and procedures, such as an electrocardiogram and echocardiogram.

PEDIATRIC POINTERS

◆ In children, Osler's nodes may result from infective endocarditis associated with congenital heart defects or rheumatic fever.

◆ Discuss measures to prevent reinfection, such as prophylactic antibiotic administration before dental or invasive procedures.
◆ Teach the patient about diagnosis and treatment plan.

Otorrhea

- Drainage from the ear
- May be bloody, purulent, clear, or serosanguineous

HISTORY

- Ask about the onset and description of drainage.
- Find out about pain, tenderness, vertigo, or tinnitus.
- Obtain a medical history, including incidence of recent upper respiratory infection or head trauma; and history of cancer, dermatitis, or immunosuppressant therapy.

PHYSICAL ASSESSMENT

- Inspect the external ear, and apply pressure on the tragus and mastoid area to elicit tenderness; then insert an otoscope.
- Observe for edema, erythema, crusts, or polyps.
- Inspect the tympanic membrane, noting color changes, perforation, absence of the normal light reflex, or a bulging membrane.
- Test hearing acuity and perform Weber's and Rinne tests.
- Palpate the neck and preauricular, parotid, and postauricular areas for lymphadenopathy.
- Test the function of cranial nerves VII, IX, X, and XI.
- Obtain vital signs.

CAUSES

MEDICAL
Allergy
- Tympanic membrane perforation may cause clear or cloudy otorrhea, rhinorrhea, and itchy, watery eyes.
- Other signs and symptoms include nasal congestion and an itchy nose and throat.

Aural polyps
- Foul, purulent, blood-streaked discharge may occur, possibly followed by partial hearing loss.

Basilar skull fracture
- Otorrhea may be clear and watery and show a positive reaction on glucose test, or it may be bloody.
- Other signs and symptoms include hearing loss, cerebrospinal fluid or bloody rhinorrhea, periorbital raccoon eyes, mastoid ecchymosis (Battle's sign), cranial nerve palsies, decreased level of consciousness, and headache.

Dermatitis of the external ear canal
- With contact dermatitis, vesicles produce clear, watery otorrhea with edema and erythema of the external ear canal.
- With infectious eczematoid dermatitis, otorrhea is purulent with erythema and crusting of the external ear canal.
- With seborrheic dermatitis, otorrhea has greasy scales and flakes.

Mastoiditis
- Thick, purulent, yellow otorrhea becomes increasingly profuse.
- Related signs and symptoms include low-grade fever, and dull aching and tenderness in the mastoid area.
- Conductive hearing loss may develop.

Myringitis, infectious
- Small, reddened, blood-filled blebs or blisters rupture, causing serosanguineous otorrhea.

- In the chronic form, purulent otorrhea, pruritus, and gradual hearing loss occur.
- Other signs and symptoms include severe ear pain and tenderness over the mastoid process.

Otitis externa

- The acute form usually causes purulent, yellow, sticky, foul-smelling otorrhea.
- Related acute signs and symptoms include edema, erythema, pain, and itching of the auricle and external ear; severe tenderness with movement of the mastoid, tragus, mouth, or jaw; tenderness and swelling of surrounding nodes; partial conductive hearing loss; and low-grade fever and headache ipsilateral to the affected ear.
- The chronic form usually causes scanty, intermittent otorrhea that may be serous or purulent, as well as edema and slight erythema.

Otitis media

- With acute otitis media, rupture of the tympanic membrane produces bloody, purulent otorrhea and conductive hearing loss that worsens over several hours.
- With acute suppurative otitis media, otorrhea may accompany signs and symptoms of upper respiratory infection, dizziness, fever, nausea, and vomiting.
- With chronic otitis media, otorrhea is intermittent, purulent, and foul-smelling, and is accompanied by gradual conductive hearing loss, pain, nausea, and vertigo.

Trauma

- Bloody otorrhea may occur and may be accompanied by partial hearing loss.

Tumor

- A benign tumor of the jugular glomus may cause bloody otorrhea.
- Related signs and symptoms include throbbing discomfort, tinnitus that resembles the sound of the patient's heartbeat, progressive stuffiness of the affected ear, vertigo, conductive hearing loss and, possibly, a reddened mass behind the tympanic membrane.
- Squamous cell carcinoma of the external ear causes purulent otorrhea with itching; deep, boring pain; hearing loss; and, in late stages, facial paralysis.
- Squamous cell carcinoma of the middle ear causes blood-tinged otorrhea that occurs early and is accompanied by hearing loss of the affected side; pain and facial paralysis are late signs.

NURSING CONSIDERATIONS

- Apply warm, moist compresses, heating pads, or hot water bottles to the ears.
- Use cotton wicks to clean the ear or to apply topical drugs.
- Keep eardrops at room temperature; instillation of cold eardrops may cause vertigo.
- If the patient has impaired hearing, make sure he understands what's explained to him.

PEDIATRIC POINTERS

- Perforation of the tympanic membrane from otitis media is the most common cause of otorrhea in infants and young children.
- Children may insert foreign bodies into their ears, resulting in infection, pain, and purulent discharge.
- Because the auditory canal of a child lies horizontal, the pinna must be pulled downward and backward to examine the ear. (See *Examining a child's ear.*)

PATIENT TEACHING

- Discuss underlying condition, diagnostic tests, and treatment options.
- Instruct the patient on safe ways to blow his nose and clean his ears.
- Stress the use of earplugs when swimming.
- Explain the signs and symptoms the patient needs to report.

Pallor

- Refers to abnormal paleness or loss of skin color
- Develops suddenly or gradually
- Can be difficult to detect in darker-skinned patients; for example, the dark skin of Blacks may appear ashen gray and the lighter-dark skin of Hispanic patients may be yellowish brown
- Can be generalized or localized
- Is caused chiefly by anemia (see *How pallor develops*)

✦ **ACTION STAT!** *If generalized pallor develops suddenly, look for signs of shock and prepare to rapidly infuse fluids or blood. Keep emergency resuscitation equipment nearby.*

HISTORY

- Obtain a medical history, including anemia, renal failure, heart failure, or diabetes.
- Ask about diet, especially intake of green vegetables.
- Ask about the onset and description of the pallor.
- Explore what aggravates and alleviates the pallor.
- Inquire about dizziness, fainting, orthostasis, weakness, fatigue, dyspnea, chest pain, palpitations, menstrual irregularities, or loss of libido.

PHYSICAL ASSESSMENT

- Assess vital signs, checking for orthostatic hypotension.
- Auscultate the heart for murmurs or gallops.
- Auscultate the lungs for crackles.
- Check skin temperature.
- Note skin ulceration.
- Palpate peripheral pulses.
- Assess oral mucous membranes.

CAUSES

MEDICAL
Anemia

- Pallor begins gradually; skin is gray or sallow.
- Other findings include fatigue, dyspnea, tachycardia, bounding pulse, atrial gallop, systolic bruit over the carotid arteries and, possibly, crackles and bleeding tendencies.

Arterial occlusion (acute)

- Pallor begins abruptly in the extremity with occlusion.
- Line of demarcation separates cool, pale, cyanotic, and mottled skin from normal skin.
- Other findings include severe pain, intense intermittent claudication, paresthesia, paresis in the affected extremity, and absent pulses below the occlusion.

Arterial occlusive disease (chronic)

- Pallor is specific to an extremity.
- Pallor develops gradually and is aggravated by elevating the extremity.

How pallor develops

Pallor may result from decreased peripheral oxyhemoglobin or decreased total oxyhemoglobin. This flowchart illustrates the progression to pallor.

◆ Other findings include intermittent claudication, weakness, cool skin, diminished pulses in the extremity and, possibly, ulceration and gangrene.

Cardiac arrhythmias
◆ Acute pallor may occur with an irregular, rapid, or slow pulse; dizziness; weakness and fatigue; hypotension; confusion; palpitations; diaphoresis; oliguria; and, possibly, loss of consciousness.

Frostbite
◆ Pallor is localized to the frostbitten area, which feels cold, waxy and, possibly, hard; sensation may be absent.
◆ Skin turns purplish blue as skin thaws; if frostbite is severe, blistering and gangrene may follow.

Orthostatic hypotension
◆ Pallor occurs abruptly on rising from a recumbent position along with a drop in blood pressure, tachycardia, and dizziness.
◆ Loss of consciousness is possible.

Raynaud's disease
◆ Upon exposure to cold or stress, the fingers abruptly turn pale (a classic sign), then cyanotic in this arteriospastic disorder.
◆ With rewarming, fingers become red and paresthetic.
◆ With chronic disease, ulceration may occur.

Shock
◆ In hypovolemic and cardiogenic shock, acute pallor occurs early with restlessness, thirst, tachycardia, tachypnea, and cool, clammy skin.
◆ As shock progresses, skin becomes increasingly clammy, pulse becomes more rapid and thready, and hypotension develops with narrowing pulse pressure.
◆ Other findings include oliguria, subnormal body temperature, and decreased level of consciousness.

Vasovagal syncope
◆ Sudden pallor immediately precedes or accompanies loss of consciousness.
◆ These fainting spells may be triggered by emotional stress or pain and usually last for a few seconds or minutes.
◆ Before loss of consciousness, diaphoresis, nausea, yawning, hyperpnea, weakness, confusion, tachycardia, and dim vision may occur followed by bradycardia, hypotension, a few clonic jerks, and dilated pupils.

NURSING CONSIDERATIONS

◆ Administer blood and fluids as well as a diuretic, cardiotonic, and an antiarrhythmic, as needed.
◆ Frequently monitor vital signs, intake and output, electrocardiogram, and hemodynamic status.

PEDIATRIC TIPS
◆ Pallor in children can also stem from a congenital heart defect or chronic lung disease.

PATIENT TEACHING

◆ For anemia, explain the importance of an iron-rich diet and rest.
◆ For frostbite and Raynaud's disease, discuss cold-protection measures.
◆ For orthostatic hypotension, explain the need to rise slowly.
◆ Discuss signs and symptoms the patient needs to report.

Palpitations

OVERVIEW

- Refers to conscious awareness of one's own heartbeat
- Usually felt over the precordium or in the throat or neck
- May be regular or irregular, fast or slow, paroxysmal or sustained
- May be described as pounding, jumping, turning, fluttering, flopping, or as skipping a beat

ACTION STAT! Ask the patient about dizziness or shortness of breath. Then inspect for pale, cool, clammy skin. Take vital signs, noting hypotension and irregular or abnormal pulse. If these signs are present, suspect cardiac arrhythmia. Begin cardiac monitoring and, if needed, prepare the patient for electrical cardioversion. Insert an I.V. catheter to administer an antiarrhythmic, if needed.

HISTORY

- Ask about the onset and description of palpitations.
- Inquire about aggravating and alleviating factors.
- Note associated signs and symptoms, such as dizziness, syncope, weakness, fatigue, angina, and pale, cool skin.
- Obtain a medical history, including cardiovascular or pulmonary disorder, or hypoglycemia.
- Obtain a drug history, including recently prescribed digoxin.
- Ask about caffeine, tobacco, and alcohol use.

PHYSICAL ASSESSMENT

- Perform a complete cardiac and pulmonary assessment.
- Auscultate the heart for gallops and murmurs.
- Auscultate the lungs for abnormal breath sounds.

CAUSES

MEDICAL

Anemia

- Palpitations occur, especially on exertion, with pallor, fatigue, and dyspnea.
- Other findings include systolic ejection murmur, bounding pulse, tachycardia, crackles, an atrial gallop, and a systolic bruit over the carotid arteries.

Anxiety attack (acute)

- Palpitations may be accompanied by diaphoresis, facial flushing, trembling, and an impending sense of doom.
- Hyperventilation may lead to dizziness, weakness, and syncope.
- Other findings include tachycardia, precordial pain, shortness of breath, restlessness, and insomnia.

Cardiac arrhythmias

- Paroxysmal or sustained palpitations may be accompanied by dizziness, weakness, and fatigue.
- Other findings include an irregular, rapid, or slow pulse rate; decreased blood pressure; confusion; pallor; chest pain; syncope; oliguria; and diaphoresis.

Hypertension

- Sustained palpitations may occur alone or with headache, dizziness, tinnitus, and fatigue.
- Blood pressure typically exceeds 140/90 mm Hg.
- Nausea, vomiting, seizures, and decreased level of consciousness (LOC) may also occur.

Hypocalcemia

- Palpitations occur with weakness and fatigue.
- Paresthesia progresses to muscle tension and carpopedal spasms.
- Related findings include muscle twitching, hyperactive deep tendon reflexes, chorea, and positive Chvostek's and Trousseau's signs.

Hypoglycemia

◆ Sustained palpitations occur with fatigue, irritability, hunger, cold sweats, tremors, tachycardia, anxiety, and headache.
◆ Eventually, blurred or double vision, muscle weakness, hemiplegia, and altered LOC develop.

Mitral prolapse

◆ Paroxysmal palpitations accompany sharp, stabbing, or aching precordial pain and midsystolic click, followed by an apical systolic murmur.
◆ Other findings include dyspnea, dizziness, severe fatigue, migraine headache, anxiety, paroxysmal tachycardia, crackles, and peripheral edema.

Mitral stenosis

◆ Early on, sustained palpitations accompany exertional dyspnea and fatigue.
◆ Loud S_1 or opening snap and a rumbling diastolic murmur at the apex are heard on auscultation.
◆ Other findings include an atrial gallop and, with advanced disease, orthopnea, dyspnea at rest, paroxysmal nocturnal dyspnea, peripheral edema, jugular vein distention, ascites, hepatomegaly, and atrial fibrillation.

Pheochromocytoma

◆ Paroxysmal palpitations occur with dramatically elevated blood pressure (the main sign of this adrenal medulla tumor).
◆ Other findings include tachycardia, headache, chest or abdominal pain, diaphoresis, warm and pale or flushed skin, paresthesia, tremors, insomnia, nausea, vomiting, and anxiety.

Thyrotoxicosis

◆ Sustained palpitations may be accompanied by tachycardia, dyspnea, diarrhea, nervousness, tremors, diaphoresis, heat intolerance, weight loss despite increased appetite, atrial or ventricular gallop and, possibly, exophthalmos.

OTHER
Drugs

◆ Drugs, including atropine, beta-adrenergic blockers, calcium channel blockers, digoxin, ganglionic blockers, minoxidil, and sympathomimetics, that precipitate cardiac arrhythmias or increase cardiac output may cause palpitations.

Exercise

◆ Exercise can cause palpitations.

Herbal remedies

◆ Herbal dietary supplements, such as ginseng and ephedra (ma huang), may cause adverse reactions including palpitations and an irregular heartbeat. (The Food and Drug Administration has banned the sale of ephedra.)

NURSING CONSIDERATIONS

◆ Monitor for signs of reduced cardiac output and cardiac arrhythmias.
◆ Prepare for procedures such as cardioversion.
◆ Provide supplemental oxygen.
◆ Provide for rest periods.

PEDIATRIC TIPS

◆ Palpitations commonly result from fever and congenital heart defects.

PATIENT TEACHING

◆ Teach about underlying disorder and treatment options.
◆ Explain diagnostic tests the patient will need.
◆ Teach the patient how to reduce anxiety.

Papular rash

OVERVIEW

- Rash that consists of small, raised, circumscribed papules
- May erupt anywhere on the body in various configurations
- May be acute or chronic

HISTORY

- Ask about onset, course of rash, and characteristics, such as itching, burning, or tenderness.
- Inquire about fever, headache, and GI distress.
- Obtain a medical history, including allergies, previous rash and skin disorder, infection, childhood disease, sexual history, sexually transmitted disease, cancer, and exposure to chemicals and pesticides.
- Obtain a drug history.
- Ask about recent insect or rodent bite, or exposure to infectious disease.

PHYSICAL ASSESSMENT

- Note rash's color, configuration, and location. (See *Recognizing common skin lesions*.)
- Perform a whole-body examination of skin, hair, and nails.

 TOP TECHNIQUE

Recognizing common skin lesions

Use these illustrations to help you identify common skin lesions. Remember to keep a centimeter ruler handy to measure the size of the lesion accurately.

MACULE

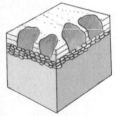

A small (usually less than 1 cm in diameter), flat blemish or discoloration that can be brown, tan, red, or white and has the same texture as the surrounding skin

VESICLE

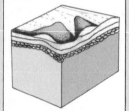

A small (less than 0.5 cm in diameter), thin-walled, raised blister containing clear, serous, purulent, or bloody fluid

WHEAL

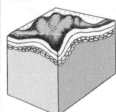

A slightly raised, firm lesion of variable size and shape that's surrounded by edema (skin may be red or pale)

PAPULE

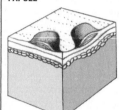

A small, solid, raised lesion less than 1 cm in diameter with red to purple skin discoloration

BULLA

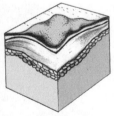

A raised, thin-walled blister greater than 0.5 cm in diameter that contains clear or serous fluid

PUSTULE

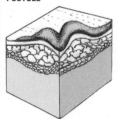

A circumscribed, pus- or lymph-filled, elevated lesion that varies in diameter; may be firm or soft and yellow or white

NODULE

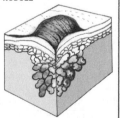

A small, firm, circumscribed, elevated lesion 1 to 2 cm in diameter with possible skin discoloration

TUMOR

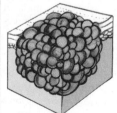

A solid, raised mass usually larger than 2 cm in diameter with possible skin discoloration

MEDICAL

Acne vulgaris
- Inflamed papules, pustules, nodules, or cysts appear on the face, shoulders, chest, and back.
- Lesions may be painful and pruritic.

Anthrax (cutaneous)
- Initially this bacterial infection appears as a small, painless, pruritic macular or papular lesion.
- A vesicle develops within 2 days and then evolves into a painless ulcer with a black necrotic center.
- Lymphadenopathy, malaise, headache, and fever may develop.

Dermatitis (perioral)
- Tiny, discrete, erythematous papules and pustules that may be pruritic and painful appear on the nasolabial fold, chin, and upper lip area.

Erythema migrans
- Papular or macular rash starts as a single lesion and spreads at margins while clearing centrally.
- Commonly appears on the thighs, trunk, or upper arms.
- Accompanying findings include fever, chills, headache, malaise, nausea, vomiting, fatigue, backache, knee pain, and stiff neck.

Gonococcemia
- Erythematous macular rash erupts sporadically on the palms and soles and rapidly becomes maculopapular, vesiculopustular, and hemorrhagic.
- Mature lesion is raised with a gray necrotic center, surrounded by erythema, and heals in 3 to 4 days.
- Eruptions may be accompanied by fever and joint pain.

Human immunodeficiency virus infection
- A generalized maculopapular rash occurs with acute infection.
- Other findings include fever, malaise, sore throat, headache, lymphadenopathy, and hepatosplenomegaly.

Insect bites
- A papular, macular, or petechial rash may be accompanied by fever, myalgia, headache, lymphadenopathy, nausea, and vomiting.

Kaposi's sarcoma
- A cancer of the lymphatic system, Kaposi's sarcoma is the most common cancer associated with acquired immunodeficiency syndrome.
- Purple or blue papules or macules of vascular origin appear on the skin, mucous membrane, and viscera.
- Lesions decrease in size with firm pressure and then return to their original size within 10 to 15 seconds.
- Lesions may become scaly and may ulcerate with bleeding.

Lichen amyloidosis
- Discrete, firm, hemispherical, pruritic papules appear on the anterior tibiae, feet, and thighs.
- Papules may be brown or yellow and smooth or scaly.

Lichen planus
- White lines or spots mark discrete, flat, angular or polygonal, violet papules.
- Papules may be linear or may coalesce into plaques and usually appear on the lumbar region, genitalia, ankles, anterior tibiae, and wrists.
- Rash usually develops first on the buccal mucosa as a lacy network of white or gray threadlike papules or plaques.
- Other findings include pruritus, distorted fingernails, and atrophic alopecia.

Mononucleosis (infectious)
- A maculopapular rash that resembles rubella is an early sign.
- Headache, malaise, and fatigue typically precede the rash.
- Other findings include sore throat, cervical lymphadenopathy, hepatosplenomegaly, and fluctuating temperature with an evening peak of 101° to 102° F (38.3° to 38.9° C).

Pityriasis rosea
- Initially, an erythematous, slightly raised, oval lesion appears anywhere on the body.
- Later, yellow to tan or erythematous patches with scaly edges appear on the trunk, arms, and legs, commonly erupting along body cleavage lines in a pine tree-shaped pattern.

Polymorphic light eruption
- Papular, vesicular, or nodular rash appears on sun-exposed areas.
- Other symptoms include pruritus, headache, and malaise.

Psoriasis
- Initially, small, erythematous pruritic and, sometimes, painful papules appear on the scalp, chest, elbows, knees, back, buttocks, and genitalia.
- Eventually, papules enlarge and coalesce, forming elevated, red, scaly plaques covered by characteristic silver scales.
- Other findings include pitted fingernails and arthralgia.

Rosacea
- Persistent erythema; telangiectasia; and recurrent eruption of papules and pustules on the forehead, malar areas, nose, and chin occur.

Sarcoidosis
- In this multisystem granulomatous disorder, small, erythematous or yellow-brown papules appear around the eyes and mouth, and on the nose, nasal mucosa, and upper back.
- Other findings include dyspnea with a nonproductive cough, fatigue, arthralgia, weight loss, lymphadenopathy, vision loss, and dysphagia.

Seborrheic keratosis
- Benign skin tumors begin as small, yellow-brown papules on the chest, back, or abdomen, eventually enlarging and becoming deeply pigmented.

Smallpox
- Maculopapular rash develops on the oral mucosa, pharynx, face, and forearms, and then spreads to the trunk and legs.

(continued)

- Within 2 days, rash becomes vesicular, and later, round firm pustules develop that are deeply embedded in the skin.
- After 8 to 9 days, pustules form a crust; later the scab separates from the skin, leaving a pitted scar.
- Initial findings include high fever, malaise, prostration, severe headache, backache, and abdominal pain.

Syphilis
- A discrete, reddish brown, mucocutaneous rash and general lymphadenopathy herald the onset of secondary syphilis.
- Rash may be papular, macular, pustular, or nodular and erupts between rolls of fat on the trunk and proximally on the arms, palms, soles, face, and scalp.
- Other findings include headache; malaise; anorexia; weight loss; nausea; vomiting; sore throat; low-grade fever; temporary alopecia; and brittle, pitted nails.

Systemic lupus erythematosus
- In this chronic connective tissue disease, a characteristic butterfly-shaped rash of erythematous maculopapules or discoid plaques in a malar distribution appears across the nose and cheeks.
- Other findings include photosensitivity, nondeforming arthritis, patchy alopecia, mucous membrane ulceration, fever, chills, lymphadenopathy, anorexia, weight loss, abdominal pain, diarrhea or constipation, dyspnea, hematuria, headache, and irritability.

OTHER
Drugs
- Allopurinol, antibiotics, benzodiazepines, gold salts, isoniazid, lithium, phenylbutazone, and salicylates may cause transient maculopapular rashes, usually on the trunk.

NURSING CONSIDERATIONS

- Apply cool compresses or an antipruritic lotion.
- Administer an antihistamine for allergic reactions and an antibiotic for infection.

PEDIATRIC TIPS
- Common causes include infectious diseases, scabies, insect bites, allergies, drug reactions, and miliaria.

GERIATRIC TIPS
- An erythematous area, sometimes with firm papules, may be the first sign of a pressure ulcer.

◆ Teach the patient appropriate skin care measures.
◆ Explain ways to reduce itching.
◆ Discuss signs and symptoms to report.

Paralysis

- Refers to total loss of voluntary motor function from severe cortical or pyramidal tract damage
- Can be local or widespread, symmetrical or asymmetrical, transient or permanent, and spastic or flaccid
- Classified as paraplegia, quadriplegia, or hemiplegia

ACTION STAT! If paralysis develops suddenly, suspect trauma or acute vascular insult. Immobilize the patient's spine, determine level of consciousness (LOC), take vital signs, and assess for signs of increasing intracranial pressure (ICP). Elevate the patient's head 30 degrees, if possible, to reduce ICP. Evaluate respiratory status, administer oxygen, and prepare the patient for intubation and mechanical ventilation, as needed.

HISTORY

- Determine the onset (and preceding events), duration, intensity, and progression of paralysis.
- Obtain a medical history, including neurologic or neuromuscular disease, recent infectious illness, sexually transmitted disease, cancer, recent injury, or recent immunizations.
- Find out about fever, headache, vision disturbances, dysphagia, nausea and vomiting, bowel or bladder dysfunction, muscle pain or weakness, and fatigue.

PHYSICAL ASSESSMENT

- Perform a complete neurologic examination.
- Test cranial nerve, motor, and sensory function, and deep tendon reflexes (DTRs).
- Assess strength in all major muscle groups, noting any muscle atrophy.

MEDICAL

Amyotrophic lateral sclerosis
- In this life-threatening progressive neurologic disorder, spastic or flaccid paralysis occurs in the major muscle groups and progresses to total paralysis.
- Early findings include progressive muscle weakness, fasciculations, hyperreflexia, and muscle atrophy.
- Later, respiratory distress, dysarthria, drooling, choking, and difficulty chewing occur.

Bell's palsy
- Transient paralysis in muscles on one side of the face.
- Increased tearing, drooling, inability to close eyelid, and a diminished or absent corneal reflex occur.

Brain tumor
- If a tumor affects the motor cortex of the frontal lobe, contralateral hemiparesis progresses to hemiplegia.
- Early findings include frontal headache and behavioral changes.
- Later findings include seizures, aphasia, and signs of increased ICP.

Conversion disorder
- Loss of voluntary movement can affect any muscle group and has no obvious physical cause.
- Paralysis appears and disappears unpredictably.

Encephalitis
- Variable paralysis develops in the late stages.
- Earlier findings include rapidly deteriorating LOC, fever, headache, photophobia, vomiting, signs of meningeal irritation, aphasia, ataxia, nystagmus, ocular palsies, myoclonus, and seizures.

Guillain-Barré syndrome
- A rapidly developing, reversible paralysis begins as leg muscle weakness and ascends symmetrically; respiratory muscle paralysis may be life-threatening.

Head trauma
- Sudden paralysis may occur; location and extent vary, depending on the injury.
- Other findings include decreased LOC, sensory disturbances, headache, blurred or double vision, nausea, vomiting, and focal neurologic disturbances.

Migraine headache
- Hemiparesis, scotomas, paresthesia, confusion, dizziness, photophobia, and other transient symptoms may precede the onset of a throbbing unilateral headache and may persist after it subsides.

Multiple sclerosis
- Paralysis waxes and wanes until the later stages, when it may become permanent; it ranges from monoplegia to quadriplegia.
- Late findings vary and may include muscle weakness and spasticity; hyperreflexia; intention tremor; gait ataxia; dysphagia; dysarthria; impotence; constipation; and urinary frequency, urgency, and incontinence.

Myasthenia gravis
- Muscle weakness and fatigue produce paralysis of certain muscle groups.
- Paralysis is usually transient in early stages but becomes more persistent as the disease progresses.
- Other findings include ptosis, diplopia, lack of facial mobility, dysphagia, dyspnea, and shallow respirations.

Neurosyphilis
- Irreversible hemiplegia may occur in the late stages, accompanied by dementia, cranial nerve palsies, meningitis, personality changes, tremors, and abnormal reflexes.

Parkinson's disease
- Extreme rigidity can progress to paralysis, particularly in the extremities.
- Tremors, bradykinesia, and "lead-pipe" or "cogwheel" rigidity are the classic signs.

Peripheral nerve trauma
- Loss of motor and sensory function in the innervated area may occur.
- Muscles become flaccid and atrophied, and reflexes are lost.

Peripheral neuropathy
- Muscle weakness may lead to flaccid paralysis and atrophy.
- Related findings include paresthesia, loss of vibration sensation, hypoactive or absent DTRs, neuralgia, and skin changes.

Rabies
- Progressive flaccid paralysis, vascular collapse, coma, and death within 2 weeks of contact with an infected animal.
- Early symptoms include fever; headache; hyperesthesia; photophobia; and excessive salivation, lacrimation, and perspiration.
- Within 2 to 10 days, agitation, cranial nerve dysfunction, cyclic respirations, high fever, urine retention, drooling, and hydrophobia occur.

Seizure disorder
- Transient local paralysis from focal seizures, which may be preceded by an aura.

Spinal cord injury
- Complete spinal cord transection results in permanent spastic paralysis below the level of the injury; reflexes may return after spinal shock resolves.

(continued)

- Partial transection causes variable paralysis and paresthesia. (See *Understanding spinal cord syndromes.*)

Understanding spinal cord syndromes

When a patient's spinal cord is incompletely severed, he experiences partial motor and sensory loss. Most incomplete cord lesions fit into one of the syndromes described here.

Anterior cord syndrome, usually resulting from a flexion injury, causes motor paralysis and loss of pain and temperature sensation below the level of injury. Touch, proprioception, and vibration sensation are usually preserved.

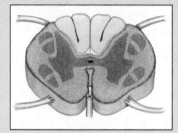

Brown-Séquard syndrome can result from flexion, rotation, or penetration injury. It's characterized by unilateral motor paralysis ipsilateral to the injury and loss of pain and temperature sensation contralateral to the injury.

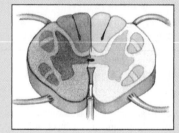

Central cord syndrome is caused by hyperextension or flexion injury. Motor loss is variable and greater in the arms than in the legs; sensory loss is usually slight.

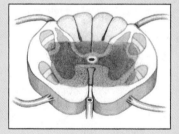

Posterior cord syndrome, produced by a cervical hyperextension injury, causes only a loss of proprioception and loss of light touch sensation. Motor function remains intact.

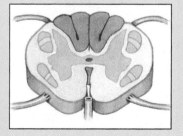

Spinal cord tumor
- Paresis, pain, paresthesia, and variable sensory loss may occur.
- Condition may progress to spastic paralysis with hyperactive DTRs, and bladder and bowel incontinence.

Stroke
- Contralateral paresis or paralysis can result if the motor cortex is involved.
- Other findings include headache, vomiting, seizures, decreased LOC, dysphagia, ataxia, contralateral paresthesia or sensory loss, apraxia, aphasia, vision disturbances, and bowel and bladder dysfunction.

Subarachnoid hemorrhage
- Sudden paralysis (temporary or permanent) may occur.
- Other findings include severe headache, mydriasis, photophobia, aphasia, decreased LOC, nuchal rigidity, vomiting, and seizures.

Thoracic aortic aneurysm
- Sudden transient paralysis may occur.
- Prominent symptoms include severe chest pain radiating to the neck, shoulders, back, and abdomen, and a sensation of tearing in the thorax.
- Other findings include diaphoresis, dyspnea, tachycardia, cyanosis, diastolic heart murmur, and abrupt loss of radial and femoral pulses, or wide variations in pulses and blood pressure between the arms and legs.

Transient ischemic attack
- Transient paresis or paralysis on one side with paresthesia, blurred or double vision, dizziness, aphasia, dysarthria, and decreased LOC may occur.

West Nile encephalitis
- Paralysis may occur in more severe infections, accompanied by fever, neck stiffness, decreased LOC, seizures, headache, rash, and lymphadenopathy.

OTHER

Drugs

◆ Neuromuscular blockers produce paralysis.

Electroconvulsive therapy (ECT)

◆ ECT can produce acute, but transient, paralysis.

◆ Change the patient's position frequently and provide skin care to prevent breakdown.
◆ Administer frequent chest physiotherapy.
◆ Perform passive range-of-motion (ROM) exercises to maintain muscle tone.
◆ Apply splints to prevent contractures.
◆ Use footboards or other devices to prevent footdrop.
◆ Arrange for physical, speech, and occupational therapy, as appropriate.

PEDIATRIC TIPS

◆ Paralysis may develop from hereditary or congenital disorders.

◆ Provide referrals to social and psychological services.
◆ Explain underlying disorder and treatment plan.
◆ Teach the patient and family how to provide care at home including passive ROM exercises, frequent turning, and chest physiotherapy.

Paresthesia

- Refers to abnormal sensation or combination of sensations—commonly described as numbness, prickling, or tingling—along peripheral nerve pathways
- May develop suddenly or gradually and may be transient or permanent

HISTORY

- Ask about the onset and nature of abnormal sensations.
- Inquire about other findings, such as sensory loss and paresis.
- Find out about recent traumatic injury, surgery, or invasive procedure.
- Take a medical history, including neurologic, cardiovascular, metabolic, renal, and chronic inflammatory disorders.

PHYSICAL ASSESSMENT

- Assess level of consciousness (LOC) and cranial nerve function.
- Test muscle strength and deep tendon reflexes (DTRs) in affected limbs.
- Evaluate light touch, pain, temperature, vibration, and position sensation.
- Note skin color and temperature, and palpate pulses.

CAUSES

MEDICAL

Arterial occlusion (acute)
- Sudden paresthesia and coldness occurs in the affected extremity; it may occur in one or both legs with a saddle embolus.
- Paresis, intermittent claudication, aching pain at rest, mottling, and absent pulses occur below the occlusion.

Arteriosclerosis obliterans
- Paresthesia may occur in the affected leg, along with intermittent claudication, pallor, paresis, coldness, and diminished or absent popliteal and pedal pulses.

Arthritis
- If the cervical spine is affected, paresthesias may occur in the neck, shoulders, and arms.
- If the lumbar spine is affected, paresthesias may occur in the legs and feet.

Brain tumor
- Progressive contralateral paresthesia may occur with tumors of the sensory cortex.
- Agnosia, apraxia, agraphia, homonymous hemianopsia, and loss of proprioception may also occur.

Buerger's disease
- In this inflammatory, occlusive vascular disorder, the feet become cold, cyanotic, and numb after exposure to cold; later they redden, become hot, and tingle.
- Other findings include intermittent claudication, weak peripheral pulses, migratory superficial thrombophlebitis and, later, ulceration, muscle atrophy, and gangrene.

Diabetes mellitus
- Paresthesia and a burning sensation may occur in the hands and legs.
- Other findings include anosmia, fatigue, polyuria, polydipsia, weight loss, and polyphagia.

Guillain-Barré syndrome
- Transient paresthesia may precede muscle weakness, which usually begins in the legs and ascends to the arms and facial nerves.
- Other findings include dysarthria, dysphagia, nasal speech, orthostatic hypotension, bladder and bowel incontinence, diaphoresis, tachycardia and, possibly, life-threatening respiratory muscle paralysis.

Head trauma
- Paresthesia may occur with a concussion or contusion.
- Other findings include variable paresis or paralysis, decreased LOC, headache, blurred or double vision, nausea, vomiting, dizziness, and seizures.

Heavy metal or solvent poisoning
- Acute or gradual paresthesia may occur.
- Mental status changes, tremors, weakness, seizures, and GI distress may occur.

Herniated disk
- Paresthesia may occur along with severe pain, muscle spasms, and weakness.

Herpes zoster
- Paresthesia occurs early in the dermatome supplied by affected spinal nerve.
- Within several days, a pruritic, erythematous, vesicular rash associated with sharp, shooting, or burning pain occurs in the affected dermatome.

Hyperventilation syndrome
◆ Transient paresthesia may occur in hands, feet, and perioral area.
◆ Other findings include agitation, vertigo, syncope, pallor, muscle twitching and weakness, carpopedal spasm and arrhythmias.

Hypocalcemia
◆ Asymmetrical paresthesia may occur in fingers, toes, and circumoral area.
◆ Other findings include muscle weakness, twitching or cramps; palpitations; hyperactive DTRs; carpopedal spasm; and positive Chvostek's and Trousseau's sign.

Migraine headache
◆ Paresthesia in hands, face, and perioral area may signal an impending migraine headache.
◆ Other early findings include scotomas, hemiparesis, confusion, dizziness, and photophobia.

Multiple sclerosis
◆ An early symptom, paresthesia commonly waxes and wanes until the later stages when it becomes permanent.
◆ Other findings include muscle weakness, spasticity, and hyperreflexia.

Peripheral nerve trauma
◆ Paresthesia and dysesthesia may occur in the area supplied by the affected nerve.
◆ Other findings include flaccid paralysis or paresis, hyporeflexia, and sensory loss.

Peripheral neuropathy
◆ Progressive paresthesia may occur in all extremities.
◆ Other findings include muscle weakness that may progress to flaccid paralysis and atrophy, loss of vibration sensation, diminished or absent DTRs, and cutaneous changes.

Rabies
◆ Paresthesia, coldness, and itching at site of an animal bite may occur in the early stage.

Raynaud's disease
◆ Exposure to cold or stress turns fingers pale, cold, and cyanotic; with rewarming, they become red, throbbing, aching, swollen, and paresthetic.

Seizure disorder
◆ Paresthesia of the lips, fingers, and toes results from seizures originating in the parietal lobe.
◆ Paresthesia may act as auras that precede tonic-clonic seizures.

Spinal cord injury
◆ Paresthesia may occur in partial spinal cord transection, after spinal shock resolves, at or below the level of the lesion.
◆ Sensory and motor loss varies.

Spinal cord tumor
◆ Paresthesia, paresis, pain, and sensory loss occur.
◆ Eventually, paresis may cause spastic paralysis with hyperactive DTRs and, possibly, bladder and bowel incontinence.

Stroke
◆ Although contralateral paresthesia may occur, sensory loss is more common.
◆ Associated findings vary and may include contralateral hemiplegia, decreased LOC, and homonymous hemianopsia.

Systemic lupus erythematosus
◆ Paresthesia may occur, but primary findings include nondeforming arthritis, photosensitivity, and a butterfly-shaped rash across the nose and cheeks.

Thoracic outlet syndrome
◆ Paresthesia occurs suddenly when the affected arm is raised and abducted.
◆ Arm becomes pale and cool, with diminished pulses.

Transient ischemic attack
◆ Abrupt paresthesia limited to an isolated body part occurs.

◆ Other findings include decreased LOC, dizziness, unilateral vision loss, nystagmus, aphasia, dysarthria, tinnitus, facial weakness, dysphagia, and ataxic gait.

Vitamin B deficiency
◆ Paresthesia and weakness may occur in the arms and legs.
◆ Other findings include burning leg pain, hypoactive DTRs, variable sensory loss, changes in mental status, and impaired vision.

OTHER
Drugs
◆ Chemotherapeutics, chloroquine, penicillamine, isoniazid, nitrofurantoin, parenteral gold therapy, and phenytoin may produce transient paresthesia.

Radiation therapy
◆ Long-term radiation therapy may cause peripheral nerve damage, resulting in paresthesia.

NURSING CONSIDERATIONS

◆ Monitor neurologic status.
◆ Help the patient perform daily activities as needed.
◆ If sensory deficits are present, protect the patient from injury.

PEDIATRIC TIPS
◆ Children usually can't describe this symptom.
◆ Hereditary polyneuropathies are first recognized in childhood.

PATIENT TEACHING

◆ Discuss safety measures.
◆ Tell the patient which signs and symptoms to report.
◆ Teach about underlying diagnosis and treatment plan.

Paroxysmal nocturnal dyspnea

- Abruptly awakens patient
- Includes common associated findings of diaphoresis, coughing, wheezing, and chest discomfort
- Abates after patient sits up or stands for several minutes, but may recur every 2 to 3 hours

- Obtain history of the patient's dyspnea including non-nocturnal episodes, triggers, timing, and frequency.
- Find out if he experiences coughing, wheezing, fatigue, or weakness during an attack.
- Ask if he has a history of lower extremity edema or jugular vein distention.
- Ask if he sleeps with his head elevated and, if so, on how many pillows or if he sleeps in a reclining chair.
- Obtain a cardiopulmonary history including history of a myocardial infarction, coronary artery disease, or hypertension or of chronic bronchitis, emphysema, asthma or cardiac surgery.

- Perform a physical examination. Begin by taking the patient's vital signs and forming an overall impression of his appearance looking for cyanosis or edema.
- Auscultate the lungs for crackles and wheezing, and the heart for gallops and arrhythmias.

CAUSES

MEDICAL

Left-sided heart failure

◆ Dyspnea—on exertion, during sleep, and eventually even at rest—is an early sign of left-sided heart failure. This sign is characteristically accompanied by Cheyne-Stokes respirations, diaphoresis, weakness, wheezing, and a persistent, nonproductive cough or a cough that produces clear or blood-tinged sputum.

◆ As the patient's condition worsens, he develops tachycardia, tachypnea, alternating pulse (commonly initiated by a premature beat), a ventricular gallop, crackles, and peripheral edema.

◆ With advanced left-sided heart failure, the patient may also exhibit severe orthopnea, cyanosis, clubbing, hemoptysis, and cardiac arrhythmias, as well as signs and symptoms of shock, such as hypotension, a weak pulse, and cold, clammy skin.

NURSING CONSIDERATIONS

◆ Prepare the patient for diagnostic tests, such as a chest X-ray, echocardiography, exercise electrocardiography, and cardiac blood pool imaging.

◆ If the hospitalized patient experiences paroxysmal nocturnal dyspnea, assist him to a sitting position or help him walk around the room. If necessary, provide supplemental oxygen. Try to calm him because anxiety can exacerbate dyspnea.

PEDIATRIC TIPS

◆ Paroxysmal nocturnal dyspnea usually stems from a congenital heart defect that precipitates heart failure.

◆ Help relieve dyspnea by elevating the patient's head and calming him.

PATIENT TEACHING

◆ Teach the patient about left-sided heart failure and its treatment plan.

◆ Tell about prescribed medications and their adverse effects.

◆ Explain to the patient what he can do during an attack to prevent exacerbation of dyspnea.

Peau d'orange

OVERVIEW

- Results from edematous thickening and pitting of breast skin that resembles an orange peel (see *Recognizing peau d'orange*)
- Usually a late sign of breast cancer

HISTORY

- Ask when peau d'orange was first noticed.
- Inquire about lumps, pain, or other breast changes.
- Find out about associated malaise, achiness, and weight loss.
- Take a lactation history.
- Obtain a history of previous breast or axillary surgery.

PHYSICAL ASSESSMENT

- Estimate the extent of peau d'orange.
- Check for breast erythema and induration.
- Assess the nipples for discharge, deviation, retraction, dimpling, and cracking.
- Palpate the area of peau d'orange for warmth or induration.
- Palpate the rest of the breast for lumps.
- Palpate the axillary lymph nodes, noting enlargement.
- Take the patient's temperature.

 TOP TECHNIQUE

Recognizing peau d'orange

In peau d'orange, the skin appears to be pitted (as shown). This condition usually indicates late-stage breast cancer.

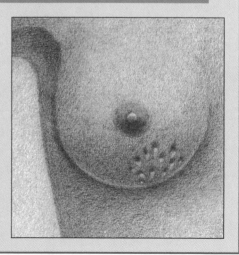

MEDICAL
Breast abscess
♦ Peau d'orange may occur with malaise, breast tenderness and erythema, and a sudden fever with shaking chills.
♦ Other findings include purulent discharge from a cracked nipple and possibly a mass.

Breast cancer
♦ Peau d'orange usually begins in dependent part of breast or areola.
♦ Palpation typically reveals a firm, immobile mass that adheres to skin above area of peau d'orange.
♦ Other findings may include changes in breast contour, size, or symmetry. Nipples may reveal deviation; erosion; retraction; and a thin and watery, bloody, or purulent discharge.

Erysipelas
♦ A well-demarcated, erythematous, elevated area, typically with a peau d'orange texture may occur due to this streptococcal infection.
♦ Other findings include pain, warmth, fever, and fatigue.

Graves' disease
♦ In this hyperthyroid disorder, raised, thickened, hyperpigmented, peau d'orange areas join together.
♦ Other findings include weight loss, palpitations, anxiety, heat intolerance, tremor, and amenorrhea.

♦ Because peau d'orange usually signals advanced breast cancer, provide emotional support.
♦ Monitor breast for nipple discharge and change in sensation.
♦ Administer prescribed pain medications as needed.

♦ Explain diagnostic tests and treatment options.
♦ Teach the patient how to do monthly breast self-examinations.
♦ Tell the patient which signs and symptoms to report.
♦ Discuss skin care if nipple discharge is present.

Pericardial friction rub

OVERVIEW

◆ Occurs when two inflamed layers of the pericardium slide over each other causing a scratching, grating, or crunching sound that ranges from faint to loud
◆ Three types: presystolic, systolic, and diastolic (see *Understanding pericardial rubs*)
◆ Is best heard along the lower left sternal border during deep inspiration

HISTORY

◆ Take a medical history, noting cancer, cardiac dysfunction, myocardial infarction, cardiac surgery, pericarditis, rheumatoid arthritis, chronic renal failure, infection, systemic lupus erythematosus, or trauma.
◆ Obtain a description of any chest pain, including character, location, and aggravating and alleviating factors.

PHYSICAL ASSESSMENT

◆ Take vital signs, noting hypotension, tachycardia, irregular pulse, tachypnea, and fever.
◆ Inspect for jugular vein distention, edema, ascites, and hepatomegaly.
◆ Auscultate heart sounds; to listen for a pericardial friction rub, have the patient sit upright, lean forward and exhale. (See *Pericardial rub or murmur?*)
◆ Auscultate the lungs for crackles. (See *Comparing auscultation findings.*)

TOP TECHNIQUE

Pericardial rub or murmur?

Is the sound you hear a pericardial rub or a murmur? Here's how to tell. The classic pericardial rub has three sound components, which are related to the phases of the cardiac cycle. In some patients, however, the rub's presystolic and early diastolic sounds may be inaudible, causing the rub to resemble the murmur of mitral insufficiency or aortic stenosis and regurgitation.

If you don't detect the classic three-component sound, you can distinguish a pericardial rub from a murmur by auscultating again and asking yourself these questions:

How deep is the sound?
A pericardial rub usually sounds superficial; a murmur sounds deeper in the chest.

Does the sound radiate?
A pericardial rub usually doesn't radiate; a murmur may radiate widely.

Does the sound vary with inspiration or changes in patient position?
A pericardial rub is usually loudest during inspiration and is best heard when the patient leans forward. A murmur varies in timing and duration with both factors.

TOP TECHNIQUE

Understanding pericardial rubs

The complete, or classic, pericardial rub is triphasic. Its three sound components are linked to phases of the cardiac cycle. The presystolic component (A) reflects atrial systole and precedes the first heart sound (S_1). The systolic component (B)—usually the loudest—reflects ventricular systole and occurs between the S_1 and the second heart sound (S_2). The early diastolic component (C) reflects ventricular diastole and follows the S_2.

Sometimes, the early diastolic component merges with the presystolic component, producing a diphasic to-and-fro sound on auscultation. In other patients, auscultation may detect only one component—a monophasic rub, typically during ventricular systole.

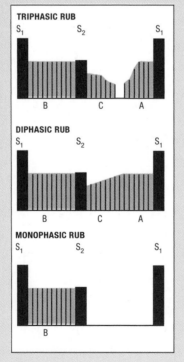

MEDICAL
Pericarditis
- Pericardial rub, the classic sign of acute pericarditis, is accompanied by sharp precordial or retrosternal pain that radiates to the left shoulder, neck, and back.
- Pain worsens with deep breathing, coughing, and lying flat.
- Pain lessens when the patient sits up and leans forward.
- Other findings of the acute condition include fever, dyspnea, tachycardia, and arrhythmias.
- In the chronic condition, a pericardial rub develops gradually and may be accompanied by peripheral edema, ascites, Kussmaul's sign, hepatomegaly, dyspnea, orthopnea, paradoxical pulse, and chest pain.

OTHER
Drugs
- Chemotherapeutics and procainamide (Pronestyl) can cause pericarditis.

Treatments
- Cardiac surgery and high-dose radiation therapy can cause pericardial friction rub.

- Monitor the patient's cardiovascular status.
- If the pericardial rub disappears, look for signs of cardiac tamponade; if the signs develop, prepare the patient for pericardiocentesis.
- Make sure that the patient gets adequate rest.
- Give an anti-inflammatory, antiarrhythmic, diuretic, or antimicrobial, as ordered, to treat the underlying cause.
- Anticipate pericardiectomy to promote cardiac filling and contraction.

PEDIATRIC TIPS
- A pericardial rub may develop with bacterial pericarditis, a life-threatening condition that usually occurs before age 6.
- A pericardial rub may occur after surgery to correct congenital cardiac anomalies.

- Teach about underlying disorder and treatments.
- Explain what the patient can do to minimize his symptoms.

 TOP TECHNIQUE

Comparing auscultation findings

During auscultation, you may detect a pleural friction rub, crackles, or a pericardial friction rub—three abnormal sounds that are commonly confused. Use this chart to help clarify auscultation findings.

FINDING	CAUSE	QUALITY	LOCATION	TIMING
Pleural rub	Inflamed visceral and parietal pleural surfaces that rub against each other	Loud and grating, creaking, or squeaking	Best heard over the low axilla or the anterior, lateral, or posterior base of the lung	Occurs in late inspiration and early expiration but ceases when the patient holds his breath; persists during coughing
Crackles	Air that suddenly enters fluid-filled airways	Nonmusical clicking or rattling	Best heard at less distended and more dependent areas of the lungs, usually at the bases	Occurs chiefly during inspiration
Pericardial rub	Inflamed layers of the pericardium that rub against each other	Hard and grating, scratching, or crunching	Best heard along the lower left sternal border	Occurs in relation to heartbeat; most noticeable during deep inspiration and continues even when the patient holds his breath

Peristaltic waves, visible

OVERVIEW

- Occur when peristalsis increases in strength and frequency as the intestine contracts to force its contents past an obstruction
- Usually, peristaltic waves not visible; if visible, appear suddenly and vanish quickly
- Best detected by stooping at the patient's side and inspecting abdominal contour while he's in a supine position

HISTORY

- Obtain a medical history, including a history of pyloric ulcer, stomach cancer, chronic gastritis, intestinal obstruction, intestinal tumors or polyps, gallstones, chronic constipation, and hernia.
- Ask about recent abdominal surgery.
- Take a drug history.
- Find out about related signs and symptoms, such as abdominal pain, nausea, and vomiting.
- Obtain a description of the vomitus, including consistency, amount, and color.

PHYSICAL ASSESSMENT

- Inspect the abdomen for distention, surgical scars, adhesions, or visible bowel loops.
- Auscultate for bowel sounds.
- Roll the patient from side to side and then auscultate for succussion splash, which is a splashing sound in the stomach from retained secretions caused by pyloric obstruction.
- Percuss for tympany. (See *Performing an abdominal assessment*.)
- Palpate abdomen for rigidity and tenderness.
- Check skin and mucous membranes for dryness and poor skin turgor.
- Take vital signs, noting tachycardia and hypotension.

TOP TECHNIQUE

Performing an abdominal assessment

When performing an abdominal assessment, use this sequence:
1. Inspection
2. Auscultation
3. Percussion
4. Palpation
   Palpating or percussing the abdomen before you auscultate can change the character of the patient's bowel sounds, resulting in an inaccurate assessment.

MEDICAL

Large-bowel obstruction
- Visible peristaltic waves in the upper abdomen are an early sign.
- Obstipation (severe constipation) may be the earliest sign.
- Other characteristic findings include nausea, colicky abdominal pain, abdominal distention, and hyperactive bowel sounds.

Pyloric obstruction
- Peristaltic waves may be detected in a swollen epigastrium or in the left upper quadrant, usually beginning near the left rib margin and rolling from left to right.
- Auscultation reveals a loud succussion splash.
- Related findings include vague epigastric discomfort or colicky pain after eating, nausea, vomiting, anorexia, and weight loss.

Small-bowel obstruction
- Peristaltic waves rolling across the upper abdomen and intermittent, cramping, periumbilical pain are early signs, along with hyperactive bowel sounds and slight abdominal distention.
- Other findings include nausea; vomiting of bilious or, later, fecal material; and constipation.
- With partial obstruction, diarrhea may occur.

- Withhold food and fluids.
- If obstruction is confirmed, perform nasogastric suctioning to decompress the stomach and small bowel as ordered.
- Provide frequent oral hygiene.
- Monitor for dehydration.
- Frequently monitor vital signs and intake and output.

PEDIATRIC TIPS
- In infants, visible peristaltic waves may indicate pyloric stenosis.
- In small children, peristaltic waves may be visible normally or may indicate bowel obstruction.

GERIATRIC TIPS
- In elderly patients, always check for fecal impaction, which is common in this age group.
- Obtain a detailed drug history; antidepressants and antipsychotics can predispose to constipation and bowel obstruction.

- Discuss diet and fluid requirements.
- Encourage the use of stool softeners and increased intake of high-fiber foods for patients with chronic constipation.
- Discuss underlying diagnosis and treatment plan.

Photophobia

OVERVIEW

- Refers to abnormal sensitivity to light
- Commonly indicates increased eye sensitivity without any underlying disease
- May indicate a systemic disorder, an ocular disorder or trauma, or the use of certain drugs

HISTORY

- Ask about the onset and severity of photophobia.
- Inquire about recent eye trauma, chemical splash, or exposure to sun lamp rays.
- Obtain a description of the location, duration, intensity, and characteristics of any pain or discomfort.
- Find out about vision changes or increased tearing.

PHYSICAL ASSESSMENT

- Take vital signs.
- Assess neurologic status.
- Inspect the eyes' external structures.
- Examine the conjunctivae and sclera, noting their color.
- Characterize the amount and consistency of any discharge.
- Check pupillary reaction to light.
- Evaluate extraocular muscle function by testing the six cardinal positions of gaze.
- Test visual acuity.

CAUSES

MEDICAL
Burns

- With a chemical burn, photophobia and eye pain may be accompanied by erythema and blistering on the face and eyelids, miosis, diffuse conjunctival injection, blurred vision, inability to keep the eyes open, and corneal changes.
- With ultraviolet radiation burn, photophobia occurs with moderate to severe eye pain.

Conjunctivitis

- Photophobia occurs when conjunctivitis affects the cornea.
- Other common findings include conjunctival injection; increased tearing; a foreign-body sensation; a feeling of fullness around the eyes; and eye pain, burning, and itching.
- Allergic conjunctivitis causes stringy eye discharge and milky red injection.
- Bacterial conjunctivitis causes brilliant red conjunctiva with copious, mucopurulent, flaky eye discharge.
- Fungal conjunctivitis produces a thick, purulent discharge; extreme redness; and crusting, sticky eyelids.
- Viral conjunctivitis causes copious tearing with little discharge and enlarged preauricular nodes.

Corneal abrasion

- Photophobia is usually accompanied by excessive tearing, conjunctival injection, visible corneal damage, blurred vision, eye pain, and foreign-body sensation in the eye.

Corneal foreign body

- Photophobia may occur with miosis, intense eye pain, foreign-body sensation, slightly impaired vision, conjunctival injection, and profuse tearing.

Corneal ulcer

- Severe photophobia and eye pain are aggravated by blinking.

- Impaired visual acuity, blurring, eye discharge, conjunctival injection, and sticky eyelids may also occur.
- A bacterial ulcer may also cause an irregularly shaped corneal ulcer and pupillary constriction.
- A fungal ulcer may be surrounded by progressively clearer rings.

Dry eye syndrome
- Photophobia may occur, but eye pain, conjunctival injection, a foreign-body sensation, itching, excessive mucus secretion and, possibly, decreased tearing and difficulty moving the eyelids are more common symptoms.

Iritis (acute)
- Severe photophobia occurs, along with conjunctival injection, moderate to severe eye pain, and blurred vision.
- Pupil may be constricted and respond poorly to light.

Keratitis (interstitial)
- Photophobia occurs along with eye pain, blurred vision, dramatic conjunctival injection, and grayish pink corneas.

Meningitis (acute bacterial)
- Photophobia occurs with such signs as nuchal rigidity, hyperreflexia, Brudzinski's and Kernig's signs, fever, chills, and opisthotonos.
- Related findings include headache, vomiting, ocular palsies, facial weakness, pupillary abnormalities, hearing loss, seizures, and altered level of consciousness.

Migraine headache
- Photophobia and noise sensitivity are prominent features.
- Other findings include fatigue, blurred vision, nausea, and vomiting.

Scleritis
- Photophobia occurs along with severe eye pain, conjunctival injection, a bluish purple sclera, and profuse tearing.

Uveitis
- Photophobia results from both anterior and posterior uveitis.
- Anterior uveitis also produces moderate to severe eye pain, severe conjunctival injection, and a small nonreactive pupil.
- Posterior uveitis develops slowly, causing visual floaters, eye pain, pupil distortion, conjunctival injection, and blurred vision.

OTHER
Drugs
- Amphetamines, cocaine, mydriatics, and ophthalmic antifungals can cause photophobia.

NURSING CONSIDERATIONS

- Darken the room and tell the patient to close his eyes.
- Administer corticosteroids and antibiotic drops or ointment as prescribed.
- Saline drops or other lubricating ointment can soothe dry eyes and improve photophobia.

PEDIATRIC TIPS
- Suspect photophobia in a child who squints, rubs his eyes frequently, or wears sunglasses indoors and outside.
- Congenital disorders such as albinism and childhood diseases, such as measles and rubella, can cause photophobia.

PATIENT TEACHING

- Teach the patient ways to increase comfort.
- Explain what diagnostic tests the patient will need.
- Discuss underlying diagnosis and treatment plan.
- Instruct the patient in the correct method of instilling eye drops or ointment.
- Stress the importance of completing antibiotic treatment if prescribed.

Pleural friction rub

- Refers to loud, coarse, grating, creaking, or squeaking sound that may be auscultated during late inspiration or early expiration
- Is indicative of inflammation of the visceral and parietal pleural lining
- Heard best over the low axilla or the anterior, lateral, or posterior bases of the lung fields with the patient in an upright position

ACTION STAT! Quickly look for signs of respiratory distress. Check for hypotension, tachycardia, and decreased level of consciousness. If you see signs of distress, open and maintain an airway. Endotracheal intubation and supplemental oxygen may be necessary. Insert a large-bore I.V. catheter to deliver drugs and fluids. Elevate the patient's head 30 degrees. Monitor cardiac status constantly, and check vital signs frequently.

HISTORY

- Obtain a description of chest pain, including onset, location, severity, duration, radiation, and aggravating and alleviating factors.
- Take a medical history, including rheumatoid arthritis, a respiratory or cardiovascular disorder, recent trauma, asbestos exposure, and radiation therapy.
- Ask about smoking history.

PHYSICAL ASSESSMENT

- Auscultate the lungs with the patient sitting upright and breathing deeply and slowly through the mouth.
- Determine whether the rub is in one lung or both.
- Listen for absent or diminished breath sounds.
- Palpate for decreased chest motion and percuss for flatness or dullness.
- Observe for clubbing and pedal edema.

CAUSES

MEDICAL
Asbestosis
- Pleural rub, exertional dyspnea, cough, chest pain, and crackles may occur.
- As the disease advances, clubbing and dyspnea develop.

Lung cancer
- A pleural rub may be heard in the area of the lung that's affected by the cancer.
- Other findings include a cough (possibly with hemoptysis), dyspnea, chest pain, weight loss, anorexia, fatigue, clubbing, fever, and wheezing.

Pleurisy
- A pleural rub occurs early.
- The main symptom is sudden, intense, unilateral chest pain in the lower and lateral parts of the chest; deep breathing, coughing, and thoracic movements aggravate the pain.
- Other findings include decreased breath sounds, inspiratory crackles, dyspnea, tachypnea, tachycardia, cyanosis, fever, and fatigue.

Pneumonia (bacterial)
- A pleural rub occurs after a dry, painful, hacking, productive cough.
- Other findings include shaking chills, high fever, headache, dyspnea, pleuritic chest pain, tachypnea, tachycardia, grunting respirations, nasal flaring, dullness to percussion, decreased breath sounds, and cyanosis.

Pulmonary embolism
- A pleural rub may occur over the affected area of the lung.
- The first symptom is usually sudden dyspnea, which may be accompanied by angina or unilateral pleuritic chest pain.
- Other findings include a nonproductive cough or a cough that produces blood-tinged sputum, tachycardia, tachypnea, low-grade fever, restlessness, and diaphoresis.

Rheumatoid arthritis
◆ A unilateral pleural rub may occur.
◆ Typical early findings include fatigue, persistent low-grade fever, weight loss, and vague arthralgia and myalgia.
◆ Later findings include warm, swollen, painful joints; joint stiffness after activity; subcutaneous nodules on the elbows; joint deformity; and muscle weakness and atrophy.

Systemic lupus erythematosus
◆ A pleural rub—accompanied by hemoptysis, dyspnea, pleuritic chest pain, and crackles—may occur with pulmonary involvement in this chronic inflammatory connective tissue disorder.
◆ More characteristic effects include a butterfly-shaped rash, nondeforming joint pain and stiffness, and photosensitivity.
◆ Fever, anorexia, weight loss, and lymphadenopathy may also occur.

Tuberculosis (pulmonary)
◆ A pleural rub may occur over the affected part of the lung.
◆ Early findings include weight loss, night sweats, low-grade fever in the afternoon, malaise, dyspnea, anorexia, and easy fatigability.
◆ Disease progression produces pleuritic chest pain, fine crackles over the upper lobes, and a productive cough with blood-streaked sputum.
◆ Advanced findings include chest wall retraction, tracheal deviation, and dullness to percussion.

OTHER
Treatments
◆ Thoracic surgery and radiation therapy can cause pleural rub.

NURSING CONSIDERATIONS
◆ Monitor the patient's respiratory status and vital signs.
◆ If the patient has a persistent dry, hacking cough that tires him, give an antitussive.
◆ Administer oxygen and an antibiotic as needed.
◆ Follow bleeding precautions in the patient on anticoagulation therapy for pulmonary embolism.

PEDIATRIC TIPS
◆ Auscultate for a pleural rub in a child who has grunting respirations, reports chest pain, or protects his chest.
◆ A pleural rub in a child is usually an early sign of pleurisy.

GERIATRIC TIPS
◆ Pleuritic chest pain may mimic cardiac chest pain.

PATIENT TEACHING
◆ Prepare the patient for diagnostic tests.
◆ Discuss pain relief measures.
◆ Explain signs and symptoms the patient needs to report.
◆ Discuss underlying disorder and treatment plan.

Polydipsia

- Refers to excessive thirst
- May reflect decreased fluid intake, increased urine output, or excessive loss of fluid

- Determine the patient's average fluid intake and output.
- Obtain a description of his urinary patterns.
- Take a personal or family history of diabetes or kidney disease.
- Take a drug history.
- Ask about recent weight loss.

- Obtain the patient's blood pressure and pulse when he's in supine and standing positions.
- Check for signs of dehydration, such as poor skin turgor and dry mucous membranes.
- Obtain urine and blood samples, as ordered.
- Perform complete physical assessment.

MEDICAL

Diabetes insipidus

- Polydipsia, excessive voiding of dilute urine, and nocturia occur.
- Fatigue and signs of dehydration occur in severe cases.

Diabetes mellitus

- Polydipsia is a classic finding.
- Polyuria, polyphagia, nocturia, and signs of dehydration may also occur.

Hypercalcemia

- In later stages, polydipsia occurs with polyuria, nocturia, constipation, paresthesia and, occasionally, hematuria and pyuria.
- If hypercalcemia is severe, vomiting, decreased level of consciousness, and renal failure develop.

Hypokalemia

- Polydipsia, polyuria, and nocturia may develop.
- Other related signs and symptoms include muscle weakness or paralysis, fatigue, decreased bowel sounds, hypoactive deep tendon reflexes, and arrhythmias.

Psychogenic polydipsia

- This psychiatric condition causes polydipsia in the absence of a physiologic stimulus to drink.
- No apparent reason for excessive thirst or fluid intake exists.
- The condition may be well-tolerated if water intoxication and hyponatremia don't occur.
- Related findings include confusion, headache, irritability, weight gain, elevated blood pressure, stupor, and coma.

Renal disorder (chronic)
- ◆ Polydipsia and polyuria signal kidney damage.
- ◆ Other related findings include nocturia, weakness, elevated blood pressure, pallor and, in later stages, oliguria.

Sickle cell anemia
- ◆ Polydipsia and polyuria occur as nephropathy develops.
- ◆ Other related signs and symptoms include abdominal pain and cramps, arthralgia and, occasionally, lower extremity skin ulcers and such bone deformities as kyphosis.

Thyrotoxicosis
- ◆ Polydipsia may occur infrequently with this disorder.
- ◆ Characteristic findings include tachycardia, palpitations, weight loss despite increased appetite, diarrhea, tremors, nervousness, heat intolerance, and enlarged thyroid.

OTHER
Drugs
- ◆ Diuretics and demeclocycline (Declomycin) may produce polydipsia.
- ◆ Phenothiazines and anticholinergics can cause dry mouth, making the patient so thirsty that he drinks compulsively.

NURSING CONSIDERATIONS
- ◆ Record total intake and output.
- ◆ Weigh the patient at the same time each day using the same scale.
- ◆ Check blood pressure and pulse in supine and standing positions.
- ◆ Give the patient ample liquids.

PEDIATRIC TIPS
- ◆ In children, polydipsia usually stems from diabetes insipidus or diabetes mellitus.
- ◆ Psychogenic polydipsia in children may reflect emotional difficulties.

PATIENT TEACHING
- ◆ Explain underlying disorder and treatments the patient will need.
- ◆ Teach about diet, exercise, and home blood-glucose monitoring.
- ◆ Stress the importance of reporting significant weight gain or loss.

Polyphagia

- Voracious or excessive eating
- Can be persistent or intermittent, resulting from endocrine or psychological disorders or from the use of certain drugs

HISTORY

- Ask about food intake during previous 24 hours, noting frequency of meals and amounts, and types of foods eaten.
- Note recent changes in food habits.
- Inquire about the pattern of overeating.
- Ask about any conditions triggering overeating, such as stress, depression, or menstruation.
- Ask the patient about vomiting or headache after overeating.
- Explore other relevant signs and symptoms, such as a recent gain or loss of weight; feeling tired, nervous, or excitable; and heat intolerance, dizziness, palpitations, diarrhea, or increased thirst or urination.
- Obtain a complete drug history, including the use of laxatives or enemas.

PHYSICAL ASSESSMENT

- Weigh the patient and observe him when you tell him his current weight.
- Inspect the patient's skin to detect dryness or poor turgor.
- Palpate for thyroid enlargement.

CAUSES

MEDICAL
Anxiety
- Polyphagia may result from mild to moderate anxiety or emotional stress.
- Mild anxiety may produce restlessness, sleeplessness, irritability, repetitive questioning, and constant seeking of attention and reassurance.
- Moderate anxiety may produce selective inattention and difficulty concentrating.
- Other effects of anxiety include muscle tension, diaphoresis, GI distress, palpitations, tachycardia, and urinary and sexual dysfunction.

Bulimia
- Polyphagia alternates with self-induced vomiting, fasting, or diarrhea.
- Bulimia most commonly occurs in women ages 18 to 29.
- The patient typically weighs less than normal but has a morbid fear of obesity, is depressed, has low self-esteem, and conceals her overeating.

Diabetes mellitus
- Polyphagia occurs with weight loss, polydipsia, and polyuria.
- Other characteristic signs and symptoms include nocturia, weakness, fatigue, and signs of dehydration, such as dry mucous membranes and poor skin turgor.

Migraine headache

◆ Polyphagia sometimes precedes a migraine headache.
◆ The patient may experience changes in appetite and food cravings.
◆ Other early signs and symptoms include fatigue, nausea, vomiting, light and noise sensitivity, and a visual aura.

Premenstrual syndrome

◆ Appetite changes, such as food cravings and binges, may occur.
◆ Other findings include abdominal bloating, depression, insomnia, headache, paresthesia, diarrhea or constipation, edema and temporary weight gain, palpitations, back pain, breast swelling and tenderness, oliguria, and easy bruising.

Thyrotoxicosis

◆ Despite constant polyphagia, weight loss occurs.
◆ Other characteristic signs and symptoms include weakness, nervousness, diarrhea, tremors, thin and brittle hair and nails, diaphoresis, dyspnea, palpitations, tachycardia, heat intolerance, exophthalmos, atrial or ventricular gallop, and an enlarged thyroid.

OTHER
Drugs

◆ Corticosteroids, antidepressants, and cyproheptadine may increase appetite, causing weight gain.

NURSING CONSIDERATIONS

◆ Monitor the patient's eating habits.
◆ Weigh the patient at least twice per week.
◆ Refer the patient to a registered dietitian for nutritional counseling, if needed.
◆ Provide emotional support.

PEDIATRIC TIPS

◆ In children, polyphagia commonly results from juvenile diabetes.
◆ In infants ages 6 to 18 months, polyphagia can result from a malabsorptive disorder.
◆ Polyphagia may also occur in a child experiencing a growth spurt.

PATIENT TEACHING

◆ Refer the patient for nutritional counseling.
◆ Provide a referral for personal or family counseling as appropriate.
◆ Give emotional support and help patient understand the disease process.

Polyuria

OVERVIEW

◆ Refers to daily production and excretion of more than 3 L of urine

HISTORY

◆ Explore the frequency and pattern of polyuria.
◆ Ask for a description of patterns and amounts of daily fluid intake.
◆ Inquire about fatigue, increased thirst, or weight loss.
◆ Obtain a medical history of vision deficits, headaches, head trauma, urinary tract obstruction, diabetes mellitus, renal disorder, chronic hypokalemia or hypercalcemia, or psychiatric disorder.
◆ Take a drug history.

PHYSICAL ASSESSMENT

◆ Take vital signs, noting increased body temperature, tachycardia, and orthostatic hypotension.
◆ Inspect for signs of dehydration.
◆ Perform a neurologic assessment, noting any change in level of consciousness.
◆ Palpate the bladder and inspect the urethral meatus.
◆ Obtain a urine specimen and check specific gravity.

CAUSES

MEDICAL

Acute tubular necrosis
◆ During the diuretic phase, urine output of more than 8 L/day gradually subsides after about 1 week.
◆ Urine specific gravity (1.101 or less) increases as polyuria subsides.
◆ Related findings include weight loss, decreasing edema, and nocturia.

Diabetes insipidus
◆ Polyuria of about 5 L/day occurs, with urine specific gravity of 1.005 or less.
◆ Accompanying findings include polydipsia, nocturia, fatigue, and signs of dehydration.

Diabetes mellitus
◆ Polyuria is seldom more than 5 L/day, and urine specific gravity is typically more than 1.020.
◆ Other findings include polydipsia, polyphagia, weight loss, frequent urinary tract infections and yeast vaginitis, fatigue, signs of dehydration, and nocturia.

Glomerulonephritis (chronic)
◆ Polyuria gradually progresses to oliguria.
◆ Urine output is usually less than 4 L/day; specific gravity is about 1.010.
◆ Related GI findings include anorexia, nausea, and vomiting.
◆ Other findings include drowsiness, fatigue, edema, headache, elevated blood pressure, dyspnea, nocturia, hematuria, frothy or malodorous urine, and proteinuria.

Hypercalcemia

◆ Polyuria of more than 5 L/day occurs with a urine specific gravity of about 1.010.
◆ Other findings include polydipsia, nocturia, constipation, paresthesia and, occasionally, hematuria, and pyuria.
◆ With severe hypercalcemia, anorexia, vomiting, stupor progressing to coma, and renal failure occur.

Hypokalemia

◆ Prolonged potassium depletion causes polyuria of less than 5 L/day with a urine specific gravity of about 1.010.
◆ Other findings include polydipsia, circumoral and foot paresthesia, hypoactive deep tendon reflexes, fatigue, hypoactive bowel sounds, nocturia, arrhythmias, and muscle cramping, weakness, or paralysis.

Postobstructive uropathy

◆ After resolution of a urinary tract obstruction, polyuria—usually more than 5 L/day with a urine specific gravity of less than 1.010—occurs for several days before gradually subsiding.
◆ Other findings include bladder distention, edema, nocturia, and weight loss.

Pyelonephritis

◆ Polyuria of less than 5 L/day with a low but variable urine specific gravity occurs in acute disease.
◆ Acute pyelonephritis findings include persistent high fever, flank pain, hematuria, costovertebral angle tenderness, chills, weakness, dysuria, urinary frequency and urgency, tenesmus, and nocturia.
◆ Chronic pyelonephritis produces polyuria of less than 5 L/day that declines as renal function worsens; urine specific gravity is usually about 1.010 but may be higher if proteinuria is present.
◆ Other effects of the chronic condition include irritability, paresthesia, fatigue, nausea, vomiting, diarrhea, drowsiness, anorexia, pyuria and, in late stages, elevated blood pressure.

Sickle cell anemia

◆ Polyuria occurs with a urinary output of less than 5 L/day with a specific gravity of about 1.020.
◆ Additional findings include polydipsia, fatigue, abdominal cramps, arthralgia, priapism and, occasionally, leg ulcers and bony deformities.

OTHER
Diagnostic tests

◆ Radiographic tests that use contrast media may cause transient polyuria.

Drugs

◆ Diuretics produce polyuria.
◆ Cardiotonics, vitamin D, demeclocycline (Declomycin), phenytoin (Dilantin), and lithium (Eskalith), can also produce polyuria.

NURSING CONSIDERATIONS

◆ Record intake and output, and weigh the patient daily.
◆ Monitor vital signs.
◆ Encourage fluid intake to maintain adequate fluid balance.

PEDIATRIC TIPS

◆ The major causes of polyuria in children are congenital nephrogenic diabetes insipidus, medullary cystic disease, polycystic renal disease, and distal renal tubular acidosis.
◆ Because a child's fluid balance is more delicate than an adult's, check urine's specific gravity at each voiding and be alert for signs of dehydration.

GERIATRIC TIPS

◆ Chronic pyelonephritis is commonly associated with an underlying disorder.

PATIENT TEACHING

◆ Teach the patient about underlying disorder.
◆ Explain fluid replacement.
◆ Instruct the patient on weight monitoring.
◆ Discuss signs and symptoms of dehydration the patient needs to report.

Priapism

- Characterized by persistent, painful erection that's unrelated to sexual excitation
- May begin during sleep and appear to be a normal erection, but may last for several hours or days
- Occurs when the veins of the corpora cavernosa fail to drain correctly, resulting in persistent engorgement of the tissues
- Without prompt treatment, penile ischemia and thrombosis occur

ACTION STAT! *If the patient has priapism, apply an ice pack to the penis, administer an analgesic, and insert an indwelling urinary catheter to relieve urine retention. Procedures to remove blood from the corpora cavernosa, such as irrigation and surgery, may be required.*

- Find out when the priapism began and if it's continuous or intermittent.
- If the patient has experienced it before, find out what he did to relieve it and how long it lasted.
- Ask about pain or tenderness during urination or change in sexual function.
- Obtain a medical history looking for a history of sickle cell anemia, and any factors that could precipitate a crisis, such as dehydration and infection, or genital trauma.
- Obtain a thorough drug history including any drugs injected or objects inserted into his penis.

- Examine the patient's penis, noting its color and temperature.
- Check for loss of sensation and signs of infection, such as redness or drainage.
- Take vital signs, particularly noting fever.

MEDICAL
Granulocytic leukemia (chronic)
- Priapism is an uncommon sign of this disorder.
- More characteristic signs and symptoms include fatigue, weakness, malaise, lymphadenopathy, pallor, dyspnea, tachycardia, and bleeding tendencies.
- Hepatosplenomegaly, bone tenderness, low-grade fever, weight loss, and anorexia may also occur.

Penile cancer
- Cancer that exerts pressure on the corpora cavernosa can cause priapism.
- Usually, the first sign is a painless ulcerative lesion or an enlarging warty growth on the glans or foreskin, which may be accompanied by localized pain, a foul-smelling discharge from the prepuce, a firm lump near the glans, and lymphadenopathy.
- Later findings include bleeding, dysuria, urine retention, and bladder distention. Phimosis and poor hygiene have been linked to the development of penile cancer.

Penile trauma
- Priapism can occur with other signs and symptoms of injury, such as bruising, abrasions, swelling, pain, and hematuria.

Sickle cell anemia

◆ With this congenital disorder, painful priapism can occur without warning, usually on awakening.

◆ The patient may have a history of priapism, impaired growth and development, and increased susceptibility to infection.

◆ Related findings include tachycardia, pallor, weakness, hepatomegaly, dyspnea, joint swelling, joint or bone aching, chest pain, fatigue, murmurs, leg ulcers and, possibly, jaundice and gross hematuria.

◆ With sickle cell crisis, signs and symptoms of sickle cell anemia may worsen and others, such as abdominal pain and low-grade fever, may appear.

Spinal cord injury

◆ With this condition, the patient may be unaware of the onset of priapism.

◆ Related effects depend on the extent and level of injury and may include autonomic signs, such as bradycardia.

Stroke

◆ A stroke may cause priapism, but sensory loss and aphasia may prevent the patient from noticing or describing it.

◆ Other findings depend on the stroke location and extent but may include contralateral hemiplegia, seizures, headache, dysarthria, dysphagia, ataxia, apraxia, and agnosia.

◆ Vision deficits include homonymous hemianopsia, blurring, decreased acuity, and diplopia.

◆ Urine retention or incontinence, fecal incontinence, constipation, and vomiting may also occur.

Thrombocytopenia

◆ This disorder uncommonly produces priapism.

◆ More typical characteristics include blood-filled bullae in the mouth and local bleeding, such as epistaxis, ecchymosis, and hematuria.

◆ Central nervous system bleeding may cause decreased level of consciousness.

◆ Fatigue, weakness, and lethargy may occur.

OTHER
Drugs

◆ Priapism can result from the use of phenothiazine, thioridazine hydrochloride, trazodone hydrochloride, an androgenic steroid, an anticoagulant, an antihypertensive, or an erectile dysfunction medication.

NURSING CONSIDERATIONS

◆ Prepare the patient for blood tests to help determine the cause of priapism.

◆ If he requires surgery, keep his penis flaccid postoperatively by applying a pressure dressing.

◆ At least once every 30 minutes, inspect the glans for signs of vascular compromise, such as coolness or pallor.

PEDIATRIC TIPS

◆ In neonates, priapism can result from hypoxia but is usually resolved with oxygen therapy.

◆ Priapism is more likely to develop in children with sickle cell disease than in adults with the disease.

PATIENT TEACHING

◆ Encourage the patient with sickle cell anemia to report episodes of priapism. Quick treatment is necessary to preserve normal sexual function.

◆ Teach about underlying diagnosis and treatment plan.

Pruritus

OVERVIEW

- Caused by unpleasant itching sensation that provokes scratching to gain relief
- Exacerbated by increased skin temperature, poor skin turgor, local vasodilation, dermatoses, and stress
- Affects the skin, mucuos membranes, and eyes

HISTORY

- Ask about onset, frequency, duration, and intensity of pruritus.
- Determine location, whether it's localized or generalized, and what aggravates and alleviates it.
- Ask about contact with irritants.
- Obtain a description of skin care practices.
- Take a drug history.
- Obtain a medical history.
- Find out about recent travel and pets in the home.

PHYSICAL ASSESSMENT

- Observe for signs of scratching, such as excoriation, purpura, scabs, scars, or lichenification.
- Look for primary lesions to help confirm dermatoses.

CAUSES

MEDICAL

Anemia (iron deficiency)

- Pruritus occasionally occurs.
- Late findings include exertional dyspnea, fatigue, listlessness, pallor, irritability, headache, tachycardia, poor muscle tone and, possibly, murmurs.
- Chronic anemia causes spoon-shaped (koilonychias) and brittle nails (cheilosis), cracked mouth corners, a smooth tongue (glossitis), and dysphagia.

Anthrax (cutaneous)

- Early infection causes small, painless or pruritic, macular or papular lesion resembling an insect bite.
- In 1 to 2 days, lesion develops into a vesicular lesion and then a painless ulcer with a black, necrotic center.
- Other findings include lymphadenopathy, malaise, headache, or fever.

Cimex lectularius

- Commonly known as *bed bugs*, the bites cause itching, burning, and purpuric spots.
- Bed bugs don't transmit disease, but skin infections and scarring can occur from scratching.

Conjunctivitis

- All forms cause eye itching, burning, and pain along with photophobia, conjunctival injection, a foreign-body sensation, and excessive tearing.

Dermatitis

- Pruritus may be accompanied by a skin lesion.
- Atopic dermatitis begins with intense, severe pruritus and an erythematous rash on dry skin at flexion points.
- In chronic atopic dermatitis, lesions may progress to dry, scaly skin with white dermatographism, blanching, and lichenification.
- In contact dermatitis, itchy, small vesicles may ooze and scale, and are surrounded by redness; localized edema may occur with a severe reaction.
- Dermatitis herpetiformis initially causes intense pruritus; 8 to 12 hours later, symmetrically distributed lesions form on the buttocks, shoulders, elbows, and knees.

Enterobiasis

- Intense perianal pruritus occurs, especially at night, due to pinworm infestation.
- Other findings include irritability, scratching, skin irritation and, sometimes, vaginitis.

Hemorrhoids

- Anal pruritus, rectal pain, and constipation may occur.

Hepatobiliary disease

- Pruritus, commonly accompanied by jaundice, may be generalized or localized to the palms and soles.
- Other findings include right-upper-quadrant pain, clay-colored stools, chills, fever, flatus, belching, a bloated feeling, epigastric burning, and bitter fluid regurgitation.
- Later findings include mental changes, ascites, bleeding tendencies, spider angiomas, palmar erythema, dry skin, fetor hepaticus, enlarged superficial abdominal veins, bilateral gynecomastia, and hepatomegaly.

Herpes zoster

- Within 4 days of fever and malaise, pruritus, paresthesia or hyperesthesia, and severe, deep pain develop in a dermatome distribution.
- Up to 2 weeks after initial symptoms, red, nodular skin eruptions appear on the painful areas and become vesicular; about 10 days later, vesicles rupture and form scabs.

Hodgkin's disease

- Severe, unexplained itching occasionally occurs.
- Early findings include persistent fever, night sweats, fatigue, weight loss, malaise, and painless lymph node swelling.
- Later findings include hepatomegaly, splenomegaly, dyspnea, dysphagia, dry cough, hyperpigmentation, jaundice, and pallor.

Lichen simplex chronicus

- Localized pruritus and a circumscribed scaling patch with sharp margins develop.
- Later, skin thickens and papules form.

Pediculosis

- Pruritus in the area of lice infestation is a prominent symptom.
- Pediculosis capitis may cause scalp excoriation from scratching; foul-

smelling, lusterless, matted hair; occipital and cervical lymphadenopathy; and oval, gray-white nits on hair shafts.
- Pediculosis corporis initially causes red papules on the body, which become urticarial from scratching; later, rashes or wheals may develop.
- Pediculosis pubis is marked by nits or adult lice and erythematous, itching papules in pubic hair or hair around the anus, abdomen, or thighs.

Pityriasis rosea
- Pruritus that's aggravated by a hot bath or shower occasionally occurs.
- An erythematous herald patch forms and progresses to scaly, yellow, erythematous patches that erupt on the trunk or extremities and persist for 2 to 6 weeks.

Controlling itching

To reduce itching and increase comfort, teach the patient to follow these simple steps:

- Avoid scratching or rubbing the itchy areas. Ask the family to let the patient know if he's scratching because he may be unaware of it. Keep fingernails short to avoid skin damage from any unconscious scratching.
- Wear cool, light, loose bedclothes. Avoid wearing rough clothing—particularly wool—over the itchy area.
- Take tepid baths, using little soap and rinsing thoroughly. Try a skin-soothing oatmeal or cornstarch bath for a change.
- Apply an emollient lotion after bathing to soften and cool the skin.
- Apply cold compresses to the itchy area.
- Use topical ointments and take prescribed medications as directed.
- Avoid prolonged exposure to excessive heat and humidity. For maximum comfort, keep room temperatures at 68° to 70° F (20° to 21.1° C) and humidity at 30% to 40%.
- Encourage the patient to take up an enjoyable hobby that distracts him from the itching during the day and leaves him tired enough to sleep at night.

Polycythemia vera
- Pruritus is generalized or localized to the head, neck, face, and extremities; hot baths and showers typically aggravate it.
- A deep, purplish red color develops on the oral mucosa, gingivae, and tongue.
- Related findings include headache, dizziness, fatigue, dyspnea, paresthesia, impaired mentation, tinnitus, double or blurred vision, scotoma, hypotension, intermittent claudication, urticaria, ruddy cyanosis, hepatosplenomegaly, and ecchymosis.

Psoriasis
- Pruritus and pain commonly occur.
- Small erythematous papules enlarge or coalesce to form red, elevated plaques with silver scales on the scalp, chest, elbows, knees, back, buttocks, and genitals.

Renal failure (chronic)
- Pruritus may develop gradually or suddenly.
- Other findings include ammonia breath odor, oliguria or anuria, fatigue, decreased mental acuity, muscle twitching and cramps, anorexia, nausea, vomiting, peripheral neuropathies, and coma.

Scabies
- Localized pruritus that awakens the patient typically occurs.
- Threadlike lesions appear with a swollen nodule or red papule.

Thyrotoxicosis
- Generalized pruritus may precede or accompany the characteristic findings of tachycardia, palpitations, weight loss despite increased appetite, tremors, diarrhea, an enlarged thyroid, dyspnea, nervousness, diaphoresis, heat intolerance and, possibly, exophthalmos.

Tinea pedis
- Severe foot pruritus typically occurs with scales and blisters between the toes and a dry, scaly squamous inflammation on the sole.

Urticaria
- Extreme pruritus and stinging occur as transient erythematous, or whitish wheals form on the skin or mucous membranes.

Vaginitis
- Localized pruritus commonly occurs with foul-smelling vaginal discharge that may be purulent, white or gray, and curdlike.
- Perineal pain and urinary symptoms may occur.

OTHER
Drugs
- When mild and localized, an allergic reaction to drugs such as penicillin and sulfonamides can cause pruritus, erythema, urticaria, and edema.

NURSING CONSIDERATIONS

- Administer a topical or oral corticosteroid, an antihistamine, or a tranquilizer.
- Prepare patient for testing related to systemic disease.
- Initiate isolation precautions as appropriate.

PEDIATRIC TIPS

- Many adult disorders also cause pruritus in children, but they may affect different parts of the body.
- Such childhood diseases as measles and chickenpox can also cause pruritus.

PATIENT TEACHING

- Discuss underlying condition.
- Teach the patient ways to control pruritus. (See *Controlling itching*.)
- Discuss appropriate hygiene and infection control techniques.

Psoas sign

OVERVIEW

- Refers to increased abdominal pain when the patient moves his leg against resistance
- Indicates direct or reflexive irritation of the psoas muscles
- Can be elicited on the right or left side

ACTION STAT! *If you elicit a positive psoas sign in a patient with abdominal pain, suspect appendicitis. Quickly check the patient's vital signs, and prepare him for possible surgery: Explain the procedure, restrict food and fluids, and withhold analgesics, which can mask symptoms. Administer I.V. fluids to prevent dehydration, but don't give a cathartic or an enema, because it can cause a ruptured appendix and lead to peritonitis.*

HISTORY

- Obtain a medical history and drug history.
- Ask about abdominal pain, when it started, what irritates it or relieves it, and ask the patient to rate it on a scale of 1 to 10.
- Find out if the patient has had a history of abdominal pain, bowel surgeries, diarrhea, constipation, or appendicitis.

PHYSICAL ASSESSMENT

- Perform an abdominal assessment including assessing for bowel sounds.
- Take vital signs.
- Check for a positive psoas sign in a patient with abdominal or lower back pain after completion of an abdominal examination to prevent spurious assessment findings. (See *Eliciting a psoas sign.*)

TOP TECHNIQUE

Eliciting a psoas sign.

You can use two techniques shown below to elicit a psoas sign in an adult with abdominal pain. With either technique, increased abdominal pain is a positive result, indicating psoas muscle irritation from an inflamed appendix or a localized abscess.

With the patient in a supine position, instruct her to move her flexed left leg against your hand to test for a left psoas sign. Then perform this maneuver on the right leg to test for a right psoas sign.

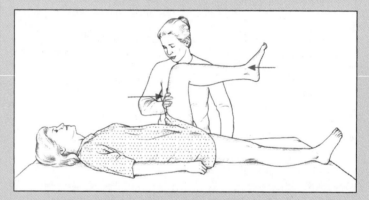

For a second method, place the patient on her right side to test for a left psoas sign. Then instruct her to push her left leg upward from the hip against your hand. Next, turn the patient onto her left side and repeat this maneuver to test for a right psoas sign.

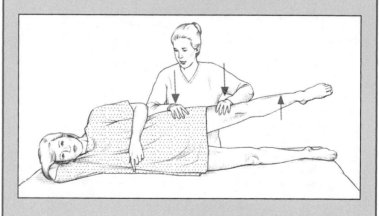

MEDICAL

Appendicitis

◆ An inflamed retrocecal appendix can cause a positive right psoas sign.

◆ Early epigastric and periumbilical pain disappears, only to worsen and localize in the right lower quadrant. This pain also worsens with walking or coughing.

◆ Related findings include nausea and vomiting, abdominal rigidity and rebound tenderness, and constipation or diarrhea. A fever, tachycardia, retractive respirations, anorexia, and malaise may also occur.

◆ If the appendix ruptures, additional findings may include sudden severe pain, followed by signs of peritonitis, such as hypoactive or absent bowel sounds, a high fever, and boardlike abdominal rigidity.

◆ A positive obturator sign may also be evident.

Retroperitoneal abscess

◆ After a lower retroperitoneal infection, an iliac or lumbar abscess can produce a positive right or left psoas sign and a fever.

◆ An iliac abscess causes iliac or inguinal pain that may radiate to the hip, thigh, flank, or knee; a tender mass in the lower abdomen or groin may be palpable.

◆ A lumbar abscess usually produces back tenderness and spasms on the affected side with a palpable lumbar mass; a tender abdominal mass without back pain may occur instead.

◆ Monitor the patient's vital signs to detect complications, such as peritonitis and pain extension along fascial planes in the abdomen, thigh, hip, subphrenic spaces, mediastinum, and pleural cavities.

◆ Promote patient comfort by helping with position changes. For example, have the patient lie down and flex his right leg. Then have him sit upright.

PEDIATRIC TIPS

◆ Elicit a psoas sign by asking the child to raise his head while you exert pressure on his forehead. Resulting right lower quadrant pain usually indicates appendicitis.

GERIATRIC TIPS

◆ In elderly patients, the psoas sign and other peritoneal signs may be decreased or absent. Make sure to differentiate pain elicited through psoas maneuvers from musculoskeletal or degenerative joint pain.

◆ Prepare the patient for diagnostic tests, such as electrolyte studies and abdominal X-rays, or surgery, if necessary.

◆ Teach the patient how to report pain using a pain rating scale.

Ptosis

OVERVIEW

- Refers to excessive drooping of one or both upper eyelids
- Can be constant, progressive, or intermittent
- Can be congenital or acquired

HISTORY

- Ask about the onset of ptosis and whether the condition has worsened or improved.
- Find out about recent traumatic eye injury.
- Inquire about eye pain or headache.
- Determine whether the patient has experienced vision changes.
- Take a drug history, noting especially the use of a chemotherapeutic drug.

PHYSICAL ASSESSMENT

- Assess the degree of ptosis.
- Check for eyelid edema, exophthalmos, and conjunctival injection.
- Evaluate extraocular muscle function.
- Examine pupil size, color, shape, and reaction to light.
- Test visual acuity.

CAUSES

MEDICAL

Alcoholism

- Ptosis, as well as such complications as severe weight loss, jaundice, ascites, and mental disturbances, can result from long-term alcohol abuse.

Botulism

- Cranial nerve dysfunction causes ptosis, dysarthria, dysphagia, and diplopia.
- Other findings include dry mouth, sore throat, weakness, vomiting, diarrhea, hyporeflexia, and dyspnea.

Cerebral aneurysm

- Sudden ptosis, diplopia, a dilated pupil, and inability to rotate the eye can occur due to compression of the oculomotor nerve and may be the first signs of this disorder.
- Ruptured aneurysm, a life-threatening condition, produces sudden severe headache, nausea, vomiting, and decreased level of consciousness (LOC).
- Other findings include nuchal rigidity, back and leg pain, fever, restlessness, irritability, seizures, blurred vision, hemiparesis, sensory deficits, dysphagia, and visual defects.

Hemangioma

- Ptosis may occur along with exophthalmos, limited extraocular movement, swollen periorbital tissue, and blurred vision.

Levator muscle maldevelopment

◆ Ptosis results from isolated dystrophy of the levator muscle.
◆ Eyelid lag on downgaze is an important clue to diagnosis.

Myasthenia gravis

◆ Gradual ptosis in both eyes is commonly the first sign of this neuromuscular disorder.
◆ Ptosis is accompanied by weak eye closure and diplopia.
◆ Other findings include muscle weakness and fatigue, masklike facies, difficulty chewing or swallowing, dyspnea, cyanosis and, possibly, paralysis.

Myotonic dystrophy

◆ Mild to severe ptosis in both eyes may occur.
◆ Distinctive cataracts with iridescent dots in the cortex, miosis, diplopia, decreased tearing, and muscular and testicular atrophy may occur.

Ocular muscle dystrophy

◆ Ptosis progresses slowly to complete closure of the eyelids.
◆ Other findings include progressive external ophthalmoplegia and muscle weakness and atrophy of the upper face, neck, trunk, and limbs.

Ocular trauma

◆ Mild to severe ptosis can result from trauma to the nerve or muscles that control the eyelids.
◆ Eye pain, eyelid swelling, ecchymosis, and decreased visual acuity may also occur.

Parinaud's syndrome

◆ Ptosis, enophthalmos, nystagmus, lid retraction, dilated pupils with absent or poor light response, and papilledema occur due to midbrain lesion.
◆ Ocular muscles fail to move voluntarily.

Subdural hematoma (chronic)

◆ Ptosis may be a late sign, along with one dilation of one pupil and sluggishness.
◆ Headache, behavioral changes, and decreased LOC commonly occur.

OTHER
Drugs

◆ Vinca alkaloids and chemotherapy medications can produce ptosis.

Lead poisoning

◆ With lead poisoning, ptosis develops over 3 to 6 months; other findings include anorexia, nausea, vomiting, diarrhea, colicky abdominal pain, a lead line in the gums, decreased LOC, tachycardia, hypotension, irritability, and peripheral nerve weakness.

NURSING CONSIDERATIONS

◆ Orient the patient with decreased visual acuity to his surroundings.
◆ Assist with special spectacle frames that suspend the eyelid by traction with a wire crutch.

PEDIATRIC TIPS

◆ In congenital ptosis, ptosis is unilateral, constant, and accompanied by lagophthalmos, which causes the infant to sleep with his eyes open.

PATIENT TEACHING

◆ Explain underlying disorder and treatment options.
◆ Discuss self-esteem issues.
◆ Prepare the patient for diagnostic tests he will need and surgery, if necessary.

Pulse, absent or weak

◆ When generalized, indicates a life-threatening condition, such as shock or arrhythmia (see *Managing an absent or weak pulse*)
◆ When localized, may indicate acute arterial occlusion

◆ Review the medical history, including heart and vascular disease.
◆ Take a drug history.
◆ Question the patient about associated signs and symptoms, such as chest pain or dyspnea.

◆ Palpate the arterial pulses for comparison. (See *Evaluating peripheral pulses*, page 468.)
◆ Obtain vital signs and electrocardiogram results.
◆ Evaluate cardiopulmonary status.

ACTION STAT!

Managing an absent or weak pulse

An absent or weak pulse can result from any one of several life-threatening disorders. Your evaluation and interventions will vary, depending on whether the weak or absent pulse is generalized or localized to one extremity. They'll also depend on associated signs and symptoms. Use this flowchart to help you establish priorities for successfully managing this emergency.

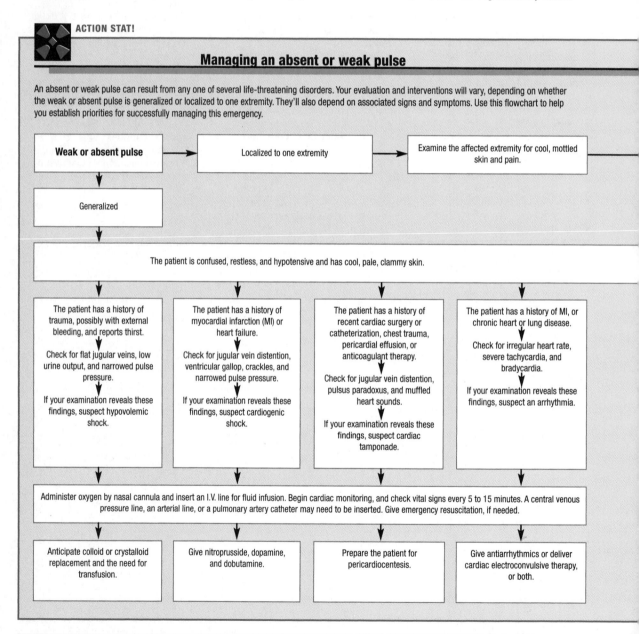

Weak or absent pulse → Localized to one extremity → Examine the affected extremity for cool, mottled skin and pain.

Generalized

The patient is confused, restless, and hypotensive and has cool, pale, clammy skin.

| The patient has a history of trauma, possibly with external bleeding, and reports thirst. | The patient has a history of myocardial infarction (MI) or heart failure. | The patient has a history of recent cardiac surgery or catheterization, chest trauma, pericardial effusion, or anticoagulant therapy. | The patient has a history of MI, or chronic heart or lung disease. |

Check for flat jugular veins, low urine output, and narrowed pulse pressure.

Check for jugular vein distention, ventricular gallop, crackles, and narrowed pulse pressure.

Check for jugular vein distention, pulsus paradoxus, and muffled heart sounds.

Check for irregular heart rate, severe tachycardia, and bradycardia.

If your examination reveals these findings, suspect hypovolemic shock.

If your examination reveals these findings, suspect cardiogenic shock.

If your examination reveals these findings, suspect cardiac tamponade.

If your examination reveals these findings, suspect an arrhythmia.

Administer oxygen by nasal cannula and insert an I.V. line for fluid infusion. Begin cardiac monitoring, and check vital signs every 5 to 15 minutes. A central venous pressure line, an arterial line, or a pulmonary artery catheter may need to be inserted. Give emergency resuscitation, if needed.

Anticipate colloid or crystalloid replacement and the need for transfusion.

Give nitroprusside, dopamine, and dobutamine.

Prepare the patient for pericardiocentesis.

Give antiarrhythmics or deliver cardiac electroconvulsive therapy, or both.

MEDICAL
Aortic aneurysm (dissecting)
◆ Weak or absent arterial pulses occur distal to the affected area when circulation to the innominate, left common carotid, subclavian, or femoral artery is affected.

◆ Tearing pain develops suddenly in the chest and neck, and may radiate to the back and abdomen.
◆ Other findings include syncope, loss of consciousness, weakness or transient paralysis of the legs or arms, diastolic murmur of aortic insufficiency, hypotension, and mottled skin below the waist.

Aortic stenosis
◆ The carotid pulse is weak.
◆ Paroxysmal or exertional dyspnea, chest pain, and syncope are common.
◆ Other findings include an atrial gallop, a harsh systolic ejection murmur, crackles, palpitations, fatigue, and narrowed pulse pressure.

(continued)

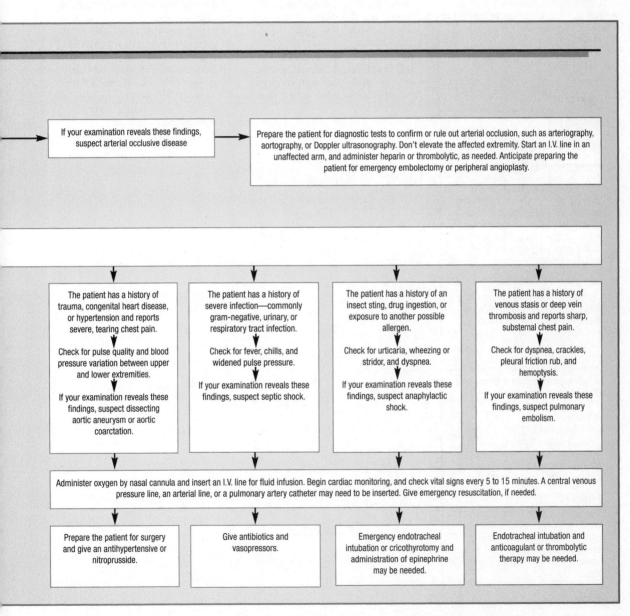

If your examination reveals these findings, suspect arterial occlusive disease

Prepare the patient for diagnostic tests to confirm or rule out arterial occlusion, such as arteriography, aortography, or Doppler ultrasonography. Don't elevate the affected extremity. Start an I.V. line in an unaffected arm, and administer heparin or thrombolytic, as needed. Anticipate preparing the patient for emergency embolectomy or peripheral angioplasty.

The patient has a history of trauma, congenital heart disease, or hypertension and reports severe, tearing chest pain.

Check for pulse quality and blood pressure variation between upper and lower extremities.

If your examination reveals these findings, suspect dissecting aortic aneurysm or aortic coarctation.

The patient has a history of severe infection—commonly gram-negative, urinary, or respiratory tract infection.

Check for fever, chills, and widened pulse pressure.

If your examination reveals these findings, suspect septic shock.

The patient has a history of an insect sting, drug ingestion, or exposure to another possible allergen.

Check for urticaria, wheezing or stridor, and dyspnea.

If your examination reveals these findings, suspect anaphylactic shock.

The patient has a history of venous stasis or deep vein thrombosis and reports sharp, substernal chest pain.

Check for dyspnea, crackles, pleural friction rub, and hemoptysis.

If your examination reveals these findings, suspect pulmonary embolism.

Administer oxygen by nasal cannula and insert an I.V. line for fluid infusion. Begin cardiac monitoring, and check vital signs every 5 to 15 minutes. A central venous pressure line, an arterial line, or a pulmonary artery catheter may need to be inserted. Give emergency resuscitation, if needed.

Prepare the patient for surgery and give an antihypertensive or nitroprusside.

Give antibiotics and vasopressors.

Emergency endotracheal intubation or cricothyrotomy and administration of epinephrine may be needed.

Endotracheal intubation and anticoagulant or thrombolytic therapy may be needed.

Arterial occlusion

◆ With acute occlusion, arterial pulses distal to the obstruction are weak and then absent.
◆ Affected limb has severe pain, varying degrees of paralysis, intermittent claudication, and paresthesia; is cool, pale, and cyanotic, with increased capillary refill time; and has a line of color and temperature demarcation at the level of obstruction.
◆ With chronic occlusion, pulses in the affected limb weaken gradually.

Cardiac arrhythmia

◆ Generalized weak pulses may accompany cool, clammy skin.
◆ Other findings include hypotension, chest pain, dyspnea, dizziness, and decreased level of consciousness.

Cardiac tamponade

◆ In this life-threatening condition, a weak rapid pulse accompanies these classic findings: paradoxical pulse, jugular vein distention, hypotension, and muffled heart sounds.
◆ Other findings include narrowed pulse pressure, pericardial friction rub, hepatomegaly, anxiety, restlessness, cyanosis, chest pain, dyspnea, tachypnea, and cold, clammy skin.

Coarctation of the aorta

◆ Bounding pulses occur in the arms and neck, with decreased pulsations and systolic pulse pressure in the lower extremities.
◆ Auscultation may reveal a systolic ejection click accompanied by a systolic ejection murmur.

Peripheral vascular disease

◆ A weakening and loss of peripheral pulses occurs.
◆ Aching pain occurs distal to the occlusion that worsens with exercise and abates with rest.
◆ Other findings include cool skin, decreased hair growth in the affected limb, and impotence with an occlusion of the descending aorta or femoral areas.

 TOP TECHNIQUE

Evaluating peripheral pulses

The rate, amplitude, and symmetry of peripheral pulses provide important clues to cardiac function and the quality of peripheral perfusion. To gather these clues, palpate peripheral pulses lightly with the pads of your index, middle, and ring fingers, as space permits.

RATE

Count all pulses for at least 30 seconds (60 seconds when recording vital signs). The normal rate is between 60 and 100 beats/minute.

AMPLITUDE

Palpate the blood vessel during ventricular systole. Describe pulse amplitude by using a scale such as this one:

  4+ = bounding
  3+ = increased
  2+ = normal
  1+ = weak, thready
  0 = absent

Use a stick figure to easily document the location and amplitude of all pulses.

SYMMETRY

Simultaneously palpate pulses (except for the carotid pulse) on both sides of the patient's body, and note any inequality. Always assess peripheral pulses methodically, moving from the arms to the legs.

Pulmonary embolism
◆ A generalized weak, rapid pulse occurs.
◆ Other features include an abrupt onset of chest pain, tachycardia, apprehension, syncope, diaphoresis, and cyanosis.
◆ Acute respiratory findings include tachypnea, dyspnea, decreased breath sounds, crackles, a pleural friction rub, and a cough, possibly with blood-tinged sputum.

Shock
◆ With anaphylactic shock, pulses become rapid and weak and then uniformly absent within seconds or minutes after exposure to an allergen.
◆ With cardiogenic shock, peripheral pulses are absent and central pulses are weak, depending on the degree of vascular collapse.
◆ With hypovolemic shock, all peripheral pulses become weak and then uniformly absent, depending on the severity of hypovolemia.
◆ With septic shock, all pulses in the extremities first become weak and then become absent.

Thoracic outlet syndrome
◆ Gradual or abrupt weakness or loss of pulses in the arms occurs.
◆ Pulse changes commonly occur after the patient works with his hands above his shoulders, lifts a weight, or abducts his arm.
◆ Other findings include paresthesia and pain along the ulnar distribution of the arm that resolves when the arm returns to a neutral position.

OTHER
Treatments
◆ Localized absent pulse may occur away from the arteriovenous shunts used for dialysis.

NURSING CONSIDERATIONS
◆ Monitor vital signs and peripheral pulses.
◆ Measure daily weight, intake and output, and central venous pressure.
◆ Maintain bleeding precautions with anticoagulation therapy.

PEDIATRIC TIPS
◆ Radial, dorsal pedal, and posterior tibial pulses aren't easily palpable in infants and small children.
◆ In children and young adults, weak or absent pulses in the legs may indicate coarctation of the aorta.

PATIENT TEACHING
◆ Discuss underlying disorder and treatment options.
◆ Explain diagnostic tests as needed.
◆ Teach the techniques for checking pulse.
◆ Explain signs and symptoms the patient needs to report.
◆ Discuss foods and fluids the patient should avoid.
◆ Emphasize avoidance of activities that reduce circulation.

Pulse, bounding

OVERVIEW

- Produced by large waves of pressure as blood ejects from the left ventricle with each contraction
- Characterized by regular recurrent expansion and contraction of the arterial walls
- Are strong and easily palpable
- Visible over superficial peripheral arteries
- Not obliterated by the pressure of palpation

HISTORY

- Ask about weakness, fatigue, shortness of breath, or other health changes.
- Take a medical history, noting hyperthyroidism, anemia, or a cardiovascular disorder.
- Ask about alcohol use.

PHYSICAL ASSESSMENT

- Check vital signs.
- Auscultate heart and lungs for abnormal sounds, rates, or rhythms.
- Complete the cardiovascular assessment. (See *Assessing peripheral pulse sites.*)

CAUSES

MEDICAL
Alcoholism (acute)

- A rapid, bounding pulse and flushed face result from vasodilation.
- An odor of alcohol on the breath and an ataxic gait are common.
- Other findings include hypothermia, bradypnea, labored and loud respirations, nausea, vomiting, diuresis, decreased level of consciousness, and seizures.

Anemia

- Bounding pulse may be accompanied by systolic ejection murmur, tachycardia, an atrial gallop, a ven-

 TOP TECHNIQUE

Assessing peripheral pulse sites

You can assess your patient's pulse rate, rhythm, and amplitude at several sites, including those shown in this illustration.

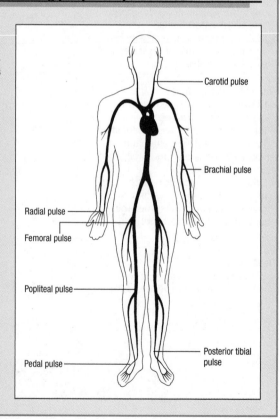

Carotid pulse

Brachial pulse

Radial pulse

Femoral pulse

Popliteal pulse

Pedal pulse

Posterior tibial pulse

tricular gallop, and a systolic bruit over the carotid artery.

♦ Other findings include fatigue, pallor, dyspnea and, possibly, bleeding tendencies.

Aortic insufficiency

♦ Bounding pulse is characterized by rapid, forceful expansion of the arterial pulse followed by rapid contraction.

♦ Widened pulse pressure also occurs.

♦ Other relevant signs and symptoms include weakness, severe dyspnea, hypotension, ventricular gallop, tachycardia, pallor, chest pain, strong and abrupt carotid pulsations, pulsus biferiens, early systolic murmur, murmur heard over the femoral artery during systole and diastole, high-pitched diastolic murmur that starts with the second heart sound, and apical diastolic rumble (Austin Flint murmur).

♦ With chronic aortic insufficiency, most patients are asymptomatic until age 40 or 50 when exertional dyspnea, increased fatigue, orthopnea, paroxysmal nocturnal dyspnea, angina, and syncope may develop.

Febrile disorder

♦ Bounding pulse may occur with fever.

♦ Accompanying findings reflect the underlying disorder and may include fatigue, chills, malaise, anorexia, tachycardia, tachypnea, and diaphoresis.

Thyrotoxicosis

♦ A rapid, full, bounding pulse occurs.

♦ Other relevant signs and symptoms include tachycardia; palpitations; an atrial or ventricular gallop; weight loss despite increased appetite; diarrhea; an enlarged thyroid; dyspnea; tremors; nervousness; chest pain; exophthalmos; heat intolerance; signs of cardiovascular collapse; and warm, moist, and diaphoretic skin.

NURSING CONSIDERATIONS

♦ If bounding pulse is accompanied by rapid or irregular heartbeat, connect the patient to a cardiac monitor for further evaluation.

♦ Provide for rest periods to reduce metabolic demands.

♦ Administer iron supplements, if indicated.

♦ Monitor intake and output.

♦ Weigh the patient daily.

♦ Restrict fluids, as necessary.

PEDIATRIC TIPS

♦ A bounding pulse can be normal in infants or children.

♦ It can also result from patent ductus arteriosus if the left-to-right shunt is large.

PATIENT TEACHING

♦ Explain underlying disorder, diagnostic tests, and treatment options.

♦ Discuss diet modifications and fluid restrictions the patient needs.

♦ Stress the need for rest periods.

♦ Emphasize the importance of avoiding alcohol, and refer the patient to cessation counseling as appropriate.

♦ Explain signs and symptoms he needs to report.

Pulse pressure, narrowed

- Refers to the difference between systolic and diastolic blood pressures of less than 30 mm Hg
- Occurs when peripheral vascular resistance increases, cardiac output declines, or intravascular volume markedly decreases (see *Understanding pulse pressure changes*)
- Is usually a sign of cardiovascular decompensation

- Ask about specific cardiac symptoms, such as chest pain, dizziness, or syncope.
- Obtain a medical history.
- Assess risk factors for heart disease.

- Check for signs of heart failure, such as hypotension, tachycardia, dyspnea, jugular vein distention, pulmonary crackles, and decreased urine output.
- Check for changes in skin temperature or color.
- Palpate peripheral pulses, noting their strength.
- Evaluate level of consciousness (LOC).
- Auscultate for heart murmurs.
- Obtain vital signs and weight.

Understanding pulse pressure changes

The amount of blood that the ventricles eject into the arteries with each beat—known as *stroke volume*—and the arteries' *peripheral resistance* to blood flow affect pulse pressure, as well as systolic and diastolic blood pressures. For example, pulse pressure narrows when systolic pressure falls (lower right), diastolic pressure rises (upper left), or both. These changes reflect decreased stroke volume, increased peripheral resistance, or both.

Pulse pressure widens when systolic pressure rises (upper right), diastolic pressure falls (lower left), or both. These changes reflect increased stroke volume, decreased peripheral resistance, or both.

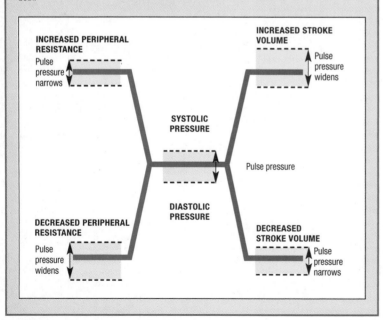

MEDICAL
Aortic stenosis
◆ Narrowed pulse pressure occurs late in significant stenosis.
◆ Other findings include atrial or ventricular gallop, chest pain, angina, crackles, fatigue, dyspnea, paroxysmal nocturnal dyspnea, syncope, and a harsh systolic ejection murmur.

Cardiac tamponade
◆ In this life-threatening disorder, pulse pressure narrows by 10 to 20 mm Hg.
◆ Paradoxical pulse, jugular vein distention, hypotension, and muffled heart sounds are classic.
◆ Other findings include anxiety, restlessness, cyanosis, clammy skin, chest pain, dyspnea, tachypnea, decreased LOC, pericardial rub, hepatomegaly, and a weak, rapid pulse.

Heart failure
◆ Narrowed pulse pressure occurs relatively late.
◆ Tachypnea, palpitations, dependent edema, steady weight gain despite nausea and anorexia, chest tightness, hypotension, diaphoresis, pallor, a ventricular gallop, inspiratory crackles, oliguria and, possibly, a tender palpable liver may also occur.
◆ Later, hemoptysis, cyanosis, marked hepatomegaly, and marked pitting edema may occur.

Shock
◆ Narrowed pulse pressure occurs late.
◆ Peripheral pulses first become weak and then uniformly absent in anaphylactic, hypovolemic, and septic shock.
◆ In cardiogenic shock, peripheral pulses are absent and central pulses are weak.
◆ Anaphylactic shock may result in hypotension, anxiety, restlessness, feelings of doom, intense itching, urticaria, dyspnea, stridor, hoarseness, chest or throat tightness, skin flushing, and seizures.
◆ Cardiogenic shock may produce hypotension; tachycardia; tachypnea; cyanosis; oliguria; restlessness; confusion; obtundation; and cold, pale, clammy skin.
◆ Deepening hypovolemia shock leads to hypotension, oliguria, confusion, decreased LOC and, possibly, hypothermia.
◆ As septic shock progresses, the patient exhibits thirst, anxiety, restlessness, confusion, hypotension, cool and cyanotic extremities, cold and clammy skin and, eventually, severe hypotension, oliguria or anuria, respiratory failure, and coma.

◆ Monitor closely for changes in pulse rate or quality and for hypotension.
◆ Assess for changes in LOC.

PEDIATRIC TIPS
◆ In children, narrowed pulse pressure can result from congenital aortic stenosis, as well as from the disorders that affect adults.

◆ Explain the disorder and its treatments.
◆ Teach about foods and fluids the patient should avoid.
◆ Stress the importance of rest periods to reduce fatigue.

Pulse pressure, widened

OVERVIEW

- Occurs when systolic pressure is more than 50 mm Hg higher than diastolic pressure
- Commonly occurs as a physiologic response to fever, hot weather, exercise, anxiety, anemia, or pregnancy

  ACTION STAT! If the patient's level of consciousness (LOC) is decreased and you suspect his widened pulse pressure comes from increased intracranial pressure (ICP), check his vital signs and oxygen saturation. Maintain a patent airway. Provide supplemental oxygen and ventilatory support to keep the patient's partial pressure of arterial oxygen above 90 mm Hg or his oxygen saturation above 95%. Give osmotic diuretics such as mannitol by I.V. infusion to decrease ICP as prescribed. Insert an indwelling urinary catheter; monitor intake and output during mannitol therapy. Start ICP monitoring. Administer analgesics as ordered.

  Hyperventilation therapy to decrease the patient's partial pressure of arterial carbon dioxide and to treat ICP remains controversial but may be needed for short intervals when ICP and neurologic deterioration increase.

  Perform a neurologic examination. Use the Glasgow Coma Scale to evaluate LOC. Check cranial nerve function—especially cranial nerves III, IV, and VI—and assess pupillary reactions, reflexes, and muscle tone. Check for edema and auscultate for murmurs.

HISTORY

- Obtain a medical history, including family history and trauma.
- Take a drug history.
- Ask about such associated signs and symptoms as chest pain, shortness of breath, weakness, fatigue, or syncope.

PHYSICAL ASSESSMENT

- Assess for signs and symptoms of heart failure, such as crackles, dyspnea, and jugular vein distention.
- Check for changes in skin temperature and color, and strength of peripheral pulses.
- Evaluate LOC.
- Auscultate the heart for murmurs.
- Check for peripheral edema.

CAUSES

MEDICAL

Aortic insufficiency

- Pulse pressure widens progressively as the valve deteriorates.
- Other relevant signs and symptoms include a bounding pulse; an atrial or ventricular gallop; chest pain; palpitations; pallor; pulsus biferiens; signs of heart failure (crackles, dyspnea, jugular vein distention); heart murmurs such as an early diastolic murmur and an apical diastolic rumble (Austin Flint murmur); and strong, abrupt carotid pulsations.

Arteriosclerosis

- Pulse pressure widens following moderate hypertension.
- Other findings include signs of vascular insufficiency, such as claudication, angina, and speech and vision disturbances.

Febrile disorders

- Fever can cause widened pulse pressure.
- Other symptoms vary by the underlying disorder but may include fatigue, chills, malaise, anorexia, tachycardia, tachypnea, and diaphoresis.

Increased ICP

- In this life-threatening condition, widening pulse pressure is an intermediate to late sign of increased ICP.
- Decreased LOC is the earliest and most sensitive indicator of increased ICP.
- Cushing's triad—bradycardia, hypertension, and respiratory pattern changes—is characteristic of increasing ICP.
- Other findings include headache, vomiting, impaired or unequal motor movement, vision disturbances, and pupillary changes.

NURSING CONSIDERATIONS

- If the patient displays increased ICP, continually reevaluate his neurologic status and vital signs.
- Be alert for restlessness, confusion, unresponsiveness, or decreased LOC.
- Watch for subtle changes in condition.

PEDIATRIC TIPS

- Widened pulse pressure is an intermediate to late sign of increased ICP.
- Widened pulse pressure can occur with patent ductus arteriosus (PDA) but may not be evident at birth; the older child with PDA experiences exertional dyspnea with pulse pressure that widens even further on exertion.

GERIATRIC TIPS

- Widened pulse pressure is a more reliable predictor of cardiovascular events in elderly patients than increased systolic and diastolic blood pressure.

PATIENT TEACHING

- Discuss underlying condition, diagnostic tests, and treatment options.
- Explain needed dietary modifications, such as restricting sodium and saturated fats.
- Stress the importance of planning rest periods.
- If the patient has decreased LOC, discuss specific safety measures.

Pulse rhythm, abnormal

OVERVIEW

◆ Irregular expansion and contraction of peripheral arterial walls
◆ May be persistent or sporadic, rhythmic or arrhythmic
◆ Reflects underlying cardiac arrhythmia (see *Abnormal pulse rhythm: A clue to cardiac arrhythmias*)

 ACTION STAT! *Quickly look for signs of reduced cardiac output, such as decreased level of consciousness (LOC), hypotension, or dizziness. Promptly obtain an electrocardiogram (ECG) and possibly a chest X-ray, and begin cardiac monitoring. Insert an I.V. catheter to give emergency cardiac drugs, and give oxygen by nasal cannula or mask. Closely monitor vital signs, pulse quality, and cardiac rhythm. Keep emergency intubation, cardioversion, and suction equipment available.*

HISTORY

◆ Ask about the onset, quality, quantity, location, and radiation of pain.
◆ Obtain a medical history, including heart disease and treatment for arrhythmias.
◆ Take a drug history and check compliance.
◆ Ask about caffeine or alcohol intake.

PHYSICAL ASSESSMENT

◆ Check apical and peripheral arterial pulses; check for a pulse deficit.
◆ Auscultate heart sounds for abnormalities.
◆ Count the apical beat for 60 seconds, noting the frequency of skipped peripheral beats.
◆ Perform complete cardiovascular assessment.

TOP TECHNIQUE

Abnormal pulse rhythm: A clue to cardiac arrhythmias

An abnormal pulse rhythm may be your only clue that the patient has a cardiac arrhythmia, but this sign doesn't help you pinpoint the specific type of arrhythmia. For that, you need a cardiac monitor or an electrocardiogram (ECG) machine.

The ECG strips below show some common cardiac arrhythmias that can cause abnormal pulse rhythms.

ARRHYTHMIA	PULSE RHYTHM AND RATE	RESULTS
Sinus arrhythmia 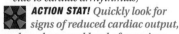	Irregular rhythm; fast, slow, or normal rate	◆ Reflex vagal tone inhibition (heart rate increases with inspiration and decreases with expiration) related to normal respiratory cycle ◆ May result from drugs, as in digoxin toxicity ◆ Occurs most often in children and young adults
Premature atrial contractions (PACs) 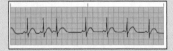	Irregular rhythm during PACs; fast, slow, or normal rate	◆ Occasional PACs may be normal ◆ Isolated PACs may indicate atrial irritation—for example, from anxiety or excessive caffeine intake; increasing PACs may herald other arrhythmias ◆ May result from heart failure, chronic obstructive pulmonary disease (COPD), or use of cardiac glycosides, aminophylline, or an adrenergic
Paroxysmal atrial tachycardia 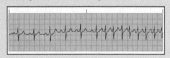	Regular rhythm with abrupt onset and termination of arrhythmia; heart rate exceeding 140 beats/minute	◆ May occur in otherwise normal, healthy people who are experiencing physical or psychological stress, hypoxia, or digoxin toxicity; who use marijuana; or who consume excessive amounts of caffeine or other stimulants ◆ May precipitate angina or heart failure

MEDICAL
Cardiac arrhythmias
- An abnormal pulse rhythm may be the only sign; pulse may be weak, rapid, or slow.
- Palpitations, a fluttering heartbeat, or weak and skipped beats may be reported by the patient.
- Dull chest pain or discomfort and hypotension may occur.
- Other findings include decreased urine output, dyspnea, tachypnea, pallor, and diaphoresis.
- Neurologic findings include confusion, dizziness, light-headedness, decreased LOC and, sometimes, seizures.

- Prepare the patient for cardioversion therapy, if needed.
- Prepare the patient for transfer to a cardiac or intensive care unit.
- Check vital signs frequently to detect bradycardia, tachycardia, hypertension, or hypotension, tachypnea, or dyspnea.
- Maintain cardiac monitor as ordered.
- Collect blood samples for serum electrolyte, cardiac enzyme, and drug level studies.
- Obtain a 12-lead ECG and compare with previous tracings.

PEDIATRIC TIPS
- Arrhythmias also produce pulse rhythm abnormalities in children.

- Tell the patient to keep a diary of activities and symptoms.
- Educate the patient on the importance of avoiding tobacco and caffeine.
- Discuss strategies to improve medication compliance.
- Instruct the patient on taking his pulse rate.
- Explain signs and symptoms he needs to report.

ARRHYTHMIA	PULSE RHYTHM AND RATE	RESULTS
Atrial fibrillation 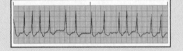	Irregular rhythm; atrial rate exceeding 400 beats/minute; ventricular rate varies	◆ May result from heart failure, COPD, hypertension, sepsis, pulmonary embolus, mitral valve disease, atrial irritation, coronary bypass, or valve replacement surgery ◆ Preload inconsistent because atria don't contract; cardiac output changes with each beat; emboli may also result
Second-degree atrioventricular heart block, type I (Wenckebach) 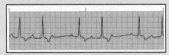	Irregular ventricular rhythm; fast, slow or normal rate	◆ Commonly transient; may progress to complete heart block ◆ May result from inferior wall myocardial infarction, digoxin or quinidine toxicity, vagal stimulation, electrolyte imbalance, or arteriosclerotic heart disease
Premature ventricular contractions (multifocal) 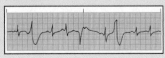	Usually irregular rhythm with a long pause after the premature beat; fast, slow, or normal rate	◆ Arise from different ventricular sites or from the same site with changing patterns of conduction ◆ May result from caffeine or stress, alcohol ingestion, myocardial ischemia or infarction, myocardial irritation by pacemaker electrodes, hypocalcemia, hypercalcemia, digoxin toxicity, or exercise

Pulsus alternans

- Refers to a beat-to-beat change in the size and intensity of a peripheral pulse
- As pulse rhythm remains regular, strong and weak contractions alternate (see *Comparing arterial pressure waves,* page 480)
- Results from the change in stroke volume that occurs with beat-to-beat alteration in the left ventricle's contractility

ACTION STAT! *Pulsus alternans indicates a critical change in the patient's status. When you detect it, be sure to quickly check other vital signs. Closely evaluate the patient's heart rate, respiratory pattern, and blood pressure. Auscultate for a ventricular gallop and increased crackles.*

- Obtain a full medical history focusing on cardiac disorders.

- Obtain vital signs.
- Assess for pulsus alternans. (See *Detecting pulsus alternans.*)

MEDICAL
Left-sided heart failure
- With this disorder, pulsus alternans is commonly initiated by a premature beat and is almost always associated with a ventricular gallop.
- Other findings include hypotension and cyanosis.
- Possible respiratory findings include exertional and paroxysmal nocturnal dyspnea, orthopnea, tachypnea, Cheyne-Stokes respirations, hemoptysis, and crackles.
- Fatigue and weakness are common.

 TOP TECHNIQUE

Detecting pulsus alternans

- Although most easily detected by sphygmomanometry, pulsus alternans can be detected by palpating the brachial, radial, or femoral artery when systolic pressure varies from beat to beat by more than 20 mm Hg. Because the small changes in arterial pressure that occur during normal respirations may obscure this abnormal pulse, you'll need to have the patient hold his breath during palpation. Apply light pressure to avoid obliterating the weaker pulse.
- When using a sphygmomanometer to detect pulsus alternans, inflate the cuff 10 to 20 mm Hg above the systolic pressure as determined by palpation, and then slowly deflate it. At first, you'll hear only the strong beats. With further deflation, all beats will become audible and palpable, and then equally intense. (The difference between this point and the peak systolic level is commonly used to determine the degree of pulsus alternans.) When the cuff is removed, pulsus alternans returns.
- Occasionally, the weak beat is so small that no palpable pulse is detected at the periphery. This produces total pulsus alternans, an apparent halving of the pulse rate.

- If left-sided heart failure develops suddenly, prepare the patient for transfer to an intensive or cardiac care unit.
- Elevate the head of the bed to promote respiratory excursion and increase oxygenation.
- Adjust the patient's current treatment plan to improve cardiac output, reduce the heart's workload, and promote diuresis.
- Monitor cardiac rhythm, vital signs, daily weight, and intake and output.

PEDIATRIC TIPS
- Pulsus alternans, which also occurs in a child with heart failure, may be difficult to assess if the child is crying or restless. Try to quiet the child by holding him, if his condition permits.

- Advise the patient about prescribed medications and adverse effects.
- Teach the patient about left-sided heart failure and its treatment plan.
- Stress the importance of follow-up care with a practitioner.

Pulsus biferiens

OVERVIEW

- Refers to hyperdynamic, double-beating pulse characterized by two systolic peaks separated by midsystolic dip
- Typically has a taller or more forceful first peak
- Occurs when a large volume of blood is rapidly ejected from the left ventricle
- Can be palpated in the peripheral arteries or observed on an arterial pressure wave recording (see *Comparing arterial pressure waves*)

HISTORY

- Obtain a medical history, including cardiac disorders.
- Take a drug history.
- Ask about associated signs and symptoms, such as dyspnea, chest pain, or fatigue.
- Find out about the onset of symptoms and aggravating or alleviating factors.

PHYSICAL ASSESSMENT

- Take vital signs.
- Auscultate for abnormal heart or breath sounds.
- Assess peripheral pulses. (See *Detecting pulsus biferiens.*)
- Complete the cardiopulmonary assessment.

TOP TECHNIQUE

Comparing arterial pressure waves

The waveforms shown here help differentiate a normal arterial pulse from pulsus alternans, pulsus biferiens, and pulsus paradoxus.

The percussion wave in a *normal arterial pulse* reflects ejection of blood into the aorta (early systole). The tidal wave is the peak of the pulse wave (later systole), and the dicrotic notch marks the beginning of diastole.

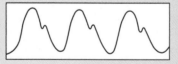

Pulsus biferiens is a double-beating pulse with two systolic peaks. The first beat reflects pulse pressure; the second, reverberation from the periphery. Pulsus biferiens commonly occurs with aortic insufficiency (aortic stenosis, aortic regurgitation), hypertrophic cardiomyopathy, or high cardiac output states.

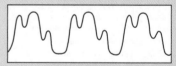

Pulsus alternans is a beat-to-beat alternation in pulse size and intensity. Although the rhythm of pulsus alternans is regular, the volume varies. If you take the blood pressure of a patient with this abnormality, you'll first hear a loud Korotkoff sound and then a soft sound, continually alternating. Pulsus alternans commonly accompanies states of poor contractility that occur with left-sided heart failure.

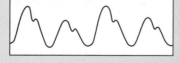

Pulsus paradoxus is an exaggerated decline in blood pressure during inspiration, resulting from an increase in negative intrathoracic pressure. A paradoxical pulse that exceeds 10 mm Hg is considered abnormal and may result from cardiac tamponade, constrictive pericarditis, or severe lung disease.

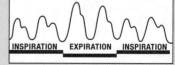

INSPIRATION   EXPIRATION   INSPIRATION

MEDICAL
Aortic insufficiency

◆ Aortic insufficiency is the most common organic cause of biferiens pulse.
◆ Other findings include exertional dyspnea; fatigue; orthopnea; paroxysmal nocturnal dyspnea; ventricular gallop; tachycardia; chest pain; palpitations; pallor; strong and abrupt carotid pulsations; widened pulse pressure; and one or more murmurs, especially an apical diastolic rumble (Austin Flint murmur).

Aortic stenosis with aortic insufficiency

◆ Pulse rate rises slowly and the second wave of the double beat is the more forceful one.
◆ Dyspnea and fatigue are common.

High cardiac output states

◆ Pulsus biferiens commonly occurs with high cardiac output states, such as anemia, thyrotoxicosis, fever, and exercise.
◆ Other findings vary with the underlying disorder and may include tachycardia, a cervical venous hum, and widened pulse pressure.

Hypertrophic obstructive cardiomyopathy

◆ Pulsus biferiens occurs with the pulse rising rapidly and the first wave being the more forceful one.
◆ Other findings include a systolic murmur, dyspnea, angina, fatigue, and syncope.

◆ Prepare the patient for diagnostic tests.
◆ Schedule regular rest periods.
◆ Monitor vital signs, intake and output, and daily weight.

PEDIATRIC TIPS
◆ Pulsus biferiens may be palpated in children with a large patent ductus arteriosus, as well as those with congenital aortic stenosis and insufficiency.

◆ Discuss the disorder and its treatment.
◆ Explain signs and symptoms of heart failure to report.
◆ Discuss the planning of rest periods.

 TOP TECHNIQUE

Detecting pulsus biferiens

To detect pulsus biferiens, lightly palpate the carotid, brachial, radial, or femoral artery. (The pulse is easiest to palpate in the carotid artery.) At the same time, listen to the patient's heart sounds to determine if the two palpable peaks occur during systole. If they do, you'll feel the double pulse between the first and second heart sounds.

Pulsus paradoxus

- An exaggerated decline in blood pressure during inspiration due to increased negative intrathoracic pressure
- Occurs when systolic pressure falls more than 10 mm Hg during inspiration (normal systolic pressure falls less than 10 mm Hg)
- With systolic pressure that falls more than 20 mm Hg, peripheral pulses may be barely palpable or may disappear during inspiration

◼ *ACTION STAT! A pulsus paradoxus may signal cardiac tamponade—a life-threatening complication of pericardial effusion that occurs when sufficient blood or fluid accumulates to compress the heart. When you detect pulsus paradoxus, quickly check the patient's other vital signs. Check for additional signs and symptoms of cardiac tamponade, such as dyspnea, tachypnea, diaphoresis, jugular vein distention, tachycardia, narrowed pulse pressure, and hypotension. Emergency pericardiocentesis to aspirate blood or fluid from the pericardial sac may be necessary. Then evaluate the effectiveness of pericardiocentesis by measuring the degree of pulsus paradoxus; it should decrease after aspiration.*

HISTORY

- Find out if the patient has a history of chronic cardiac or pulmonary disease.
- Ask about recent trauma or cardiac surgery.
- Ask about the development of associated signs and symptoms, such as a cough or chest pain.

PHYSICAL ASSESSMENT

- Auscultate for abnormal breath sounds.
- Obtain vital signs. (See *Detecting pulsus paradoxus.*)
- Perform cardiopulmonary assessment.
- Obtain electrocardiogram and blood samples for cardiac enzymes, coagulation studies, electrolytes, and blood count.

CAUSES

MEDICAL
Cardiac tamponade

- Pulsus paradoxus commonly occurs with this disorder, but it may be difficult to detect if intrapericardial pressure rises abruptly and profound hypotension occurs.
- With severe tamponade, assessment also reveals these classic findings: hypotension, diminished or muffled heart sounds, and jugular vein distention.
- Related findings include chest pain, pericardial friction rub, narrowed pulse pressure, anxiety, restlessness, clammy skin, and hepatomegaly.
- Characteristic respiratory signs and symptoms include dyspnea, tachypnea, and cyanosis; the patient typically sits up and leans forward to facilitate breathing.
- If cardiac tamponade develops gradually, pulsus paradoxus may be accompanied by weakness, anorexia, and weight loss. The patient may also report chest pain, but he won't have muffled heart sounds or severe hypotension.

Chronic obstructive pulmonary disease (COPD)

- The wide fluctuations in intrathoracic pressure that characterize this disorder produce pulsus paradoxus and possibly tachycardia.
- Other findings may include dyspnea, tachypnea, wheezing, productive or nonproductive cough, accessory muscle use, barrel chest, and clubbing.
- The patient may show labored, pursed-lip breathing after exertion or even at rest. He typically sits up and leans forward to facilitate breathing.
- Auscultation reveals decreased breath sounds, rhonchi, and crackles.
- Weight loss, cyanosis, and edema may occur.

Pericarditis (chronic constrictive)

- Pulsus paradoxus can occur in up to 50% of patients with this disorder.

- Other findings include pericardial friction rub, chest pain, exertional dyspnea, orthopnea, hepatomegaly, and ascites.
- The patient also exhibits peripheral edema and Kussmaul's sign—jugular vein distention that becomes more prominent on inspiration.

Pulmonary embolism (massive)
- Decreased left ventricular filling and stroke volume in massive pulmonary embolism produce pulsus paradoxus, as well as syncope and severe apprehension, dyspnea, tachypnea, and pleuritic chest pain.
- The patient appears cyanotic, with jugular vein distention.
- He may succumb to circulatory collapse, with hypotension and a weak rapid pulse.
- Pulmonary infarction may produce hemoptysis along with decreased breath sounds and a pleural friction rub over the affected area.

Right ventricular infarction
- This infarction may produce pulsus paradoxus and elevated jugular venous or central venous pressure.
- Other findings are similar to those of myocardial infarction.

- Prepare the patient for an echocardiogram to visualize cardiac motion and to help determine the causative disorder.
- Monitor vital signs and frequently check the degree of paradox. An increase in the degree of paradox may indicate recurring or worsening cardiac tamponade or impending respiratory arrest in severe COPD.
- Vigorous respiratory treatment, such as chest physiotherapy, may avert the need for endotracheal intubation.

PEDIATRIC TIPS
- Pulsus paradoxus commonly occurs in children with chronic pulmonary disease, especially during an acute asthma attack.
- Children with pericarditis may also develop pulsus paradoxus due to cardiac tamponade, although this disorder more commonly affects adults.
- A pulsus paradoxus above 20 mm Hg is a reliable indicator of cardiac tamponade in children; a change of 10 to 20 mm Hg is equivocal.

- Explain about all hospital procedures and required tests.
- Teach about underlying diagnosis and treatment plan.
- Emphasize the importance of prescribed medications and their adverse effects.

TOP TECHNIQUE

Detecting pulsus paradoxus

- To accurately detect and measure pulsus paradoxus, use a sphygmomanometer or an intra-arterial monitoring device. Inflate the blood pressure cuff 10 to 20 mm Hg beyond the peak systolic pressure. Then deflate the cuff at a rate of 2 mm Hg/second until you hear the first Korotkoff sound during expiration. Note the systolic pressure.
- As you continue to slowly deflate the cuff, observe the patient's respiratory pattern. If a pulsus paradoxus is present, the Korotkoff sounds will disappear with inspiration and return with expiration.
- Continue to deflate the cuff until you hear Korotkoff sounds during both inspiration and

expiration and, again, note the systolic pressure. Subtract this reading from the first one to determine the degree of pulsus paradoxus. A difference of more than 10 mm Hg is abnormal.
- You can also detect pulsus paradoxus by palpating the radial pulse over several cycles of slow inspiration and expiration. Marked pulse diminution during inspiration indicates pulsus paradoxus.
- When you check for pulsus paradoxus, remember that irregular heart rhythms and tachycardia cause variations in pulse amplitude and must be ruled out before a true pulsus paradoxus can be identified.

Pupils, nonreactive

OVERVIEW

- Refers to failure of pupils to constrict in response to light or dilate when light is removed
- May signal a life-threatening emergency or brain death (see *Understanding pupillary changes*)
- Can occur with optic drug use

  ACTION STAT! *If the patient is unconscious and develops nonreactive pupils, quickly take his vital signs. Look for decerebrate or decorticate posture, bradycardia, elevated systolic blood pressure, and widened pulse pressure. One dilated, nonreactive pupil may be an early sign of uncal brain herniation. Emergency surgery to decrease intracranial pressure (ICP) may be necessary. Insert an I.V. line to administer a diuretic, an osmotic agent, or a corticosteroid to treat increased ICP as ordered. The patient may need controlled hyperventilation.*

HISTORY

- Obtain medical history including recent infection.
- Ask about the use of eyedrops and when they were last instilled.
- Find out about pain and its location, intensity, and duration.
- Ask about recent trauma.
- Obtain information from family if patient is unable to respond.

PHYSICAL ASSESSMENT

- Assess neurologic status.
- Check visual acuity in both eyes.
- Test the pupillary reaction to accommodation. (See *Assessing pupillary reaction*.)
- Examine the cornea and iris for abnormalities.

TOP TECHNIQUE

Understanding pupillary changes

Use this chart as a guide when observing your patient for pupillary changes.

PUPILLARY CHANGE	POSSIBLE CAUSES
Unilateral, dilated (9 mm), fixed, and nonreactive 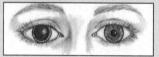	• Uncal herniation with oculomotor nerve damage • Brain stem compression • Increased intracranial pressure • Tentorial herniation • Head trauma with subdural or epidural hematoma • May be normal in some people
Bilateral, dilated (9 mm), fixed, and nonreactive 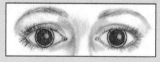	• Severe midbrain damage • Cardiopulmonary arrest (hypoxia) • Anticholinergic poisoning
Bilateral, midsize (2 mm), fixed, and nonreactive 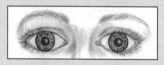	• Midbrain involvement caused by edema, hemorrhage, infarctions, lacerations, contusions
Bilateral, pinpoint (<1 mm), and usually nonreactive 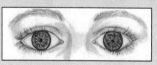	• Lesions of pons, usually after hemorrhage
Unilateral, small (1.5 mm), and nonreactive 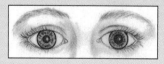	• Disruption of sympathetic nerve supply to the head caused by spinal cord lesion above the first thoracic vertebra

---

CAUSES

MEDICAL
Botulism
◆ Nonreactive pupils and mydriasis in both eyes usually appear 12 to 36 hours after ingestion of tainted food.
◆ Other early findings include blurred vision, diplopia, ptosis, strabismus, extraocular muscle palsies, anorexia, nausea, vomiting, diarrhea, and dry mouth.
◆ Vertigo, deafness, hoarseness, nasal voice, dysarthria, and dysphagia follow.
◆ Progressive muscle weakness and absent deep tendon reflexes evolve over 2 to 4 days, resulting in severe constipation and paralysis of respiratory muscles with respiratory distress.

Encephalitis
◆ Initially sluggish pupils become dilated and nonreactive.
◆ Decreased accommodation and other symptoms of cranial nerve palsies develop.
◆ A decreased level of consciousness (LOC), high fever, headache, vomiting, and nuchal rigidity occur within 48 hours.
◆ Aphasia, ataxia, nystagmus, hemiparesis, and photophobia may occur with seizures.

Glaucoma (acute angle-closure)
◆ A moderately dilated, nonreactive pupil occurs in the affected eye in this ophthalmic emergency.
◆ Sudden blurred vision, followed by excruciating pain in and around the affected eye occurs.
◆ Other findings include seeing halos around white lights at night, conjunctival injection, corneal clouding, and decreased visual acuity.
◆ Nausea and vomiting occur with severely elevated intraocular pressure (IOP).

Ocular trauma
◆ A transient or permanent nonreactive, dilated pupil may result from severe damage to the iris or optic nerve.

◆ Eye pain, eye edema, and ecchymoses may occur.
◆ A V-shaped notch in the pupillary rim, indicating a tear in the iris sphincter muscle, may be seen on slit-lamp examination.

Oculomotor nerve palsy
◆ A dilated, nonreactive pupil and loss of the accommodation reaction is the first sign.
◆ This sign may signal life-threatening brain herniation.

Uveitis
◆ In anterior uveitis, a small, nonreactive pupil appears suddenly and is accompanied by severe eye pain, conjunctival injection, and photophobia.
◆ With posterior uveitis, similar features develop insidiously, along with blurred vision and distorted pupil shape.

Wernicke's disease
◆ Nonreactive pupils occur late in this disease associated with thiamine deficiency.
◆ Initial findings include an intention tremor accompanied by a sluggish pupillary reaction.
◆ Other ocular findings include diplopia, gaze paralysis, nystagmus, ptosis, decreased visual acuity, and conjunctival injection.
◆ Orthostatic hypotension, tachycardia, ataxia, apathy, and confusion may also occur.

OTHER
Drugs
◆ Instillation of a topical mydriatic or cycloplegic may induce a temporarily nonreactive pupil in the affected eye.
◆ Opiates cause pinpoint pupils with a minimal light response that can be seen only with a magnifying glass.
◆ Atropine (AtroPen) poisoning produces widely dilated, nonreactive pupils.

NURSING CONSIDERATIONS

◆ Monitor vital signs and LOC.
◆ If the patient is conscious, monitor his pupillary light reflex.
◆ If the patient is unconsciousness, close his eyes to prevent corneal exposure.

PEDIATRIC TIPS
◆ The most common cause of nonreactive pupils in children is oculomotor nerve palsy from increased IOP.

PATIENT TEACHING

◆ Discuss underlying condition, diagnostic tests, and treatment options.
◆ Teach proper methods for instilling eye drops.
◆ Explain methods of reducing photophobia.
◆ Stress the importance of follow-up care to check IOP.

 TOP TECHNIQUE

Assessing pupillary reaction

To evaluate pupillary reaction to light, first test the patient's direct light reflex. Darken the room and cover one of the patient's eyes while you hold open the opposite eyelid. Using a bright penlight, bring the light toward the patient from the side and shine it directly into his opened eye. If normal, the pupil will promptly constrict. Next, test the consensual light reflex. Hold the patient's eyelids open and shine the light into one eye while watching the pupil of the opposite eye. If normal, both pupils will promptly constrict. Repeat both procedures in the opposite eye.

Pupils, sluggish

- Refers to abnormally slow pupillary response to light
- Can occur in one pupil or both; a normal pupillary reaction always occurs bilaterally
- Indicates dysfunction of cranial nerves II and III, which mediate the light reflex
- Accompanies degenerative disease of the central nervous system and diabetic neuropathy

HISTORY

- Obtain a medical history.
- Find out about the use of eyedrops and when they were last used.
- Ask about pain and other ocular symptoms.

PHYSICAL ASSESSMENT

- Test visual acuity.
- Assess pupillary reaction to accommodation.
- Examine the cornea and iris for irregularities, scars, and foreign bodies.
- Perform neurologic assessment.

CAUSES

MEDICAL

Adie's syndrome
- Sluggish pupillary response with abrupt onset of mydriasis progresses to a nonreactive pupil in this idiopathic neurologic condition.
- Other findings include blurred vision, and hypoactive or absent deep tendon reflexes in the arms and legs.

Diabetic neuropathy
- Sluggish pupillary response occurs with long-standing disease.
- Other findings include orthostatic hypotension, syncope, dysphagia, episodic constipation or diarrhea, painless bladder distention with overflow incontinence, retrograde ejaculation, and impotence.

Encephalitis
- Sluggish response in both pupils is an initial symptom.
- Later, dilated nonreactive pupils, decreased accommodation, and other cranial nerve palsies may occur.
- Other findings include decreased level of consciousness, headache, high fever, vomiting, nuchal rigidity, aphasia, ataxia, nystagmus, hemiparesis, photophobia, and seizures.

Herpes zoster
- A sluggish pupillary response may occur if the nasociliary nerve is affected.
- Examination of the conjunctive reveals follicles.
- Other ocular findings include a serous discharge, absence of tears, ptosis, and extraocular muscle palsy.

Iritis (acute)
- A sluggish pupillary response and conjunctival injection occur in the affected eye.
- The pupil may remain constricted; pupil will be irregularly shaped if posterior synechiae have formed.
- Sudden onset of eye pain, photophobia, and blurred vision may also occur.

Multiple sclerosis

◆ Small, irregularly shaped pupils react better to accommodation than to light in this neurologic disorder of the brain and spinal cord.
◆ Other findings include ptosis, nystagmus, diplopia, and blurred vision.
◆ Early findings include vision problems and sensory impairment.
◆ Later findings include muscle weakness and paralysis; intention tremor, spasticity, hyperreflexia, and gait ataxia; dysphagia and dysarthria; constipation; urinary urgency, frequency, and incontinence; impotence; and emotional instability.

Myotonic dystrophy

◆ Myotonic dystrophy may cause sluggish pupillary reaction with lid lag, ptosis, miosis and, possibly, diplopia.
◆ Other findings include decreased visual acuity from cataract formation; muscle weakness and atrophy; and testicular atrophy.

Tertiary syphilis

◆ Sluggish pupillary reaction occurs in the late stage of neurosyphilis.
◆ Marked weakness of extraocular muscles, visual field defects, and decreased visual acuity also occur in this disorder.

Wernicke's disease

◆ Early findings related to this thiamine deficiency disorder include an intention tremor with a sluggish pupillary reaction; later findings include nonreactive pupils.
◆ Other ocular findings include diplopia, gaze paralysis, nystagmus, ptosis, decreased visual acuity, and conjunctival injection.
◆ Orthostatic hypotension, tachycardia, ataxia, apathy, and confusion are also possible.

NURSING CONSIDERATIONS

◆ A sluggish pupillary reaction isn't diagnostically significant.
◆ Treat the underlying disorder.
◆ If vision is affected, provide for the patient's safety.
◆ Monitor for eye pain and changes in vision.

PEDIATRIC TIPS

◆ Children experience sluggish pupillary reactions for the same reasons as adults.

GERIATRIC TIPS

◆ A sluggish pupillary response may occur normally in elderly people, whose pupils become smaller and less responsive with age.

PATIENT TEACHING

◆ Stress the importance of regular ophthalmologic examinations.
◆ Teach about underlying disorder, diagnostic tests, and treatment options.
◆ Explain ways of reducing photophobia.
◆ Teach the patient self-care for diabetes, if needed.

Purple striae

OVERVIEW

- Thin, purple streaks on the skin
- Occur from the catabolic action of excess glucocorticoids on skin, fat, and muscle thereby inhibiting fibroblast activity; this results in loss of collagen and connective tissue, causing extreme thinning of the skin, which, along with erythrocytosis, causes purple color
- Occur most commonly over the abdominal area, but also over the breasts, hips, buttocks, thighs, and axillae

HISTORY

- Ask the patient when—and on what part of his body—he first noticed purple striae.
- Obtain a complete drug history.
- If the patient is receiving glucocorticoid therapy, find out the drug's name, the daily dose and schedule, and the reason for treatment. Ask if the dosage has been altered recently and if the drug is given intramuscularly.
- Ask the patient if he uses a topical corticosteroid, especially a fluorinated product; ask about concomitant use of occlusive dressings and, with large skin surface areas, the amount of corticosteroid applied.

PHYSICAL ASSESSMENT

- Examine the patient and note all areas where purple striae appear.
- When checking for striae, remember that the patient's skin is extremely thin and susceptible to bruising.

CAUSES

MEDICAL
Hypercortisolism
◆ Although hypercortisolism can be caused by adrenocortical carcinoma, adrenal adenoma, and pituitary adenoma, it usually results from excessive use of glucocorticoids.
◆ With this disorder, purple striae—usually more than 1 cm wide—develop gradually over the abdomen and possibly the breasts, hips, buttocks, thighs, and axillae.
◆ Inspection reveals the cardinal signs of moon face, buffalo hump, and truncal obesity.
◆ Other findings include acne, ecchymoses, petechiae, muscle weakness and wasting, poor wound healing, excessive perspiration, hypertension, fatigue, and personality changes.
◆ Women may develop hirsutism, menstrual irregularities, and inability to achieve orgasm. Men may become impotent.

OTHER
Drugs
◆ Excessive use of a glucocorticoid can cause purple striae and other cushingoid effects.

NURSING CONSIDERATIONS

◆ Expect to collect 24-hour urine specimens before and during the 2-day low-dose and 2-day high-dose dexamethasone tests.
◆ Explain to the patient that purple striae develop gradually and, with treatment, may gradually fade or decrease in size.

PEDIATRIC TIPS
◆ Although relatively rare in children, hypercortisolism may occur at any age.
◆ In infancy and early childhood, it usually results from adrenal tumor, systemic absorption of a topical corticosteroid applied excessively, or oral administration of a glucocorticoid.
◆ After age 7, it usually stems from inappropriate pituitary secretion of corticotropin, with bilateral adrenal hyperplasia.

PATIENT TEACHING

◆ Help the patient cope with changes in his body image by clearly explaining the disease process and allowing him to openly express his concerns.
◆ Prepare for diagnostic tests to confirm hypercortisolism and determine its cause.
◆ Explain the importance of follow-up tests.

Purpura

- Results from extravasation of red blood cells from the blood vessels into the skin, subcutaneous tissue, or mucous membranes
- Involves easily visible purplish or brownish red discoloration
- Causes discoloration that fails to blanch with pressure
- Purpuric lesions that include petechiae, ecchymoses, and hematomas (see *Identifying purpuric lesions*)

HISTORY

- Ask about the onset and location of lesions.
- Take a drug and diet history.
- Find out about a personal or family history of bleeding disorders or easy bruising.
- Inquire about recent illnesses, trauma, and transfusions.
- Ask about other signs, such as epistaxis, bleeding gums, hematuria, hematochezia, fever, and heavy menstrual flow.

PHYSICAL ASSESSMENT

- Inspect the entire skin surface and mucous membranes to determine the type, size, location, distribution, and severity of purpuric lesions.

CAUSES

MEDICAL

Cholesterol emboli

- Purpura typically occurs in the lower extremities of patients with atherosclerotic vascular disease, or after anticoagulation therapy or an invasive arterial procedure.
- Other findings include livedo reticularis, cyanosis, gangrene, nodules, and ulceration of the skin.

Disseminated intravascular coagulation

- Purpura occurs in different degrees.
- Cutaneous oozing, hematemesis, or bleeding from incision or needle insertion sites may occur.
- Other findings include acrocyanosis; nausea; dyspnea; seizures; oliguria; and severe muscle, back, and abdominal pain.

Dysproteinemias

- Petechiae and ecchymoses occur along with bleeding tendencies in multiple myeloma and cryoglobulinemia.
- Hyperglobulinemia typically begins insidiously with occasional outbreaks of purpura over the lower legs and feet.

Fat emboli

- Petechiae occur on the upper body a few days after a major injury.
- Other findings include fever, tachycardia, tachypnea, blood-tinged sputum, cyanosis, anxiety, altered level of consciousness, seizures, coma, or rash.

Idiopathic thrombocytopenic purpura

- Scattered petechiae on the distal arms and legs are an early sign.
- Deep-lying ecchymoses may also occur.
- Other findings include epistaxis, easy bruising, hematuria, hematemesis, and menorrhagia.

Leukemia

- Widespread persistent petechiae appear on the skin, mucous membranes, retina, and serosal surfaces.
- Other findings include fever, abdominal or bone pain, lymphadenopathy, splenomegaly, swollen and bleeding gums, epistaxis, and other bleeding tendencies.

Liver disease

- Purpura, particularly ecchymoses, and other bleeding tendencies may occur.

Meningococcemia

- Cutaneous and oropharyngeal petechiae and purpura are initially discrete but become confluent, developing into hemorrhagic bullae and ulcerations.
- Sudden severe infection results in extensive purpura and ecchymosis with irregular borders, most notably on the extremities.
- Other findings include spiking fevers, chills, myalgia, and arthralgia progressing to headache, neck stiffness, and nuchal rigidity.

Myeloproliferative disorder

- Hemorrhage accompanied by ecchymoses and ruddy cyanosis can occur.
- The oral mucosa takes on a deep purplish red hue, and slight trauma causes swollen gums to bleed.
- Other findings include pruritus, urticaria, lethargy, fatigue, weight loss, headache, dizziness, vertigo, dyspnea, paresthesia, visual alterations, intermittent claudication, hypertension, hepatosplenomegaly, and impaired mentation.

Nutritional deficiencies

- With vitamin C deficiency, purpura patches join together to form ecchymoses on the inner thighs and lower buttocks.
- With vitamin K deficiency, abnormal bleeding tendencies, such as ecchymosis, gum bleeding, epistaxis, and hematuria occur.
- With vitamin B_{12} and folic acid deficiencies, varying degrees of purpura occur.

Identifying purpuric lesions

Purpuric lesions fall into three categories: petechiae, ecchymoses, and hematomas. Use these illustrations to help you accurately identify purpuric lesions in your patients.

PETECHIAE

Petechiae are painless, round, pinpoint lesions, 1 to 3 mm in diameter. Caused by extravasation of red blood cells into cutaneous tissue, these red or brown lesions usually arise on dependent portions of the body. They appear and fade in crops and can group to form ecchymoses.

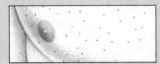

ECCHYMOSES

Ecchymoses, another form of blood extravasation, are larger than petechiae. These purple, blue, or yellow-green bruises vary in size and shape, and can arise anywhere on the body as a result of trauma. Ecchymoses usually appear on the arms and legs of patients with bleeding disorders.

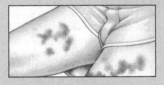

HEMATOMAS

Hematomas are palpable ecchymoses that are painful and swollen. Usually the result of trauma, superficial hematomas are red, whereas deep hematomas are blue. Hematomas commonly exceed 1 cm in diameter, but their size varies widely.

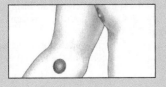

Rocky Mountain spotted fever

◆ Initial skin lesions are small pink macules that evolve into blatant petechiae and palpable purpura; palms and soles are particularly affected.
◆ Other findings include fever, severe headache, myalgia, photophobia, nausea, and vomiting; later, shock and even death may occur.

Septicemia

◆ Purpura, especially petechiae, may occur with septicemia.
◆ Other findings include fever, chills, headache, tachycardia, lethargy, diaphoresis, anorexia, and signs of specific infection.

Systemic lupus erythematosus

◆ Purpura may occur with other cutaneous findings.
◆ Characteristic butterfly-shaped rash appears in the connective disorder's acute phase.
◆ Common findings include nondeforming joint pain and stiffness, Raynaud's phenomenon, seizures, psychotic behavior, photosensitivity, fever, anorexia, weight loss, and lymphadenopathy.

Trauma

◆ Local or widespread purpura may occur.

OTHER
Diagnostic tests and procedures

◆ Invasive diagnostic tests may produce local ecchymoses and hematomas.
◆ Procedures that disrupt circulation, coagulation, or platelet activity or production can cause purpura.

Drugs

◆ Anticoagulants may cause purpura.

NURSING CONSIDERATIONS

◆ Maintain bleeding precautions, as appropriate.
◆ Apply pressure and cold compresses to hematomas for the first 24 hours to reduce bleeding; then apply hot compresses to speed absorption of blood.
◆ Monitor skin condition frequently.

PEDIATRIC TIPS

◆ Neonates commonly exhibit petechiae—particularly on the head, neck, and shoulders—after vertex deliveries.
◆ The most common type of purpura in children is allergic purpura.
◆ When assessing a child with purpura, be alert for signs of possible child abuse.

GERIATRIC TIPS

◆ Purpura can be a consequence of aging.
◆ Chronic stasis produces dusky reddish purpura on the legs after prolonged standing.

PATIENT TEACHING

◆ Explain treatment of the underlying disease.
◆ Discuss the avoidance of fade creams.

Pustular rash

- Characterized by rash consisting of crops of pustules—visible collections of pus within or beneath the epidermis—commonly in hair follicles or sweat glands
- Pustules vary in size and shape; can be generalized or localized
- Rash that results from other skin eruptions if secondary infection develops

HISTORY

- Ask about the appearance, location, and onset of the first pustular lesion.
- Find out about occurrence of different preceding lesions.
- Determine how the lesions spread.
- Take a drug history, including the use of topical medications.
- Ask about a family history of skin disorders.

PHYSICAL ASSESSMENT

- Assess entire skin surface, noting if it's dry, oily, or moist.
- Record the exact location and distribution of skin lesions, noting color, shape, and size.

CAUSES

MEDICAL

Acne vulgaris
- Pustules accompany papules, nodules, cysts, and open and closed comedones.
- Lesions commonly appear on the face, shoulders, back, and chest.
- Other findings include pain on pressure, pruritus, burning and, if chronic, scars.

Blastomycosis
- Small, painless, nonpruritic macules or papules can enlarge to well-circumscribed, verrucous, crusted, or ulcerated lesions edged by pustules in this fungal infection.
- Other findings include pleuritic chest pain and a dry, hacking or productive cough with occasional hemoptysis.

Folliculitis
- Individual pustules occur, each pierced by a hair.
- Pruritus occurs with folliculitis.
- If the condition progresses, hard painful nodules of furunculosis may occur.

Furunculosis
- Acute, deep-seated, red, hot, tender abscess evolves from a staphylococcal folliculitis at the base of hair follicles.
- Most commonly occur in areas prone to repeated infection, such as the face, neck, forearms, groin, axillae, buttocks, and legs.
- Pustules remain tense for 2 to 4 days and then become fluctuant.
- With rupture, pus and necrotic material are discharged and pain subsides, but erythema and edema may persist.

Gonococcemia
- A rash of scanty, pinpoint erythematous macules rapidly becomes vesiculopustular, maculopapular and, frequently, hemorrhagic.
- Mature lesions are elevated, with dirty gray necrotic centers and surrounding erythema.
- Rash occurs on palms and soles, usually during the first day that other signs and symptoms, such as fever and joint pain, occur.
- Rash disappears after 3 or 4 days but may recur with each episode of fever.

Impetigo contagiosa
- Vesicles form and break, and a crust forms from the exudate: a thick yellow crust in streptococcal impetigo, and a thin clear crust in staphylococcal impetigo.
- Painless itching occurs in both forms.

Nummular or annular dermatitis
- Numerous coinlike or ringed pustular lesions appear, usually on the extensor surfaces of the extremities, posterior trunk, buttocks, and lower legs.
- Lesions commonly ooze a purulent exudate, itch severely, and become crusted and scaly rapidly.

Pustular miliaria
- Pustular lesions begin as tiny erythematous papulovesicles at sweat glands.
- Diffuse erythema may radiate from the lesion.
- Rash and associated burning and pruritus worsen with sweating.

Rosacea
- Acute episodes of pustules, papules, and edema occur with telangiectasia.
- Rosacea is characterized by persistent erythema.
- It may begin as a flush covering the forehead, malar region, nose, and chin.
- Intermittent episodes gradually become more persistent, and the skin develops varying degrees of erythema.

Scabies
- Threadlike channels or burrows under the skin characterize scabies; pustules, vesicles, and excoriations may also occur.
- Lesions have a swollen nodule or red papule that contains the itch mite.

Smallpox

- A maculopapular rash develops on the mucosa of the mouth, pharynx, face, and forearms, and then spreads to the trunk and legs.
- Initial findings include high fever, malaise, prostration, severe headache, and abdominal pain.
- Within 2 days, the rash becomes vesicular and later, pustular.
- Pustules are round, firm, and deeply embedded in the skin.
- After 8 to 9 days the pustules form a crust, and later the scab separates from the skin, leaving a pitted scar.

Varicella zoster

- Extremely painful and pruritic vesicles and pustules occur along a dermatome.
- Chronic pain may persist for months.

OTHER

Drugs

- Bromides and iodides commonly cause a pustular rash.
- Anabolic steroids, androgens, corticosteroids, dactinomycin (Cosmegen), isoniazid, hormonal contraceptives, lithium (Eskalith), phenobarbital, phenytoin (Dilantin), and trimethadione (Tridione) may also cause a pustular rash.

NURSING CONSIDERATIONS

- Until infection is ruled out, follow wound and skin isolation precautions.
- If the organism is infectious, don't allow any drainage to touch unaffected skin.

PEDIATRIC TIPS

- Varicella, erythema toxicum neonatorum, candidiasis, impetigo, infantile acropustulosis, and acrodermatitis enteropathica may produce a pustular rash in children.

PATIENT TEACHING

- Discuss underlying disorder, diagnostic tests, and treatment options.
- Explain methods to prevent the spread of infection.
- Give emotional support.
- Provide information about relieving pain and itching.

Pyrosis

OVERVIEW

- Refers to substernal burning sensation that rises in the chest and may radiate to the neck or throat
- Also called *heartburn*
- Caused by reflux of gastric contents into the esophagus
- Commonly accompanied by regurgitation
- Usually develops after meals or when the patient lies down, bends over, lifts heavy objects, or exercises vigorously; improves when the patient sits upright or takes an antacid (see *How pyrosis occurs*)

HISTORY

- Ask about medical history including diet, medication, and alcohol use.
- Find out about factors that aggravate, alleviate, or trigger heartburn.
- Determine the location of pain and whether it radiates.
- Ask about other signs and symptoms, including regurgitation.

PHYSICAL ASSESSMENT

- Perform an abdominal assessment.
- Examine the mouth and throat.

CAUSES

MEDICAL
Esophageal cancer
- Painless dysphagia that progressively worsens is an early symptom.
- Regurgitation and aspiration commonly occur at night.
- Other findings include rapid weight loss, steady pain in the front and back of chest, hoarseness, sore throat, nausea, vomiting, and a feeling of substernal fullness.

Esophageal diverticula
- Pyrosis, regurgitation, and dysphagia may occur, although the disorder usually causes no symptoms.
- Other findings include chronic cough, halitosis, chest pain, a bad taste in the mouth, and a gurgling in the esophagus when liquids are swallowed.

How pyrosis occurs

Serving as a barrier to reflux, the lower esophageal sphincter (LES) normally relaxes only to allow food to pass from the esophagus into the stomach. However, hormonal fluctuations, mechanical stress, and the effects of certain foods and drugs can lower LES pressure. When LES pressure falls and intra-abdominal or intragastric pressure rises, the normally contracted LES relaxes inappropriately and allows reflux of gastric acid or bile secretions into the lower esophagus. There, the acids or secretions irritate and inflame the esophageal mucosa, producing pyrosis (as shown here).

Persistent inflammation can cause LES pressure to decrease even more and may trigger a cycle of reflux and pyrosis.

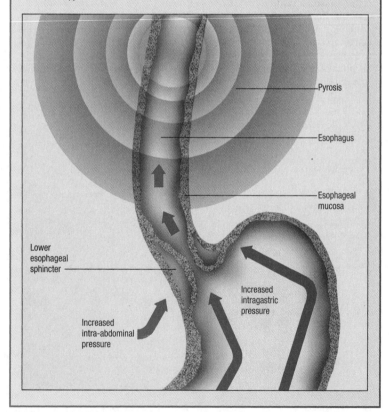

Labels: Pyrosis, Esophagus, Esophageal mucosa, Lower esophageal sphincter, Increased intra-abdominal pressure, Increased intragastric pressure

Gastroesophageal reflux disease

◆ Pyrosis, which is typically severe, is the most common symptom.
◆ Pyrosis tends to be chronic, occurs 30 to 60 minutes after eating, and may be triggered by certain foods or beverages.
◆ Pyrosis worsens when the patient lies down or bends, and abates when he sits upright or takes an antacid.
◆ Other findings include postural regurgitation, dysphagia, flatulent dyspepsia, and dull retrosternal pain that may radiate.

Hiatal hernia

◆ Eructation after eating, with heartburn, regurgitation of sour-tasting fluid, and abdominal distention.
◆ Dull substernal or epigastric pain, radiating to the shoulder.
◆ Dysphagia, nausea, weight loss, dyspnea, tachypnea, a cough, and halitosis.

Obesity

◆ Reflux and resulting pyrosis occur from increased intra-abdominal pressure.
◆ Other findings include hypertension, cardiovascular disease, diabetes mellitus, renal disease, gallbladder disease, and psychosocial difficulties.

Peptic ulcer disease

◆ Pyrosis and indigestion usually signal the start of a peptic ulcer attack.
◆ Gnawing, burning pain in the left epigastrium may occur 2 or 3 hours after eating or when the stomach is empty (usually at night) and is relieved by eating or taking an antacid or antisecretory.

Scleroderma

◆ Reflux with pyrosis occurs from esophageal dysfunction in this connective tissue disease.
◆ Other GI findings include a sensation of food sticking behind the breastbone, odynophagia, bloating after meals, weight loss, abdominal distention, constipation or diarrhea, and maladorous floating stool.

◆ Early findings include blanching, pruritus, cyanosis, and stress- or cold-induced erythema of the fingers and toes.
◆ Later findings include finger and joint pain, stiffness, and swelling; skin thickening on the hands and forearms; masklike facies; and flexion contractures.
◆ With advanced disease, arrhythmias, dyspnea, cough, malignant hypertension, and signs of renal failure may occur.

OTHER

Drugs

◆ Anticholinergics, aspirin, drugs that have anticholinergic effects, and tolbutamide may cause or aggravate pyrosis.

Lifestyle

◆ Large meals or pregnancy may cause or aggravate pyrosis.

NURSING CONSIDERATIONS

◆ Prepare the patient for diagnostic tests.
◆ Position the patient to alleviate pyrosis.
◆ Give antacids, if needed.

PEDIATRIC TIPS

◆ Help a child describe the sensation to aid differentiation between esophageal pain and pyrosis.

GERIATRIC TIPS

◆ Elderly patients with peptic ulcer disease commonly present with nonspecific abdominal discomfort or weight loss.
◆ Elderly patients are at greater risk for complications from nonsteroidal anti-inflammatories.
◆ Many elderly patients develop pyrosis caused by intolerance to spicy foods.

PATIENT TEACHING

◆ Explain underlying disorder, diagnostic studies, and treatment options.
◆ Discuss lifestyle changes, such as eating frequent small meals and sitting upright for 2 hours after meals.
◆ Explain dietary restrictions and guidelines the patient needs to use.
◆ Discuss measures to prevent increased intra-abdominal pressure.
◆ Stress the importance of stopping smoking and drugs that reduce sphincter control.

Raccoon eyes

OVERVIEW

- Refers to periorbital ecchymoses that don't result from facial soft-tissue trauma (see *Recognizing raccoon eyes*)
- Usually an indicator of basilar skull fracture
- Develops when damage at the time of fracture tears the meninges and causes the venous sinuses to bleed into the arachnoid villi and cranial sinuses
- May be only indicator of basilar skull fracture

HISTORY

- Find out when the head injury occurred and the nature of the injury.
- Obtain a medical history.

PHYSICAL ASSESSMENT

- Take vital signs.
- Evaluate level of consciousness (LOC) using the Glasgow Coma Scale.
- Evaluate function of the cranial nerves, especially I (olfactory), III (oculomotor), IV (trochlear), VI (abducens), and VII (facial).
- Assess for signs and symptoms of increased intracranial pressure.
- Test visual acuity.
- Assess gross hearing.
- Note irregularities in the facial or skull bones.
- Observe for swelling, localized pain, a Battle's sign (ecchymosis over the mastoid process or the temporal lobe), or lacerations of the face or scalp.
- Inspect for hemorrhage or cerebrospinal fluid (CSF) leakage from the nose or ears.
- Test any drainage with a sterile gauze pad and note whether a halo sign is present, indicating CSF.
- Use a glucose reagent strip to test any clear drainage for glucose indicative of CSF.

TOP TECHNIQUE

Recognizing raccoon eyes

It's usually easy to differentiate "raccoon eyes" from the "black eye" associated with facial trauma. Raccoon eyes (as shown) are always bilateral. They develop within 2 or 3 days of a closed-head injury that results in basilar skull fracture. In contrast, the periorbital ecchymosis that occurs with facial trauma can affect one eye or both. A black eye usually develops within hours of injury.

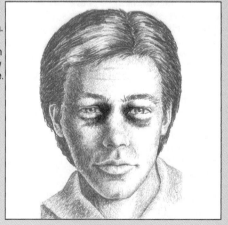

CAUSES

MEDICAL
Basilar skull fracture
◆ Raccoon eyes are produced after head trauma that doesn't involve the orbital area.
◆ Other findings vary with the fracture site and may include pharyngeal hemorrhage, epistaxis, rhinorrhea, otorrhea, and a bulging tympanic membrane from blood or CSF.
◆ Additional findings include difficulty hearing, headache, nausea, vomiting, cranial nerve palsies, a positive Battle's sign, and altered LOC.

OTHER
Surgery
◆ Raccoon eyes occurring after craniotomy may indicate a meningeal tear and bleeding into the sinuses.

NURSING CONSIDERATIONS

◆ Keep the patient on complete bedrest.
◆ Perform frequent neurologic evaluations to reevaluate his LOC.
◆ Check vital signs frequently; look for changes such as bradycardia, bradypnea, hypertension, and fever.
◆ Instruct the patient not to blow his nose, cough vigorously, or strain to avoid worsening a dural tear.
◆ If otorrhea or rhinorrhea is present, don't attempt to stop the flow; instead, place a sterile loose gauze pad under the nose or ear to absorb the drainage.
◆ Monitor the amount of drainage and test it with a glucose reagent strip to confirm or rule out CSF.
◆ To prevent further tearing of the mucous membranes and infection, never suction or pass a nasogastric tube through the patient's nose.
◆ Observe for signs and symptoms of meningitis, such as Brudzinski's sign, Kernig's sign, fever and nuchal rigidity, and expect to administer a prophylactic antibiotic.
◆ Prepare the patient for diagnostic studies such as skull X-rays and computed tomography scan of the head.
◆ If the dural tear doesn't heal spontaneously, contrast cisternography may be performed to locate the tear, possibly followed by corrective surgery.

PEDIATRIC TIPS
◆ Raccoon eyes are usually caused by a basilar skull fracture after a fall.

PATIENT TEACHING

◆ Explain which signs and symptoms of neurologic deterioration the patient should report.
◆ Discuss activity limitations the patient needs to follow.
◆ Give instructions for care of a scalp wound.

Rebound tenderness

OVERVIEW

- Refers to intense, elicited abdominal pain caused by rebound of the palpated tissues (see *Eliciting rebound tenderness*)
- Also called *Blumberg's sign*
- Is a reliable indicator of peritonitis or peritoneal inflammation
- May be localized, as in an abscess, or generalized, as in perforation of an intra-abdominal organ
- Occurs usually with abdominal pain, tenderness, and rigidity

 ***ACTION STAT!** If you elicit rebound tenderness in a patient who's experiencing constant, severe abdominal pain, quickly take his vital signs. Insert a large-bore I.V. catheter and begin administering I.V. fluids. Insert an indwelling urinary catheter, and monitor intake and output. Give supplemental oxygen as needed, and continue to monitor the patient for signs of shock, such as hypotension and tachycardia.*

HISTORY

- Ask about events that led up to the tenderness.
- Inquire about what aggravates and alleviates the tenderness.
- Find out about other signs and symptoms, such as nausea, vomiting, fever, or abdominal bloating or distention, or changes in bowel and bladder function.
- Take a medical history.

PHYSICAL ASSESSMENT

- Inspect the abdomen for distention, visible peristaltic waves, and scars.
- Auscultate for bowel sounds and characterize their motility.
- Palpate for associated rigidity or guarding, starting with light palpation and, if needed, progressing to deep palpation.
- Percuss the abdomen noting any tympany.

TOP TECHNIQUE

Eliciting rebound tenderness

To elicit rebound tenderness, help the patient into a supine position, and push your fingers deeply and steadily into his abdomen (as shown). Quickly release the pressure. Pain that results from the rebound of palpated tissue (rebound tenderness) indicates peritoneal inflammation or peritonitis.

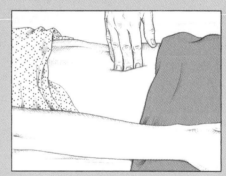

You can also elicit this symptom on a miniature scale by percussing the patient's abdomen lightly and indirectly (as shown). Better still, simply ask the patient to cough. This allows you to elicit rebound tenderness without having to touch the patient's abdomen and may also increase his cooperation because he won't associate exacerbation of his pain with your actions.

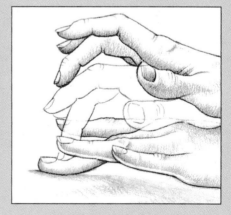

CAUSES

MEDICAL
Peritonitis
- A life-threatening disorder; rebound tenderness is accompanied by sudden and severe abdominal pain, which may be diffuse or localized.
- Pain may worsen with movement.
- Typical findings include weakness, pallor, excessive sweating, and cold skin.
- Other findings include hypoactive or absent bowel sounds, tachypnea, tachycardia, hypotension, nausea, vomiting, positive psoas and obturator signs, high fever, and abdominal distention, rigidity, and guarding.
- Shoulder pain and hiccups suggest inflammation of the diaphragmatic peritoneum.

NURSING CONSIDERATIONS

- Promote comfort by helping the patient flex his knees or assume a semi-Fowler's position in order to relax the abdominal muscles.
- Know that an analgesic may mask other symptoms.
- Give an antiemetic, antipyretic, and antibiotic as prescribed.
- Withhold oral drugs and fluids because of decreased intestinal motility and the probability that the patient may require surgery.
- Insert a nasogastric tube, if needed.
- Give continuous parenteral fluid or nutrition.

PEDIATRIC TIPS
- Because eliciting rebound tenderness may be difficult in young children, look for such clues as an anguished facial expression or intensified crying.
- When eliciting this symptom, use assessment techniques that produce minimal tenderness.

GERIATRIC TIPS
- Rebound tenderness may be diminished or absent in elderly patients.

PATIENT TEACHING

- Explain signs and symptoms the patient needs to report immediately.
- Teach the patient about required tests and procedures.
- Instruct the patient in postoperative care.

Rectal pain

OVERVIEW

- Refers to discomfort arising in the anorectal area
- Is a common symptom of anorectal disorders
- May result from or be aggravated by diarrhea, constipation, or passage of stool
- May be aggravated by intense pruritus associated with drainage of mucus, blood, or feces that irritates the skin and nerve endings

HISTORY

- Obtain a description of pain, including quality and intensity, and what aggravates and alleviates the pain.
- Find out about other signs and symptoms, such as rectal bleeding, presence of mucus or pus, and constipation or diarrhea.
- Ask the date of last bowel movement and bowel habits.
- Obtain a dietary history.

PHYSICAL ASSESSMENT

- Inspect the rectal area for bleeding, drainage, or protrusions.
- Check for inflammation and other lesions.
- Perform a rectal examination, if needed.
- Assess stool for occult blood.

CAUSES

MEDICAL

Abscess

- A superficial abscess produces constant, throbbing, local pain that's exacerbated by sitting or walking.
- With a deep abscess, the pain may begin insidiously high in the rectum or even in the lower abdomen and be accompanied by an indurated anal mass, fever, malaise, anal swelling and inflammation, purulent drainage, and local tenderness.
- A prostatic abscess occasionally produces rectal pain and may be accompanied by urine frequency with retention, dysuria, and fever.

Anal fissure

- Sharp rectal pain occurs on defecation.
- A tearing, cutting, or burning sensation and gnawing pain may continue up to 4 hours after defecation.
- Fear of provoking pain may lead to acute constipation.
- Other findings include anal pruritus and extreme tenderness, and the patient may report finding spots of blood on the toilet tissue after defecation.

Anorectal fistula

- Pain develops when a tract formed between the anal canal and skin temporarily seals.
- Other findings include pruritus and drainage of pus, mucus, blood and, occasionally, stool.

Cryptitis
◆ Particles of stool lodged in anal folds decay, resulting in infection.
◆ Dull anal pain or discomfort occurs with anal pruritus.
◆ Intense pain may occur when the anal sphincter contracts.

Hemorrhoids
◆ Rectal pain worsens during defecation and subsides after it.
◆ Usually, rectal pain is accompanied by severe itching.
◆ Fear of provoking pain may lead to constipation.
◆ With internal hemorrhoids, mild, intermittent bleeding characteristically occurs as spotting on toilet tissue or on the stool surface.

Proctalgia fugax
◆ Muscle spasms of the rectum and pelvic floor produce sudden episodes of severe rectal pain that last several minutes and then subside.
◆ The pain is sometimes associated with stress or anxiety, and relieved by food and drink.
◆ The pain may awaken the patient.

Rectal cancer
◆ Rectal pain, bleeding, tenesmus, and a hard, nontender mass are typical findings in this rare form of cancer.

OTHER
Anal intercourse
◆ Shearing forces may cause inflammation or tearing of the mucous membranes and discomfort.

NURSING CONSIDERATIONS
◆ Apply analgesic ointment or give suppositories.
◆ Give a stool softener, if needed.
◆ Apply cold compresses to help shrink protruding hemorrhoids, prevent thrombosis, and reduce pain.
◆ If the patient's condition permits, place him in Trendelenburg's position with his buttocks elevated to further relieve pain.
◆ Provide emotional support and privacy.

PEDIATRIC TIPS
◆ Observe any child with rectal pain for bleeding, drainage, and signs of infection.
◆ Acute anal fissure is a common cause of rectal pain and bleeding in children, whose fear of provoking the pain may lead to constipation.
◆ Infants who seem to have pain on defecation should be evaluated for congenital rectal anomalies.
◆ Look for other indicators of sexual abuse in all children who complain of rectal pain.

GERIATRIC TIPS
◆ Perform a thorough evaluation because elderly patients typically underreport their symptoms and have an increased risk of neoplastic disorders.

PATIENT TEACHING
◆ Instruct the patient on how to ease discomfort.
◆ Explain about proper diet, adequate fluid intake, and exercise to alleviate constipation.
◆ Discuss stool softeners.

Respirations, grunting

OVERVIEW

- A deep, low-pitched grunting sound at the end of each breath
- Occurs as the glottis closes
- Indicates intrathoracic disease with lower respiratory involvement
- May be soft and heard only on auscultation, or loud and clearly audible without a stethoscope
- Intensity of grunting reflects severity of respiratory distress
- Most common in children but can signal severe respiratory distress in adults.

> **ACTION STAT!** *Quickly place the patient in a comfortable position and check for signs of respiratory distress. Monitor oxygen saturation, and administer oxygen and drugs such as bronchodilators. Have emergency equipment available to intubate the patient if necessary. Obtain arterial blood gas (ABG) analysis to determine oxygenation.*

HISTORY

- Ask about the onset of grunting respirations.
- Find out the gestational age of a premature infant.
- Ask if anyone in the home has recently had an upper respiratory tract infection.
- Inquire about a personal history of frequent colds or upper respiratory tract infections.
- Ask about a history of respiratory syncytial virus.
- Note changes in activity level or feeding pattern.

PHYSICAL ASSESSMENT

- Obtain vital signs
- Observe for use of accessory muscles and retractions during respiration.
- Check for cyanosis, diaphoresis, and edema.
- Auscultate the lungs, noting diminished or abnormal sounds.
- Characterize the color, amount, and consistency of any discharge or sputum.
- Note the characteristics of the cough, if any.

CAUSES

MEDICAL
Asthma

- Grunting respirations may be apparent during a severe attack.
- As the attack progresses, dyspnea, audible wheezing, chest tightness, and coughing occur.

Heart failure

- Grunting respirations accompany increasing pulmonary edema as a late sign of left-sided heart failure.
- Other findings include productive cough, crackles, and chest wall retractions.
- Cyanosis may also be evident, depending on the underlying congenital cardiac defect.

Pneumonia

- Grunting respirations accompany diminished breath sounds, scattered crackles, sibilant rhonchi, high fever, tachypnea, a productive cough, anorexia, and lethargy.
- As the disorder progresses, severe dyspnea, substernal and subcostal retractions, nasal flaring, cyanosis, and increasing lethargy may occur.
- GI signs, such as vomiting, diarrhea, and abdominal distention may also be seen.

Respiratory distress syndrome

- Initially, audible expiratory grunting occurs with intercostal, subcostal, or substernal retractions; tachycardia; and tachypnea.
- Later, as the infant tires, apnea or irregular respirations replace grunting.
- Cyanosis, frothy sputum, dramatic nasal flaring, lethargy, bradycardia, and hypotension characterize severe distress.

◆ Closely monitor the patient's condition.
◆ Keep emergency equipment nearby.
◆ Administer oxygen using an oxygen hood or tent.
◆ Frequently monitor ABG levels and deliver the minimum amount of oxygen possible to avoid causing retinopathy of prematurity.
◆ Begin inhalation therapy with a bronchodilator as ordered.
◆ If the patient has pneumonia, give an I.V. antimicrobial as ordered.
◆ Perform chest physiotherapy, if appropriate.
◆ Provide emotional support to the patient and family.

PEDIATRIC TIPS
◆ Grunting respirations are a chief sign of respiratory distress in infants and children. An infant with grunting respirations may need chest physiotherapy to mobilize and drain excess lung secretions. (See *Positioning an infant for chest physical therapy*.)

◆ Explain the sights and sounds of the intensive care unit. including the patient's family.
◆ Teach techniques for home respiratory care and therapy.
◆ Give instructions on the proper use of prescribed drugs, especially bronchodilators.
◆ Explain signs and symptoms to report.

Positioning an infant for chest physical therapy

Auscultate first to locate congested areas and determine the best drainage position. The illustrations here show various drainage positions and where to place your hands for percussion. When you percuss the infant, use the fingers of one hand. Vibrate these fingers and move them toward the infant's head to facilitate drainage.

Hold the infant upright and about 30 degrees forward to percuss and drain the apical segments of the upper lobes. Repeat with the infant in a supine position to drain the anterior segments of the upper lobes.

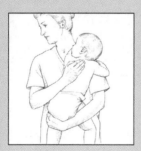

Hold the infant at a 45-degree angle on his side with his head down about 15 degrees to percuss and drain the right middle lobe.

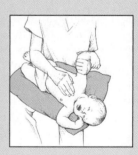

Place the infant in a supine position with his head 30 degrees lower than his feet to percuss and drain the anterior segments of the lower lobes. Repeat in the prone and both lateral positions to drain the posterior and lateral segments of the lower lobes.

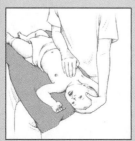

Use a prone position to percuss and drain the superior segments of the lower lobes.

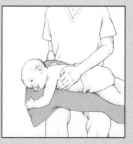

Respirations, shallow

OVERVIEW

- Refers to a diminished volume of air during inspiration
- Trigger accelerated respiratory rate as the patient attempts to obtain enough oxygen
- Lead to inadequate gas exchange as muscles tire and compensatory increase in respirations diminishes
- May develop suddenly or gradually and may last briefly or become chronic
- Are key signs of respiratory distress and neurologic deterioration

 ACTION STAT! *Look for impending respiratory failure or arrest. Look for signs of airway obstruction. If the patient is choking, perform the Heimlich maneuver or back blows for infants to try to expel the foreign object. If secretions occlude the patient's airway, use suction.*

If the patient is also wheezing, check for stridor, nasal flaring, and the use of accessory muscles. Administer oxygen with a face mask or handheld resuscitation bag. Attempt to calm the patient. If the patient loses consciousness, insert an artificial airway and prepare for endotracheal intubation, ventilatory support, and cardiopulmonary resuscitation. Measure his tidal volume and minute volume with a Wright respirometer to determine the need for mechanical ventilation. (See Measuring lung volumes.) Check arterial blood gas (ABG) levels, heart rate, blood pressure, and oxygen saturation.

HISTORY

- If the patient isn't in severe respiratory distress, take a complete medical history, including chronic respiratory disorders or respiratory tract infection, neurologic or neuromuscular disease, surgery, and trauma.
- Ask if the patient has had a tetanus booster within the past 10 years.
- Ask about smoking history.
- Take a drug history and explore the possibility of drug abuse.
- Determine the onset and duration of shallow respirations.
- Ask about factors that exacerbate or relieve shallow respirations.
- Note any changes in appetite, weight, activity level, and behavior.

PHYSICAL ASSESSMENT

- Evaluate the patient's level of consciousness (LOC) and his orientation to time, person, and place.
- Observe for spontaneous movements.
- Test muscle strength and deep tendon reflexes.
- Inspect the chest for deformities or abnormal movements.
- Inspect the extremities for cyanosis, edema, and digital clubbing.
- Palpate for expansion and diaphragmatic tactile fremitus.
- Percuss for hyperresonance or dullness.
- Auscultate for diminished, absent, or adventitious breath sounds, and for abnormal or distant heart sounds.
- Examine the abdomen for distention, tenderness, or masses.

TOP TECHNIQUE

Measuring lung volumes

Use a Wright respirometer to measure tidal volume (the amount of air inspired with each breath) and minute volume (the volume of air inspired in a minute—or tidal volume multiplied by respiratory rate). You can connect the respirometer to an intubated patient's airway using an endotracheal tube (shown here) or a tracheostomy tube. If the patient isn't intubated, connect the respirometer to a face mask, making sure the seal over the patient's mouth and nose is airtight.

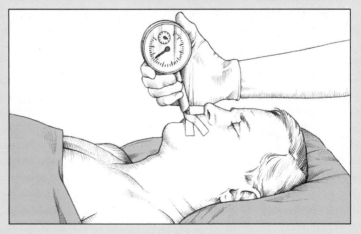

MEDICAL

Acute respiratory distress syndrome
- A life-threatening disorder; rapid, shallow respirations and dyspnea appear initially, sometimes after the patient appears stable.
- Other findings include intercostal and suprasternal retractions, diaphoresis, rhonchi, crackles, restlessness, apprehension, decreased LOC, cyanosis, and tachycardia.

Amyotrophic lateral sclerosis
- Progressive degenerative respiratory muscle weakness leads to shallow, ineffective respirations.
- Initial findings include upper extremity muscle weakness and wasting.
- Other findings include muscle cramps and atrophy, hyperreflexia, slight spasticity of the legs, coarse fasciculations of the affected muscle, impaired speech, and difficulty chewing and swallowing.

Asthma
- Rapid, shallow respirations result from bronchospasm and decreased alveolar gas exchange.
- Related respiratory findings include wheezing, rhonchi, a dry cough, dyspnea, prolonged expirations, intercostal and supraclavicular retractions on inspiration, nasal flaring, chest tightness, tachycardia, diaphoresis, flushing or cyanosis, and the use of accessory muscles.

Atelectasis
- Decreased lung expansion or pleuritic pain causes sudden onset of rapid, shallow respirations.
- Other findings include a dry cough, dyspnea, tachycardia, anxiety, cyanosis, diaphoresis, dullness to percussion, decreased breath sounds and vocal fremitus, inspiratory lag, and substernal or intercostal retractions.

Bronchiectasis
- Increased secretions obstruct airflow in the bronchi, leading to shallow respirations and a productive cough with copious, foul-smelling, mucopurulent sputum (a classic finding).
- Other findings include hemoptysis, wheezing, rhonchi, coarse crackles during inspiration, weight loss, fatigue, dyspnea on exertion, fever, and late-stage clubbing.

Chronic bronchitis
- Shallow respirations result from chronic airway inflammation and obstruction.
- A nonproductive, hacking cough that later becomes productive is an early sign.
- Other findings include prolonged expirations, wheezing, dyspnea, accessory muscle use, barrel chest, cyanosis, tachypnea, scattered rhonchi, coarse crackles, and late-stage clubbing.

Emphysema
- Increased breathing effort causes muscle fatigue, leading to chronic shallow respirations.
- Other findings include dyspnea, anorexia, malaise, tachypnea, diminished breath sounds, cyanosis, pursed-lip breathing, accessory muscle use, barrel chest, chronic productive cough, and late-stage clubbing.

Flail chest
- Decreased air movement results in rapid, shallow respirations; and paradoxical chest wall motion.
- Other findings include tachycardia, hypotension, ecchymoses, cyanosis, and pain over the affected area.

Fractured ribs
- Sharp, severe pain on inspiration may cause shallow respirations.
- Other findings include dyspnea, cough, splinting, and tenderness and edema at the fracture site.

Guillain-Barré syndrome
- Progressive ascending paralysis causes rapid or progressive onset of shallow respirations.
- Muscle weakness begins in the lower limbs and extends to the face.
- Other findings include paresthesia, dysarthria, diminished or absent corneal reflex, nasal speech, dysphagia, ipsilateral loss of facial muscle control, and flaccid paralysis.

Kyphoscoliosis
- Skeletal cage distortion causes rapid, shallow respirations from reduced lung capacity.
- Accompanying features include back pain, fatigue, tracheal deviation, ineffective coughing, and dyspnea.

Multiple sclerosis
- Muscle weakness causes progressively shallow respirations.
- Early findings include diplopia, blurred vision, and paresthesia.
- Other possible findings include nystagmus, constipation, paralysis, spasticity, hyperreflexia, intention tremor, ataxic gait, dysphagia, dysarthria, urinary dysfunction, impotence, and emotional lability.

Muscular dystrophy
- Progressive thoracic deformity and muscle weakness cause shallow respirations to occur.
- Other findings include waddling gait, contractures, scoliosis, lordosis, and muscle atrophy or hypertrophy.

Myasthenia gravis
- Progressive respiratory muscle weakness leads to shallow respirations, dyspnea, and cyanosis.
- Other findings include fatigue, weak eye closure, ptosis, diplopia, and difficulty chewing and swallowing.

Obesity
- Due to excess weight, the work of breathing may cause shallow respirations.

(continued)

Parkinson's disease
- Fatigue and weakness lead to progressively shallow respirations.
- Disorder slowly progresses to increased rigidity, masklike facies, stooped posture, shuffling gait, dysphagia, drooling, dysarthria, and pill-rolling tremor.

Pleural effusion
- Restricted lung expansion causes shallow respirations.
- Other findings include nonproductive cough, weight loss, dyspnea, pleural friction rub, tachycardia, tachypnea, decreased chest motion, decreased or absent breath sounds, and pleuritic chest pain.

Pneumonia
- Pulmonary consolidation results in rapid, shallow respirations.
- Accompanying findings include dyspnea, fever, shaking chills, chest pain, cough, tachycardia, decreased breath sounds, crackles, rhonchi, myalgia, abdominal pain, fatigue, anorexia, headache, and cyanosis.

Pneumothorax
- Shallow respirations and dyspnea begin suddenly.
- Related findings include tachycardia; tachypnea; nonproductive cough; cyanosis; accessory muscle use; asymmetrical chest expansion; anxiety; restlessness; subcutaneous crepitation; diminished or absent breath sounds on the affected side; and sudden, sharp, severe unilateral chest pain that worsens with movement.

Pulmonary edema
- Pulmonary vascular congestion causes rapid, shallow respirations.
- Early findings include angina or pleurtic chest pain, exertional dyspnea, paroxysmal nocturnal dyspnea, nonproductive cough, tachycardia, tachypnea, crackles, and a ventricular gallop.

- Severe pulmonary edema produces more rapid, labored respirations; widespread crackles; a productive cough with frothy, bloody sputum; worsening tachycardia; arrhythmias; cold, clammy skin; cyanosis; hypotension; and thready pulse.

Pulmonary embolism
- Rapid, shallow respirations and severe dyspnea begin suddenly.
- Other findings include tachycardia, tachypnea, a nonproductive cough or a productive cough with blood-tinged sputum, low-grade fever, restlessness, pleural friction rub, crackles, diffuse wheezing, chest pain, and signs of circulatory collapse.

Spinal cord injury
- Diaphragmatic breathing and shallow respirations may occur in injury to the C5 to C8 cervical vertebrae.
- Other findings include quadriplegia with flaccidity followed by spastic paralysis, areflexia, hypotension, sensory loss below the level of injury, and bowel and bladder incontinence.

Upper airway obstruction
- Partial airway obstruction causes acute shallow respirations with sudden gagging and dry, paroxysmal coughing; hoarseness; stridor; and tachycardia.
- Other findings include dyspnea, decreased breath sounds, wheezing, and cyanosis.

OTHER
Drugs
- Anesthetics, hypnotics and sedatives, magnesium sulfate, neuromuscular blockers, opioids, and tranquilizers can produce slow, shallow respirations.

Surgery
- After abdominal or chest surgery, pain from chest splinting and decreased chest wall motion may cause shallow respirations.

NURSING CONSIDERATIONS
- Position the patient upright to ease his breathing.
- Ensure adequate hydration and the use of humidification, as needed.
- Give oxygen, a bronchodilator, a mucolytic, an expectorant, or an antibiotic as prescribed
- Turn the patient frequently.
- Monitor the patient for increasing lethargy, which may indicate rising carbon dioxide levels.

PEDIATRIC TIPS
- In children, shallow respirations commonly indicate a life-threatening condition.
- Airway obstruction can occur rapidly because of the narrow passageways; if it does, administer back blows or chest thrusts but not abdominal thrusts, which can damage internal organs.

GERIATRIC TIPS
- Stiffness or deformity of the chest wall may cause shallow respirations.

- Explain the importance of coughing and deep breathing (See *Teaching coughing and deep-breathing exercises.*)
- Provide emotional support and teach the caregiver to do so as well.
- Teach about underlying diagnosis and treatment plan.

Teaching coughing and deep-breathing exercises

The exercises described below will speed your patient's recovery and reduce his risk of respiratory complications.

COUGHING EXERCISES

Patients who risk developing excess secretions should perform coughing exercises. Patients who have ear or eye surgery or repair of hiatal or large abdominal hernias should avoid coughing. Also, patients undergoing neurosurgery shouldn't cough postoperatively because intracranial pressure will rise.

- If the patient's condition permits, instruct him to sit on the edge of his bed. Provide a stool if his feet don't touch the floor. Tell him to bend his legs and lean slightly forward.
- If the patient is scheduled for chest or abdominal surgery, teach him how to splint his incision before he coughs.
- Instruct the patient to take a slow, deep breath; he should breathe in through his nose and concentrate on fully expanding his chest. Then he should breathe out through his mouth, and concentrate on feeling his chest sink downward and inward. Then he should take a second breath in the same manner.
- Next, tell him to take a third deep breath and hold it. He should then cough two or three times in a row (once isn't enough). This will clear his breathing passages. Encourage him to concentrate on feeling his diaphragm force out all the air in his chest. Then he should take three to five normal breaths, exhale slowly, and relax.
- The patient should repeat the exercise at least every 2 hours to help keep his lungs free from secretions. Reassure the surgical patient that his stitches are very strong and won't split during coughing.

DEEP-BREATHING EXERCISES

Advise the patient that performing deep-breathing exercises several times per hour helps keep lungs expanded. To deep-breathe correctly, he must use his diaphragm and abdominal muscles, not just his chest muscles.

- Have him lie on his back in a comfortable position with one hand placed on his chest and the other over his upper abdomen. Instruct him to relax, and bend his legs slightly.
- Instruct him to exhale normally. He should then close his mouth and inhale deeply through his nose, concentrating on feeling his abdomen rise. His chest shouldn't expand. Have him hold his breath and slowly count to five.
- Next, have the patient purse his lips as though about to whistle, then exhale completely through his mouth, with letting his cheeks puff out. His ribs should sink downward and inward.
- After resting several seconds, the patient should repeat the exercise 5 to 10 times. He should also do this exercise while lying on his side, sitting, standing, or turning in bed.

Respirations, stertorous

- Are characterized by harsh, rattling, or snoring sound
- Result from the vibration of relaxed oropharyngeal structures during sleep or coma, causing partial airway obstruction
- May be aggravated by the ingestion of alcohol or sedatives which increases oropharyngeal flaccidity before bed and by sleeping in a supine position which allows the relaxed tongue to slip back into the airway.

ACTION STAT! Check the patient's mouth and throat for edema, redness, masses, or foreign objects. If edema is marked, take vital signs, including oxygen saturation levels. Observe for signs and symptoms of respiratory distress, such as dyspnea, tachypnea, using accessory muscles, intercostal muscle retractions, and cyanosis. Elevate the head of the bed 30 degrees to help ease the patient's breathing and reduce edema. Administer supplemental oxygen and prepare for intubation, tracheostomy, or mechanical ventilation as needed. Insert an I.V. catheter for fluid and drug access, and begin cardiac monitoring.

- Ask the patient's sleeping partner about his snoring habits.
- Find out about factors that decrease snoring.
- Inquire about sleeptalking and sleepwalking.
- Ask about signs of sleep deprivation, such as personality changes, headaches, daytime somnolence, or decreased mental acuity.

- Perform a complete respiratory assessment.
- Examine the head, nose, and throat.
- If you detect stertorous respirations while the patient is sleeping, observe his breathing pattern for 3 to 4 minutes.
- Watch for periods of apnea and note their length.

CAUSES

MEDICAL
Airway obstruction
◆ With partial obstruction, stertorous respirations may be accompanied by wheezing, dyspnea, tachypnea, intercostal retractions, and nasal flaring.
◆ In complete obstruction, the patient abruptly loses ability to talk and displays diaphoresis, tachycardia, and inspiratory chest movement but absent breath sounds; severe hypoxemia rapidly ensues, resulting in cyanosis, loss of consciousness, and cardiopulmonary collapse.

Obstructive sleep apnea
◆ Loud and disruptive snoring is a major characteristic, commonly affecting the obese.
◆ Snoring alternates with periods of sleep apnea, which usually end with loud gasping sounds.
◆ Alternating tachycardia and bradycardia, ankle edema, and hypertension may occur.
◆ Sleep disturbances such as somnambulism and talking during sleep may occur.
◆ Other relevant findings may include a generalized headache, feeling tired and unrefreshed, daytime sleepiness, depression, hostility, and decreased mental acuity.

Pickwickian syndrome
◆ Syndrome is defined as a group of symptoms that primarily affect extremely obese patients.
◆ Obstructive sleep apnea with disruptive snoring and disturbed sleep at night results from excessive fatty tissue surrounding the chest muscles.
◆ Related signs and symptoms include excessive sleepiness during the day, shortness of breath, flushed face or bluish tinge to the face, elevated blood pressure, and enlarged liver.

OTHER
Procedures
◆ Endotracheal intubation, suction, or surgery may cause significant palatal or uvular edema, resulting in stertorous respirations.

NURSING CONSIDERATIONS

◆ Give a corticosteroid or an antibiotic as prescribed.
◆ To reduce palatal and uvular inflammation and edema, provide cool, humidified oxygen.
◆ Monitor the patient's respiratory status.
◆ Prepare patient for diagnostic tests such as laryngoscopy and sleep studies.

PEDIATRIC TIPS
◆ The most common cause of stertorous respirations is nasal or pharyngeal obstruction from tonsillar or adenoid hypertrophy or the presence of a foreign body.

GERIATRIC TIPS
◆ Encourage the patient to seek treatment for sleep apnea or significant hypertrophy of tonsils or adenoids.

PATIENT TEACHING

◆ Discuss underlying condition, diagnostic tests and treatment options.
◆ Discuss importance and methods of weight loss.
◆ Explain set-up and use of continuous or bilevel positive airway pressure device.
◆ Teach the patient how to elevate his head while sleeping.
◆ Give information and recommend a smoking cessation program if the patient smokes.

Retractions, costal and sternal

OVERVIEW

◆ Characterized by visible indentations of soft tissue covering chest wall
◆ Occur as suprasternal, intercostal, subcostal, or substernal
◆ Are a classic sign of respiratory distress in infants and children

 ACTION STAT! *If you detect retractions in a child, check quickly for other signs of respiratory distress. Prepare the child for suctioning, insertion of an artificial airway, and administration of oxygen. Observe the depth and location of retractions. Also note the rate, depth, and quality of respirations. Look for accessory muscle use, nasal flaring during inspiration, or grunting during expiration. Note whether the child appears restless or lethargic. Auscultate the child's lungs to detect abnormal breath sounds. Check oxygen saturation. (See* Observing retractions.*)*

HISTORY

◆ Ask the parents about the child's medical and birth history.
◆ Find out about recent signs of upper respiratory infection.
◆ Determine the frequency of respiratory problems during the past year.
◆ Ask about recent exposure to cold, flu, or respiratory ailment.
◆ Find out about aspiration of food, liquid, or foreign body.
◆ Inquire about a personal or family history of allergies or asthma.

PHYSICAL ASSESSMENT

◆ If the child isn't in severe distress, complete a cardiopulmonary assessment.
◆ Take the child's vital signs, including his temperature.

TOP TECHNIQUE

Observing retractions

When you observe retractions in infants and children, note their exact location (as shown here)—an important clue to the cause and severity of respiratory distress. For example, subcostal and substernal retractions usually result from lower respiratory tract disorders; suprasternal retractions result from upper respiratory tract disorders.

Mild intercostal retractions alone may be normal. However, intercostal retractions with subcostal and substernal retractions may indicate moderate respiratory distress. Deep suprasternal retractions typically indicate severe distress.

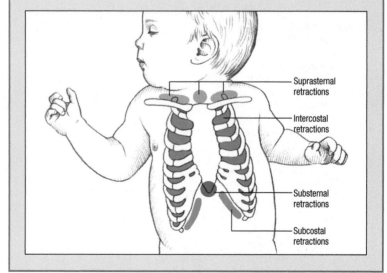

MEDICAL

Asthma attack

- Intercostal and suprasternal retractions may accompany acute attack.
- Retractions are preceded by dyspnea, wheezing, a hacking cough, and pallor.
- Related findings include cyanosis or flushing, crackles, rhonchi, diaphoresis, tachycardia, tachypnea, a frightened, anxious expression and, with severe distress, nasal flaring.

Bronchiolitis

- Intercostal and subcostal retractions, nasal flaring, tachypnea, dyspnea, cough, restlessness, and a slight fever may occur, most commonly in children younger than age 2.

Croup (spasmodic)

- Attacks of a barking cough, hoarseness, dyspnea, and restlessness occur.
- As distress worsens, findings include suprasternal, substernal, and intercostal retractions; nasal flaring; tachycardia; cyanosis; and an anxious, frantic expression.

Epiglottiditis

- This life-threatening disorder may precipitate severe respiratory distress with suprasternal, substernal, and intercostal retractions.
- Early findings include sudden onset of a barking cough, stridor, cyanosis, nasal flaring,tachycardia, a high fever, sore throat, hoarseness, dysphagia, drooling, dyspnea, and restlessness.

Heart failure

- Intercostal and substernal retractions occur along with nasal flaring, progressive tachypnea, grunting respirations, edema, and cyanosis.
- Other findings include productive cough, crackles, jugular vein distention, tachycardia, right-upper-quadrant pain, anorexia, and fatigue.

Laryngotracheobronchitis (acute)

- Substernal and intercostal retractions follow low to moderate fever, runny nose, poor appetite, a barking cough, hoarseness, and inspiratory stridor.
- Other findings include tachycardia; shallow, rapid respirations; restlessness; irritability; and pale, cyanotic skin.

Pneumonia (bacterial)

- Subcostal and intercostal retractions follow signs and symptoms of acute infection.
- Other findings include nasal flaring; dyspnea; tachypnea; high fever; lethargy; grunting respirations; cyanosis; a productive cough; and diminished breath sounds, crackles, and sibilant rhonchi over the affected lung.

Respiratory distress syndrome

- In this life-threatening disorder, substernal and subcostal retractions are early signs.
- Other early findings include tachypnea, tachycardia, and expiratory grunting.
- As respiratory distress worsens, intercostal and suprasternal retractions occur, and apnea or irregular respirations replace grunting.
- Other findings include nasal flaring, cyanosis, lethargy, and eventual unresponsiveness, bradycardia, and hypotension.

Other

Aspiration of foreign body
- A potentially life-threatening situation, the severity of retractions is related to the degree of obstruction.
- Other findings include diminished breath sounds over the obstructed area, rhonchi, wheezing, fever, pain and cough.

- Monitor vital signs frequently.
- Keep suction equipment and an airway at the bedside.
- If the infant weighs less than 15 lb (6.8 kg), place him in an oxygen hood; if he weighs more, place him in a cool mist tent.
- Perform chest physical therapy with postural drainage.
- Give a bronchodilator and a steroid as prescribed.
- Prepare patient for diagnostic tests, such as X-rays, pulmonary function tests and arterial blood gases (ABG).

PEDIATRIC TIPS

- When examining a child for retractions, know that crying may accentuate the contractions.

GERIATRIC TIPS

- Retractions are more difficult to assess in an older patient who is obese or has chronic chest wall stiffness or deformity.

- Discuss underlying condition, diagnostic studies and treatment options.
- Instruct the patient or his family in how to take prescribed drugs properly at home especially completing full antiobiotic course.
- Give instructions for providing a humidified environment.
- Stress the importance of ensuring adequate hydration and infection control techniques.

Rhinorrhea

OVERVIEW

- Refers to free discharge of thin nasal mucus
- Is self-limiting or chronic
- Produces clear, purulent, bloody, or serosanguineous discharge, depending on the cause

HISTORY

- Obtain a description of the onset and characteristics of the rhinorrhea.
- Find out about aggravating and alleviating factors.
- Take a drug history, especially the use of nose drops or sprays.
- Inquire about exposure to nasal irritants at home or at work.
- Take a medical history, including seasonal allergies.
- Determine whether the patient recently had a head injury.

PHYSICAL ASSESSMENT

- Examine the nose, checking airflow from each nostril.
- Evaluate the size, color, and condition of the turbinate mucosa.
- Note if the mucosa is red, pale, blue, or gray.
- Examine the area beneath each turbinate. (See *Using a nasal speculum.*)
- Palpate over the frontal, ethmoid, and maxillary sinuses for tenderness.
- Collect a small amount of drainage on a glucose reagent strip to differentiate nasal mucus from cerebrospinal fluid (CSF).
- Test for anosmia (loss of the sense of smell)

CAUSES

MEDICAL
Basilar skull fracture
- Produces CSF rhinorrhea that increases when the head is lowered.
- Other findings include epistaxis, otorrhea, a bulging tympanic membrane, headache, facial paralysis, nausea, vomiting, impaired eye movement, ocular deviation, vision and hearing loss, depressed level of consciousness, Battle's sign, and raccoon eyes.

Common cold
- Initial watery nasal discharge may become thicker and mucopurulent.
- Related findings include sneezing, nasal congestion, a dry and hacking cough, sore throat, mouth breathing, and transient loss of smell and taste.
- Other findings include malaise, fatigue, myalgia, arthralgia, a slight headache, low-grade fever, dry lips, and a red upper lip and nose.

Headache (cluster)
- Rhinorrhea may accompany a cluster headache.
- Related ocular effects include miosis, ipsilateral tearing, conjunctival injection, and ptosis.
- Other findings include flushing, facial diaphoresis, bradycardia, and restlessness.

Nasal or sinus tumors
- Intermittent, bloody or serosanguineous discharge is produced, which may be purulent and foul-smelling.
- Nasal congestion, postnasal drip, and headache may also occur.
- A cheek mass or eye displacement, facial paresthesia or pain, and nasal obstruction may occur in the advanced stages of a paranasal sinus tumor.

 TOP TECHNIQUE

Using a nasal speculum

To visualize the interior of the nares, use a nasal speculum and a good light source, such as a penlight. Hold the speculum in the palm of one hand and the penlight in the other hand. Have the patient tilt the head back slightly and rest it against a wall or other firm support, if possible. Insert the speculum blades about ½" (1.3 cm) into the nasal vestibule, as shown.

Place your index finger on the tip of the patient's nose for stability. Carefully open the speculum blades. Shine the light source in the direction of the nares. Now, inspect the nares. The mucosa should be deep pink. Note any discharge, masses, lesions, or mucosal swellings. Check the nasal septum for perforation, bleeding, or crusting. Bluish turbinates suggest allergy. A rounded, elongated projection suggests a polyp.

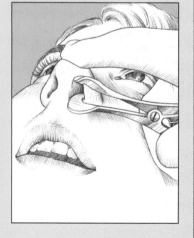

Rhinitis

◆ Allergic rhinitis produces an episodic, profuse watery discharge with increased tearing; nasal congestion; itchy eyes, nose, and throat; postnasal drip; sneezing; mouth breathing; impaired sense of smell; frontal or temporal headache; pale, engorged turbinates; and pale, boggy mucosa.

◆ Atrophic rhinitis produces scanty, purulent, and foul-smelling nasal discharge with nasal obstruction and pale pink, shiny mucosa.

◆ Vasomotor rhinitis produces a profuse watery nasal discharge accompanied by chronic nasal obstruction, sneezing, recurrent postnasal drip, blue nasal mucosa, and pale swollen turbinates.

Sinusitis

◆ With acute sinusitis, a thick and purulent nasal discharge leads to a purulent postnasal drip that results in throat pain and halitosis; accompanying features include nasal congestion, severe pain and tenderness over the involved sinuses, fever, headache, and malaise.

◆ With chronic sinusitis, the nasal discharge is scant, thick, and intermittently purulent, with nasal congestion, discomfort or pressure over the involved sinuses, a chronic sore throat, and nasal polyps.

Wegener's granulomatosis

◆ This disorder is characterized by vasculitis affecting small vessels primarily of the upper respiratory tract, lungs, and kidneys.

◆ Bloody, mucopurulent discharge is accompanied by conductive hearing loss, crusting, epistaxis, and tissue necrosis of the nose due to inflammation of blood vessels primarily of the upper respiratory tract, lungs, and kidneys.

OTHER
Drugs

◆ Nasal sprays or nose drops containing vasoconstrictors that are used longer than 5 days may cause rebound rhinorrhea.

Surgery

◆ Cerebrospinal rhinorrhea may occur after sinus or cranial surgery.

NURSING CONSIDERATIONS

◆ Give an antihistamine, a decongestant, an analgesic, or an antipyretic.

◆ Encourage increased fluid intake to thin secretions.

◆ Prepare patient for diagnostic tests such as X-rays and computed tomography scan.

PEDIATRIC TIPS

◆ Rhinorrhea may stem from choanal atresia, allergic or chronic rhinitis, acute ethmoiditis, or congenital syphilis.

◆ Assume that rhinitis and nasal obstruction in one nostril is caused by a foreign body in the nose until proven otherwise.

GERIATRIC TIPS

◆ Increased adverse reactions to drugs used to treat rhinorrhea may occur, such as elevated blood pressure or confusion.

PATIENT TEACHING

◆ Explain proper use of over-the-counter nasal sprays.

◆ Teach about underlying diagnosis and treatment plan.

◆ Advise the patient about prescribed medications and adverse effects.

Rhonchi

OVERVIEW

- Are continuous adventitious breath sounds detected by auscultation
- Are louder and lower-pitched than crackles
- May be described as rattling, sonorous, bubbling, rumbling, or musical (see *Comparing adventitious breath sounds*)
- Are heard over large airways such as the trachea
- Can occur when air flows through passages that have been narrowed by secretions, a tumor or foreign body, bronchospasm, or mucosal thickening

HISTORY

- Take a smoking history.
- Ask about a history of asthma or other pulmonary disorder.
- Obtain a drug history.

PHYSICAL ASSESSMENT

- Take vital signs, including oxygen saturation.
- Characterize the patient's respirations as rapid or slow, shallow or deep, and regular or irregular.
- Inspect the chest, noting the use of accessory muscles.
- Listen for audible wheezing or gurgling.
- Auscultate for other abnormal breath sounds and note location.
- Percuss the chest, and note frequency and productivity of cough.

CAUSES

MEDICAL

Acute respiratory distress syndrome
- A life-threatening disorder; initial features include dyspnea, rhonchi, crackles, and rapid shallow respirations.
- Intercostal and suprasternal retractions, diaphoresis, and fluid accumulation occur with developing hypoxemia.
- As hypoxemia worsens, findings include difficulty breathing, restless-

---

TOP TECHNIQUE

Comparing adventitious breath sounds

The characteristics of discontinuous and continuous adventitious breath sounds are compared in the chart below. Note the timing of each sound during inspiration and expiration on the corresponding graphs.

SOUND	CHARACTERISTICS

Discontinuous sounds

Fine crackles

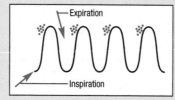

- Intermittent
- Nonmusical
- Soft
- High-pitched
- Short, cracking, popping
- Heard during inspiration (5 to 10 msec)

Coarse crackles

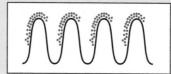

- Intermittent
- Nonmusical
- Loud
- Low-pitched
- Bubbling, gurgling
- Heard during early inspiration and possibly during expiration (20 to 30 msec)

Continuous sounds

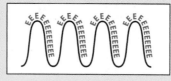

- Musical
- High-pitched
- Squeaking
- Mainly heard during expiration but may also occur during inspiration

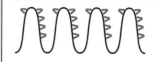

- Musical
- Low-pitched
- Snoring, moaning
- Heard during both inspiration and expiration, but are more prominent during expiration

---

ness, apprehension, decreased level of consciousness, cyanosis, motor dysfunction, and tachycardia.

Asthma
♦ An asthma attack can cause rhonchi, crackles and, commonly, wheezing.
♦ Other findings include apprehension, a dry cough that later becomes productive, prolonged expirations, accessory muscle use, nasal flaring, tachypnea, tachycardia, diaphoresis, flushing or cyanosis, and intercostal and supraclavicular retractions on inspiration.

Bronchiectasis
♦ Lower-lobe rhonchi and crackles occur.
♦ Classic sign is a cough that produces mucopurulent, foul-smelling sputum.
♦ Other findings include fever, weight loss, exertional dyspnea, fatigue, malaise, halitosis, weakness, and late-stage clubbing.

Bronchitis
♦ Sonorous rhonchi and wheezing occur in acute tracheobronchitis; other features include chills, sore throat, fever, muscle and back pain, substernal tightness, and a cough that becomes productive as secretions increase.
♦ Scattered rhonchi, coarse crackles, wheezing, high-pitched piping sounds, and prolonged expirations occur with chronic bronchitis; accompanying findings include exertional dyspnea, increased accessory muscle use, barrel chest, cyanosis, tachypnea, and late-stage clubbing.

Emphysema
♦ Sonorous rhonchi may occur, but faint, high-pitched wheezing is more typical.
♦ Other findings include weight loss; anorexia; malaise; barrel chest; peripheral cyanosis; exertional dyspnea; accessory muscle use on inspiration; tachypnea; grunting expirations; late-stage clubbing; and a mild, chronic, cough with scant sputum.

Pneumonia
♦ Bacterial pneumonias can cause rhonchi and a dry cough that later becomes productive.
♦ Related findings include shaking chills, high fever, myalgia, headache, pleuritic chest pain, tachypnea, tachycardia, dyspnea, cyanosis, diaphoresis, decreased breath sounds, and fine crackles.

OTHER
Aspiration of foreign body
♦ Inspiratory and expiratory rhonchi and wheezing occur because of increased secretions.
♦ Other findings include diminished breath sounds over the obstructed area, fever, pain, and cough.

Diagnostic tests
♦ Pulmonary function tests or bronchoscopy can loosen secretions and mucus, causing rhonchi.

Respiratory therapy
♦ Respiratory therapy may produce rhonchi from loosened secretions and mucus.

NURSING CONSIDERATIONS

♦ To ease breathing, place the patient in semi-Fowler's position.
♦ Give an antibiotic, a bronchodilator, and an expectorant as prescribed.
♦ Provide humidification to thin secretions, relieve inflammation, and preventing drying.
♦ Promote coughing, deep breathing, and incentive spirometry.
♦ Provide pulmonary physiotherapy with postural drainage and percussion to loosen secretions.
♦ Use tracheal suctioning, if necessary, to clear secretions.

PEDIATRIC TIPS
♦ Rhonchi can result from bacterial pneumonia, cystic fibrosis, and croup syndrome.
♦ Because a respiratory tract disorder may begin abruptly and progress rapidly in an infant or a child, observe closely for signs of airway obstruction.

PATIENT TEACHING

♦ Explain deep-breathing and coughing techniques.
♦ Stress the need for increasing fluid intake.
♦ Discuss increasing activity levels.
♦ Discuss underlying condition, diagnostic tests, and treatment plan.

Romberg's sign

- Refers to inability to maintain balance when standing erect with feet together and eyes closed (see *Assessing Romberg's sign*)
- Indicates a vestibular or proprioceptive disorder or a disorder of the spinal tracts when sign is positive

HISTORY

- Obtain a medical history including previous neurologic symptoms and disorders.
- Ask about sensory changes and their onset.

PHYSICAL ASSESSMENT

- Obtain vital signs
- Test the patient's awareness of body part position.
- Test the patient's direction of movement.
- Test sensation and two-point discrimination in all dermatomes.
- Test and characterize the patient's deep tendon reflexes (DTRs).
- Test the patient's vibratory sense.
- Assess for hearing loss.
- Observe for nystagmus.

CAUSES

MEDICAL
Multiple sclerosis

- A positive Romberg's sign may occur in multiple sclerosis.
- Early findings may include vision changes, diplopia, and paresthesia.
- Other findings include nystagmus, constipation, muscle weakness and spasticity, hyperreflexia, intention tremors, gait ataxia, dysphagia, dysarthria, incontinence, urinary frequency and urgency, impotence, and emotional instability.

 TOP TECHNIQUE

Assessing Romberg's sign

Observe the patient's balance as he stands with his eyes open, feet together, and arms at his sides. Then ask him to close his eyes. Hold your arms out on either side of him to protect him if he sways. If he falls to one side, the result of the Romberg's test is positive.

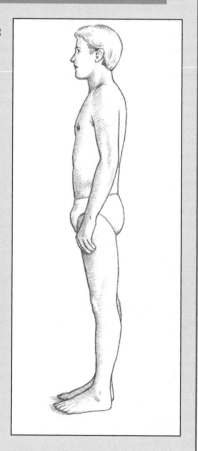

Peripheral nerve disease

◆ Positive Romberg's sign may be accompanied by impotence, fatigue, and paresthesia, hyperesthesia, or anesthesia in the hands and feet.
◆ Related findings include incoordination, ataxia, burning in the affected area, progressive muscle weakness and atrophy, hypoactive DTRs, and loss of vibration sense.

Pernicious anemia

◆ A positive Romberg's sign and loss of proprioception in the lower limbs reflect peripheral nerve and spinal cord damage.
◆ Gait changes (usually ataxia), muscle weakness, impaired coordination, paresthesia, and sensory loss may be present.
◆ Other findings include a sore tongue, a positive Babinski's reflex, fatigue, blurred vision, diplopia, and light-headedness.

Spinal cerebellar degeneration

◆ Positive Romberg's sign accompanies decreased visual acuity, fatigue, paresthesia, loss of vibration sense, incoordination, ataxic gait, hypoactive DTRs, and muscle weakness and atrophy.

Spinal cord disease

◆ Positive Romberg's sign may accompany pain, fasciculations, muscle weakness and atrophy, and loss of sphincter tone, proprioception, and vibration sense.
◆ DTRs may be hypoactive at the level of the lesion and hyperactive above it.

Vestibular disorders

◆ Positive Romberg's sign may accompany vertigo, nystagmus, nausea, tinnitus, hearing loss, and vomiting.

NURSING CONSIDERATIONS

◆ Help the patient with ambulation.
◆ Keep a night-light on and raise the side rails of the bed for safety.

PEDIATRIC TIPS

◆ Romberg's sign can't be tested until a child can stand without support and follow commands.
◆ A positive sign in children commonly results from spinal cord disease.

PATIENT TEACHING

◆ Teach about underlying diagnosis and treatment plan.
◆ Provide instruction on safety measures to avoid injury.
◆ Discuss the proper use of assistive devices.

Salivation, decreased

OVERVIEW

- Refers to diminished production or excretion of saliva
- Also called *xerostomia*

HISTORY

- Ask about the onset and course of dry mouth.
- Take a drug history.
- Determine what aggravates or alleviates the condition.
- Ask about burning or itching eyes and changes in sense of smell or taste.
- Inquire about recent dental or oral procedures.

PHYSICAL ASSESSMENT

- Inspect the mouth for abnormalities.
- Observe the eyes for conjunctival irritation, matted lids, and corneal epithelial thickening.
- Perform simple tests of smell and taste to detect impairment.
- Check for enlarged parotid and submaxillary glands. (See *Examining salivary glands and ductal openings*.)
- Palpate for tender or enlarged areas along the neck.

CAUSES

MEDICAL
Dehydration

- Decreased saliva production causes dry oral mucous membranes.
- Other findings include decreased skin turgor, reduced urine output, hypotension, tachycardia, and a low-grade fever.

Facial nerve paralysis

- Diminished saliva production, decreased sense of taste, and decreased facial muscle movement occur.

 TOP TECHNIQUE

Examining salivary glands and ductal openings

When a patient reports decreased salivation, assess the parotid and submaxillary glands for enlargement and the ductal openings for salivary flow.

To detect an enlarged parotid gland, ask the patient to clench his teeth, thereby tensing the masseter muscle. Then palpate the parotid duct (about 2″ [5 cm] long); you should be able to feel it against the tensed muscle, on the cheek just below the zygomatic arch. Next, check the ductal orifice, opposite the second molar. Using a gloved finger, palpate the orifice for enlargement, and observe for drainage.

Palpate the submaxillary gland. About the size of a walnut, this gland is located under the mandible, anterior to the angle of the jaw. Using a gloved finger, palpate the floor of the mouth for enlargement of the submaxillary ductal orifice.

Finally, test both ductal openings for salivary flow. Place cotton under the patient's tongue, have him sip pure lemon juice, and then remove the cotton and observe salivary flow from each opening. Document your findings.

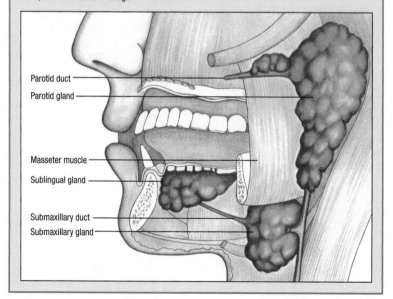

◆ Affected side of the face may sag and appear masklike.

Salivary duct obstruction
◆ Reduced salivation occurs with local pain and swelling of the face or neck.
◆ Symptoms are most noticeable when eating or drinking.

Sjögren's syndrome
◆ Diminished secretions from the lacrimal, parotid, and submaxillary glands produce the characteristic findings of decreased or absent salivation and dry eyes with a persistent burning, gritty sensation.
◆ Dryness of the nose, respiratory tract, vagina, and skin may also occur.
◆ Related oral findings include difficulty chewing, talking, and swallowing as well as ulcers and soreness of the lips and mucosa.
◆ Other findings include parotid and submaxillary gland enlargement, nasal crusting, epistaxis, fatigue, lethargy, nonproductive cough, abdominal discomfort, and polyuria.
◆ Signs and symptoms of rheumatoid arthritis and other connective tissue disorders may also occur.

OTHER
Drugs
◆ Anticholinergics, antihistamines, clonidine (Catapres), opioid analgesics, phenothiazines, and tricyclic antidepressants can decrease salivation; this effect disappears after stopping therapy.

Radiation
◆ Excessive irradiation of the mouth or face from radiation therapy or dental X-rays may cause transient decreased salivation.

NURSING CONSIDERATIONS
◆ Monitor intake and output.
◆ Allow the patient extra time for speaking, eating, and swallowing.

PEDIATRIC TIPS
◆ Mouth breathing and anticholinergics are causes of decreased salivation in children.

PATIENT TEACHING
◆ Describe ways to relieve dry mouth.
◆ Instruct the patient in proper oral hygiene and dental care.
◆ Explain the proper use of pilocarpine for symptom relief, if prescribed.
◆ Teach the patient to chew slowly and thoroughly to help increase saliva production.

Salivation, increased

- Also known as *ptyalism* or *sialism*
- Is an uncommon symptom that results from GI disorders, systemic disorders, use of certain drugs, or exposure to certain toxins
- May be due to difficulty swallowing

HISTORY

- Ask about fatigue, fever, headache, or sore throat.
- Inquire about recent exposure to toxins.
- Take a drug history, noting use of iodides, cholinergics, and miotics.
- Take a medical history.

PHYSICAL ASSESSMENT

- Test for a gag reflex.
- Observe ability to swallow and chew.
- Note any drooling.
- Inspect the mouth for lesions; note their appearance.
- Palpate any mouth lesions and describe their appearance.
- Inspect the uvula, gingivae, and pharynx.
- Palpate lymph nodes, and determine if parotid glands are swollen or sore.

CAUSES

MEDICAL
Bell's palsy
- Facial nerve paralysis causes an inability to control salivation or close the eye on the affected side.
- Affected side of the face sags and is expressionless, the nasolabial fold flattens, and the palpebral fissure (the distance between the upper and lower eyelids) widens.
- Other findings include diminished or absent corneal reflex and partial loss of taste or abnormal taste sensation.

Motion sickness
- Hypersalivation may occur with vertigo, nausea, vomiting, and headache in response to rhythmic or erratic motions.
- Dizziness, fatigue, diaphoresis, and dyspnea may also occur.

Pregnancy
- In early months, increased salivation, nausea, gum swelling, and breast tenderness may occur.

Rabies
- Excessive salivation occurs after initial symptoms of fever, headache, nausea, sore throat, and cough.
- Other findings include trismus, restlessness, cranial nerve dysfunction, localized pain at bite site, and hydrophobia.
- If not promptly treated, generalized, flaccid paralysis occurs leading to peripheral vascular collapse, coma, and death.

Stomatitis
- Mucosal ulcers may be accompanied by moderately increased salivation, mouth pain, fever, and erythema.
- Spontaneous healing usually occurs in 7 to 10 days, but scarring and recurrence are possible.

Syphilis
- With secondary syphilis, mucosal ulcers cause increased salivation that may persist up to 1 year.

- Related findings include fever, malaise, headache, anorexia, weight loss, nausea, vomiting, sore throat, and lymphadenopathy.
- A symmetrical rash appears on the arms, trunk, palms, soles, face, and scalp.
- Condylomata develop in the genital and perianal areas.

Tuberculosis
- Certain forms may produce solitary, irregularly shaped mouth or tongue ulcers, covered with exudate, that cause increased salivation.
- Other findings include weight loss, anorexia, fever, fatigue, malaise, dyspnea, cough, night sweats (a common sign), and hemoptysis.

OTHER
Arsenic poisoning
- Common effects of arsenic poisoning are diarrhea, diffuse skin hyperpigmentation, and edema of the face, eyelids and ankles; increased salivation occurs infrequently.
- Other findings include garlicky breath odor, pruritus, headache, drowsiness, confusion, and weakness.

Drugs
- Increased salivation may occur with iodide toxicity, but the earliest symptoms are a brassy taste and a burning sensation in the mouth and throat; other findings include sneezing, irritated eyelids, and pain in the frontal sinus.
- Pilocarpine hydrochloride and other miotics used to treat glaucoma may be absorbed systemically, increasing salivation.
- Cholinergics such as bethanechol chloride (Duvoid) may cause increased salivation.

Mercury poisoning
- Stomatitis, characterized by increased salivation and a metallic taste, commonly occurs.
- Teeth may be loose with painful, swollen gums that are prone to bleeding.
- Blue line appears on the gingivae.

- Other findings include personality changes, memory loss, abdominal cramps, diarrhea, paresthesia, and tremors of the eyelids, lips, tongue, and fingers.

NURSING CONSIDERATIONS

- Increased salivation doesn't require treatments beyond those needed to correct the underlying disorder.
- If the patient has difficulty swallowing, suction the mouth as needed.

PEDIATRIC TIPS
- Increased salivation in children may stem from the same conditions that affect adults or from congenital esophageal atresia.

GERIATRIC TIPS
- Drooling is common in an elderly patient with Parkinson's disease, stroke, or transient ischemic attacks.

PATIENT TEACHING

- Instruct the patient in proper oral hygiene.
- Emphasize the importance of obtaining proper dental care.
- Teach about underlying diagnosis and treatment plan.

Scrotal swelling

- Occurs when a condition affecting the testicles, epididymis, or scrotal skin produces edema or a mass
- Can occur in one or both testicles and be painful or painless

◼ **ACTION STAT!** *If the patient also has severe pain, ask when the swelling began. Using a Doppler stethoscope, evaluate blood flow to the testicle. If it's decreased or absent, suspect testicular torsion and prepare the patient for surgery. Withhold food and fluids. Insert an I.V. catheter and apply an ice pack to the scrotum to reduce pain and swelling. An attempt may be made to untwist the cord manually, but even if this is successful, the patient may still require surgery for stabilization.*

HISTORY

- Ask about a history of injury to the scrotum, urethral discharge, cloudy urine, increased urinary frequency, dysuria, sexually transmitted disease, prostate surgery, or prolonged catheterization.
- Find out about recent illness, particularly mumps.
- Obtain a history of sexual activity.
- Ask which body positions alleviate or aggravate swelling.

PHYSICAL ASSESSMENT

- Take vital signs, especially noting fever.
- Palpate the abdomen for tenderness and swelling.
- Examine the genital area.
- Assess the scrotum with the patient in a supine position and then standing.
- Check the testicles' position in the scrotum.
- Palpate the scrotum for a cyst or lump, note tenderness or firmness.
- Transilluminate the scrotum to distinguish a fluid-filled cyst from a solid mass.

CAUSES

MEDICAL

Epididymal cysts
- Painless scrotal swelling occurs.

Epididymitis
- Inflammation, pain, extreme tenderness, and swelling develop in the groin and scrotum.
- Other findings include high fever, malaise, urethral discharge and cloudy urine, lower abdominal pain on the affected side, and hot, red, dry, flaky, and thin scrotal skin.

Hernia
- Swelling and a soft or unusually firm scrotum are produced by herniation of the bowel into the scrotum.
- Nausea, anorexia, vomiting, and reduced bowel sounds may occur if the bowel is obstructed.

Hydrocele
- Fluid accumulation produces gradual scrotal swelling that's usually painless.
- The scrotum may be soft and cystic or firm and tense.
- Palpation reveals a round, nontender scrotal mass.

Orchitis (acute)
- Sudden painful swelling of one or both testicles occurs.
- Related findings include hot, reddened scrotum; fever; chills; lower abdominal pain; nausea; vomiting; and extreme weakness.

Scrotal trauma
- Scrotal swelling, bruising, and severe pain may result.
- The scrotum may appear dark blue.
- Nausea, vomiting, and difficult urination may also occur.

Spermatocele
- A movable, painless cystic mass develops that may be transilluminated.

Testicular torsion
- Scrotal swelling; sudden, severe pain; and, possibly, elevation of the affect-

ed testicle within the scrotum occur with this urologic emergency.
♦ Disorder occurs most commonly before puberty.
♦ Other findings include possible nausea and vomiting.

Testicular tumor
♦ Scrotum swells and produces a local sensation of excessive weight.
♦ Typically, these tumors are painless, smooth, and firm.
♦ With ureteral obstruction, urinary complaints are common.

OTHER
Surgery
♦ Blood effusion from surgery can produce a hematocele, leading to scrotal swelling.

NURSING CONSIDERATIONS

♦ Place the patient on bed rest.
♦ Give an antibiotic, as prescribed.
♦ Provide fluids, fiber, and stool softeners.
♦ Place a rolled towel under the scrotum to help reduce swelling.
♦ For moderate swelling, suggest a loose-fitting athletic supporter.
♦ Apply heat or ice packs to decrease inflammation.
♦ Administer an analgesic, as needed.

PEDIATRIC TIPS
♦ In children up to age 1, a hernia or hydrocele of the spermatic cord may cause scrotal swelling.
♦ In infants, scrotal swelling may stem from ammonia-related dermatitis if diapers aren't changed often enough.
♦ In prepubescent boys, scrotal swelling usually results from torsion of spermatic cord.

PATIENT TEACHING

♦ Explain the importance of performing testicular self-examination, and teach the technique, if needed. (See *Teaching testicular self-examination.*)
♦ Teach about underlying diagnosis and treatment plan.

Teaching testicular self-examination

To help your patient detect abnormalities early, tell him that he should examine his testicles once a month on the same date. Explain that the best time to examine his testicles is during or after a hot bath or shower. The heat causes the testicles to descend and relaxes the scrotum, which makes finding abnormalities easier.

Have the patient follow these simple instructions for performing self-examination, using the illustration (upper right) to locate anatomic landmarks.

CHECK THE SCROTUM
First, ask him to lift his penis, with one hand, and check his scrotum (the pouch of skin containing the testicles and parts of the spermatic cords) for any change in shape or size and for reddened, distended veins. Tell him to expect the scrotum's left side to hang slightly lower than the right.

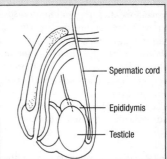

CHECK EACH TESTICLE
Next, have the patient place his left thumb on the front of his left testicle and his index and middle fingers behind it (as shown middle right). Tell him to gently but firmly roll the testicle between his thumb and fingers. Then ask him to use his right hand to examine his right testicle in the same manner. Explain that his testicles should feel smooth, rubbery, slightly tender, and movable within the scrotum.

If the patient notices any lumps, masses, or other changes, tell him to notify his physician.

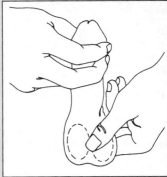

CHECK EACH SPERMATIC CORD
Finally, have the patient locate the epididymis, the cordlike structure at the back of his testicles. Then have him locate the spermatic cord extending upward from it (as shown bottom right).

Ask the patient to gently squeeze the spermatic cord above his left testicle between his thumb and the first two fingers of his left hand. Then have him repeat this step on the right side, using his right hand to check for lumps and masses along the entire length of the cords.

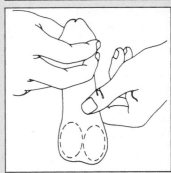

Seizures, complex partial

OVERVIEW

- Occur when focal seizures begin in the temporal lobe and cause partial alterations of consciousness
- Often preceded by an aura—usually a complex hallucination, illusion, or sensation—in a psychomotor seizure
- Cause hallucinations that may be audiovisual, auditory, or olfactory
- Produce other types of auras that include sensations of déjà vu, unfamiliarity with surroundings, or depersonalization
- Cause confusion, drowsiness, and amnesia after seizure occurs (see *Understanding seizure types*)

HISTORY

- Ask about the occurrence of an aura.
- Ask witnesses for a description of the seizure.
- Find out about previous seizures or therapies.
- Ask about history of head trauma.

PHYSICAL ASSESSMENT

- Examine the patient for injury after the seizure.
- Ensure a patent airway.
- Perform a complete neurologic assessment.

Understanding seizure types

The various types of seizures—partial, generalized, status epilepticus, and unclassified—have distinct signs and symptoms.

PARTIAL SEIZURES

Arising from a localized area of the brain, partial seizures cause focal symptoms. These seizures are classified by their effect on consciousness and whether they spread throughout the motor pathway, causing a generalized seizure.

- A *simple partial seizure* begins locally and generally doesn't cause an alteration in consciousness. It may present with sensory symptoms (lights flashing, smells, and auditory hallucinations), autonomic symptoms (sweating, flushing, and pupil dilation), and psychic symptoms (dream states, anger, and fear). The seizure lasts for a few seconds and occurs without preceding or provoking events. This type can be motor or sensory.
- A *complex partial seizure* alters consciousness. Amnesia for events that occur during and immediately after the seizure is a differentiating characteristic. During the seizure, the patient may follow simple commands. This type of seizure usually lasts for 1 to 3 minutes.

GENERALIZED SEIZURES

As the term suggests, generalized seizures cause a generalized electrical abnormality within the brain. They can be convulsive or nonconvulsive and include several types:

- *Absence seizures* occur most commonly in children, although they may affect adults. They usually begin with a brief change in level of consciousness, indicated by a blinking or rolling of the eyes, a blank stare, and slight mouth movements. The patient retains his posture and continues preseizure activity without difficulty. Typically, each seizure lasts from 1 to 10 seconds. If not properly treated, seizures can recur as frequently as 100 times per day. An absence seizure is a nonconvulsive seizure, but it may progress to a generalized tonic-clonic seizure.
- *Myoclonic seizures* are brief, involuntary muscular jerks of the body or extremities, commonly occurring in the early morning.
- *Clonic seizures* are characterized by rhythmic movements.

- *Tonic seizures* are characterized by a sudden stiffening of muscle tone, usually of the arms, but possibly including the legs.
- *Generalized tonic-clonic seizures* typically begin with a loud cry, precipitated by air rushing from the lungs through the vocal cords. The patient then loses consciousness and falls to the ground. The body stiffens (tonic phase) and then alternates between episodes of muscle spasm and relaxation (clonic phase). Tongue biting, incontinence, labored breathing, apnea, and subsequent cyanosis may occur. The seizure stops in 2 to 5 minutes, when abnormal electrical conduction ceases. When the patient regains consciousness, he's confused and may have difficulty talking. If he can talk, he may complain of drowsiness, fatigue, headache, muscle soreness, and arm or leg weakness. He may fall into a deep sleep after the seizure.
- *Atonic seizures* are characterized by a general loss of postural tone and a temporary loss of consciousness. They occur in young children and are sometimes called drop attacks because they cause the child to fall.

STATUS EPILEPTICUS

Status epilepticus is a continuous seizure state that can occur in all seizure types. The most life-threatening example is generalized tonic-clonic status epilepticus, a continuous generalized tonic-clonic seizure. Status epilepticus is accompanied by respiratory distress leading to hypoxia or anoxia and can result from abrupt withdrawal of anticonvulsants, hypoxic encephalopathy, acute head trauma, metabolic encephalopathy, or septicemia caused by encephalitis or meningitis.

UNCLASSIFIED SEIZURES

The unclassified seizures category is reserved for seizures that don't fit the characteristics of partial or generalized seizures or status epilepticus. Events that lack the data necessary for making a definitive diagnosis are included in the category of unclassified seizures.

CAUSES

MEDICAL
Brain abscess
◆ If the temporal lobe is affected, complex partial seizures commonly occur after the abscess resolves.
◆ Related findings include headache, nausea, vomiting, generalized seizures, and a decreased level of consciousness (LOC).
◆ Central facial weakness, auditory receptive aphasia, hemiparesis, and ocular disturbances may also occur.

Head trauma
◆ Trauma to the temporal lobe can produce complex partial seizures months or years later.
◆ Seizures may decrease in frequency and eventually stop.
◆ Generalized seizures and behavior and personality changes may also occur.

Temporal lobe tumor
◆ Complex partial seizures may be the first sign.
◆ Other findings include headache, pupillary changes, and mental dullness.
◆ Increased intracranial pressure may cause a decreased LOC, vomiting, and papilledema.

NURSING CONSIDERATIONS

◆ After the seizure, reorient the patient to his surroundings and protect him from injury.
◆ Keep the patient in bed until he's fully alert.
◆ Remove harmful objects from the area.
◆ Provide emotional support to the patient and his family.
◆ Monitor for therapeutic drug levels.

PEDIATRIC TIPS
◆ Complex partial seizures in children may resemble absence seizures and can result from birth injury, abuse, infection, or cancer.
◆ Repeated complex partial seizures commonly lead to generalized seizures.

PATIENT TEACHING

◆ Discuss methods for coping with seizures.
◆ Instruct the patient and his family in safety measures to take during a seizure.
◆ Emphasize compliance with drug therapy.
◆ Tell the patient to carry medical identification.

Seizures, generalized tonic-clonic

OVERVIEW

- Also known as *grand mal seizures*
- Are caused by paroxysmal, uncontrolled discharge of central nervous system neurons, leading to neurologic dysfunction (see *How to respond to a seizure*)
- Extend to the entire brain

HISTORY

- Obtain a description of the seizure, including onset, duration, body area affected, characteristics, and progression. (See *Recognizing a generalized tonic-clonic seizure.*)
- Ask about unusual sensations before the seizure.
- Find out about a personal and family history of seizures.
- Take a drug history and determine compliance.
- Ask about head trauma, sleep deprivation, or emotional or physical stress at time of seizure.
- Obtain a medical history.

PHYSICAL ASSESSMENT

- If the patient may have sustained a head injury, observe him closely for loss of consciousness, unequal or nonreactive pupils, and focal neurologic signs.
- Examine the arms, legs, and face (including tongue) for injury, residual paralysis, or limb weakness.
- Take vital signs.
- Complete a neurologic assessment.
- Observe for adequate oxygenation.

 ACTION STAT!

How to respond to a seizure

If you witness the beginning of the seizure, first check the patient's airway, breathing, and circulation, and ensure that the cause isn't asystole or a blocked airway. Stay with the patient and ensure a patent airway. Focus your care on observing the seizure and protecting the patient. Place a towel under his head to prevent injury, loosen his clothing, and move any sharp or hard objects out of his way. Never try to restrain the patient or force a hard object into his mouth; you might chip his teeth or fracture his jaw.

PREVENTING ASPIRATION

If possible, turn the patient to one side *during* the seizure to allow secretions to drain and to prevent aspiration. Otherwise, do this at the end of the clonic phase when respirations return. (If they fail to return, check for airway obstruction and suction the patient, if needed. Cardiopulmonary resuscitation, intubation, and mechanical ventilation may be needed.)

ADMINISTERING CARE

If the seizure lasts longer than 4 minutes or if a second seizure occurs before full recovery from the first, suspect status epilepticus. Establish an airway, insert an I.V. catheter, give supplemental oxygen, and begin cardiac monitoring. Draw blood for appropriate studies. Turn the patient on his side, with his head in a semi-dependent position, to drain secretions and prevent aspiration. Periodically turn him to the opposite side, check his arterial blood gas levels for hypoxemia, and administer oxygen by

mask, increasing the flow rate if necessary. Administer diazepam or lorazepam by slow I.V. push, repeat two or three times at 10- to 20-minute intervals, as ordered, to stop the seizures. If the patient isn't known to have epilepsy, an I.V. bolus of dextrose 50% (50 ml) with thiamine (100 mg) may be given. If the patient has hypoglycemia, dextrose may stop the seizures. If his thiamine level is low, also give thiamine to guard against further damage.

If the patient is intubated, expect to insert a nasogastric (NG) tube to prevent vomiting and aspiration. If the patient hasn't been intubated, the NG tube itself can trigger the gag reflex and cause vomiting.

PROVIDING PROTECTION

Protect the patient after the seizure by providing a safe area in which he can rest. As he awakens, reassure and reorient him. Check his vital signs and neurologic status. Carefully record these data as well as your observations of the seizure.

CAUSES

MEDICAL

Alcohol withdrawal syndrome

◆ Seizures as well as status epilepticus may occur 7 to 48 hours after sudden alcohol withdrawal.
◆ Other findings include restlessness, hallucinations, profuse diaphoresis, and tachycardia.

Arsenic poisoning

◆ Generalized seizures may occur with a garlicky breath odor, increased salivation, generalized pruritus, diarrhea, nausea, vomiting, and abdominal pain.
◆ Related findings include diffuse hyperpigmentation; sharply defined edema of the eyelids, face, and ankles; paresthesia of the extremities; alopecia; irritated mucous membranes; weakness; muscle aches; and peripheral neuropathy.

Brain abscess

◆ Generalized seizures may occur in the acute stage of abscess formation or after the abscess disappears.
◆ Constant headache, nausea, vomiting, and focal seizures are early signs and symptoms.
◆ Other findings include decreased LOC, ocular disturbances, aphasia, hemiparesis, abnormal behavior, and personality changes.

Brain tumor

◆ Generalized seizures may occur, depending on the tumor's location and type.
◆ Other findings include a slowly decreasing LOC, morning headache, dizziness, confusion, focal seizures, vision loss, motor and sensory disturbances, aphasia, and ataxia.
◆ Later findings include papilledema, vomiting, increased systolic blood pressure, widening pulse pressure and, eventually, decorticate posture.

Cerebral aneurysm

◆ Generalized seizures may occur.
◆ Onset is typically abrupt with severe headache, nausea, vomiting, and decreased LOC.
◆ Related findings vary with the site and amount of bleeding, but may include nuchal rigidity, irritability, hemiparesis, hemisensory defects, dysphagia, photophobia, diplopia, ptosis, and unilateral pupil dilation.

Eclampsia

◆ Generalized seizures are a hallmark sign.
◆ Related findings include severe frontal headache, nausea, vomiting, vision disturbances, increased blood pressure, fever, peripheral edema, oliguria, irritability, hyperactive deep tendon reflexes (DTRs), decreased LOC, and sudden weight gain.

Encephalitis

◆ Seizures are an early sign, indicating a poor prognosis.
◆ Seizures may also occur after recovery as a result of residual damage.
◆ Other findings include fever, headache, photophobia, nuchal rigidity, neck pain, vomiting, aphasia, ataxia, hemiparesis, nystagmus, irritability, cranial nerve palsies, and myoclonic jerks.

Head trauma

◆ Generalized seizures may occur at the time of injury; focal seizures may occur months later.

 TOP TECHNIQUE

Recognizing a generalized tonic-clonic seizure

BEFORE THE SEIZURE

Prodromal signs and symptoms, such as myoclonic jerks, throbbing headache, and mood changes, may occur over several hours or days. The patient may have premonitions of the seizure. For example, he may report an aura, such as seeing a flashing light or smelling a characteristic odor.

DURING THE SEIZURE

If a generalized seizure begins with an aura, this indicates that irritability in a specific area of the brain quickly became widespread. Common auras include palpitations, epigastric distress rapidly rising to the throat, head or eye turning, and sensory hallucinations.

Next, loss of consciousness occurs as a sudden discharge of intense electrical activity overwhelms the brain's subcortical center. The patient falls and experiences brief, bilateral myoclonic contractures. Air forced through spasmodic vocal cords may produce a birdlike, piercing cry.

During the *tonic phase*, skeletal muscles contract for 10 to 20 seconds. The patient's eyelids are drawn up, his arms are flexed, and his legs are extended. His mouth opens wide, then snaps shut; he may bite his tongue. His respirations cease because of respiratory muscle spasm, and initial pallor of the skin and mucous membranes (the result of impaired venous return) changes to cyanosis caused by apnea. The patient arches his back and slowly lowers his arms. Other effects include dilated, nonreactive pupils; greatly increased heart rate and blood pressure; increased salivation and tracheobronchial secretions; and profuse diaphoresis.

During the *clonic phase*, lasting about 60 seconds, mild trembling progresses to violent contractures or jerks. Other motor activity includes facial grimaces (with possible tongue biting) and violent expiration of bloody, foamy saliva from clonic contractures of thoracic cage muscles. Clonic jerks slowly decrease in intensity and frequency. The patient is still apneic.

AFTER THE SEIZURE

The patient's movements gradually cease, and he becomes unresponsive to external stimuli. Other postseizure features include stertorous respirations from increased tracheobronchial secretions, equal or unequal pupils (but becoming reactive), and urinary incontinence due to brief muscle relaxation. After about 5 minutes, the patient's level of consciousness increases, and he appears confused and disoriented. His muscle tone, heart rate, and blood pressure return to normal.

After several hours' sleep, the patient awakens exhausted and may have a headache, sore muscles, and amnesia about the seizure.

(continued)

- Related findings include decreased LOC; soft-tissue injury of the face, head, or neck; clear or bloody drainage from the mouth, nose, or ears; facial edema; bony deformity of the face, head, or neck; Battle's sign; and lack of response to oculocephalic and oculovestibular stimulation.
- Other findings include motor and sensory deficits, altered respirations, and signs of increasing ICP.

Hepatic encephalopathy
- Generalized seizures may occur late.
- Other findings include fetor hepaticus, asterixis, hyperactive DTRs, and a positive Babinski's sign.

Hypertensive encephalopathy
- Seizures with increased blood pressure, decreased LOC, intense headache, vomiting, transient blindness, paralysis, and Cheyne-Stokes respirations occur with this life-threatening disorder.

Hypoglycemia
- Generalized seizures usually occur in severe cases.
- Other findings include blurred or double vision, motor weakness, hemiplegia, trembling, excessive diaphoresis, tachycardia, myoclonic twitching, and decreased LOC.

Hyponatremia
- Seizure develops when sodium level falls below 125 mEq/L, especially if the decrease is rapid.
- Other findings include orthostatic hypotension, headache, muscle twitching and weakness, fatigue, oliguria or anuria, cold and clammy skin, decreased skin turgor, irritability, lethargy, confusion, and stupor or coma.
- Excessive thirst, tachycardia, nausea, vomiting, and abdominal cramps may also occur.

Hypoparathyroidism
- Generalized seizures occur as a result of worsening tetany.
- Chronic condition produces neuromuscular irritability, Chvostek's sign, dysphagia, tetany, and hyperactive DTRs.

Hypoxic encephalopathy
- Generalized seizures, myoclonic jerks, and coma occur.
- Later, dementia, visual agnosia, choreoathetosis, and ataxia may occur.

Neurofibromatosis
- Focal and generalized seizures occur.
- Other findings include café-au-lait spots, multiple skin tumors, scoliosis, kyphoscoliosis, dizziness, ataxia, monocular blindness, and nystagmus.

Porphyria
- Generalized seizures are a late sign of this disorder and indicate severe central nervous system involvement.
- Other related findings include severe abdominal pain, tachycardia, muscle weakness, and psychotic behavior.

Renal failure (chronic)
- Onset of twitching, trembling, myoclonic jerks, and generalized seizures is rapid.
- Related signs and symptoms include anuria or oliguria, fatigue, malaise, irritability, decreased mental acuity, muscle cramps, peripheral neuropathies, pruritus, uremic frost, anorexia, and constipation or diarrhea.
- Other findings include ammonia breath odor, nausea and vomiting, ecchymoses, petechiae, GI bleeding, mouth and gum ulcers, hypertension, and Kussmaul's respirations.

Sarcoidosis
- Lesions may affect the brain, causing focal or generalized seizures.
- Other related findings include nonproductive cough with dyspnea, substernal pain, malaise, fatigue, myalgia, weight loss, tachypnea, dysphagia, skin lesions, and impaired vision.

Stroke
- Seizures (focal more often than generalized) may occur within 6 months of an ischemic stroke.
- Other findings vary but may include decreased LOC, contralateral hemiplegia, dysarthria, dysphagia, ataxia, sensory loss on one side, apraxia, agnosia, aphasia, visual deficits, memory loss, personality changes, emotional lability, and incontinence.

OTHER
Diagnostic tests
◆ Contrast agents used in radiologic tests may cause generalized seizures.

Drugs
◆ In chronically intoxicated patients, barbiturate withdrawal may produce generalized seizures 2 to 4 days after the last dose.
◆ Amphetamines, isoniazid, phenothiazines, tricyclic antidepressants, and vincristine sulfate may cause seizures in patients with preexisting epilepsy.
◆ Toxic levels of some drugs, such as cimetidine (Tagamet), lidocaine (Xylocaine), meperidine (Demerol), penicillins, and theophylline, may cause generalized seizures.

NURSING CONSIDERATIONS
◆ Support respiratory status, if indicated.
◆ Protect the patient from injury.
◆ Monitor the patient after the seizure for recurring seizure activity.
◆ Monitor for therapeutic drug levels.

PEDIATRIC TIPS
◆ Common in children, generalized seizures may stem from fever, epilepsy, inborn errors of metabolism, perinatal injury, brain infection, Reye's syndrome, Sturge-Weber syndrome, arteriovenous malformation, lead poisoning, hypoglycemia, and idiopathic causes.

PATIENT TEACHING
◆ Teach the patient's family how to observe and record seizure activity and explain the reasons for doing so.
◆ Emphasize the importance of compliance with drug regimen and follow-up appointments.
◆ Explain the possible adverse reactions of prescribed drugs.
◆ Tell the patient to carry medical identification.

Seizures, simple partial

- Result from an irritable focus in the cerebral cortex
- Last about 30 seconds and don't alter level of consciousness (LOC)
- Vary in type and pattern depending on location of the irritable focus
- Are classified as motor (including jacksonian seizures and epilepsia partialis continua) or somatosensory (including visual, olfactory, and auditory seizures) (see *Identifying body functions affected by focal seizures*)

HISTORY

- Obtain a description of the seizure activity.
- Ask about events before the seizure.
- Ask if the patient can describe an aura or recognize its onset.
- Inquire about loss of consciousness, tonicity and clonicity, cyanosis, tongue biting, and urinary incontinence.
- Explore any history of head trauma, stroke, or infection with fever, headache, or stiff neck.

PHYSICAL ASSESSMENT

- Perform a complete physical assessment, focusing on the neurologic assessment.
- Check LOC.
- Test for residual deficits and sensory disturbances.

CAUSES

MEDICAL
Brain abscess
- Seizures can occur in the acute stage of abscess formation or after resolution of the abscess.
- Decreased LOC varies from drowsiness to deep stupor.
- Early findings reflect increased ICP, such as a constant, intractable headache, nausea, and vomiting.
- Later findings include ocular disturbances, such as nystagmus, decreased visual acuity, and unequal pupils.
- Other findings vary with the abscess site and may include aphasia, hemiparesis, and personality changes.

Brain tumor
- Focal seizures are commonly the earliest indicators.
- Morning headache, dizziness, confusion, vision loss, and motor and sensory disturbances may occur.
- Other findings include aphasia, generalized seizures, ataxia, decreased LOC, papilledema, vomiting, increased systolic blood pressure, widening pulse pressure and, eventually, decorticate posture.

Head trauma
- Penetrating wounds are associated with focal seizures.
- Seizures usually begin 3 to 15 months after injury, decrease in frequency after several years, and eventually stop.
- Generalized seizures and a decreased LOC may progress to coma.

Multiple sclerosis
- Focal or generalized seizures may occur in the late stages.

TOP TECHNIQUE

Identifying body functions affected by focal seizures

The site of the irritable focus determines which body functions are affected by a focal seizure, as shown in this illustration.

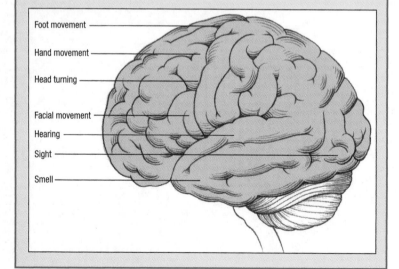

Foot movement
Hand movement
Head turning
Facial movement
Hearing
Sight
Smell

- Other findings include visual deficits, paresthesia, constipation, muscle weakness, spasticity, paralysis, hyperreflexia, intention tremor, gait ataxia, dysphagia, dysarthria, emotional lability, impotence, and urinary frequency, urgency, and incontinence.

Neurofibromatosis
- Multiple brain lesions cause focal seizures and, at times, generalized seizures.
- Other findings include café-au-lait spots, multiple skin tumors, scoliosis, kyphoscoliosis, dizziness, ataxia, progressive monocular blindness, nystagmus, and endocrine abnormalities.

Stroke
- Focal seizures may occur up to 6 months after a stroke's onset; generalized seizures may also occur.
- Accompanying effects vary and may include decreased LOC, contralateral hemiplegia, dysarthria, dysphagia, ataxia, unilateral sensory loss, apraxia, agnosia, and aphasia.
- Other findings include vision deficits, memory loss, poor judgment, personality changes, emotional lability, headache, urinary incontinence or retention, and vomiting.

NURSING CONSIDERATIONS
- Remain with the patient during the seizure, maintain his safety, and reassure him.
- Give anticonvulsants, as prescribed.
- Provide emotional support.
- Monitor for therapeutic drug levels.

PEDIATRIC TIPS
- Focal seizures affect more children than adults and are likely to spread and become generalized; they typically cause the child's eyes, or his head and eyes, to turn to the side; in neonates, they cause mouth twitching, staring, or both.
- Focal seizures in children can result from hemiplegic cerebral palsy, head trauma, child abuse, arteriovenous malformation, or Sturge-Weber syndrome.

PATIENT TEACHING
- Teach the patient's family how to record seizures.
- Emphasize the importance of complying with the prescribed drug regimen.
- Provide information on maintaining a safe environment.
- Tell the patient to carry medical identification.

Skin, bronze

OVERVIEW

- Results from excessive circulating melanin (see *Evaluating skin color variations*)
- Tends to appear at pressure points and increases on the palms and soles
- May extend to the buccal mucosa and gums before covering the entire body

HISTORY

- Ask about the onset of bronze skin.
- Determine whether the hue has changed.
- Inquire about the last exposure to the sun or a tanning source.
- Find out about a history of infection, illness, surgery, or trauma.
- Ask about abdominal pain, weakness, fatigue, diarrhea, constipation, or weight loss.
- Ask about the patient's current maintenance therapy for adrenal insufficiency.
- Take a nutritional history.

PHYSICAL ASSESSMENT

- Examine the mucosa, gums, and scars for hyperpigmentation.
- Check pressure points—such as the knuckles, elbows, toes, and knees—for color changes.
- Look for signs of dehydration.
- Observe the abdomen for distention.
- Examine the entire body for loss of body hair and tissue and muscle wasting.
- Palpate for hepatosplenomegaly.

TOP TECHNIQUE

Evaluating skin color variations

To quickly interpret your findings of skin color variations, refer to this chart.

COLOR	DISTRIBUTION	POSSIBLE CAUSE
Absent	◆ Small circumscribed areas ◆ Generalized	◆ Vitiligo ◆ Albinism
Blue	◆ Around lips or generalized	◆ Cyanosis (*Note:* In blacks, blue gingivae are normal.)
Deep red	◆ Generalized	◆ Polycythemia vera (increased red blood cell count)
Pink	◆ Local or generalized	◆ Erythema (superficial capillary dilation and congestion)
Tan to brown	◆ Facial patches	◆ Chloasma of pregnancy; butterfly rash of lupus erythematosus
Tan to brown-bronze	◆ Generalized (not related to sun exposure)	◆ Addison's disease
Yellow to yellowish brown	◆ Sclera or generalized	◆ Jaundice from liver dysfunction (*Note:* In blacks, yellowish brown pigmentation of sclera is normal.)
Yellowish orange	◆ Palms, soles, and face; not sclera	◆ Carotenemia (carotene in the blood)

CAUSES

MEDICAL

Adrenal hyperplasia
◆ A dark bronze tone develops within a few months.
◆ Other findings include visual field deficits; headache; signs of masculinization in females, such as clitoral enlargement and male distribution of hair, fat, and muscle mass.

Biliary cirrhosis
◆ Bronze skin develops on exposed areas of jaundiced skin, including the eyelids, palms, neck, and chest or back.
◆ Other findings include pruritus, weakness, fatigue, jaundice, dark urine, pale stools with steatorrhea, decreased appetite with weight loss, and hepatomegaly.

Hemochromatosis
◆ Progressive, generalized bronzing, accentuated by metallic gray-bronze skin on sun-exposed areas, genitalia, and scars, is an early sign.
◆ Other early associated effects include weakness, lethargy, weight loss, abdominal pain, loss of libido, polydipsia, and polyuria.

Malnutrition
◆ Bronzing, apathy, lethargy, anorexia, weakness, and slow pulse and respiratory rates occur.
◆ Other findings include paresthesia in the extremities; dull, sparse, dry hair; brittle nails; dark, swollen cheeks; dry, flaky skin; red, swollen lips; muscle wasting; and gonadal atrophy in males.

Primary adrenal insufficiency
◆ Bronze skin is a classic sign.
◆ Other findings include axillary and pubic hair loss, vitiligo, progressive fatigue, weakness, anorexia, nausea, vomiting, weight loss, orthostatic hypotension, weak and irregular pulse, abdominal pain, irritability, diarrhea or constipation, amenorrhea, and syncope.

Renal failure (chronic)
◆ The skin becomes pallid, yellowish bronze, dry, and scaly.
◆ Other findings include ammonia breath odor, oliguria, fatigue, decreased mental acuity, seizures, muscle cramps, peripheral neuropathy, bleeding tendencies, pruritus and, occasionally, uremic frost and hypertension.

OTHER

Drugs
◆ Prolonged therapy with high doses of phenothiazines may cause a gradual bronzing of the skin.

NURSING CONSIDERATIONS

◆ Prepare the patient for diagnostic tests.
◆ Encourage the patient to discuss concerns about changes in body image.
◆ If fatigue is a problem, encourage frequent rest periods.

PEDIATRIC TIPS
◆ Celiac disease can cause bronze skin in young children, beginning with the introduction of cereals and usually subsiding later in childhood.

PATIENT TEACHING

◆ Emphasize the importance of rest periods.
◆ Provide referral to nutritional counseling, if appropriate.
◆ Discuss underlying condition and treatment plan.

Skin, clammy

OVERVIEW

- Is characterized by moist, cool, and usually pale skin
- Refers to a sympathetic response involving the release of epinephrine and norepinephrine, which causes cutaneous vasoconstriction and secretion of cold sweat from eccrine glands
- Usually occurs on the palms, forehead, and soles
- May occur possibly with shock, acute hypoglycemia, anxiety reactions, arrhythmias, and heat exhaustion (see *Clammy skin: A key finding*)

HISTORY

- Ask about a history of type 1 diabetes or cardiac disorder.
- Take a drug history, noting use of an antiarrhythmic.
- Find out about pain, chest pressure, nausea, epigastric distress, weakness, diarrhea, increased urination, or dry mouth.

PHYSICAL ASSESSMENT

- Take vital signs.
- Perform a cardiovascular assessment; then complete the physical assessment.
- Examine the pupils for dilation.
- Check for abdominal distention.
- Check blood glucose level.
- Test for increased muscle tension.

ACTION STAT!

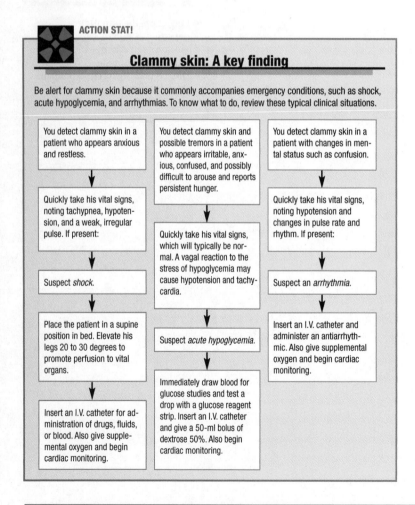

Clammy skin: A key finding

Be alert for clammy skin because it commonly accompanies emergency conditions, such as shock, acute hypoglycemia, and arrhythmias. To know what to do, review these typical clinical situations.

You detect clammy skin in a patient who appears anxious and restless.
↓
Quickly take his vital signs, noting tachypnea, hypotension, and a weak, irregular pulse. If present:
↓
Suspect *shock.*
↓
Place the patient in a supine position in bed. Elevate his legs 20 to 30 degrees to promote perfusion to vital organs.
↓
Insert an I.V. catheter for administration of drugs, fluids, or blood. Also give supplemental oxygen and begin cardiac monitoring.

You detect clammy skin and possible tremors in a patient who appears irritable, anxious, confused, and possibly difficult to arouse and reports persistent hunger.
↓
Quickly take his vital signs, which will typically be normal. A vagal reaction to the stress of hypoglycemia may cause hypotension and tachycardia.
↓
Suspect *acute hypoglycemia.*
↓
Immediately draw blood for glucose studies and test a drop with a glucose reagent strip. Insert an I.V. catheter and give a 50-ml bolus of dextrose 50%. Also begin cardiac monitoring.

You detect clammy skin in a patient with changes in mental status such as confusion.
↓
Quickly take his vital signs, noting hypotension and changes in pulse rate and rhythm. If present:
↓
Suspect an *arrhythmia.*
↓
Insert an I.V. catheter and administer an antiarrhythmic. Also give supplemental oxygen and begin cardiac monitoring.

MEDICAL
Anxiety
◆ With anxiety, clammy skin is present on the forehead, palms, and soles.
◆ Pallor, dry mouth, tachycardia or bradycardia, palpitations, and hypertension or hypotension also occur.
◆ Other findings include possible tremors, breathlessness, headache, muscle tension, nausea, vomiting, abdominal distention, diarrhea, increased urination, and sharp chest pain.

Cardiac arrhythmias
◆ Generalized clammy skin occurs with mental status changes, dizziness, and hypotension.
◆ Pulse rate may be rapid, slow, or irregular.
◆ Other findings include palpitations, chest pain, diaphoresis, light-headedness, and weakness.

Cardiogenic shock
◆ Generalized clammy skin accompanies confusion, restlessness, hypotension, tachycardia, tachypnea, narrowing pulse pressure, cyanosis, and oliguria.
◆ Other signs and symptoms include anginal pain, dyspnea, jugular vein distention, ventricular gallop, and a bounding (early) or weak (late) pulse.

Heat exhaustion
◆ In heat exhaustion, generalized clammy skin, an ashen appearance, headache, confusion, syncope, giddiness and, possibly, a subnormal temperature develop with mild heat exhaustion.
◆ Other findings include a rapid and thready pulse, nausea, vomiting, tachypnea, oliguria, thirst, muscle cramps, and hypotension.

Hypoglycemia (acute)
◆ Generalized cool, clammy skin or diaphoresis may accompany irritability, tremors, palpitations, hunger, headache, tachycardia, and anxiety.

◆ Central nervous system findings include blurred vision, diplopia, confusion, motor weakness, hemiplegia, and coma.

Hypovolemic shock
◆ Generalized pale, cold, clammy skin accompanies subnormal body temperature, hypotension with narrowing pulse pressure, tachycardia, tachypnea, and rapid, thready pulse.
◆ Other findings are flat neck veins, increased capillary refill time, decreased urine output, poor skin turgor, confusion, and decreased level of consciousness.

Septic shock
◆ The cold shock stage of septic shock causes generalized cold, clammy skin.
◆ Other findings include rapid and thready pulse, severe hypotension, persistent oliguria or anuria, and respiratory failure.

◆ Take vital signs frequently.
◆ Monitor urine output.
◆ Provide measures to correct the underlying cause.
◆ Give emotional support to the patient and his family.
◆ Provide frequent skin care and dry bed linens, as appropriate.

PEDIATRIC TIPS
◆ Infants in shock don't have clammy skin because of immature sweat glands.

GERIATRIC TIPS
◆ Elderly patients develop clammy skin easily because of decreased tissue perfusion.
◆ Consider bowel ischemia in the differential diagnosis of older patients with cool, clammy skin, especially if abdominal pain or bloody stools occur.

◆ Explain the underlying illness, diagnostic tests, and treatment options.
◆ Provide orientation to the intensive care unit, if applicable.

Skin, mottled

- Refers to patchy discoloration of the skin
- Indicates changes of deep, middle, or superficial dermal blood vessels
- May indicate an emergency condition (see *Mottled skin: Knowing what to do*)

HISTORY

- Ask about the onset of mottled skin (sudden or gradual).
- Determine precipitating, aggravating, and alleviating factors.
- Inquire about associated pain, numbness, or tingling in the extremity.

PHYSICAL ASSESSMENT

- Obtain vital signs.
- Observe the patient's skin color.
- Palpate the arms and legs for skin texture, swelling, and temperature differences.
- Check capillary refill time.
- Palpate for pulses and note their quality.
- Note breaks in the skin, muscle appearance, and hair distribution.
- Assess motor and sensory function.

ACTION STAT!

Mottled skin: Knowing what to do

If your patient's skin is pale, cool, clammy, and mottled at the elbows and knees or all over, he may be developing hypovolemic shock. Quickly take his vital signs and be sure to note tachycardia or a weak, thready pulse. Observe the neck for flattened veins. Does the patient appear anxious? If you detect these signs and symptoms, place the patient in a supine position in bed with his legs elevated 20 to 30 degrees. Administer oxygen by nasal cannula or face mask and begin cardiac monitoring. Insert a large-bore I.V. catheter for rapid fluid or blood product administration and prepare to insert a central line or a pulmonary artery catheter. Also prepare to insert a catheter to monitor urine output.

Localized mottling in a pale, cool extremity that the patient says feels painful, numb, and tingling may signal acute arterial occlusion. Immediately check the patient's distal pulses. If they're absent or diminished, you'll need to insert an I.V. catheter in an unaffected extremity and prepare the patient for arteriography, thrombolytic therapy, or immediate surgery.

MEDICAL

Arterial occlusion (acute)

◆ Temperature and color changes that develop at the level of obstruction are initial signs of this disorder.
◆ Pallor may change to blotchy cyanosis and livedo reticularis (mottling).
◆ Color and temperature demarcation develop at the level of obstruction.
◆ Other findings include sudden onset of pain in the extremity, diminished or absent pulses, cool extremity, increased capillary refill time, pallor, diminished reflexes and, possibly, paresthesia, paresis, and a sensation of cold in the affected area.

Arteriosclerosis obliterans

◆ Leg pallor, cyanosis, blotchy erythema, and livedo reticularis develop.
◆ Other findings include intermittent claudication, diminished or absent pedal pulses, paresthesia, increased capillary refill time, and leg coolness.

Buerger's disease

◆ Color changes and mottling, particularly livedo networking in the lower extremities, occur.
◆ Also intermittent claudication and erythema along extremity blood vessels can occur.
◆ During cold exposure, feet become cold, cyanotic, and numb; later, they become hot, red, and tingling.
◆ Other possible findings include impaired peripheral pulses and peripheral neuropathy.

Hypovolemic shock

◆ Vasoconstriction commonly produces skin mottling, initially in the knees and elbows.
◆ As shock worsens, mottling becomes generalized.
◆ Early signs include sudden onset of pallor, cool skin, restlessness, thirst, tachypnea, and slight tachycardia.
◆ As shock progresses, other findings include cool, clammy skin; rapid, thready pulse; hypotension; narrowed pulse pressure; decreased urine output; subnormal temperature; confusion; and decreased level of consciousness.

Livedo reticularis (idiopathic or primary)

◆ Symmetrical, diffuse mottling can involve the hands, feet, arms, legs, buttocks, and trunk.
◆ Initially, networking is intermittent and most pronounced on exposure to cold or stress; eventually, mottling persists even with warming.

Polycythemia vera

◆ Livedo reticularis, hemangiomas, purpura, rubor, ulcerative nodules, and scleroderma-like lesions are produced in this disorder.
◆ Other symptoms include headache, a vague feeling of fullness in the head, dizziness, vertigo, vision disturbances, dyspnea, and aquagenic pruritus.

Rheumatoid arthritis

◆ Skin mottling may occur.
◆ Early findings include joint pain and stiffness with subcutaneous nodules on the elbows.

Systemic lupus erythematosus

◆ Livedo reticularis occurs most commonly on the outer arms.
◆ Other findings include a butterfly rash, nondeforming joint pain and stiffness, photosensitivity, Raynaud's phenomenon, patchy alopecia, seizures, fever, anorexia, weight loss, lymphadenopathy, and emotional lability.

OTHER

Immobility

◆ Prolonged immobility may cause bluish mottling, most noticeably in dependent extremities.

Thermal exposure

◆ Prolonged thermal exposure, such as from a heating pad or hot water bottle, may cause localized, reticulated, brown-to-red mottling.

◆ Monitor vital signs, intake and output, and peripheral pulses.
◆ Provide care to treat the underlying condition.

PEDIATRIC TIPS

◆ A common cause of mottled skin in children is systemic vasoconstriction from shock.

GERIATRIC TIPS

◆ Decreased tissue perfusion can easily cause mottled skin.
◆ Conditions producing mottled skin in older patients include arterial occlusion, polycythemia vera, and bowel ischemia.

◆ Encourage the avoidance of tight clothing and overexposure to cold or heating devices.
◆ Teach the patient to recognize flare-up of the underlying condition.
◆ Explain to the patient about prescribed mediations.

Skin turgor, decreased

OVERVIEW

- Refers to pinched skin that tents or holds for up to 30 seconds, then slowly returns to its normal contour
- Is commonly assessed over the hand, arm, or sternum (see *Evaluating skin turgor*)
- Results from dehydration or volume depletion, which moves interstitial fluid into the vascular bed to maintain circulating blood volume, leading to slackness in the skin's dermal layer

HISTORY

- Ask about food and fluid intake and fluid loss.
- Find out about recent vomiting, diarrhea, draining wounds, fever with sweating, or increased urination.
- Take a drug history, noting use of diuretics.
- Ask about use of alcohol.

PHYSICAL ASSESSMENT

- Take vital signs, noting orthostatic hypotension and tachycardia.
- Evaluate level of consciousness.
- Inspect the oral mucosa, the furrows of the tongue, and axillae for dryness.
- Check jugular vein distention.
- Check capillary refill.

TOP TECHNIQUE

Evaluating skin turgor

To evaluate skin turgor in an adult, pick up a fold of skin over the sternum or the arm, as shown at left. (In an infant, roll a fold of loosely adherent skin on the abdomen between your thumb and forefinger.) Then release it. Normal skin will immediately return to its previous contour. In decreased skin turgor, the skin fold will "tent," or "hold," as shown at right for up to 30 seconds.

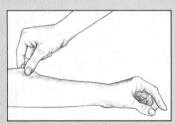
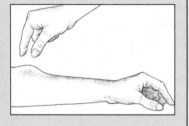

MEDICAL

Cholera

◆ Abrupt watery diarrhea and vomiting, leading to severe water and electrolyte loss that causes decreased skin turgor, characterize this disorder.

◆ Other findings include intense thirst, weakness, muscle cramps, cyanosis, oliguria, tachycardia, falling blood pressure, fever, and hypoactive bowel sounds.

Dehydration

◆ Decreased skin turgor occurs with moderate to severe dehydration.

◆ Other findings include dry oral mucosa, decreased perspiration, resting tachycardia, orthostatic hypotension, dry and furrowed tongue, increased thirst, weight loss, oliguria, fever, and fatigue.

◆ As dehydration worsens, findings include enophthalmos, lethargy, weakness, confusion, delirium or obtundation, anuria and shock.

◆ Monitor intake and output.
◆ Assess vital signs.
◆ Turn the patient every 2 hours to prevent skin breakdown.
◆ Administer I.V. fluid replacement, and frequently offer oral fluids.
◆ Weigh the patient daily.
◆ Monitor electrolyte levels.

PEDIATRIC TIPS

◆ Diarrhea from gastroenteritis is the most common cause of dehydration, which causes decreased skin turgor, in children, especially up to age 2.

GERIATRIC TIPS

◆ Decreased skin turgor is a normal finding in elderly patients, making it an unreliable indicator of dehydration.

◆ Explain fluid replacement and its importance.
◆ Tell the patient or caregiver which signs and symptoms to report.

Splenomegaly

- Refers to enlargement of the spleen
- May be detected by light palpation under the left costal margin (see *Palpating for splenomegaly*)
- Can result from any process that triggers lymphadenopathy, such as infection or inflammation, cancer, increased blood cell destruction, or vascular congestion from portal hypertension (because spleen functions as the body's largest lymph node)

 ACTION STAT! *If the patient has a history of abdominal or thoracic trauma, don't palpate the abdomen because this may aggravate internal bleeding. Instead, examine for left-upper-quadrant pain and signs of shock. If you detect these signs, suspect splenic rupture. Insert an I.V. catheter for emergency fluid and blood replacement, and administer oxygen. Catheterize the patient to evaluate urine output and begin cardiac monitoring. Prepare the patient for possible surgery.*

HISTORY

- Inquire about fatigue; frequent colds, sore throats, or other infections; bruising; left-upper-quadrant pain; abdominal fullness; and early satiety.
- Obtain a complete medical history.
- Ask about recent trauma or surgery.

PHYSICAL ASSESSMENT

- Complete an abdominal assessment.
- Examine the skin for pallor and ecchymoses.
- Palpate the axillae, groin, and neck for lymphadenopathy.

CAUSES

MEDICAL
Cirrhosis
- Moderate to severe splenomegaly occurs with advanced cirrhosis.
- Late findings also include jaundice, hepatomegaly, leg edema, hematemesis, and ascites.
- Signs of hepatic encephalopathy may also occur, such as asterixis, fetor hepaticus, slurred speech, and decreased level of consciousness that may progress to coma.
- Other findings include jaundice, pruritus, bleeding tendencies, menstrual irregularities or testicular atrophy, gynecomastia, and right-upper abdominal pain.

Endocarditis (subacute infective)
- Spleen is enlarged but nontender in this disorder.
- A suddenly changing murmur or the discovery of a new murmur in the presence of a fever is a classic sign.
- Other findings include anorexia, pallor, weakness, fever, night sweats, fatigue, tachycardia, weight loss, arthralgia, petechiae, hematuria, Osler's nodes, and Janeway lesions.

Hepatitis
- Splenomegaly may occur with hepatitis.
- Characteristic findings include dark urine, clay-colored stools, anorexia, malaise, pruritus, hepatomegaly, vomiting, jaundice, and fatigue.

Histoplasmosis
- Splenomegaly and hepatomegaly occur with this disorder.
- Other findings include lymphadenopathy, jaundice, fever, anorexia, and signs and symptoms of anemia.

 TOP TECHNIQUE

Palpating for splenomegaly

Detecting splenomegaly requires skillful and gentle palpation to avoid rupturing the enlarged spleen. Follow these steps carefully:
- Place the patient in the supine position and stand at his right side. Place your left hand under the left costovertebral angle and push lightly to move the spleen forward. Then press your right hand gently under the left front costal margin.
- Have the patient take a deep breath and then exhale. As he exhales, move your right hand along the tissue contours under the border of the ribs, feeling for the spleen's edge. The enlarged spleen should feel like a firm mass that bumps against your fingers. Remember to begin palpation low enough in the abdomen to catch the edge of a massive spleen.
- Grade the splenomegaly as slight (½" to 1½" [1 to 4 cm] below the costal margin), moderate (1½" to 3" [4 to 8 cm] below the costal margin), or great (greater than or equal to 3" below the costal margin).
- Reposition the patient on his right side with his hips and knees flexed slightly to move the spleen forward. Then repeat the palpation procedure.

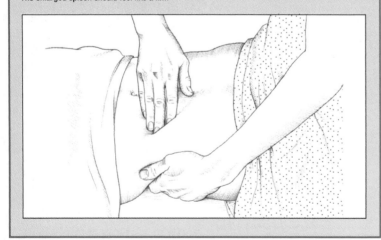

Hypersplenism (primary)

- Splenomegaly accompanies anemia, neutropenia, or thrombocytopenia.
- Left-sided abdominal pain may occur.
- With anemia, findings include weakness, fatigue, malaise, and pallor.
- With severe neutropenia, findings include frequent infections.
- With thrombocytopenia, easy bruising or spontaneous, widespread hemorrhage may occur.

Leukemia

- Moderate to severe splenomegaly is an early sign of leukemia.
- With chronic granulocytic leukemia, findings include hepatomegaly, lymphadenopathy, fatigue, malaise, pallor, fever, gum swelling, bleeding tendencies, weight loss, anorexia, and abdominal, bone, and joint pain.
- Acute leukemia may produce dyspnea, tachycardia, and palpitations.

Lymphoma

- Moderate to massive splenomegaly is late sign of lymphoma.
- Other late findings include hepatomegaly, painless lymphadenopathy, night sweats, fever, fatigue, weight loss, malaise, and scaly dermatitis with pruritus.

Mononucleosis (infectious)

- Splenomegaly, a common sign, is most pronounced during second and third weeks of illness.
- Triad includes sore throat, cervical lymphadenopathy, and fluctuating temperature with an evening peak.
- Hepatomegaly, jaundice, and a maculopapular rash may also develop.

Pancreatic cancer

- Moderate to severe splenomegaly may occur if a tumor compresses the splenic vein.
- Other characteristic findings include abdominal or back pain, anorexia, nausea, vomiting, weight loss, GI bleeding, jaundice, pruritus, skin lesions, emotional lability, weakness, and fatigue.

Polycythemia vera

- Enlarged spleen resulting in easy satiety, abdominal fullness, and left-upper-quadrant abdominal pain or pleuritic chest pain occur late in the disease.
- Also occurring with polycythemia vera are finger and toe paresthesia, impaired mentation, tinnitus, blurred or double vision, scotoma, increased blood pressure, pruritus, epigastric distress, weight loss, hepatomegaly, bleeding tendencies, and intermittent claudication.
- Other possible findings include deep purplish red oral mucous membranes, headache, dyspnea, dizziness, vertigo, weakness, and fatigue.

Splenic rupture

- Splenomegaly may result from massive abdominal or thoracic hemorrhage that predisposes the spleen to rupture.
- Other findings include left-upper-quadrant pain, abdominal rigidity, Kehr's sign, and signs of shock.

NURSING CONSIDERATIONS

- Monitor the patient's vital signs and blood count.
- Prepare the patient for diagnostic tests.
- Provide measures to treat the underlying disorder.

PEDIATRIC TIPS

- Children may develop splenomegaly in congenital hemolytic anemia, Gaucher's disease, or sickle cell disease.
- Splenic abscess is the most common cause of splenomegaly in immunocompromised children.

PATIENT TEACHING

- Instruct the patient to avoid infection.
- Emphasize the importance of complying with drug therapy.
- Teach about underlying diagnosis and treatment plan.

Stools, clay-colored

- Result from hepatocellular degeneration or biliary obstruction that interferes with the formation or release of bile pigments
- Are commonly associated with jaundice and dark "cola-colored" urine

- Ask about the onset of clay-colored stools.
- Explore associated abdominal or back pain, nausea and vomiting, fatigue, anorexia, weight loss, and dark urine.
- Inquire about difficulty digesting fatty foods or heavy meals.
- Note whether the patient bruises easily.
- Take a medical history, noting gallbladder, hepatic, or pancreatic disorders.
- Ask about recent barium studies or use of antacids.
- Note a history of alcoholism.
- Find out about exposure to toxic substances.

- Take vital signs.
- Check for jaundice.
- Inspect the abdomen for distention and ascites.
- Auscultate for hypoactive bowel sounds.
- Percuss and palpate for masses and rebound tenderness.

CAUSES

MEDICAL

Bile duct cancer
◆ Clay-colored stools may be accompanied by jaundice, pruritus, anorexia, weight loss, bleeding tendencies, and palpable mass in bile duct cancer.
◆ Pain may develop in the epigastrium or right upper quadrant.

Biliary cirrhosis
◆ Clay-colored stools typically follow unexplained pruritus that worsens at bedtime, weakness, fatigue, weight loss, and vague abdominal pain.
◆ Other findings include jaundice; hyperpigmentation; signs of malabsorption; bone and back pain, hematemesis; ascites; edema; firm, nontender hepatomegaly; and xanthomas on the palms, soles, and elbows.

Cholangitis (sclerosing)
◆ Clay-colored stools, chronic or intermittent jaundice, pruritus, right-upper-quadrant pain, weakness, fatigue, chills, and fever occur.

Cholelithiasis
◆ Obstruction of the common bile duct may result in clay-colored stools.
◆ Associated symptoms include dyspepsia and biliary colic.
◆ Right-upper-quadrant pain intensifies over several hours, may radiate to the epigastrium or shoulder blades, and is relieved by antacids.
◆ Pain is accompanied by tachycardia, restlessness, nausea, intolerance to certain foods, vomiting, upper abdominal tenderness, fever, chills, and jaundice.

Hepatic cancer
◆ Weight loss, weakness, and anorexia precede clay-colored stools in hepatic cancer.
◆ Later, nodular, firm hepatomegaly; jaundice; right-upper-quadrant pain; ascites; dependent edema; and fever develop.

Hepatitis
◆ Clay-colored stools signal the start of the icteric phase of hepatitis.
◆ Associated signs include mild weight loss, dark urine, anorexia, jaundice, and tender hepatomegaly.
◆ Findings during the icteric phase include irritability, right-upper-quadrant pain, splenomegaly, enlarged cervical lymph nodes, and severe pruritus.

Pancreatic cancer
◆ Common bile duct obstruction may cause clay-colored stools in pancreatic cancer.
◆ Classic associated findings include abdominal or back pain, jaundice, pruritus, nausea and vomiting, anorexia, weight loss, fatigue, weakness, and fever.
◆ Other findings include diarrhea, skin lesions, emotional lability, splenomegaly, and signs of GI bleeding.

Pancreatitis (acute)
◆ Clay-colored stools, dark urine, jaundice, and severe epigastric pain that's aggravated by lying down occur with acute pancreatitis.
◆ Other findings include nausea, vomiting, fever, abdominal rigidity and tenderness, hypoactive bowel sounds, and crackles at the lung bases.

OTHER

Surgery
◆ Biliary surgery may cause bile duct stricture, resulting in clay-colored stools.

NURSING CONSIDERATIONS

◆ Prepare the patient for diagnostic tests.
◆ Encourage rest periods.
◆ Administer analgesics, as prescribed.
◆ Give vaccines for hepatitis A and B, as ordered.

PEDIATRIC TIPS
◆ Clay-colored stools may occur in infants with biliary atresia.

GERIATRIC TIPS
◆ Because elderly patients with cholelithiasis, which causes clay-colored stools, have a greater risk of developing its complications, surgery should be considered.

PATIENT TEACHING

◆ Discuss underlying disorder and treatment options.
◆ Explain ways to reduce abdominal pain.
◆ Discuss the dietary modifications the patient needs.
◆ Stress the need for a restful environment.
◆ Emphasize the importance of avoiding alcohol.

Stridor

OVERVIEW

- Refers to a loud, harsh, musical respiratory sound
- Results from an obstruction in the trachea or larynx
- Usually heard during inspiration, but may also occur during expiration in severe upper airway obstruction
- May begin as a low-pitched croaking and progress to high-pitched crowing as respirations become more vigorous

 ACTION STAT! *Check vital signs, including oxygen saturation, and examine the patient for signs of partial airway obstruction. Abrupt end of stridor signals complete airway obstruction. If you detect airway obstruction, clear the airway with back blows or abdominal thrusts. Give oxygen or prepare to assist with emergency endotracheal (ET) intubation or tracheostomy and mechanical ventilation. (See Assisting with emergency ET intubation.) Suction any aspirated vomitus or blood. Connect the patient to a cardiac monitor and position him upright.*

HISTORY

- Ask about the onset of stridor.
- Inquire about any previous instances of stridor.
- Note any current respiratory tract infection.
- Ask about a history of allergies, tumors, or respiratory and vascular disorders.
- Note recent exposure to smoke or noxious fumes or gases.
- Inquire about associated pain or cough.

PHYSICAL ASSESSMENT

- Examine the mouth for excessive secretions, foreign matter, inflammation, and swelling.
- Assess the neck for swelling, masses, subcutaneous crepitation, and scars.
- Observe the chest for decreased or asymmetrical expansion.
- Auscultate for wheezes, rhonchi, crackles, rubs, and other abnormal breath sounds.
- Percuss for dullness, tympany, or flatness.
- Note burns or signs of trauma.

CAUSES

MEDICAL
Airway trauma

- Acute airway obstruction is common and results in the sudden onset of stridor.
- Other findings include dysphonia, dysphagia, hemoptysis, cyanosis, accessory muscle use, intercostal retractions, nasal flaring, tachypnea, progressive dyspnea, and shallow respirations.

Anaphylaxis

- Upper airway edema and laryngospasm cause stridor and other signs of respiratory distress.
- Typically, these respiratory effects are preceded by a feeling of impending doom or fear, weakness, diaphoresis, sneezing, nasal pruritus, urticaria, erythema, and angioedema.
- Other common findings include chest or throat tightness, dysphagia and, possibly, signs of shock.

Anthrax (inhalation)

- The second stage develops abruptly with rapid deterioration marked by stridor, fever, dyspnea, and hypotension generally leading to death within 24 hours.
- Initial findings include fever, chills, weakness, cough, and chest pain.

ACTION STAT!

Assisting with emergency ET intubation

For a patient with stridor, you may have to assist with emergency endotracheal (ET) intubation to establish a patent airway and administer mechanical ventilation. Follow these essential steps:

- Gather the necessary equipment.
- Explain the procedure to the patient (if he's alert).
- Place the patient flat on his back with a small blanket or pillow under his head. This position aligns the axis of the oropharynx, posterior pharynx, and trachea.
- Check the cuff on the ET tube for leaks before to insertion by the physician.
- After intubation, inflate the cuff, using the minimal leak technique.
- Check tube placement by auscultating for bilateral breath sounds or using a capnometer; observe the patient for chest expansion and feel for warm exhalations at the ET tube's opening.
- Insert an oral airway or bite block.
- Secure the tube and airway with tape applied to skin treated with compound benzoin tincture.

- Suction secretions from the patient's mouth and the ET tube as needed.
- Administer oxygen or initiate mechanical ventilation (or both).

After the patient has been intubated, suction secretions as needed and check cuff pressure once every shift. Provide mouth care every 2 to 3 hours and as needed. Prepare the patient for chest X-rays to check tube placement, and restrain and reassure him as needed.

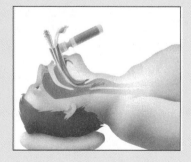

Aspiration of foreign body

- Sudden stridor is characteristic in this life-threatening situation.
- Other findings include abrupt onset of dry, paroxysmal coughing, gagging, or choking; hoarseness; tachycardia; wheezing; dyspnea; tachypnea; intercostal muscle retractions; diminished breath sounds; cyanosis; anxiety; and shallow respirations.

Epiglottiditis

- Stridor, caused by an erythematous, edematous epiglottis that obstructs the upper airway, occurs along with fever, sore throat, and a croupy cough in this life-threatening situation.
- Other findings include cough that may progress to severe respiratory distress with sternal and intercostal retractions, nasal flaring, cyanosis, and tachycardia.

Hypocalcemia

- Laryngospasm can cause stridor in hypocalcemia.
- Other findings include paresthesia, carpopedal spasm, hyperactive deep tendon reflexes, muscle twitching and cramping, and positive Chvostek's and Trousseau's signs.

Inhalation injury

- Laryngeal edema and bronchospasms, resulting in stridor, may develop within 48 hours after inhalation of smoke or noxious fumes.
- Other findings include singed nasal hairs, orofacial burns, coughing, hoarseness, sooty sputum, crackles, rhonchi, wheezes, dyspnea, accessory muscle use, intercostal retractions, and nasal flaring.

Laryngeal tumor

- This type of tumor is a late sign, occurring with possible dysphagia, dyspnea, enlarged cervical nodes, and pain that radiates to the ear.
- Laryngeal tumor is preceded by hoarseness, minor throat pain, and a mild, dry cough.

Laryngitis (acute)

- Severe laryngeal edema, resulting in stridor and dyspnea, may occur.
- Mild to severe hoarseness is the chief sign.
- Other findings include sore throat, dysphagia, dry cough, malaise, and fever.

Mediastinal tumor

- Compression of the trachea and bronchi results in stridor.
- Other findings include hoarseness, brassy cough, tracheal shift or tug, dilated neck veins, swelling of the face and neck, stertorous respirations, dyspnea, dysphagia, suprasternal retractions on inspiration, and pain in the chest, shoulder, or arm.

Thoracic aortic aneurysm

- If the trachea is compressed, stridor, dyspnea, wheezing, and a brassy cough may result.
- Other findings include hoarseness or complete voice loss, dysphagia, jugular vein distention, prominent chest veins, tracheal tug, paresthesia or neuralgia, and edema of the face, neck, and arms.

OTHER
Diagnostic tests

- Bronchoscopy or laryngoscopy may precipitate laryngospasm and stridor due to airway irritation.

Treatments

- Neck surgery, such as thyroidectomy, may cause laryngeal paralysis and stridor.
- After prolonged intubation, the patient may exhibit laryngeal edema and stridor when the tube is removed.

NURSING CONSIDERATIONS

- Continue to monitor vital signs and oxygen saturation and for signs of respiratory distress.
- Prepare the patient for diagnostic tests.
- Offer reassurance and calm the patient.
- Administer antibiotics and respiratory treatments, as ordered.

PEDIATRIC TIPS

- Causes of stridor in children include foreign-body aspiration, croup syndrome, laryngeal diphtheria, pertussis, retropharyngeal abscess, and congenital abnormalities of the larynx.

PATIENT TEACHING

- Explain all procedures and treatments.
- Teach about underlying diagnosis.

Syncope

- Is characterized by a transient loss of consciousness
- Can be associated with impaired cerebral blood supply or cerebral hypoxia
- May be abrupt and last for seconds to minutes

ACTION STAT! *If you see a patient faint, ensure a patent airway and patient safety. Take vital signs. Place the patient in a supine position, elevate his legs, and loosen any tight clothing. Be alert for tachycardia, bradycardia, or an irregular pulse. Place the patient on a cardiac monitor to detect arrhythmias. If an arrhythmia appears, give oxygen and insert an I.V. catheter for drug or fluid administration. Be ready to begin cardiopulmonary resuscitation. Cardioversion, defibrillation, or insertion of a temporary pacemaker may also be required.*

HISTORY

- Obtain a description of the fainting episode and its duration.
- Inquire about precipitating factors.
- Ask about preceding symptoms, including weakness, light-headedness, nausea, or diaphoresis.
- Ask about associated headache.
- Obtain a history of previous fainting.

PHYSICAL ASSESSMENT

- Take vital signs.
- Examine the patient for any injuries from falling during syncope.
- Perform a complete cardiac and neurologic assessment.

CAUSES

MEDICAL
Aortic arch syndrome

- Syncope may be accompanied by weak or abruptly absent carotid pulses and unequal or absent radial pulses.
- Early findings include night sweats, pallor, nausea, anorexia, weight loss, arthralgia, and Raynaud's phenomenon.
- Other findings include hypotension in the arms; neck, shoulder, and chest pain; paresthesia; intermittent claudication; bruits; vision disturbances; and dizziness.

Aortic stenosis

- A classic late sign, syncope is accompanied by exertional dyspnea and angina.
- Fatigue, orthopnea, paroxysmal nocturnal dyspnea, palpitations, atrial and ventricular gallops, and diminished carotid pulses occur.
- A harsh, crescendo-decrescendo systolic ejection murmur that's loudest at the right sternal border of the second intercostal space may be heard.

Cardiac arrhythmias

- Decreased cardiac output and impaired cerebral circulation may cause syncope.

Carotid sinus hypersensitivity

- Syncope is triggered by compression of the carotid sinus.
- Preceding findings include palpitations, pallor, confusion, diaphoresis, dyspnea, and hypotension.
- Syncope may develop without warning in Stokes-Adams syndrome; asystole during syncope may precipitate spasm and myoclonic jerks if prolonged.

Hypoxemia

- Syncope, confusion, tachycardia, restlessness, tachypnea, dyspnea, cyanosis, and incoordination may occur.

Orthostatic hypotension

♦ Syncope occurs when the patient rises quickly from a recumbent position.
♦ Other findings include tachycardia, pallor, dizziness, blurred vision, nausea, and diaphoresis.

Transient ischemic attack

♦ Syncope and decreased level of consciousness may result.
♦ Other findings vary with the affected artery but may include vision loss, nystagmus, aphasia, dysarthria, unilateral numbness, hemiparesis or hemiplegia, tinnitus, facial weakness, dysphagia, and staggering or uncoordinated gait.

Vagal glossopharyngeal neuralgia

♦ Localized pressure may trigger pain in the base of the tongue, pharynx, larynx, tonsils, and ear, resulting in syncope.

OTHER
Diagnostic tests

♦ Tilt table tests cause syncope to help identify a cardiogenic source of the symptom.

Drugs

♦ Occasionally, griseofulvin, indomethacin (Indocin), and levodopa (Sinemet) can produce syncope.
♦ Prazosin hydrochloride (Minipress) may cause severe orthostatic hypotension and syncope, usually after the first dose.
♦ Other medications that cause orthostatic hypotension and syncope include antihypertensives, diuretics, levodopa, monoamine oxidase inhibitors, morphine, nitrates, phenothiazines, spinal anesthesia, and tricyclic antidepressants.
♦ Quinidine may cause syncope—and possibly death—associated with ventricular fibrillation.

NURSING CONSIDERATIONS

♦ Continue to monitor vital signs, oxygenation, and heart rhythm, as appropriate.
♦ Prepare the patient for diagnostic studies.

PEDIATRIC TIPS

♦ Syncope in children may result from a cardiac or neurologic disorder, allergies, or emotional stress.

PATIENT TEACHING

♦ Discuss underlying condition.
♦ Encourage the patient to pace his activities.
♦ Explain that he should avoid standing for prolonged periods of time and to make position changes slowly.
♦ Tell him what measures to take if he's feeling faint.
♦ Discuss medications and their adverse effects.

Tachycardia

OVERVIEW

- Refers to a heart rate greater than 100 beats/minute (see *What happens in tachycardia*)
- Detected by counting the apical, carotid, or radial pulse

 ACTION STAT! *If the patient has tachycardia, increased or decreased blood pressure, drowsiness, and confusion, obtain an electrocardiograph (ECG). Give oxygen, and begin cardiac monitoring. Insert an I.V. catheter for fluid, blood, and drug administration, and keep resuscitation equipment nearby.*

HISTORY

- Explore palpitations, dizziness, shortness of breath, weakness, fatigue, syncope, and chest pain.
- Ask about a history of trauma, diabetes, and cardiac, pulmonary, or thyroid disorders.
- Obtain an alcohol and drug history.

What happens in tachycardia

Tachycardia represents the heart's effort to deliver more oxygen to body tissues by increasing the rate at which blood passes through the vessels. This sign can also reflect overstimulation within the sinoatrial node, the atrium, the atrioventricular node, or the ventricles.

Because heart rate affects cardiac output (cardiac output = heart rate x stroke volume), tachycardia can lower cardiac output by reducing ventricular filling time and stroke volume (the output of each ventricle at every contraction). As cardiac output plummets, arterial pressure and peripheral perfusion decrease. Tachycardia further aggravates myocardial ischemia by increasing the heart's demand for oxygen while reducing the duration of diastole—the period of greatest coronary blood flow.

PHYSICAL ASSESSMENT

- Inspect for pallor or cyanosis.
- Assess pulses and blood pressure and note peripheral edema.
- Auscultate the heart and lungs for abnormal sounds and rhythms.

CAUSES

MEDICAL

Acute respiratory distress syndrome
- Tachycardia, crackles, rhonchi, dyspnea, tachypnea, nasal flaring, and grunting respirations occur with this disorder.
- Other findings include cyanosis, anxiety, and decreased level of consciousness (LOC).

Adrenocortical insufficiency
- A rapid, weak pulse with progressive weakness and fatigue occur.
- Other findings include abdominal pain, nausea, vomiting, altered bowel habits, weight loss, orthostatic hypotension, irritability, bronze skin, decreased libido, and syncope.

Anemia
- Tachycardia and bounding pulse occur with anemia.
- Related findings include fatigue, pallor, dyspnea, bleeding tendencies, atrial gallop, crackles, and a systolic bruit over the carotid arteries.

Anxiety
- Tachycardia, tachypnea, chest pain, cold and clammy skin, dry mouth, nausea, and light-headedness are signs and symptoms of anxiety.

Aortic insufficiency
- Tachycardia with a bounding pulse and a large, diffuse apical heave occurs with aortic insufficiency.
- A high-pitched, blowing diastolic murmur starting with the second heart sound occurs.
- Other findings include angina, dyspnea, palpitations, strong and abrupt carotid pulsations, pallor, syncope, and signs of heart failure.

Aortic stenosis
- Tachycardia, a weak and thready pulse, and an atrial gallop occur with aortic stenosis.
- Chiefly, dyspnea, angina, dizziness, and syncope occur.
- Other findings include palpitations, crackles, fatigue, a harsh systolic ejection murmur and signs of heart failure or pulmonary edema.

Cardiac arrhythmias
- Tachycardia with hypotension, dizziness, palpitations, weakness, and fatigue occur with cardiac arrhythmias.
- Related findings include tachypnea; decreased LOC; and pale, cool, clammy skin.

Cardiac contusion
- With a cardiac contusion, tachycardia, substernal pain, dyspnea, hypotension, palpitations, sternal ecchymoses, and a pericardial rub or tamponade occur.

Cardiac tamponade
- A life-threatening disorder, cardiac tamponade causes tachycardia commonly with paradoxical pulse, dyspnea, and tachypnea.
- Other findings include anxiety, cyanosis, clammy skin, hypotension, jugular vein distention, narrowed pulse pressure, pericardial rub, muffled heart sounds, chest pain, and hepatomegaly.

Chronic obstructive pulmonary disease
- Tachycardia with cough, tachypnea, pursed-lip breathing, accessory muscle use, cyanosis, diminished breath sounds, rhonchi, crackles, wheezing and, in the late stages, barrel chest and clubbing occur in this disorder.

Diabetic ketoacidosis
- A rapid, thready pulse with Kussmaul's respirations is the cardinal sign of this disorder.
- Other findings include decreased LOC, dehydration, oliguria with ketosis.

Febrile illness
◆ Fever can cause tachycardia, chills, diaphoresis, headache, and weakness.

Heart failure
◆ Tachycardia with a ventricular gallop, fatigue, dyspnea, orthopnea, and leg edema occur.

Hyperosmolar hyperglycemic nonketotic syndrome
◆ This syndrome causes a rapidly deteriorating LOC with tachycardia, hypotension, tachypnea, seizures, oliguria without ketosis, and severe dehydration.

Hypertensive crisis
◆ A life-threatening disorder, hypertensive crisis causes tachycardia with diastolic blood pressure over 120 mm Hg and systolic blood pressure that may exceed 200 mm Hg.
◆ Related findings include tachypnea, signs of pulmonary edema, chest pain, oliguria, severe headache, confusion, anxiety, tinnitus, epistaxis, muscle twitching, seizures, nausea, vomiting, and progressive loss of conciousness.

Hypoglycemia
◆ Tachycardia with nervousness, mental confusion, weakness, headache, hunger, nausea, diaphoresis, and moist, clammy skin occur with hypoglycemia.

Hypovolemia
◆ With hypovolemia, tachycardia with hypotension, decreased urine output, fatigue, muscle weakness, decreased skin turgor, sunken eyeballs, thirst, syncope, and dry skin and tongue occur.

Hypoxemia
◆ Tachycardia with dyspnea, tachypnea, and cyanosis occur with hypoxemia.
◆ Other findings include confusion, restlessness, and disorientation, progressing to coma.

Myocardial infarction
◆ A life-threatening disorder, myocardial infarction causes tachycardia or bradycardia with crushing substernal chest pain that may radiate to the left arm, jaw, neck, or shoulder.
◆ Related findings include pallor, clammy skin, dyspnea, diaphoresis, atrial gallop, a new murmur, crackles, nausea, vomiting, anxiety, restlessness, and increased or decreased blood pressure.

Orthostatic hypotension
◆ Tachycardia with dizziness, syncope, pallor, blurred vision, diaphoresis, and nausea occur with this disorder.
◆ Dim vision, spots before the eyes, and signs of dehydration may also occur.

Pneumothorax
◆ Pneumothorax is a life-threatening disorder that causes tachycardia and other signs and symptoms of distress, such as severe dyspnea and chest pain, tachypnea, and cyanosis.
◆ Other findings include dry cough, subcutaneous crepitation, absent or decreased breath sounds, reduced or absent chest movement on the affected side, and decreased vocal fremitus.

Pulmonary embolism
◆ Tachycardia preceded by sudden dyspnea, angina, or pleuritic chest pain occurs with a pulmonary embolism.
◆ Weak peripheral pulse, tachypnea, low-grade fever, restlessness, diaphoresis, and a dry cough or a cough with blood-tinged sputum may also occur.

Shock
◆ With shock, tachycardia, tachypnea, skin temperature changes, hypotension, apprehension, and decreased LOC occur before cardiac collapse.
◆ It can be a life-threatening disorder whether the source is cardiac, hypovolemic, neurologic, or septic.

Thyrotoxicosis
◆ Tachycardia, an enlarged thyroid, nervousness, heat intolerance, weight loss despite increased appetite, diaphoresis, tremors, palpitations and, possibly, exophthalmos are classic findings.

OTHER
Diagnostic tests
◆ Cardiac catheterization and electrophysiologic studies may induce transient tachycardia.

Drugs and alcohol
◆ Acetylcholinesterase inhibitors, alpha blockers, anticholinergics, beta-adrenergic bronchodilators, nitrates, phenothiazines, sympathomimetics, and vasodilators may cause tachycardia.
◆ Excessive caffeine intake and alcohol intoxication may also cause tachycardia.

Surgery and pacemakers
◆ Cardiac surgery and pacemaker malfunction or wire irritation may cause tachycardia.

NURSING CONSIDERATIONS

◆ Continue to monitor the patient.
◆ Explain ordered diagnostic tests.
◆ Obtain a resting 12-lead ECG.

PEDIATRIC TIPS
◆ Normal heart rates for children are higher than those for adults: 130 beats/minute for a neonate, 100 beats/minute for a child age 4, 90 beats/minute for a child age 8, and 75 to 80 beats/minute for an adolescent age 16.

PATIENT TEACHING

◆ Explain the possibility of tachyarrhythmia recurrence and signs and symptoms to report.
◆ Discuss the use of antiarrhythmics, pacemaker, internal defibrillator, or ablation therapy.
◆ Teach about underlying diagnosis and treatment plan.
◆ Teach the patient how to take his pulse.

Tachypnea

- Refers to an abnormally fast respiratory rate—20 or more breaths/minute in an adult

◆ **ACTION STAT!** *Evaluate cardiopulmonary status. Obtain vital signs, including oxygen saturation; check for cyanosis, chest pain, dyspnea, tachycardia, and hypotension. If the patient has paradoxical chest movement, suspect flail chest and immediately splint the chest with your hands or with sandbags. Administer supplemental oxygen, and, if possible, place the patient in semi-Fowler's position. If respiratory failure occurs, intubation and mechanical ventilation may be needed. Insert an I.V. catheter for fluid and drug administration and begin cardiac monitoring.*

HISTORY

- Ask about the onset, precipitating factors, and description of tachypnea.
- Inquire about a history of pulmonary or cardiac conditions or anxiety attacks.
- Find out about other signs and symptoms, such as diaphoresis, chest pain, or recent weight loss.
- Take a drug history.

PHYSICAL ASSESSMENT

- Take vital signs, including oxygen saturation.
- Auscultate the chest for abnormal heart and breath sounds.
- Record the color, amount, and consistency of any sputum.
- Check for jugular vein distention.
- Examine the skin for pallor, cyanosis, edema, and warmth or coolness.

CAUSES

MEDICAL

Acute respiratory distress syndrome
- Tachypnea, an early finding, gradually worsens as fluid accumulates in the lungs.
- Other findings include accessory muscle use, grunting expirations, suprasternal and intercostal retractions, crackles, and rhonchi.

Anemia
- Tachypnea may occur, depending on the disorder.
- Other findings include fatigue, pallor, dyspnea, tachycardia, postural hypotension, bounding pulse, atrial gallop, and a systolic bruit over the carotid arteries.

Anxiety
- Tachypnea may occur with tachycardia, restlessness, chest pain, nausea, and light-headedness.

Aspiration of a foreign body
- With partial obstruction, a dry, paroxysmal cough with rapid, shallow respirations develops abruptly.
- Other findings include dyspnea, gagging or choking, intercostal retraction, nasal flaring, cyanosis, decreased or absent breath sounds, hoarseness, and stridor or coarse wheezing.

Asthma
- Tachypnea is common along with mild wheezing and a dry cough in initial stages.
- If left untreated, this disorder progresses to productive cough, prolonged expirations, intercostal and supraclavicular retractions on inspiration, severe wheezing, rhonchi, flaring nostrils, tachycardia, diaphoresis, and flushing or cyanosis.

Bronchitis (chronic)
- Mild tachypnea may occur, accompanied by a dry, hacking cough, which later produces copious amounts of sputum.
- Other findings include dyspnea, prolonged expirations, wheezing, scattered rhonchi, accessory muscle use, cyanosis, and late-stage clubbing and barrel chest.

Cardiac arrhythmias
- Tachypnea may occur along with hypotension, dizziness, palpitations, weakness, fatigue and, possibly, decreased level of consciousness (LOC).

Cardiac tamponade
- A life-threatening disorder, cardiac tamponade may cause tachypnea that's accompanied by tachycardia, dyspnea, and paradoxical pulse.
- Related findings include muffled heart sounds, pericardial rub, chest pain, hypotension, narrowed pulse pressure, hepatomegaly, anxiety, cyanosis, clammy skin, and neck vein distention.

Emphysema
- Tachypnea is accompanied by exertional dyspnea.
- Accompanying findings include anorexia, malaise, peripheral cyanosis, pursed-lip breathing, accessory muscle use, chronic productive cough, and late-stage clubbing and barrel chest.

Febrile illness
- Fever can cause tachypnea, tachycardia, chills, diaphoresis, headache, and weakness.

Flail chest
- In this life-threatening disorder tachypnea usually appears early.

◆ Other findings include paradoxical chest wall movement, rib bruises and palpable fractures, localized chest pain, hypotension, diminished breath sounds, dyspnea, and accessory muscle use.

Head trauma
◆ When trauma affects the brain stem, central neurogenic hyperventilation may produce a form of tachypnea marked by rapid, even, and deep respirations.
◆ Other signs of life-threatening neurogenic dysfunction include coma, unequal and nonreactive pupils, seizures, hemiplegia, flaccidity, and hypoactive or absent deep tendon reflexes.

Hyperosmolar hyperglycemic nonketotic syndrome
◆ Rapidly deteriorating LOC occurs with tachypnea, tachycardia, hypotension, seizures, oliguria, and signs of dehydration.

Hypoxia
◆ Tachypnea occurs, possibly with restlessness, impaired judgment, tachycardia, dyspnea, and cyanosis.

Interstitial fibrosis
◆ Tachypnea develops gradually and may become severe.
◆ Other findings include exertional dyspnea, pleuritic chest pain, a paroxysmal, dry cough, crackles, late inspiratory wheezing, cyanosis, fatigue, weight loss, and late-stage clubbing.

Lung abscess
◆ Tachypnea occurs with dyspnea and worsens with fever.
◆ The chief sign of lung abscess is a productive cough with copious amounts of purulent, foul-smelling, usually bloody sputum.

Plague
◆ Plague causes tachypnea, productive cough, chest pain, dyspnea, hemoptysis, and increasing respiratory distress and cardiopulmonary insufficiency.

Pneumonia (bacterial)
◆ Tachypnea is usually preceded by a painful, hacking, dry cough that rapidly becomes productive.
◆ Other findings include high fever, shaking chills, headache, dyspnea, pleuritic chest pain, tachycardia, grunting respirations, nasal flaring, and cyanosis.

Pneumothorax
◆ A life-threatening disorder, pneumothorax causes tachypnea and is typically accompanied by severe, sharp, one-sided chest pain.
◆ Other findings include dyspnea, tachycardia, accessory muscle use, asymmetrical chest expansion, dry cough, cyanosis, anxiety, and restlessness.
◆ Deviated trachea occurs with tension pneumothorax.

Pulmonary edema
◆ Tachypnea, an early sign, is accompanied by exertional dyspnea, paroxysmal nocturnal dyspnea and, later, orthopnea.
◆ Other findings include productive cough with pink frothy sputum, crackles, tachycardia, and a ventricular gallop.

Pulmonary embolism (acute)
◆ Sudden tachypnea occurs with dyspnea.
◆ Related findings include angina or pleuritic pain, tachycardia, a dry or productive cough with blood-tinged sputum, fever, restlessness, and diaphoresis.

Shock
◆ With shock, tachypnea, tachycardia, skin temperature changes, hypotension, apprehension, and decreased LOC occur before cardiac collapse.

Tumor
◆ A lung, pleural, or mediastinal tumor, causes tachypnea along with exertional dyspnea, cough, hemoptysis, and pleuritic chest pain.
◆ Related findings include tracheal shift, neck vein distention, weight loss, anorexia, and fatigue.

OTHER
Drugs
◆ Tachypnea may result from an overdose of salicylates.

NURSING CONSIDERATIONS

◆ Continue to monitor vital signs and oxygenation status.
◆ Keep suction and emergency equipment nearby.
◆ Prepare for intubation and mechanical ventilation if needed.

PEDIATRIC TIPS
◆ Normal respiratory rate varies with the child's age.
◆ Other causes include congenital heart defects, meningitis, metabolic acidosis, cystic fibrosis, hunger, and anxiety.

GERIATRIC TIPS
◆ In the older adult patient, heart failure, chronic obstructive pulmonary disease, anxiety, or failure to take cardiac and respiratory drugs appropriately may cause tachypnea.

PATIENT TEACHING

◆ Explain that slight increases in respiratory rate may be normal.
◆ Teach about underlying diagnosis and treatment plan.
◆ Discuss importance of compliance with drug therapy.

Taste abnormalities

OVERVIEW

- Include a loss of taste (ageusia), partial loss of taste (hypogeusia), a distorted sense of taste (dysgeusia), or an unpleasant sense of taste (cacogeusia)
- Refer to abnormal function of sensory receptors for taste (the taste buds)

that are concentrated over the tongue's surface and scattered over the palate, pharynx, and larynx
- Complex flavors perceived by taste and olfactory receptors
- Caused by any factor that interrupts the transmission of taste stimuli to receptors in the brain (see *Tracing taste pathways to the brain*)

HISTORY

- Ask about the onset of taste abnormality.
- Find out about a history of oral or other disorders.
- Note recent flu, head trauma, or radiation treatments.
- Ask about smoking habits.
- Take a drug history.

PHYSICAL ASSESSMENT

- Evaluate taste: Withdraw the tongue with a gauze sponge, apply various flavors (such as salt or sugar) on the tongue, and ask the patient to identify the tastes.
- Inspect the oral cavity for lesions, sores, and mucosal or taste bud abnormalities.
- Evaluate sense of smell: Pinch one nostril and ask the patient to close his eyes and sniff through the open nostril to identify nonirritating odors such as coffee. Repeat test on the other nostril.

CAUSES

MEDICAL
Basilar skull fracture
- If the first cranial nerve is involved, the patient usually can't detect aromatic flavors.
- Other findings include epistaxis, rhinorrhea, otorrhea, Battle's sign, raccoon eyes, headache, nausea, vomiting, hearing and vision loss, and a decreased level of consciousness.

Bell's palsy
- Taste loss in the anterior two-thirds of the tongue is common along with hemifacial muscle weakness or paralysis.
- Affected side of the face sags and is masklike.
- Associated signs include drooling and tearing, diminished or absent corneal reflex, and difficulty blinking the affected eye.

Tracing taste pathways to the brain

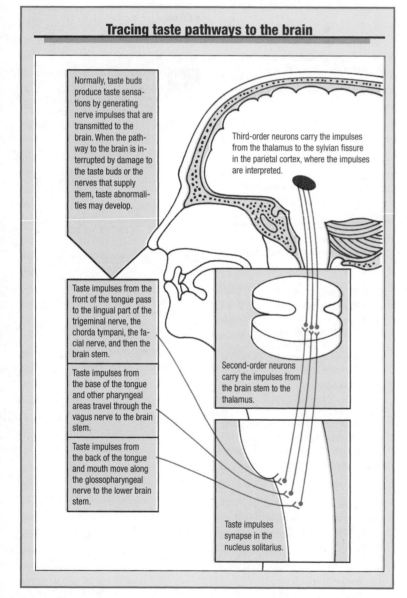

Normally, taste buds produce taste sensations by generating nerve impulses that are transmitted to the brain. When the pathway to the brain is interrupted by damage to the taste buds or the nerves that supply them, taste abnormalities may develop.

Third-order neurons carry the impulses from the thalamus to the sylvian fissure in the parietal cortex, where the impulses are interpreted.

Taste impulses from the front of the tongue pass to the lingual part of the trigeminal nerve, the chorda tympani, the facial nerve, and then the brain stem.

Taste impulses from the base of the tongue and other pharyngeal areas travel through the vagus nerve to the brain stem.

Taste impulses from the back of the tongue and mouth move along the glossopharyngeal nerve to the lower brain stem.

Second-order neurons carry the impulses from the brain stem to the thalamus.

Taste impulses synapse in the nucleus solitarius.

Common cold

- Impaired taste is usually from loss of smell due to congestion.
- Other common findings include rhinorrhea with sore throat, headache, fatigue, myalgia, arthralgia, malaise, and a dry, hacking cough.

Geographic tongue

- Taste abnormalities occur with areas of loss and regrowth of filiform papillae.
- Affected areas are continually changing and produce a maplike appearance with denuded red patches surrounded by thick white borders.

Influenza

- The patient may have hypogeusia, dysgeusia, or both as well as an impaired sense of smell.
- Common complaints include sore throat, fever with chills, headache, weakness, malaise, muscle aches, cough and, occasionally, hoarseness and rhinorrhea.

Oral cancer

- Tumors involving the tongue may destroy or damage taste buds.
- Other findings include difficulty chewing and speaking, and halitosis.

Sjögren's syndrome

- Impaired sense of taste results from extreme dry mouth and occurs with ocular dryness, burning, and pain around the eyes and under the lids.
- Other findings include photosensitivity; impaired vision; eye redness; mouth soreness; difficulty chewing, swallowing, and talking; a dry cough; hoarseness; epistaxis; dry, scaly skin; decreased sweating; abdominal distress; and polyuria.

Thalamic syndrome

- A distorted sense of taste is preceded by contralateral sensory loss, transient hemiparesis, and homonymous hemianopia.
- Later, sensation is gradually regained, and pain or hyperpathia may then be experienced.

Thrush

- Cream-colored or bluish white patches of exudate on the tongue, mouth, or pharynx cause altered taste, pain, and burning.

Viral hepatitis (acute)

- Hypogeusia commonly precedes jaundice by 1 to 2 weeks.
- Associated preicteric findings include altered sense of smell, anorexia, nausea, vomiting, fatigue, malaise, headache, photophobia, muscle and joint aches, sore throat, and a cough.

Vitamin B_{12} deficiency

- Hypogeusia is accompanied by impaired sense of smell, anorexia, weight loss, abdominal discomfort, and glossitis.
- Yellow skin, peripheral neuropathy, dyspnea, ataxic gait, and dementia may also occur.

Zinc deficiency

- Idiopathic hypogeusia may occur with cacogeusia.
- Other findings include a distorted sense of smell, anorexia, soft and misshapen nails, hepatosplenomegaly, and sparse hair growth.

OTHER
Drugs

- Antibiotics, antithyroid drugs, captopril (Capoten), griseofulvin, lithium (Eskalith), penicillamine (Cuprimine), procarbazine hydrochloride (Matulane), rifampin (Rifadin), vincristine sulfate, and vinblastine sulfate may distort the sense of taste.

Radiation therapy

- Irradiation of the head or neck may cause excessive dryness of the mouth, resulting in impaired taste sensation.

NURSING CONSIDERATIONS

- Modify the patient's diet if needed.
- Encourage oral hygiene before and after meals.

PEDIATRIC TIPS

- Children may be unable to differentiate between abnormal taste sensation and taste dislike.

GERIATRIC TIPS

- Aging reduces the number of taste buds, leading to impaired taste.

PATIENT TEACHING

- Emphasize proper oral hygiene.
- Discuss the use of spices to enhance flavors.
- Provide referral to a dietitian as needed.
- Discuss underlying condition, diagnostic tests, and treatment plan.

Tearing, increased

OVERVIEW

- Refers to excessive lacrimation or tear production
- Also known as epiphora
- Usually results from inadequate tear drainage because of obstruction of the lacrimal drainage system or malposition of the lower lid
- May occur in response to emotional or physical stress (psychic lacrimation)
- May be neurogenic—lacrimation triggered by reflex stimulation associated with ocular trauma or inflammation or with exposure to environmental irritants
- Tearing can also be decreased resulting from aging, vitamin A deficiency, eye trauma, and certain drugs (see *Causes of decreased tearing*)

HISTORY

- Ask about the onset and description of tearing.
- Find out about accompanying pain, irritation, or discharge.
- Inquire about a history of eye trauma or ocular and systemic disorders.
- Take a drug history.
- Discuss possible occupational hazards.

PHYSICAL ASSESSMENT

- Examine the external structures of both eyes.
- Examine the eyelids for lesions and edema.
- Determine whether the eyeballs appear shrunken or swollen.
- Check for ptosis.
- Examine the conjunctiva for redness and abnormal drainage.
- Note the color of the sclera.
- Using a flashlight, examine the cornea and iris for scars, irregularities, and foreign bodies.
- Evaluate extraocular muscle function by testing the six cardinal fields of gaze.
- Test visual acuity.

CAUSES

MEDICAL
Conjunctival foreign bodies and abrasions
- Increased tearing may occur with localized conjunctival injection, eye pain, and photophobia.
- A foreign-body sensation may be present.

Conjunctivitis
- With conjunctivitis, increased tearing, conjunctival injection, and itching occur.
- With allergic conjunctivitis, a stringy discharge occurs.
- With bacterial conjunctivitis, copious, purulent discharge; burning; a foreign-body sensation; and eye pain if the cornea is involved may occur.
- With fungal conjunctivitis, lid edema; burning; photophobia; pain if the cornea is involved; and a copious, thick, purulent discharge that may form sticky crusts on the lids occur.
- With viral conjunctivitis, a foreign-body sensation, slight exudate, and lid edema occur.

Corneal abrasion
- Corneal pain with increased tearing and severe pain is aggravated by itching and blinking.
- A foreign-body sensation, blurred vision, conjunctival injection, and photophobia may also occur.

Corneal foreign body
- Increased tearing, blurred vision, a foreign-body sensation, photophobia, eye pain, miosis, and conjunctival injection occur.
- Dark specks may be visible in the cornea.

Corneal ulcers
- Increased tearing, severe photophobia, and eye pain aggravated by blinking occur.
- Related findings include blurred vision, conjunctival injection, and a white, opaque cornea.

Causes of decreased tearing

Decreased tearing makes the patient's eyes uncomfortably dry. This symptom is usually associated with aging, but it may also result from:

- *Anticholinergics.* Decreased tearing commonly follows use of an anticholinergic (mydriatic), such as atropine, scopolamine, cyclopentolate, and tropicamide.
- *Keratoconjunctivitis sicca (dry eye syndrome).* With dry eye syndrome, atrophy of the lacrimal glands curtails tear production.
- *Ocular trauma.* Decreased tearing during healing and scar formation follows acute ocular trauma.
- *Sarcoidosis.* Decreased tearing results from inflammation of the lacrimal and salivary glands in this syndrome.
- *Stevens-Johnson syndrome.* With Stevens-Johnson syndrome, decreased tearing is accompanied by purulent conjunctivitis and severe eye pain.
- *Turner's syndrome.* Characterized by congenital absence of the lacrimal gland, Turner's syndrome causes decreased tearing.
- *Vitamin A deficiency.* Typically, vitamin A deficiency causes decreased tearing and poor night vision.

Nontraumatic decreased tearing is usually treated with artificial tears as either drops or ointment.

- With bacterial ulcers, a copious, purulent discharge that may form sticky crusts on the lids occurs.

Dacryocystitis
- Increased tearing and a purulent discharge are the chief complaints.
- Other findings include pain and tenderness around the tear sac with marked eyelid edema and redness near the lacrimal punctum.
- Pressing the tear sac produces a thick, purulent discharge or, in chronic cases, a mucoid discharge.

Dry eye syndrome
- Excess tearing from excessive dryness of the cornea and conjunctiva occurs.
- Other findings include eye pain, conjunctival injection, and itching.

Episcleritis
- Increased tearing and photophobia occur.
- If the sclera is inflamed, eye pain and tenderness on palpation may also occur.
- Related findings include conjunctival injection and edema, a purplish pink sclera, and episcleral edema.

Herpes zoster
- If the trigeminal nerve is affected, increased tearing occurs.
- Severe one-sided facial and eye pain is followed by the eruption of vesicles within several days.
- Associated findings include red and swollen eyelids, scanty serous discharge, conjunctival injection, and a white, cloudy cornea.

Lid contractions
- Increased tearing from stricture of the canaliculi occurs.

Psoriasis vulgaris
- Lesions that affect the eyelids and extend into the conjunctiva may cause irritation, increased tearing, and a foreign-body sensation.
- Early signs include chronic conjunctivitis and conjunctival injection.

Punctum misplacement
- Increased tearing with keratitis occurs.

Thyrotoxicosis
- Increased tearing in both eyes occurs.
- In the eyes, ptosis, lid edema, photophobia, a foreign-body sensation, conjunctival injection, chemosis, diplopia, and, at times, exophthalmos may also occur.
- Related findings include weight loss despite increased appetite, heat intolerance, nervousness, sweating, diarrhea, tremors, tachycardia, palpitations, and an enlarged thyroid.

OTHER
Drugs
- Cholinergic drugs, such as miotics and pilocarpine hydrochloride (Salagen), may cause increased tearing.

NURSING CONSIDERATIONS

- Obtain a tear specimen for culture.
- Prepare the patient for Schirmer's test and irrigation of lacrimal drainage system.
- Follow standard precautions to prevent transmitting the infection.

PEDIATRIC TIPS
- The most common causes of increased tearing in children are allergies, conjunctivitis, and the common cold.

PATIENT TEACHING

- Explain the importance of avoiding cross-contamination and correct application of eye drops or ointments.
- Teach the patient good hand-washing techniques.
- Explain underlying diagnosis and treatment plan.

Throat pain

OVERVIEW

- Refers to discomfort in pharynx
- Ranges from sensation of scratchiness to severe pain
- Typically accompanied by ear pain because cranial nerves IX and X innervate the pharynx as well as the middle and external ear (see *Anatomy of the throat*)

HISTORY

- Ask about the onset of throat pain.
- Find out about fever, ear pain, or dysphagia.
- Take a medical history, including throat problems, mouth breathing, and allergies.
- Ask about vocal strain, alcohol consumption, and inhalation of smoke or chemicals such as ammonia.

PHYSICAL ASSESSMENT

- Examine the pharynx, oropharynx, nasopharynx and tonsils, noting redness, exudate, and swelling.
- Examine the nose, using a nasal speculum.
- Check the ears using an otoscope.
- Palpate neck and oropharynx for nodules or lymph node enlargement.

CAUSES

MEDICAL
Agranulocytosis
- Sore throat occurs after progressive fatigue and weakness.
- Related findings include nausea, vomiting, anorexia, bleeding tendencies and, possibly, ulcers on the gums, palate, or perianal area.

Allergic rhinitis
- Sore throat occurs with nasal congestion with a thin nasal discharge, postnasal drip, paroxysmal sneezing, decreased sense of smell, headache, and itchy eyes, nose, and throat.

Avian flu
- Throat pain, muscle aches, cough, and fever are common early symptoms of this disorder.
- Other findings include pneumonia and acute respiratory distress.

Bronchitis (acute)
- Lower throat pain occurs with fever, chills, productive cough, and muscle and back pain.
- Other findings include rhonchi, wheezing, and crackles.

Chronic fatigue syndrome
- Incapacitating fatigue with sore throat, myalgia, lymphadenopathy, and cognitive dysfunction occur.

Common cold
- Sore throat occurs with cough, sneezing, nasal congestion, mouth breathing, rhinorrhea, fatigue, headache, myalgia, and arthralgia.

Anatomy of the throat

The throat, or pharynx, is divided into three areas: the nasopharynx (the soft palate and the posterior nasal cavity), the oropharynx (the area between the soft palate and the upper edge of the epiglottis), and the hypopharynx (the area between the epiglottis and the level of the cricoid cartilage). A disorder affecting any of these areas may cause throat pain. Pinpointing the causative disorder begins with accurate assessment of the throat structures illustrated here.

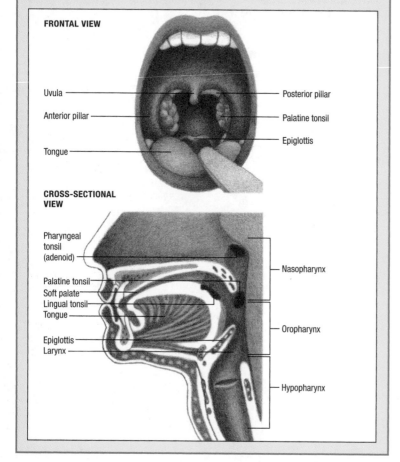

FRONTAL VIEW

Uvula
Anterior pillar
Tongue
Posterior pillar
Palatine tonsil
Epiglottis

CROSS-SECTIONAL VIEW

Pharyngeal tonsil (adenoid)
Palatine tonsil
Soft palate
Lingual tonsil
Tongue
Epiglottis
Larynx
Nasopharynx
Oropharynx
Hypopharynx

Contact ulcers
- Ulcers appear symmetrically on the posterior vocal cords, resulting in sore throat.
- Pain is aggravated by talking and may occur with referred ear pain and, occasionally, hemoptysis.

Gastroesophageal reflux disease
- Chronic sore throat and hoarseness occur.
- Pyrosis is common.

Glossopharyngeal neuralgia
- Knifelike throat pain occurs on one side in the tonsillar fossa, possibly radiating to the ear.
- Sore throat may also result from yawning, chewing, swallowing, or eating spicy foods.

Herpes simplex virus
- Sore throat may result from lesions on the oral mucosa.
- Lesions erupt into erythematous vesicles that eventually rupture and leave a painful ulcer, followed by a yellowish crust.

Influenza
- Sore throat with fever, chills, headache, weakness, malaise, cough, muscle aches and, occasionally, hoarseness and rhinorrhea may occur.

Laryngeal cancer
- With extrinsic laryngeal cancer, pain or burning in the throat when drinking citrus juice or hot liquids occurs, or the patient feels a lump in the throat.
- With intrinsic laryngeal cancer, hoarseness lasts for longer than 3 weeks.

Laryngitis (acute)
- Sore throat with mild to severe hoarseness is the chief sign.
- Related findings include malaise, fever, dysphagia, dry cough, and tender, enlarged lymph nodes.

Mononucleosis (infectious)
- Sore throat, cervical lymphadenopathy, and fluctuating temperature occur.

- Possible findings include hepatomegaly and splenomegaly.

Necrotizing ulcerative gingivitis (acute)
- Abrupt sore throat occurs, and gums ulcerate and bleed.
- Gray exudate on the gums and pharyngeal tonsils also may occur.
- Related findings include a foul taste in the mouth, halitosis, cervical lymphadenopathy, headache, malaise, and fever.

Oral cancer
- Localized pain occurs around lesion or ulcer of throat, tongue, or tonsils.
- Pain may radiate to the ear, and dysphagia may occur.

Peritonsillar abscess
- Severe throat pain, radiating to the ear may occur.
- Related findings include dysphagia, drooling, dysarthria, halitosis, fever with chills, malaise, and nausea.

Pharyngeal burns
- Throat pain and dysphagia occur.
- If the larynx is involved, laryngeal edema, bronchospasm, and stridor may also occur.

Pharyngitis
- The bacterial form causes abrupt sore throat on one side.
- The fungal form causes a diffuse, burning sore throat.
- The viral form causes a diffuse sore throat, malaise, fever, and mild erythema and edema of the posterior oropharyngeal wall.

Pharyngomaxillary space abscess
- Mild throat pain with a bulge in the medial wall of the pharynx and swelling of the neck on the affected side occur.
- Related findings include fever, dysphagia, trismus and, possibly, signs of respiratory distress or toxemia.

Sinusitis (acute)
- Sore throat with purulent nasal discharge and postnasal drip occur with acute sinusitis.

- Other findings include halitosis, headache, malaise, cough, fever, and facial pain and swelling associated with nasal congestion.

Tonsillitis
- With acute tonsillitis, mild-to-severe throat pain occurs.
- With chronic tonsillitis, mild sore throat occurs.
- With lingual tonsillitis, throat pain on one or both sides, just above the hyoid bone occurs.

Uvulitis
- Throat pain or a sensation of something in the throat occurs.
- Related findings include swollen and red uvula; in allergic uvulitis, pale uvula.

OTHER
Treatments
- Endotracheal intubation and local surgery, such as tonsillectomy and adenoidectomy, may cause throat pain.
- Radiation therapy to the head and neck may cause throat pain.

NURSING CONSIDERATIONS
- Provide analgesic sprays or lozenges to relieve throat pain.
- Prepare the patient for throat culture, blood work, and a monospot test.

PEDIATRIC TIPS
- Causes of sore throat in children include acute epiglottiditis, herpangina, scarlet fever, acute follicular tonsillitis, and retropharyngeal abscess.

PATIENT TEACHING
- Explain the importance of completing the full course of antibiotic treatment.
- Discuss ways to soothe the throat.
- Teach about underlying diagnosis and treatment plan.

Thyroid enlargement

OVERVIEW

- Caused by inflammation, physiologic changes, iodine deficiency, and thyroid tumors or hormone imbalance
- Results from either hyperfunction or hypofunction, depending on the medical cause, with resulting excess or deficiency of the hormone thyroxine
- May cause goiter, an enlarged thyroid that causes visible swelling in the front of the neck

HISTORY

- Ask about the onset of enlargement.
- Inquire about the use of thyroid hormone replacement drugs.
- Ask about previous irradiation of the thyroid gland or the neck and about recent infections.
- Take a personal and family history, including thyroid disease.

PHYSICAL ASSESSMENT

- Inspect the trachea for midline deviation.
- Palpate the enlarged gland; note the size, shape, consistency of gland, and the presence or absence of nodules. (See *Palpating the thyroid gland.*)
- Using bell of stethoscope, listen over the lobes of the thyroid gland for a bruit.

 TOP TECHNIQUE

Palpating the thyroid gland

To palpate the thyroid gland, you'll need to stand behind the patient. Give the patient a cup of water and have him extend his neck slightly. Place the fingers of both hands on the patient's neck, just below the cricoid cartilage and just alongside the trachea. Tell the patient to take a sip of water and swallow. The thyroid gland should rise as he swallows. Use your fingers to palpate on the sides and downward to feel the whole thyroid gland. Palpate over the midline to feel the isthmus of the thyroid as shown here.

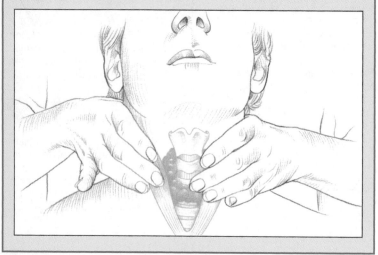

CAUSES

MEDICAL

Hypothyroidism

- Enlarged thyroid occurs with weight gain despite anorexia; fatigue; cold intolerance; constipation; menorrhagia; slowed intellectual and motor activity; dry, pale, cool skin; dry, sparse hair; and thick, brittle nails.
- Eventually, the face assumes a dull expression with periorbital edema.

Thyroiditis

- Autoimmune thyroiditis may not produce symptoms other than thyroid enlargement.
- In subacute granulomatous thyroiditis, thyroid enlargement may follow an upper respiratory infection or a sore throat; other findings may include a painful and tender thyroid and dysphagia.

Thyrotoxicosis

- An enlarged thyroid gland is a classic finding.
- Other findings include nervousness; heat intolerance; fatigue; weight loss despite increased appetite; diarrhea; sweating; palpitations; tremors; smooth, warm, flushed skin; fine, soft hair; exophthalmos; nausea and vomiting; and oligomenorrhea or amenorrhea.

Tumors

- An enlarged thyroid may be accompanied by hoarseness, loss of voice, and dysphagia.
- A malignant tumor usually appears as a single nodule in the neck.
- A nonmalignant tumor may appear as multiple nodules in the neck.

OTHER

Drugs

- Certain drugs, including aminosalicylic acid (Paser), lithium (Eskalith), phenylbutazone, and sulfonamides may decrease thyroxine production.

Goitrogens

- Foods containing goitrogens include peanuts, cabbage, soybeans, strawberries, spinach, rutabagas, and radishes and may cause an enlarged thyroid.

NURSING CONSIDERATIONS

- Prepare the patient for diagnostic tests and surgery or radiation therapy, if needed.
- Specific interventions depend on whether the patient is hypothyroid, has thyroiditis, or is recovering from a thyroidectomy.

PEDIATRIC TIPS

- Congenital goiter, a syndrome of infantile myxedema or cretinism, is characterized by mental retardation, growth failure, and other signs and symptoms of hypothyroidism; early treatment can prevent mental retardation.

PATIENT TEACHING

- Explain the signs and symptoms of hypothyroidism or hyperthyroidism to report.
- Describe posttreatment precautions to a patient undergoing radioactive iodine therapy.
- Teach about thyroid hormone replacement therapy and signs of thyroid hormone overdose.

Tinnitus

OVERVIEW

- Refers to abnormal ringing, sizzling, buzzing, or humming in the ear
- Can be classified as subjective or objective and as tinnitus aurium (the patient hears noise in his ears) or tinnitus cerebri (the patient hears noise in his head)
- Usually associated with neural injury in the auditory pathway (see *Common causes of tinnitus*)

HISTORY

- Ask about the onset, location, and description of the sound.
- Inquire about other symptoms, such as vertigo, headache, or hearing loss.
- Take a health and drug history.

PHYSICAL ASSESSMENT

- Inspect the ears and examine the tympanic membrane, using an otoscope.
- Perform Weber's test and the Rinne tests to check for hearing loss.
- Auscultate for bruits in the neck.
- Compress the jugular or carotid artery to see if this affects the tinnitus.
- Examine the nasopharynx for masses that might cause eustachian tube dysfunction and tinnitus.

CAUSES

MEDICAL
Acoustic neuroma
- Tinnitus in one ear precedes sensorineural hearing loss and vertigo in the same ear.
- Facial paralysis, headache, nausea, vomiting, and papilledema may occur.

Anemia
- Mild tinnitus may occur, if anemia is severe.
- Other findings include pallor, weakness, fatigue, exertional dyspnea, tachycardia, bounding pulse, atrial gallop, and a systolic bruit over the carotid arteries.

Atherosclerosis of the carotid artery
- Constant tinnitus can be stopped by applying pressure over the carotid artery.
- Auscultation over the upper part of the neck, on the auricle, or near the ear on the affected side may detect a bruit.
- Palpation may reveal a weak carotid pulse.

Cervical spondylosis
- Osteophytic growths may compress the vertebral arteries, resulting in tinnitus.
- A stiff neck and pain aggravated by activity accompany tinnitus.
- Other findings include brief vertigo, nystagmus, hearing loss, paresthesia, weakness, and pain that radiates down the arms.

Ear canal obstruction
- Tinnitus with conductive hearing loss, itching, blockage, and a feeling of fullness or pain in the ear may occur.

Eustachian tube patency
- Tinnitus, audible breath sounds, loud and distorted voice sounds, and

---

Common causes of tinnitus

Tinnitus usually results from a disorder that affects the external, middle, or inner ear. Below are some of its more common causes and their locations.

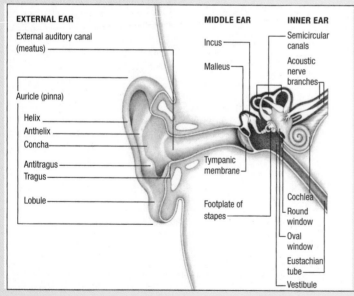

EXTERNAL EAR
- External auditory canal (meatus)
- Auricle (pinna)
- Helix
- Anthelix
- Concha
- Antitragus
- Tragus
- Lobule

MIDDLE EAR
- Incus
- Malleus
- Tympanic membrane
- Footplate of stapes

INNER EAR
- Semicircular canals
- Acoustic nerve branches
- Cochlea
- Round window
- Oval window
- Eustachian tube
- Vestibule

EXTERNAL EAR
- Ear canal obstruction by cerumen or a foreign body
- Otitis externa
- Tympanic membrane perforation

MIDDLE EAR
- Ossicle dislocation
- Otitis media
- Otosclerosis

INNER EAR
- Acoustic neuroma
- Atherosclerosis of carotid artery
- Labyrinthitis
- Ménière's disease

---

a sense of fullness in the ear can occur.

◆ Use a pneumatic otoscope to see if the tympanic membrane moves with respiration.

Hypertension
◆ High-pitched tinnitus in both ears may occur with severe hypertension.
◆ Diastolic blood pressure over 120 mm Hg may also cause severe, throbbing headache; restlessness; nausea; vomiting; blurred vision; seizures; and decreased level of consciousness.

Intracranial arteriovenous malformation
◆ A large malformation may cause tinnitus accompanied by a bruit over the mastoid process.
◆ Other findings include severe headache, seizures, and progressive neurologic deficits.

Labyrinthitis (suppurative)
◆ Tinnitus occurs with sudden, severe attacks of vertigo, sensorineural hearing loss in one or both ears, nystagmus, dizziness, nausea, and vomiting.

Ménière's disease
◆ Attacks of tinnitus occur with vertigo, a feeling of fullness or blockage in the ear, and fluctuating sensorineural hearing loss for 10 minutes to several hours.
◆ Other findings include severe nausea, vomiting, diaphoresis, and nystagmus.

Ossicle dislocation
◆ Tinnitus and sensorineural hearing loss occur.
◆ Possible bleeding from the middle ear may also occur.

Otitis externa (acute)
◆ If debris in the external ear canal invades the tympanic membrane, tinnitus may result.
◆ More typical findings include pruritus, foul-smelling purulent discharge, and severe ear pain that are aggravated by manipulation of the

tragus or auricle, teeth clenching, mouth opening, and chewing.
◆ External ear canal appears red and edematous and may be occluded by debris, causing partial hearing loss.

Otitis media
◆ Tinnitus and conductive hearing loss may occur.
◆ More typical findings include ear pain, a red and bulging tympanic membrane, high fever, chills, and dizziness.

Otosclerosis
◆ The patient may describe ringing, roaring, or whistling tinnitus or a combination of these sounds.
◆ Progressive hearing loss and vertigo may occur.

Presbycusis
◆ Tinnitus and a progressive, symmetrical, sensorineural hearing loss in both ears, usually of high frequency tones occur.

Tympanic membrane perforation
◆ Tinnitus is usually the chief complaint in a small perforation; hearing loss, in a larger perforation.
◆ Other findings include pain, vertigo, and a feeling of fullness in the ear.

OTHER
Drugs and alcohol
◆ Alcohol, indomethacin (Indocin), and quinine sulfate may also cause reversible tinnitus.
◆ Common drugs that may cause irreversible tinnitus include the aminoglycoside antibiotics and vancomycin.
◆ Overdose of salicylates commonly causes reversible tinnitus.

Noise
◆ Chronic exposure to noise, especially high-pitched sounds, can damage the ear's hair cells, causing temporary or permanent tinnitus and total hearing loss.

◆ Take steps to communicate clearly with patients with hearing loss.
◆ Address safety concerns in patients with vertigo.
◆ A hearing aid may be used to amplify environmental sounds, thereby obscuring tinnitus.

PEDIATRIC TIPS
◆ Maternal use of ototoxic drugs during the third trimester of pregnancy can cause labyrinthine damage in the fetus, resulting in tinnitus.

PATIENT TEACHING
◆ Educate the patient about strategies for adapting to the tinnitus.
◆ Provide information about avoidance of excessive noise, ototoxic agents, and other factors that may cause cochlear damage.
◆ Teach the patient about the treatment plan.
◆ Prepare the patient for diagnostic testing.

Tracheal deviation

OVERVIEW

◆ Signals an underlying condition that can compromise pulmonary function and possibly cause respiratory distress (see *Detecting slight tracheal deviation*)
◆ Occurs with disorders that produce mediastinal shift from asymmetrical thoracic volume or pressure
◆ Is a classic sign of life-threatening tension pneumothorax

 ACTION STAT! *Look for signs and symptoms of respiratory distress. If possible, place the patient in semi-Fowler's position to aid chest expansion and improve oxygenation. Give supplemental oxygen, and prepare for intubation if needed. Insert an I.V. catheter for fluid and drug administration. Palpate for subcutaneous crepitation in the neck and chest, a sign of tension pneumothorax. Chest tube insertion may be needed to release trapped air or fluid and to restore normal intrapleural and intrathoracic pressure gradients.*

HISTORY

◆ Take a history of pulmonary or cardiac disorders, surgery, trauma, or infection.
◆ Ask about smoking habits.
◆ Find out about other signs and symptoms, such as breathing difficulty, pain, and cough.

PHYSICAL ASSESSMENT

◆ Take vital signs.
◆ Observe for respiratory distress.
◆ Perform a complete cardiopulmonary assessment.

CAUSES

MEDICAL
Atelectasis
◆ Extensive lung collapse can produce tracheal deviation toward the affected side.
◆ Respiratory findings include dyspnea, tachypnea, pleuritic chest pain, dry cough, dullness on percussion, decreased vocal fremitus and breath sounds, inspiratory lag, and substernal or intercostal retractions.

Hiatal hernia
◆ Intrusion of abdominal viscera into the pleural space causes tracheal deviation toward the unaffected side.
◆ Other findings include pyrosis, regurgitation or vomiting, chest or abdominal pain, and respiratory distress.

Kyphoscoliosis
◆ Rib cage distortion and mediastinal shift produces tracheal deviation toward the compressed lung.
◆ Respiratory findings include dry cough, dyspnea, asymmetrical chest expansion and, possibly, asymmetrical breath sounds.
◆ Backache and fatigue are common.

Mediastinal tumor
◆ If large, a mediastinal tumor can press against the trachea and nearby structures, causing tracheal deviation and dysphagia.
◆ Other late findings include stridor, dyspnea, brassy cough, hoarseness, and stertorous respirations with suprasternal retraction.
◆ Shoulder, arm, or chest pain, and edema of the neck, face, or arm may develop.
◆ Neck and chest wall veins may be dilated.

Pleural effusion
◆ If the effusion is large, the mediastinum can shift to the contralateral side, producing tracheal deviation.
◆ Related findings include dry cough, dyspnea, pleuritic pain, pleural friction rub, tachypnea, decreased chest

TOP TECHNIQUE

Detecting slight tracheal deviation

Although gross tracheal deviation is visible, detection of slight deviation requires palpation and perhaps even an X-ray. Try palpation first.

With the tip of your index finger, locate the patient's trachea by palpating between the sternocleidomastoid muscles, as shown here. Then compare the trachea's position to an imaginary line drawn vertically through the suprasternal notch. Any deviation from midline is usually considered abnormal.

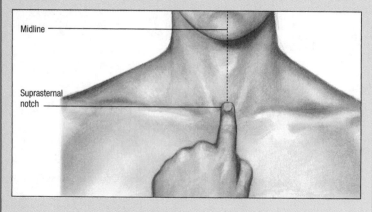

Midline

Suprasternal notch

motion, decreased or absent breath sounds, egophony, flatness on percussion, decreased tactile fremitus, fever, and weight loss.

Pulmonary fibrosis

◆ Tracheal deviation occurs as the mediastinum shifts toward the affected side.
◆ Other possible findings include dyspnea, cough, clubbing, malaise, and fever.

Pulmonary tuberculosis

◆ Tracheal deviation occurs toward the affected side with asymmetrical chest excursion, and inspiratory crackles.
◆ Insidious early findings include anorexia, weight loss, fever, chills, and night sweats.
◆ Productive cough, hemoptysis, pleuritic chest pain, and dyspnea occur as the disease progresses.

Tension pneumothorax

◆ A life-threatening disorder, tension pneumothorax causes tracheal deviation toward the unaffected side.
◆ Related findings include sudden onset of respiratory distress, sharp chest pain, dry cough, severe dyspnea, tachycardia, wheezing, cyanosis, accessory muscle use, nasal flaring, air hunger, and asymmetrical chest movement.
◆ Other findings include restlessness, anxiety, subcutaneous crepitation in the neck and upper chest, decreased or absent breath sounds on the affected side, jugular vein distention, and hypotension.

Thoracic aortic aneurysm

◆ The trachea usually deviates to the right.
◆ Findings may include stridor; dyspnea; wheezing; brassy cough; hoarseness; dysphagia; edema of the face, neck, or arm; jugular vein distention; and substernal, neck, shoulder, or lower back pain.

NURSING CONSIDERATIONS

◆ Monitor respiratory and cardiac condition constantly.
◆ Make sure that emergency equipment is readily available.
◆ Give analgesics for comfort if needed.
◆ Provide emotional support.

PEDIATRIC TIPS

◆ Respiratory distress typically develops more rapidly in children than in adults.

GERIATRIC TIPS

◆ Tracheal deviation to the right commonly stems from an elongated, atherosclerotic aortic arch, but this deviation isn't considered abnormal.

PATIENT TEACHING

◆ Teach the patient how to perform coughing and deep-breathing exercises.
◆ Explain signs and symptoms of respiratory difficulty to report.
◆ Teach about underlying diagnosis and treatment plan.

Tremors

- Refer to rhythmic, involuntary, oscillatory trembling that result from alternating contraction of opposing muscle groups
- Are characterized by their location, amplitude, and frequency
- Are classified as resting (occurs in extremity at rest, subsides with movement), intention (occurs with movement, subsides at rest) or postural (occurs when extremity or trunk is actively held in a particular position)

HISTORY

- Ask about the onset, duration, and progression of tremors.
- Determine what aggravates or alleviates tremors.
- Find out about other symptoms, such as behavioral changes or memory loss.
- Explore personal and family history of neurologic, endocrine, or metabolic disorders.
- Obtain a drug history, especially use of phenothiazines.
- Ask about alcohol use.

PHYSICAL ASSESSMENT

- Assess overall appearance and demeanor, noting mental condition.
- Test range of motion and strength in all major muscle groups while observing for chorea, athetosis, dystonia, and other involuntary movements.
- Check deep tendon reflexes (DTRs).
- Observe the patient's gait.

CAUSES

MEDICAL
Alcohol withdrawal syndrome
- Resting and intention tremors occur as soon as 7 hours after the last drink and progressively worsen.
- Early findings include diaphoresis, tachycardia, elevated blood pressure, anxiety, restlessness, irritability, insomnia, headache, nausea, and vomiting.
- In severe withdrawal, profound tremors, agitation, confusion, hallucinations, and seizures occur.

Alkalosis
- A severe intention tremor occurs with twitching, carpopedal spasms, agitation, diaphoresis, and hyperventilation.
- Other findings include dizziness, tinnitus, palpitations, and peripheral and circumoral cyanosis.

Cerebellar tumor
- An intention tremor is a classic sign.
- Related findings include ataxia, nystagmus, incoordination, muscle weakness and atrophy, and hypoactive or absent DTRs.

Graves' disease
- Fine hand tremors occur along with nervousness, weight loss, fatigue, palpitations, dyspnea, heat intolerance, an enlarged thyroid gland and, possibly, exophthalmos.

Hypercapnia
- A rapid, fine intention tremor occurs.

- Associated findings include headache, fatigue, blurred vision, weakness, lethargy, and decreased level of consciousness (LOC).

Hypoglycemia
- A rapid, fine intention tremor occurs with confusion, weakness, tachycardia, diaphoresis, and cold, clammy skin.
- Possible disappearing tremor as hypoglycemia worsens and hypotonia and decreased LOC become evident.
- Early findings include headache, profound hunger, nervousness, and blurred or double vision.

Kwashiorkor
- In the advanced stages of this protein deficiency disorder, coarse intention and resting tremors occur.
- Related findings include myoclonus, rigidity of all extremities, hyperreflexia, hepatomegaly, and pitting edema in the hands, feet, and sacral areas.
- Other findings include flat affect, pronounced hair loss, and dry, peeling skin.

Multiple sclerosis
- An intention tremor that waxes and wanes may be an early sign along with visual and sensory impairments.
- Other findings may include nystagmus, muscle weakness, paralysis, spasticity, hyperreflexia, ataxic gait, dysphagia, dysarthria, constipation, urinary frequency and urgency, incontinence, impotence, and emotional lability.

Parkinson's disease
- Tremors, a classic early sign, usually begin in the fingers and may eventually affect the foot, eyelids, jaw, lips, and tongue.
- Other characteristic findings include cogwheel rigidity, bradykinesia, propulsive gait with forward-leaning posture, monotone voice, masklike facies, drooling, dysphagia, dysarthria, and occasionally oculogyric crisis or blepharospasm.

Porphyria
- Resting tremor and rigidity with chorea and athetosis occur.
- As the disease progresses, generalized seizures with aphasia and hemiplegia occur.

Thalamic syndrome
- Contralateral ataxic tremors and other abnormal movements occur along with Weber's syndrome, paralysis of vertical gaze, and stupor or coma occur with central midbrain syndromes.
- Tremor, deep sensory loss, hemiataxia, and extrapyramidal dysfunction may occur with anteromedial-inferior syndrome.

Thyrotoxicosis
- A rapid, fine intention tremor of the hands and tongue with clonus, and hyperreflexia occur.
- Other findings include tachycardia, cardiac arrhythmias, palpitations, anxiety, dyspnea, diaphoresis, heat intolerance, weight loss despite increased appetite, diarrhea, an enlarged thyroid and, possibly, exophthalmos.

Wernicke's disease
- An intention tremor is an early sign of thiamine deficiency.
- Other findings include ocular abnormalities, ataxia, apathy, confusion, orthostatic hypotension, and tachycardia.

West Nile encephalitis
- In severe infections, headache, high fever, neck stiffness, stupor, disorientation, coma, tremors, occasional seizures, and paralysis occur.

OTHER
Drugs
- Antipsychotics and phenothiazines, and infrequently metoclopramide hydrochloride (Reglan) and metyrosine (Demser), may cause resting and pill-rolling tremors.
- Amphetamines, lithium (Eskalith) toxicity, phenytoin (Dilantin), and sympathomimetics can cause

tremors that disappear with dose reduction.

Manganese toxicity
- Early signs of manganese toxicity include resting tremor, chorea, propulsive gait, cogwheel rigidity, personality changes, amnesia, and masklike facies.

Mercury poisoning
- Mercury poisoning is characterized by irritability, copious amounts of saliva, loose teeth, gum disease, slurred speech, and tremors.

NURSING CONSIDERATIONS

- Assist the patient with activities as needed.
- Take precautions against possible injury during activities.
- Encourage the patient to talk about changes in body image.

PEDIATRIC TIPS
- Causes of pathologic tremors in children include cerebral palsy, fetal alcohol syndrome, and maternal drug addiction.
- A normal neonate may display coarse tremors with stiffening—an exaggerated hypocalcemic startle reflex—in response to noises and chills.

PATIENT TEACHING

- Reinforce the patient's independence.
- Instruct the patient in the use of assistive devices as needed.
- Teach about underlying diagnosis and treatment plan.

Trismus

OVERVIEW

- Commonly known as *lockjaw*
- Results from prolonged and painful tonic spasm of the masticatory jaw muscles

HISTORY

- Obtain a pertinent history inquiring about a recent injury (even a slight wound), infection, animal bite or a history of epilepsy, neuromuscular disease, or endocrine or metabolic disorders.
- Obtain a complete drug history, including self-injected drugs because the use of a contaminated needle may produce tetanus.
- Ask about paresthesia or pain in the throat, jaw, neck, or shoulders.
- Ask about last tetanus vaccination or booster.

PHYSICAL ASSESSMENT

- Examination of the oral cavity may be difficult or impossible to perform. If possible, examine the pharynx, tonsils, oral mucosa, gingivae, and teeth.
- Perform a neurologic assessment, evaluating cranial nerve, motor, and sensory function and deep tendon reflexes.
- Check the jaw jerk reflex. An extremely hyperactive response and a careful patient history usually establish the diagnosis. (See *Performing the jaw jerk test*.)

CAUSES

MEDICAL

Hypocalcemia

- Severe hypocalcemia can produce trismus and cramping spasms in virtually all muscle groups, except those of the eye.
- It also causes fatigue, weakness, chorea, and palpitations.
- Chvostek's and Trousseau's signs may be elicited.

Peritonsillar abscess

- This disorder occurs after an episode of acute tonsillitis when infection penetrates the tonsillar capsule and surrounding deeper tissues.
- Symptoms include severe sore throat, trismus, odynophagia, deviation of the uvula, and fever.

Rabies

- Trismus commonly develops after a prodromal period of fever, headache, photophobia, hyperesthesia, and increasing restlessness and agitation.
- Other neuromuscular effects include excessive salivation, painful laryngeal and pharyngeal muscle spasms and, possibly, respiratory distress.

Seizure disorder

- Trismus commonly occurs during a generalized tonic-clonic seizure along with spasms of other facial muscles, the limbs, and the trunk.

Temporomandibular joint syndrome

- This syndrome causes trismus, mandibular dysfunction, and facial pain.
- The pain may range from a severe dull ache to an intense spasm that radiates to the cheek, temple, lower jaw, ear, mastoid area, neck, or shoulders.
- Earache occurs without involvement of the tympanic membrane or external auditory canal.

Tetanus

- This acute, life-threatening infection is heralded by trismus, which typical-

TOP TECHNIQUE

Performing the jaw jerk test

If your patient reports difficulty in opening her mouth, perform the jaw jerk test because even slight trismus may indicate an otherwise asymptomatic mild localized tetanus.

Here's how to elicit and interpret this important reflex: Ask the patient to relax her jaw and open her mouth slightly. Then place your index finger over the middle of her chin, and firmly tap it with a reflex hammer.

Normally, this tap produces sudden jaw closing; then an inhibitory mechanism abruptly halts motor nerve activity, and the mouth remains closed. In trismus, however, this inhibitory mechanism fails and motor activity increases, causing immediate spasm of jaw muscles.

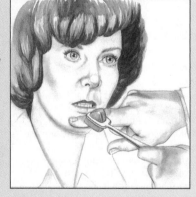

ly appears within 14 days of the initial infection.

◆ The painful spasms increase in frequency and intensity during the initial disease stage, then gradually subside.

◆ Although trismus is commonly the first sign of tetanus, it occasionally follows a short prodromal period of headache, restlessness, irritability, slight fever, chills, swelling at the wound site, and dysphagia.

◆ As the disease progresses, painful involuntary muscle spasms spread to other areas, such as the abdomen, producing boardlike rigidity; the back, resulting in opisthotonos; the face, producing a characteristic grotesque grin (risus sardonicus); or possibly the laryngeal or chest wall muscles.

◆ Tachycardia, diaphoresis, hyperactive deep tendon reflexes, and seizures may also develop.

OTHER
Drugs

◆ Phenothiazines (particularly the piperazine derivatives such as fluphenazine hydrochloride [Prolixin]) and other antipsychotics may produce an acute dystonic reaction marked by trismus, involuntary facial movements, and tonic spasms in the limbs. These complications usually occur early in drug therapy, sometimes after the initial dose.

Strychnine poisoning

◆ In this potentially fatal condition, tonic seizures characterized by trismus, leg muscle rigidity, and respiratory muscle spasm follow early symptoms of irritability and twitching.

NURSING CONSIDERATIONS

◆ Maintain a quiet environment for the patient with trismus; darken his room and keep all stimulation to a minimum.

◆ Administer a sedative as needed.

◆ Constantly assess the patient's respiratory status and make sure that oxygen and emergency airway equipment are readily available.

◆ To treat tetanus, expect to administer human tetanus immune globulin, which neutralizes unbound toxin.

◆ Administer I.V. fluids to prevent dehydration if the patient can't drink fluids.

◆ If trismus is prolonged enough to affect his nutritional status, the patient may require parenteral nutrition.

◆ If the patient can't speak, make sure that he has a pen and paper and that his call bell is within reach at all times.

PEDIATRIC TIPS

◆ Trismus in a neonate can result from tetanus neonatorum, which occurs when the tetanus toxin is introduced through the umbilical cord.

◆ Trismus usually develops within 10 days of birth.

PATIENT TEACHING

◆ Teach the patient with tetanus about the importance of booster injections to ensure immunization.

◆ Explain underlying diagnosis and treatment plan.

Urethral discharge

◆ Occurs as a purulent, mucoid or thin, sanguineous discharge from the urinary meatus

◆ Ask about the onset and description of the discharge.
◆ Inquire about other pain or burning on urination, difficulty starting a urine stream, urinary frequency, fever, chills, and perineal fullness.
◆ Obtain a medical history, including prostate problems, sexually transmitted disease, or urinary tract infection.
◆ Find out about recent sexual contacts or a new sex partner.

◆ Inspect the urethral meatus for inflammation and swelling.
◆ Obtain a culture specimen. (See *Collecting a urethral discharge specimen*.)
◆ Obtain a urine specimen for urinalysis and culture.

Collecting a urethral discharge specimen

To obtain a urethral specimen from a male patient, follow these steps:

Instruct the patient not to void for 1 hour before specimen collection to prevent flushing secretions from the urethra.

↓

Provide privacy for the patient. Explain the procedure. Help him into a supine position, and expose his penis. Have him grasp and raise his penis to allow you to see the urethra.

↓

Wash your hands, and put on sterile gloves. Clean the urethral meatus with sterile gauze or a cotton swab. Then insert a thin, sterile urogenital alginate swab no more than ¾" (2 cm) into the urethra. Rotate the swab, and leave it in place for 10 to 30 seconds to absorb organisms.

↓

Remove the swab and send the specimen to the laboratory. Provide perineal care and cover the patient.

To obtain a urethral specimen from a female patient, follow these steps:

Instruct the patient not to void for 1 hour before specimen collection to prevent flushing of secretions from the urethra.

↓

Provide privacy for the patient. Explain the procedure. Help her onto an examination table and into the lithotomy position or into a supine position with knees bent.

↓

Wash your hands, and put on sterile gloves. Clean the urethral meatus with sterile gauze or a cotton swab. Then insert a thin, sterile urogenital alginate swab into the urethral meatus. Gently rotate the swab, and leave it in place for 10 to 30 seconds to absorb organisms. Take care not to touch the swab to the area around the urethral meatus.

↓

Remove the swab and send the specimen to the laboratory. Assist the patient off the table or reposition her. Provide perineal care and cover the patient.

CAUSES

MEDICAL
Prostatitis
◆ In the acute form, findings include purulent urethral discharge, sudden fever, chills, lower back pain, myalgia, perineal fullness, arthralgia, frequent and urgent urination, dysuria, nocturia, and a tense, boggy, tender, and warm prostate.
◆ In the chronic form, findings include a persistent urethral discharge that's thin, milky, or clear at the meatus after not voiding for a long time; dull aching in the prostate or rectum; sexual dysfunction such as ejaculatory pain; and urinary disturbances, such as frequency, urgency, and dysuria.

Reiter's syndrome
◆ Urethral discharge and other signs of acute urethritis occur 1 or 2 weeks after sexual contact.
◆ Other findings include asymmetrical arthritis, conjunctivitis, and ulcerations on the oral mucosa, glans penis, palms, and soles.

Urethritis
◆ This finding can be secondary to urinary tract infection or sexually transmitted diseases (STDs), such as chlamydia, gonorrhea, or trichomoniasis.
◆ Scant or profuse urethral discharge occurs that's thin and clear, mucoid, or thick and purulent.
◆ Related findings include urinary hesitancy, urgency, and frequency and itching and burning around the meatus.

NURSING CONSIDERATIONS

◆ To relieve prostatitis symptoms, suggest that the patient take hot sitz baths several times daily, increase his fluid intake, void frequently, and avoid caffeine, tea, and alcohol.
◆ Monitor for urine retention.

PEDIATRIC TIPS
◆ Evaluate a child with urethral discharge for evidence of sexual and physical abuse.

GERIATRIC TIPS
◆ Urethral discharge in elderly patients isn't usually related to a sexually transmitted disease.

PATIENT TEACHING

◆ Advise the patient with active prostatitis of the importance of avoiding sexual activity until acute symptoms subside.
◆ Explain that chronic prostatitis symptoms can be relieved by engaging in regular sexual activity.
◆ Teach about prescribed medications, their importance and adverse effects.
◆ Advise the patient to avoid sexual contact until the test results are available if evaluating for an STD.
◆ Teach perineal hygiene and infection control techniques, as appropriate.

Urinary frequency

OVERVIEW

- Refers to increased incidence of the urge to void without an increase in the total volume of urine produced
- Is a classic sign of urinary tract infection (UTI)

HISTORY

- Ask about current and previous voiding patterns.
- Determine the onset and duration of urinary frequency.
- Find out about fever, chills, dysuria, urgency, incontinence, hematuria, discharge, or lower abdominal pain with urination.
- Obtain a medical history, especially of UTI, other urologic problems or recent urologic procedures, and neurologic disorders.
- Inquire about a history of prostatic enlargement in men.
- Ask about the possibility of pregnancy in women.

PHYSICAL ASSESSMENT

- Obtain a clean-catch midstream specimen.
- Palpate the suprapubic area, abdomen, and flanks, noting any tenderness.
- Examine the urethral meatus for redness, discharge, or swelling.
- Palpate the prostate gland.
- Perform a neurologic assessment if the history reveals symptoms or a history of neurologic diseases.
- Obtain temperature reading.

CAUSES

MEDICAL
Benign prostatic hyperplasia

- Urinary frequency with nocturia and, possibly, incontinence and hematuria occur with this disorder.
- Initial findings include reduced caliber and force of the urine stream, urinary hesitancy, tenesmus, inability to stop the stream of urine, a feeling of incomplete voiding, and occasionally urine retention.

Bladder calculus

- Urinary frequency and urgency, dysuria, hematuria at the end of micturition, and suprapubic pain from bladder spasms occur.
- If the calculus lodges in the bladder neck, overflow incontinence occurs with greatest discomfort at the end of micturition.

Bladder cancer

- Urinary frequency, urgency, dribbling, and nocturia may develop.
- The first sign commonly is gross, painless, intermittent hematuria (with clots).
- Suprapubic or pelvic pain commonly occurs with invasive lesions.

Multiple sclerosis

- Urinary frequency, urgency, and incontinence are common.
- Vision problems (such as diplopia and blurred vision) and sensory impairment (such as paresthesia) are the earliest symptoms.
- Other findings include constipation, muscle weakness, paralysis, spasticity, hyperreflexia, intention tremor, ataxic gait, dysarthria, impotence, and emotional lability.

Prostate cancer

- In advanced stages, urinary frequency along with hesitancy, dribbling, nocturia, dysuria, bladder distention, perineal pain, constipation, and a hard, irregularly shaped prostate occur.

Prostatitis

- In the acute form, urinary frequency, urgency, dysuria, nocturia, and purulent urethral discharge are produced.
- Other acute findings include fever, chills, lower back pain, myalgia, arthralgia, perineal fullness and, possibly, a tense, boggy, tender, and warm prostate.
- In the chronic form, pain on ejaculation may occur as well as the same findings as in the acute form, but to a lesser degree.

Rectal tumor

- Pressure from the tumor on the bladder may cause urinary frequency.
- Early findings include changed bowel habits, commonly starting with an urgent need to defecate on arising or obstipation alternating with diarrhea; blood or mucus in the stool; and a sense of incomplete evacuation.

Reiter's syndrome

- Urinary frequency occurs 1 or 2 weeks after sexual contact.
- Other findings include asymmetrical arthritis of knees, ankles, and metatarsophalangeal joints; conjunctivitis; and small, painless ulcers on the mouth, tongue, glans penis, palms, and soles.

Reproductive tract tumor

- A tumor may compress the bladder, causing urinary frequency.
- Other findings may include abdominal distention, menstrual disturbances, vaginal bleeding, weight loss, pelvic pain, and fatigue.

Spinal cord lesion

- Urinary frequency, continuous overflow, dribbling, urgency, urinary hesitancy, and bladder distention from incomplete spinal cord transection occur with this type of lesion.
- Other findings below the level of the lesion may occur, such as weakness, paralysis, sensory disturbances, hyperreflexia, and impotence.

Urethral stricture

- Bladder decompensation produces urinary frequency, along with urgency and nocturia.
- Early signs include hesitancy, tenesmus, and reduced caliber and force of the urine stream.
- Overflow incontinence, urinoma, and urosepsis may also develop.

Urinary tract infection

- With UTI, urinary frequency, urgency, dysuria, hematuria, cloudy urine, and discharge occur.
- Related findings include fever, bladder spasms, and a feeling of warmth during urination.

Uterine prolapse

- Urinary frequency, hesitancy, infection, leakage, and retention occur.
- Associated findings include abdominal, vaginal, or lower back pain; and dyspareunia (painful intercourse).
- Signs and symptoms often occur gradually as pelvic muscles and ligaments weaken from age, childbirth, or abdominal surgery.

OTHER

Diuretics

- Diuretics, including caffeine, reduce the body's total volume of water and salt by increasing urine excretion.

Treatments

- Radiation therapy may cause bladder inflammation, leading to urinary frequency.

Urinary hesitancy

- Refers to difficulty starting a urine stream generally followed by a decrease in the force of the stream
- Usually arises gradually, commonly going unnoticed until urine retention causes bladder distention and discomfort

- Obtain a history about the patient's urinary problems asking when he first noticed hesitancy and if he has ever had the problem before, and other urinary problems, especially reduced force or interruption of the urine stream.
- Find out if he has ever been treated for a prostate problem (male patient), a urinary tract infection (UTI), or a urinary tract obstruction.
- Obtain a drug history.

PHYSICAL ASSESSMENT

- Inspect the patient's urethral meatus for inflammation, discharge, and other abnormalities.
- Examine the anal sphincter and test sensation in the perineum.
- Obtain a clean-catch urine specimen for urinalysis and culture and sensitivity tests.
- A male patient requires prostate gland palpation. A female patient requires a gynecologic examination.

MEDICAL
Benign prostatic hyperplasia
- Signs and symptoms of this disorder depend on the extent of prostatic enlargement and the lobes affected.
- Characteristic early findings include urinary hesitancy, reduced caliber and force of the urine stream, perineal pain, a feeling of incomplete voiding, inability to stop the urine stream, and occasionally urine retention.
- As the obstruction increases, the patient may develop urinary frequency, nocturia, urinary overflow, incontinence, bladder distention and, possibly, hematuria.

Prostate cancer
- In advanced cancer, urinary hesitancy may occur along with frequency, dribbling, nocturia, dysuria, bladder distention, perineal pain, and constipation.
- Digital rectal examination commonly reveals a hard, nodular prostate.

Spinal cord lesion
- A lesion below the micturition center that has destroyed the sacral nerve roots causes urinary hesitancy, tenesmus, and constant dribbling from urine retention and overflow incontinence.
- Associated findings are urinary frequency and urgency, dysuria, and nocturia.

Urethral stricture
- Partial obstruction of the lower urinary tract secondary to trauma or infection produces urinary hesitancy, tenesmus, and decreased force and caliber of the urine stream.
- Urinary frequency and urgency, nocturia, and eventually overflow incontinence may develop.
- Pyuria usually indicates accompanying infection. Increased obstruction may lead to urine extravasation and formation of urinomas.

Urinary tract infection

◆ Urinary hesitancy may be associated with UTIs.
◆ Characteristic urinary changes include frequency, dysuria, nocturia, cloudy urine and, possibly, hematuria.
◆ Associated findings include bladder spasms; costovertebral angle tenderness; suprapubic, low back, pelvic, or flank pain; urethral discharge in males; fever; chills; malaise; nausea; and vomiting.

OTHER
Drugs

◆ Anticholinergics and drugs with anticholinergic properties (such as tricyclic antidepressants and some nasal decongestants and cold remedies) may cause urinary hesitancy.
◆ Hesitancy also may occur in patients recovering from general anesthesia.

NURSING CONSIDERATIONS

◆ Monitor the patient's voiding pattern, and palpate the abdomen frequently for bladder distention.
◆ Apply local heat to the perineum or the abdomen to enhance muscle relaxation and aid urination.

PEDIATRIC TIPS

◆ The most common cause of urinary obstruction in male infants is posterior strictures.
◆ Infants with this problem may have a less forceful urine stream and may also exhibit a fever due to UTI, failure to thrive, and a palpable bladder.

PATIENT TEACHING

◆ Teach the patient how to perform a clean, intermittent self-catheterization, if indicated. (See *Teaching self-catheterization*.)
◆ Prepare the patient for tests, such as cystometrography or cystourethrography.
◆ Explain about underlying diagnosis and treatment plan.

Teaching self-catheterization

Following sterile technique, teach a female patient to hold the catheter in her dominant hand as if it were a pencil or a dart, about ½" (1.3 cm) from its tip. Keeping the vaginal folds separated, she should slowly insert the lubricated catheter about 3" (7.6 cm) into the urethra. Tell her to press down with her abdominal muscles to empty the bladder, allowing all urine to drain through the catheter and into the toilet or drainage container.

Following sterile technique, teach a male patient to hold his penis in his nondominant hand, at a right angle to his body. He should hold the catheter in his dominant hand as if it were a pencil and slowly insert it 7" to 10" (17.5 to 25 cm) into the urethra until urine begins flowing. Then he should gently advance the catheter about 1" (2.5 cm) farther, allowing all urine to drain into the toilet or drainage container.

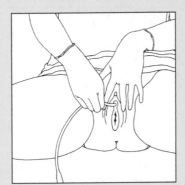

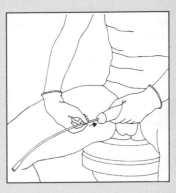

Urinary incontinence

- Refers to the uncontrollable passage of urine
- May be transient or permanent
- May involve large volumes of urine or scant dribbling
- Is classified as stress, overflow, urge, or total

- Ask about the onset and description of incontinence.
- Obtain a description of normal urinary pattern and fluid intake.
- Inquire about other urinary problems, such as hesitancy, frequency, urgency, nocturia, and decreased force or interruption of the urine stream.
- Ask about a history of urinary tract infection (UTI), prostate conditions, spinal injury or tumor, stroke, or surgery involving the bladder, prostate, or pelvic floor.
- Ask a female patient about the number of pregnancies and childbirths.

- Have the patient empty his bladder.
- Inspect the urethral meatus for inflammation or defect.
- Have the female patient bear down; note any urine leakage.
- Gently palpate the abdomen for bladder distention.
- Perform a complete neurologic assessment, noting motor and sensory function and obvious muscle atrophy.
- Assess post-void residual urine volume with a straight catheter.

MEDICAL
Benign prostatic hyperplasia
- Overflow incontinence results from urethral obstruction and urine retention.

- Reduced caliber and force of the urine stream, urinary hesitancy, and a feeling of incomplete voiding constitute prostatism and are early findings.
- Urination becomes more frequent, with nocturia and, possibly, hematuria as the obstruction increases.
- Bladder distention and an enlarged prostate are revealed by examination.

Bladder calculus
- Overflow incontinence may occur if the calculus lodges in the bladder neck.
- Other findings may include those of an irritable bladder, such as urinary frequency and urgency, dysuria, hematuria, and suprapubic pain from bladder spasms.
- Pelvic pain and pain referred to the tip of the penis, vulva, lower back, or heel pain may occur.

Bladder cancer
- Urge incontinence and hematuria are early signs.
- Obstruction by a tumor may produce overflow incontinence.
- Other findings include frequency, dysuria, nocturia, dribbling, and suprapubic pain from bladder spasms after voiding.
- A mass may be palpable on bimanual examination.

Diabetic neuropathy
- Bladder distention with overflow incontinence may occur.
- Related findings include episodic constipation or diarrhea (which is commonly nocturnal), impotence and retrograde ejaculation, orthostatic hypotension, syncope, and dysphagia.

Guillain-Barré syndrome
- Urinary incontinence may occur early.
- Profound muscle weakness, which typically starts in the legs and extends to the arms and facial nerves within 24 to 72 hours, is the most prominent sign.

- Other findings include paresthesia, dysarthria, nasal speech, dysphagia, orthostatic hypotension, fecal incontinence, diaphoresis, drooling, tachycardia, and pain in the shoulders, thighs, or lumbar region.

Multiple sclerosis
- Urinary incontinence, urgency, and frequency are common urologic findings.
- Early findings include vision problems and sensory impairment.
- Other findings include constipation, muscle weakness, paralysis, spasticity, hyperreflexia, intention tremor, ataxic gait, dysarthria, impotence, and emotional lability.

Prostate cancer
- Urinary incontinence usually appears only in advanced stages.
- Other late findings include urinary frequency and hesitancy, nocturia, dysuria, bladder distention, perineal pain, constipation, and a hard, irregularly shaped, nodular prostate.

Prostatitis (chronic)
- Urinary incontinence may occur as well as urinary frequency and urgency, dysuria, hematuria, bladder distention, persistent urethral discharge, dull perineal pain that may radiate, ejaculatory pain, and decreased libido.

Spinal cord injury
- Overflow incontinence follows rapid bladder distention.
- Other findings include paraplegia, sexual dysfunction, sensory loss, muscle atrophy, anhidrosis, and loss of reflexes far from the injury.

Stroke
- Transient or permanent urinary incontinence occurs with stroke.
- Related findings include impaired mentation, emotional lability, behavioral changes, altered level of consciousness, and seizures.
- Other findings include headache, vomiting, vision deficits, and decreased visual acuity.

- Sensorimotor findings include contralateral hemiplegia, dysarthria, dysphagia, ataxia, apraxia, agnosia, aphasia, and unilateral sensory loss.

Urethral stricture
- Eventually, overflow incontinence occurs with urethral stricture.
- Urinomas and urosepsis occur as obstruction increases.

Urinary tract infection
- Incontinence, urinary urgency, dysuria, hematuria, and cloudy urine occur with UTI.
- Possible bladder spasms or a feeling of warmth during urination may occur.

OTHER
Surgery
- Urinary incontinence after prostatectomy as a result of urethral sphincter damage may occur.

NURSING CONSIDERATIONS

- Obtain a urine specimen.
- Start bladder retraining. (See *Correcting incontinence with bladder retraining.*)
- If incontinence is neurologic, monitor the patient for urine retention.

PEDIATRIC TIPS
- Causes of incontinence in children include infrequent or incomplete voiding and an ectopic ureteral orifice.

GERIATRIC TIPS
- Elderly patients with UTIs may present only with urinary incontinence or changes in mental status, anorexia, or malaise.

PATIENT TEACHING

- Instruct the patient in performing Kegel exercises. (See *Teaching Kegel exercises.*)

- Teach the patient self-catheterization techniques. (See *Teaching self-catheterization,* page 573.)

 TOP TECHNIQUE

- Review drug therapy with the patient.
- Discuss underlying disorder, diagnostic tests, and treatment plan.

Correcting incontinence with bladder retraining

The incontinent patient typically feels frustrated, embarrassed, and sometimes hopeless. Fortunately, though, the problem may be corrected by bladder retraining—a program that aims to establish a regular voiding pattern. Here are some guidelines for establishing such a program:
- Before you start bladder retraining, assess the patient's intake pattern, voiding pattern, and behavior (for example, restlessness or talkativeness) before each voiding episode.
- Encourage the patient to use the toilet 30 minutes before he's usually incontinent. If this isn't successful, readjust the schedule. Once he's able to stay dry for 2 hours, increase the time between voidings by 30 minutes each day until he achieves a 3- to 4-hour voiding schedule.
- When your patient voids, make sure that the sequence of conditioning stimuli is always the same.
- Make sure that the patient has privacy while voiding; any inhibiting stimuli should be avoided.
- Keep a record of continence and incontinence for 5 days; this may reinforce your patient's efforts to remain continent.

TIPS FOR SUCCESS
Remember that you and your patient need a positive attitude to ensure his successful bladder retraining. Here are some additional tips that may help your patient succeed:
- Make sure the patient is close to a bathroom or portable toilet. Leave a light on at night and ensure a clear pathway to the bathroom.
- If your patient needs assistance getting out of his bed or chair, promptly answer his call for help.
- Encourage the patient to wear his usual clothing as an indication that you're confident he can remain continent. Acceptable alternatives to diapers include condoms for the male patient and incontinence pads or panties for the female patient.
- Urge the patient to drink 2 to 2½ qt (2 to 2.5 L) of fluid each day. Less fluid doesn't prevent incontinence but does promote bladder infection. Limiting his intake after 5 p.m., however, will help him remain continent during the night.
- Reassure your patient that episodes of incontinence don't signal a failure of the program. Encourage him to maintain a positive attitude.

Teaching Kegel exercises

Kegels are isometric exercises that will strengthen the pubococcygeus (PC) muscle to increase voluntary control over urination. Teach your patient these techniques.
- Begin by asking her to sit on the toilet with her legs spread. Then, without moving her legs, instruct her to start and stop the flow of urine. Tell her that the PC muscle is the one that contracts to help control urine flow.
- Now that she's identified the PC muscle, she can exercise it regularly. Kegel exercises can be performed almost anywhere—sitting at a desk, lying in bed, standing in line, and especially while urinating. Tell her to remember to breathe naturally—not to hold her breath.

- Have her contract the PC muscle as she did to stop the urine flow. Ask her to count slowly to three, then relax the muscle.
- Next, have her contract and relax the PC muscle as quickly as possible, without using her stomach or buttock muscles.
- Ask her to slowly contract the entire vaginal area. Tell her to bear down, using her abdominal muscles and her PC muscle.
- For the first week, tell the patient to repeat each exercise 10 times (1 set) for 5 sets daily. Then each week, add 5 repetitions of each exercise (15, 20, and so forth). Advise her to keep doing 5 sets daily.

Finally, let her know that after about 2 weeks of practice, she'll notice improvement.

Urinary urgency

- Refers to a sudden, compelling urge to urinate
- Occurs with bladder pain as a classic symptom of urinary tract infection (UTI)
- May occur without bladder pain that may point to an upper motor neuron lesion that has disrupted bladder control

HISTORY

- Ask about the onset and history of urgency.
- Inquire about other urologic symptoms, such as dysuria and cloudy urine.
- Ask about neurologic symptoms, such as paresthesia.
- Obtain a medical history, especially of UTIs and surgery or procedures involving the urinary tract.
- Obtain a prescription and nonprescription drug history.

PHYSICAL ASSESSMENT

- Obtain a clean-catch specimen for urinalysis and culture.
- Note urine character, color, and odor; use a reagent strip to test for pH, glucose, and blood.
- Palpate the suprapubic area and both flanks for distention and tenderness.
- If the history or symptoms suggest neurologic dysfunction, perform a neurologic examination.

CAUSES

Bladder calculus

- Urinary urgency and frequency, dysuria, chills, fever, hematuria at the end of micturition, and suprapubic pain may occur.
- Pain may pass on to the penis, vulva, or lower back.

Multiple sclerosis

- Urinary urgency can occur with or without frequent UTIs.
- Vision and sensory impairments are the earliest findings.
- Other findings include urinary frequency, incontinence, constipation, muscle weakness, paralysis, spasticity, intention tremor, hyperreflexia, ataxic gait, dysphagia, dysarthria, impotence, and emotional lability.

Reiter's syndrome

- Urgency occurs with other symptoms of acute urethritis 1 or 2 weeks after sexual contact primarily in men.
- Asymmetrical arthritis of knees, ankles, or metatarsal phalangeal joints; conjunctivitis; and ulcers on the penis, or skin, or in the mouth usually develop within several weeks after sexual contact.

Spinal cord lesion

- Urinary urgency can occur along with urinary frequency and difficulty initiating and inhibiting a urine stream; bladder distention and discomfort may also occur.

◆ Neuromuscular findings far from the lesion include weakness, paralysis, hyperreflexia, sensory disturbances, and impotence.

Urethral stricture
◆ Bladder decompensation produces urinary urgency, frequency, and nocturia.

Urinary tract infection
◆ Urinary urgency, frequency, and hesitancy; hematuria; dysuria; nocturia; and cloudy urine occur with UTI.
◆ Related findings include bladder spasms; costovertebral angle tenderness; suprapubic, low back, or flank pain; urethral discharge in males; fever; chills; malaise; nausea; and vomiting.

OTHER
Treatments
◆ Radiation therapy may irritate and inflame the bladder, causing urinary urgency.

NURSING CONSIDERATIONS

◆ Increase the patient's fluid intake.
◆ Give an antibiotic and a urinary anesthetic, as prescribed.

PEDIATRIC TIPS
◆ In young children, urinary urgency may appear as a change in toilet habits.
◆ Urgency may also result from urethral irritation caused by bubble bath salts.

PATIENT TEACHING

◆ Instruct the patient in safe sex practices.
◆ Explain proper genital hygiene to female patients.
◆ Discuss adequate fluid intake and frequent daily voiding.
◆ Instuct the patient with a noninfective cause of urgency how to do Kegel exercises. (See *Teaching Kegel exercises,* page 575.)
◆ Discuss underlying disorder and treatment plan.

Urticaria

OVERVIEW

- Referes to a vascular skin reaction
- Also known as *hives*
- Is characterized by the eruption of transient pruritic wheals—smooth, slightly elevated patches with well-defined erythematous margins and pale centers of various shapes and sizes
- May be produced in response to the local release of histamine or other vasoactive substances as part of a hypersensitivity reaction
- Acute urticaria: evolves rapidly and usually has a detectable cause
- Angioedema, or giant urticaria: is characterized by the acute eruption of wheals involving the mucous membranes and, occasionally, the arms, legs, or genitals (see *Urticaria or angioedema?*)

ACTION STAT! *In acute urticaria, quickly evaluate respiratory status and take vital signs. Ensure patent I.V. access if respiratory difficulty or signs of impending anaphylactic shock are present. As needed, give local epinephrine or apply ice to the affected site to decrease absorption through vasoconstriction. Maintain a patent airway, give oxygen as needed, and institute cardiac monitoring. Have resuscitation equipment available, and begin cardiopulmonary resuscitation if needed. Intubation or a tracheostomy may be required.*

HISTORY

- Ask about any known allergies and allergen exposure.
- Inquire about a pattern of urticaria and what aggravates it.
- Find out about exposure to chemicals on the job or at home.
- Obtain a detailed drug history.
- Note any history of chronic or parasitic infection, skin disease, or a GI disorder.

PHYSICAL ASSESSMENT

- Obtain vital signs.
- Perform a complete cardiopulmonary assessment, noting signs and symptoms of shock or respiratory distress.
- Assess for urticaria in other areas because new crops may continue to appear.

Urticaria or angioedema?

The illustration below shows typical urticarial lesions: red, raised plaques that are surrounded by a white halo and can appear on any skin surface.

Angioedema is an urticarial swelling that occurs in the subcutaneous tissue. The skin over the angioedema may appear to be normal or may be reddened. Although it occurs frequently on the face and mucous membranes, angioedema can occur on other areas of the body, as shown below.

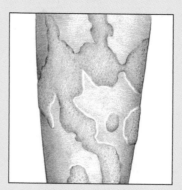

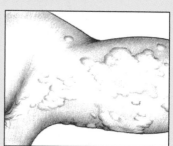

MEDICAL

Anaphylaxis

◆ Rapid eruption of diffuse urticaria and angioedema develops; wheals range from pinpoint to palm-size or larger in this potentially life-threatening disorder.

◆ Lesions are usually pruritic and stinging; paresthesia commonly precedes their eruption.

◆ Other acute findings include profound anxiety; weakness; diaphoresis; sneezing; shortness of breath; profuse rhinorrhea; nasal congestion; dysphagia; and warm, moist skin.

Hereditary angioedema

◆ This nonallergenic type of angioedema occurs as recurrent episodes in many cases after trauma or stress.

◆ Patches of nonpitting, nonpruritic edema develop on the arms, legs, or face.

◆ Respiratory mucosal involvement can produce life-threatening acute laryngeal edema.

◆ GI tract involvement may cause severe abdominal pain, nausea, and vomiting.

Lyme disease

◆ Urticaria may result from erythema chronicum migrans.

◆ Later findings include constant malaise and fatigue, intermittent headache, fever, chills, lymphadenopathy, neurologic and cardiac abnormalities, and arthritis.

OTHER

Drugs

◆ Various drugs (most commonly aspirin, atropine [Atropen], codeine, dextrans, immune serums, insulin, morphine, penicillin, quinine sulfate, sulfonamides, and vaccines) can produce urticaria.

◆ Radiographic contrast medium commonly produces urticaria, especially when given I.V.

NURSING CONSIDERATIONS

◆ Apply a bland skin emollient or one containing menthol and phenol to help relieve discomfort.

◆ Give an antihistamine, a systemic corticosteroid, or a tranquilizer, as prescribed.

◆ Tepid baths and cool compresses may decrease pruritus.

PEDIATRIC TIPS

◆ Acute papular urticaria (especially after insect bites) and urticaria pigmentosa (rare) may occur in children.

PATIENT TEACHING

◆ Emphasize the importance of wearing medical identification for allergies.

◆ Discuss the signs and symptoms to report.

◆ Stress ways to prevent anaphylaxis.

◆ Teach the patient the proper use of an anaphylaxis kit.

Vaginal bleeding, postmenopausal

OVERVIEW

- Refers to bleeding that occurs 6 or more months after menopause
- Presents as slight, brown or red spotting; oozing of fresh blood; or bright red hemorrhage
- Is an important indicator of gynecologic cancer; may also result from other causes, such as infection, local pelvic disorder, atrophy of endometrium, and physiologic thinning and drying of vaginal mucosa

HISTORY

- Determine the patient's current age and age at menopause.
- Ask about the onset of bleeding.
- Obtain a thorough obstetric, gynecologic, and sexual history.
- Find out all drugs used presently or within the time symptoms began, including douches and estrogen products.
- Obtain a history of sexually transmitted disease.

PHYSICAL ASSESSMENT

- Observe the external genitalia, noting the character of any vaginal discharge and the appearance of the labia, vaginal rugae, and clitoris.
- Palpate the breasts and lymph nodes for nodules or enlargement.
- The patient will need pelvic and rectal examinations.

MEDICAL

Atrophic vaginitis

- Bloody staining may normally follow coitus or douching, but must be evaluated to rule out cancer.
- Characteristic white, watery discharge may be accompanied by pruritus, dyspareunia, and a burning sensation in the vagina and labia.
- Sparse pubic hair, a pale vagina with decreased rugae and small hemorrhagic spots, clitoral atrophy, and shrinking of the labia minora may also occur.

Cervical cancer

- Spotting or heavier bleeding occurs early in invasive cervical cancer; bleeding may also normally follow coitus or douching.
- Related findings include persistent, pink-tinged, and foul-smelling discharge, and postcoital pain.
- As the cancer spreads, back and sciatic pain, leg swelling, anorexia, weight loss, hematuria, dysuria, rectal bleeding, and weakness may occur.

Cervical or endometrial polyps

- Spotting (possibly mucopurulent and pink) may occur after coitus, douching, or straining at stool.

Endometrial hyperplasia or cancer

- Early, bleeding is brownish and scant or red and profuse and usually follows coitus or douching.
- Later, bleeding becomes heavier and more frequent, leading to clotting and anemia.
- Pelvic, rectal, lower back, and leg pain may accompany bleeding.
- Uterus may be enlarged.

Ovarian tumor (feminizing)

- Endometrial shedding may occur and cause heavy bleeding.
- A palpable pelvic mass, increased cervical mucus, breast enlargement, and spider angiomas may be present.

Vaginal cancer

- Characteristic spotting or bleeding may be preceded by a thin, watery discharge.
- Bleeding may be spontaneous but usually follows coitus or douching.
- A firm, ulcerated vaginal lesion may be present.
- Dyspareunia, urinary frequency, bladder and pelvic pain, rectal bleeding, and vulvar lesions may develop later.

Vulvar cancer

- Bleeding, itching, groin pain, unusual lumps or sores, and abnormal urination and defecation may occur.

OTHER

Drugs

- Unopposed estrogen replacement therapy may cause abnormal vaginal bleeding, but cancer must always be ruled out.
- Antibiotics may change the normal vaginal pH and flora.

- Until a diagnosis is made, estrogen replacement is stopped.
- Prepare the patient for diagnostic tests.

GERIATRIC TIPS

- Endometrial atrophy may cause postmenopausal bleeding, but malignancy should be ruled out.

- Reassure the patient that postmenopausal vaginal bleeding may be benign, but careful assessment is still needed.
- Teach about underlying diagnosis and treatment plan.

Vaginal discharge

OVERVIEW

- Appears mucoid, clear or white, non-bloody, and odorless
- Occurs abnormally when a marked increase or change in color, odor, or consistency occurs that may signal disease

HISTORY

- Ask about the onset and description of the discharge.
- Find out about other symptoms, such as dysuria and perineal pruritus and burning.
- Determine recent changes in sexual habits or hygiene practices.
- Ask about previous discharge or infection and treatment used.
- Take a drug history, including use of antibiotics, oral estrogens, and contraceptives.
- Ask about the possibility of pregnancy.

PHYSICAL ASSESSMENT

- Examine the external genitalia and note the character of the discharge. (See *Identifying causes of vaginal discharge.*)
- Observe vulvar and vaginal tissues for redness, edema, and excoriation.
- Palpate the inguinal nodes for tenderness or enlargement.
- Palpate the abdomen for tenderness.
- A pelvic examination may be needed.
- Obtain vaginal discharge specimens for testing.

CAUSES

MEDICAL

Atrophic vaginitis

- A thin, scant, watery white vaginal discharge may be accompanied by pruritus, burning, and tenderness.
- Sparse pubic hair, a pale vagina with decreased rugae and small hemorrhagic spots, clitoral atrophy, and shrinking of the labia minora may also occur.

Bacterial vaginosis

- Thin, foul-smelling, green or gray-white discharge adheres to the vaginal walls and can be easily wiped away.
- Pruritus, redness, and other signs of vaginal irritation may occur.

Candidiasis

- A profuse, white, curdlike discharge with a yeasty, sweet odor is produced.
- Onset of discharge is abrupt, usually just before menses or during a course of antibiotics.
- Exudate may be lightly attached to the labia and vaginal walls and is commonly accompanied by vulvar redness and edema.
- The inner thighs may be covered with a fine, red dermatitis and weeping erosions.
- Intense labial itching and burning and external dysuria may also occur.

Chlamydial infection

- A yellow, mucopurulent, odorless, or acrid vaginal discharge is produced.
- Other findings include dysuria, dyspareunia, and vaginal bleeding after douching or coitus, especially following menses.

Endometritis

- A scant, serosanguineous discharge with a foul odor can result.
- Other findings include fever, lower back and abdominal pain, abdominal muscle spasm, malaise, dysmenorrhea, and an enlarged uterus.

 TOP TECHNIQUE

Identifying causes of vaginal discharge

The color, consistency, amount, and odor of your patient's vaginal discharge provide important clues about the underlying disorder. For quick reference, use this chart to match common characteristics of vaginal discharge and their possible causes.

CHARACTERISTICS	POSSIBLE CAUSES
Thin, scant, watery white discharge	Atrophic vaginitis
Thin, green or gray-white, foul-smelling discharge	Bacterial vaginosis
White, curdlike, profuse discharge with yeasty, sweet odor	Candidiasis
Yellow, mucopurulent, odorless, or acrid discharge	Chlamydial infection
Scant, serosanguineous, or purulent discharge with foul odor	Endometritis
Profuse, mucopurulent discharge, possibly foul-smelling	Genital warts
Yellow or green, foul-smelling discharge from the cervix or occasionally from Bartholin's or Skene's ducts	Gonorrhea
Chronic, watery, bloody, or purulent discharge, possibly foul-smelling	Gynecologic cancer
Copious mucoid discharge	Herpes simplex (genital)
Frothy, green-yellow, and profuse (or thin, white, and scant) foul-smelling discharge	Trichomoniasis

Genital warts

◆ A profuse, mucopurulent vaginal discharge, which may be foul-smelling if the warts are infected, may be produced.
◆ Mosaic, papular vulvar lesions occur, frequently with burning or paresthesia around the vaginal opening.
◆ Genital warts can also appear around the anus or on the cervix.

Gonorrhea

◆ Occasionally, yellow or green, foul-smelling discharge can be expressed from Bartholin's or Skene's ducts, but 80% of women have no symptoms.
◆ Other findings include dysuria, urinary frequency and incontinence, bleeding, vaginal redness and swelling, fever, and severe pelvic and abdominal pain.

Gynecologic cancer

◆ Chronic, watery, bloody or purulent vaginal discharge may be foul-smelling.
◆ Other findings include abnormal vaginal bleeding and, later, weight loss; pelvic, back, and leg pain; fatigue; urinary frequency; and abdominal distention.

Herpes simplex (genital)

◆ Copious mucoid discharge results, but the initial complaint is painful, indurated vesicles and ulcerations on the labia, vagina, cervix, anus, thighs, or mouth.
◆ Erythema, marked edema, and tender inguinal lymph nodes may occur with fever, malaise, and dysuria.

Trichomoniasis

◆ A foul-smelling discharge, which may be frothy, green-yellow, and profuse or thin, white, and scant, may be produced, although about 70% of patients are asymptomatic.
◆ Other findings include pruritus; a red, inflamed vagina with tiny petechiae; dysuria and urinary frequency; and dyspareunia, postcoital spotting, menorrhagia, or dysmenorrhea.

OTHER

Contraceptive creams and jellies

◆ Contraceptive creams and jellies can increase vaginal secretions.

Drugs

◆ Drugs that contain estrogen can cause increased mucoid vaginal discharge.
◆ Antibiotics may increase the risk of candidal vaginal infection and discharge.

Radiation therapy

◆ Irradiation of the reproductive tract can cause a watery, odorless, vaginal discharge.

NURSING CONSIDERATIONS

◆ Obtain cultures of the discharge.
◆ Give antibiotics, antivirals, or other drugs, if ordered.
◆ Observe standard precautions to prevent the spread of infection.

PEDIATRIC TIPS

◆ Female neonates who have been exposed to their mother's estrogens in utero may have a white, mucous, vaginal discharge for the first month after birth; a yellow mucous discharge indicates disease.
◆ In an older child, purulent, foul-smelling, and possibly bloody vaginal discharge commonly results from a foreign object placed in the vagina. Consider the possibility of sexual abuse.

GERIATRIC TIPS

◆ Incidence of vaginitis increases in elderly patients.

PATIENT TEACHING

◆ Explain the importance of keeping the perineum clean and dry and avoiding tight-fitting clothing.
◆ Suggest douching with vinegar and water to relieve discomfort, if appropriate.
◆ Stress compliance with prescribed drugs.
◆ Instruct the patient to avoid intercourse until symptoms of infection clear.
◆ Provide information on safer sex practices.

Vertigo

- Refers to an illusion of movement in which the patient feels that he's revolving in space (subjective) or the feeling of the surroundings revolving around the individual (objective)
- May be temporary or permanent, mild or severe
- Commonly occurs with nausea, vomiting, nystagmus, and tinnitus or hearing loss
- May worsen with movement and subside when lying down

- Ask about the onset and description of vertigo.
- Note what aggravates and alleviates vertigo.
- Ask about motion sickness and hearing loss.
- Obtain a recent drug history.
- Find out about alcohol use.

- Obtain vital signs.
- Perform a neurologic assessment, focusing particularly on eighth cranial nerve function.
- Observe gait and posture.
- Perform a hearing test.

MEDICAL

Acoustic neuroma

- Mild, intermittent vertigo occurs with sensorineural hearing loss in one ear.
- Other findings include tinnitus, postauricular or suboccipital pain, and—with cranial nerve compression—facial paralysis.

Benign positional vertigo

- Debris in a semicircular canal produces vertigo on head position change, lasting a few minutes.

Brain stem ischemia

- Sudden, severe vertigo may become episodic and later persistent.
- Other findings include ataxia, nausea, vomiting, increased blood pressure, tachycardia, nystagmus, and lateral deviation of the eyes toward the side of the lesion.
- Hemiparesis and paresthesia may also occur.

Head trauma

- Persistent vertigo occurs soon after injury along with spontaneous or positional nystagmus and, if the temporal bone is fractured, hearing loss.
- Other findings include headache, nausea, vomiting, and decreased level of consciousness (LOC).
- Behavioral changes, diplopia or visual blurring, seizures, motor or sensory deficits, and signs of increased intracranial pressure may also develop.

Herpes zoster

- Infection of the eighth cranial nerve produces sudden onset of vertigo, facial paralysis, hearing loss in the affected ear, and herpetic vesicular lesions in the auditory canal.

Labyrinthitis

- Severe vertigo begins abruptly and may occur in a single episode or recur over months or years.
- Associated findings include nausea, vomiting, progressive sensorineural hearing loss, and nystagmus.

Ménière's disease
◆ Labyrinthine dysfunction causes abrupt onset of vertigo, lasting minutes, hours, or days.
◆ Unpredictable episodes of severe vertigo and unsteady gait may cause the patient to fall.
◆ During an attack, any sudden motion of the head or eyes can precipitate nausea or vomiting.

Motion sickness
◆ Vertigo, nausea, vomiting, and headache occur in response to rhythmic or erratic motions.
◆ Dizziness, fatigue, diaphoresis, hypersalivation, and dyspnea may also occur.

Multiple sclerosis
◆ Episodic vertigo may occur early and become persistent.
◆ Other early findings include diplopia, visual blurring, and paresthesia.
◆ Nystagmus, constipation, muscle weakness, paralysis, spasticity, hyperreflexia, intention tremor, and ataxia may also occur.

Posterior fossa tumor
◆ Positional vertigo occurs and lasts a few seconds.
◆ Other findings include papilledema, headache, memory loss, nausea, vomiting, nystagmus, apneustic respirations, and elevated blood pressure.

Seizures
◆ Temporal lobe seizures may produce vertigo, usually associated with other symptoms of partial complex seizures.
◆ Seizures may be heralded by an aura and followed by several minutes of mental confusion.

Vestibular neuritis
◆ Severe vertigo usually begins abruptly and lasts several days, without tinnitus or hearing loss.
◆ Other findings include nausea, vomiting, and nystagmus.

OTHER
Diagnostic tests
◆ Caloric testing (irrigating the ears with warm or cold water) can induce vertigo.

Drugs and alcohol
◆ High or toxic doses of certain drugs (such as aminoglycosides, antibiotics, hormonal contraceptives, quinine, and salicylates) or alcohol may produce vertigo.

Surgery and procedures
◆ Use of overly warm or cold eardrops or irrigating solutions can cause vertigo.
◆ Ear surgery may cause vertigo that lasts for several days.

NURSING CONSIDERATIONS

◆ Place the patient in a comfortable position.
◆ Monitor vital signs and LOC.
◆ Keep the bed's side rails up; if the patient is standing, help him to a chair.
◆ Darken the room and keep the patient calm.
◆ Give drugs to control nausea and vomiting and decrease labyrinthine irritability.

PEDIATRIC TIPS
◆ Ear infection and vestibular neuritis may cause vertigo.

PATIENT TEACHING

◆ Explain the need for moving around with assistance.
◆ Stress the need to avoid sudden position changes and dangerous tasks.
◆ Teach about underlying diagnosis and treatment plan.
◆ Teach about prescribed medications and precautions.

Vesicular rash

OVERVIEW

- Appears as a scattered or linear distribution of sharply circumscribed, blisterlike lesions that are usually less than 0.5 cm in diameter
- May be filled with clear, cloudy, or bloody fluid
- May be mild or severe and temporary or permanent

HISTORY

- Ask about the onset and characteristics of rash.
- Take a drug history.
- Ask about other signs and symptoms.
- Find out about a family history of skin disorders.
- Ask about a history of allergies.
- Inquire about recent infections, insect bites, or exposure to allergens.

PHYSICAL ASSESSMENT

- Note if skin is dry, oily, or moist.
- Observe the distribution of the lesions; record their location.
- Note the color, shape, and size of the lesions.
- Check for crusts, scales, scars, macules, papules, or wheals.
- Palpate the vesicles or bullae to determine if they're flaccid or tense.

CAUSES

MEDICAL

Burns (second-degree)
- Vesicles and bullae, erythema, swelling, pain, and moistness occur with second-degree burns.

Dermatitis
- With contact dermatitis, small vesicles are surrounded by redness and marked edema; vesicles may ooze, scale, and cause severe pruritus.
- With dermatitis herpetiformis, vesicular, papular, bullous, pustular, or erythematous lesions form; severe pruritus, burning, and stinging may also occur.
- With nummular dermatitis, groups of pinpoint vesicles and papules appear on erythematous or pustular lesions; pustular lesions may ooze a purulent exudate, itch severely, and rapidly become crusted and scaly.

Dermatophytid
- Pruritic and tender vesicular lesions develop on the hands.
- Other findings include fever, anorexia, generalized adenopathy, and splenomegaly.

Erythema multiform
- This disorder is heralded by a sudden eruption of erythematous macules, papules, and occasionally vesicles and bullae.
- Vesiculobullous lesions usually appear on the mucous membranes, especially the lips and buccal mucosa—where they may rupture and ulcerate producing thick, yellow or white exudate.
- A characteristic rash appears symmetrically over the hands, arms, feet, legs, face and neck.

Herpes simplex
- Vesicles that are 2 to 3 mm in size and on an inflamed base most commonly appear on the lips and lower face.
- Vesicles are preceded by itching, tingling, burning, or pain.

Eventually, vesicle rupture forms a painful ulcer followed by a yellowish crust.

Herpes zoster

- A vesicular rash is preceded by erythema and, occasionally, by a nodular skin eruption and sharp pain along a dermatome.
- About 5 days later, lesions erupt and the pain becomes burning; vesicles dry and scab about 10 days after eruption.
- Other findings include fever, malaise, pruritus, and paresthesia or hyperesthesia of the involved area.
- If the cranial nerves are involved, facial palsy, hearing loss, dizziness, loss of taste, eye pain, and impaired vision occur.

Insect bites

- Vesicles appear on red papules and may become hemorrhagic.
- Other findings include fever, myalgia, headache, lymphadenopathy, nausea, and vomiting.

Pemphigus

- Groups of tiny vesicles erupt on normal skin or mucous membranes.
- Vesicles are thin-walled, flaccid, and easily broken, producing small denuded areas that eventually form crusts; itching and burning of the skin may also occur.

Pompholyx (dyshidrosis or dyshidrosis eczema)

- Symmetrical vesicular lesions occur that can become pustular appear on the palms and soles.
- Pruritic lesions are more common on the palms than on the soles with possible minimal erythema.

Scabies

- Small vesicles erupt on an erythematous base and may be at the end of a threadlike burrow.
- Pustules and excoriations may occur.
- Pruritus occurs and may worsen with inactivity, warmth, and nightfall.

Smallpox

- A maculopapular rash on the mucosa of the mouth, pharynx, face, and forearms spreads to the trunk and legs, then turns vesicular within 2 days and later pustular.
- Initial findings include high fever, malaise, prostration, severe headache, backache, and abdominal pain.
- After 8 to 9 days, the pustules form a crust; later, the scab separates from the skin, leaving a pitted scar.

Tinea pedis

- Vesicles and scaling develop between the toes.
- Inflammation, pruritus, and difficulty walking occur with severe infection.

- If skin eruptions cover a large skin surface, insert an I.V. catheter to replace fluid and electrolytes.
- Keep the environment warm and free from drafts.
- Obtain cultures to determine the standard causative organism.
- Look for signs of secondary infection.
- Give the patient an antibiotic and apply corticosteroid or antimicrobial ointment to the lesions, as prescribed.

PEDIATRIC TIPS

- Vesicular rash may be caused by staphylococcal infections, varicella, hand-foot-and-mouth disease, contact dermatitis, and prickly heat in children.

- Explain the importance of frequent hand-washing and other infection-control techniques.
- Instruct the patient to avoid touching the lesions.
- Explain the use of tepid baths or cold compresses to relieve itching and discomfort.
- Discuss underlying condition and treatment.

Vision loss

OVERVIEW

- Refers to an inability to perceive visual stimuli that ranges from slight impairment to total blindness
- Can be sudden or gradual, temporary or permanent
- If sudden, can be an ocular emergency (see *Managing sudden vision loss*)

HISTORY

- Ask about the characteristics of vision loss.
- Find out about associated photosensitivity or eye pain.
- Obtain an ocular history and family history of eye problems or systemic diseases that may lead to eye problems, such as hypertension; diabetes mellitus; thyroid, rheumatic, or vascular disease; infections; and cancer.
- Determine current medications, especially eye drops.

PHYSICAL ASSESSMENT

- If the patient has perforating or penetrating ocular trauma, don't touch his eye.
- Assess visual acuity, with best available correction in each eye. (See *Testing visual acuity.*)
- Inspect the eyes, noting edema, foreign bodies, drainage, or conjunctival or scleral redness.
- Observe whether lid closure is complete or incomplete and check for ptosis.
- Using a flashlight, examine the cornea and iris for scars, irregularities, and foreign bodies.
- Observe the size, shape, and color of the pupils.
- Test the direct and consensual light reflex and the effect of accommodation.

 ACTION STAT!

Managing sudden vision loss

Sudden vision loss can signal central retinal artery occlusion or acute angle-closure glaucoma—ocular emergencies that require immediate intervention. If your patient reports sudden vision loss, immediately notify an ophthalmologist for an emergency examination, and perform these interventions:

FOR SUSPECTED CENTRAL RETINAL ARTERY OCCLUSION

Perform light massage over the patient's closed eyelid. Increase his carbon dioxide level by administering a set flow of oxygen and carbon dioxide through a Venturi mask, as ordered, or have the patient rebreathe in a paper bag to retain exhaled carbon dioxide. These steps will dilate the artery and, possibly, restore blood flow to the retina.

FOR SUSPECTED ACUTE ANGLE-CLOSURE GLAUCOMA

Measure the patient's intraocular pressure (IOP) with a tonometer. (You can also estimate IOP without a tonometer by placing your fingers over the patient's closed eyelid. A rock-hard eyeball usually indicates increased IOP.) Instill timolol drops and administer I.V. acetazolamide, as ordered, to help decrease IOP.

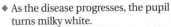

CAUSES

MEDICAL

Amaurosis fugax
- Recurrent attacks of vision loss in one eye may last from a few seconds to a few minutes.

 TOP TECHNIQUE

Testing visual acuity

Use a Snellen letter chart (as shown at bottom left) to test visual acuity in the literate patient older than age 6. Have the patient sit or stand 20' (6 m) from the chart. Tell him to cover his left eye and read aloud the smallest line of letters that he can see. Record the fraction assigned to that line on the chart (the numerator indicates distance from the chart; the denominator indicates the distance at which a normal eye can read the chart). Normal vision is 20/20. Repeat the test with the patient's right eye covered.

If your patient can't read the largest letter from a distance of 20', have him approach the chart until he can read it. Then, record the distance between him and the chart as the numerator of the fraction. For example, if he can see the top line of the chart at a distance of 3' (1 m), record the test result as 3/20.

Use a Snellen symbol chart (as shown at bottom right) to test children ages 3 to 6 and illiterate patients. Follow the same procedure as for the Snellen letter chart, but ask the patient to indicate the direction of the E's fingers as you point to each symbol.

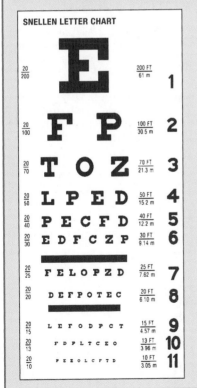

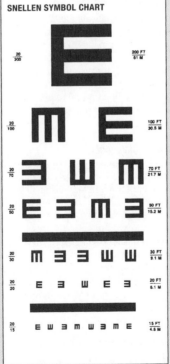

- Vision is normal at other times.
- Transient one-sided weakness, hypertension, and elevated intraocular pressure (IOP) in the affected eye may also develop.

Cataract
- Painless and gradual blurring of vision precedes vision loss.

- As the disease progresses, the pupil turns milky white.
- Night blindness and halo vision may be early signs.

Concussion
- Vision may be temporarily blurred, doubled, or lost.
- Other findings include headache, anterograde and retrograde amnesia, transient loss of consciousness, nausea, vomiting, dizziness, irritability, confusion, lethargy, and aphasia.

Diabetic retinopathy
- Retinal edema and hemorrhage lead to blurred vision, which may progress to blindness.
- Loss of central vision and color vision may also occur.
- This disorder is usually a sign of poorly controlled, brittle, or advanced diabetes.

Endophthalmitis
- Permanent unilateral vision loss may result as well as headache, photophobia, and ocular discharge.

Glaucoma
- Gradual blurring of vision may progress to total blindness.
- Acute angle-closure glaucoma, an ocular emergency, may produce blindness within 3 to 5 days, inflammation, and pain in one eye; eye pressure; moderate pupil dilation; nonreactive pupillary response; a cloudy cornea; reduced visual acuity, photophobia; nausea; vomiting; and perception of blue or red halos around lights.
- Chronic open-angle glaucoma typically causes a slowly progressive peripheral vision loss, aching eyes, halo vision, and reduced visual acuity especially at night.

(continued)

Herpes zoster

* When the nasociliary nerve is affected, vision loss with eyelid lesions, conjunctivitis, skin lesions, and ocular muscle palsies may occur.

Hyphema

* Blood in the anterior chamber can reduce vision to light perception only.
* Other findings include moderate pain, conjunctival injection, and eyelid edema.

Keratitis

* Complete vision loss occurs in one eye with an opaque cornea, increased tearing, irritation, and photophobia.

Ocular trauma

* Vision loss is sudden, total or partial, permanent or temporary, and in one or both eyes.
* Eyelids may be reddened, edematous, and lacerated; intraocular contents may be extruded.

Optic atrophy

* Irreversible loss of the visual field and changes in color vision result.
* Pupillary reactions are sluggish, and optic disk pallor is evident.

Optic neuritis

* Vision loss in one eye is temporary but severe.
* Pain around the eye occurs, especially with movement of the globe.
* Visual field defects and a sluggish pupillary response may also occur.

Paget's disease

* Vision loss may develop because of bony impingements on the cranial nerves.
* Hearing loss, tinnitus, vertigo, and severe, persistent bone pain also occur. Cranial enlargement may be noticeable frontally and occipitally, and headaches may occur.
* Sites of bone involvement are warm and tender, and impaired mobility and pathologic fractures are common.

Papilledema

* Acute papilledema may lead to momentary blurring or transiently obscured vision; chimeric papilledema may cause vision loss.

Pituitary tumor

* Blurred vision progresses to hemianopsia and, possibly, unilateral blindness as the tumor grows.
* Double vision, nystagmus, ptosis, limited eye movement, and headaches may also occur.

Retinal artery occlusion (central)

* An ocular emergency—partial or complete vision loss in one eye is sudden.
* Permanent blindness may occur within hours.
* A sluggish direct pupillary response and a normal consensual response occur.

Retinal detachment

* Painless vision loss may be gradual or sudden and total or partial.
* With partial vision loss, visual field defects or a shadow or curtain over the visual fields, and visual floaters may be reported.
* Total blindness occurs with macular involvement.

Retinal vein occlusion (central)

* Decrease in visual acuity in one eye may occur with variable vision loss.
* IOP may be elevated in both eyes.

Senile macular degeneration

* Painless blurring or loss of central vision occurs.
* Vision loss may proceed slowly or rapidly, may eventually affect both eyes, and may be worse at night.

Temporal arteritis

* Vision blurring and loss with a throbbing headache are characteristic findings.
* Other findings include malaise, anorexia, weight loss, weakness, low-grade fever, generalized muscle aches, and confusion.

Uveitis

* Inflammation of the uveal tract may cause unilateral vision loss.
* Anterior uveitis produces moderate to severe eye pain, severe conjunctival injection, photophobia, and a small, nonreactive pupil.
* Posterior uveitis may produce insidious onset of blurred vision, conjunctival injection, visual floaters, pain, and photophobia.

Vitreous hemorrhage

* Vision loss in one eye is sudden.
* Visual floaters and partial vision with a reddish haze may occur.

OTHER
Drugs
- Digoxin derivatives, ethambutol, indomethacin (Indocin), methanol toxicity, and quinine sulfate may cause vision loss.
- Chloroquine phosphate (Aralen) therapy may cause patchy retinal pigmentation that typically leads to blindness.

NURSING CONSIDERATIONS
- If the patient has photophobia, darken the room and suggest wearing sunglasses during the day.
- Obtain cultures of eye drainage.
- Get the patient a referral to an ophthalmologist for evaluation.

PEDIATRIC TIPS
- Optic nerve gliomas and retinoblastomas may cause vision loss in children.
- Congenital rubella and syphilis may cause vision loss in infants.

GERIATRIC TIPS
- Reduced visual acuity may be caused by morphologic changes in the choroid, pigment epithelium, and retina or by decreased function of the rods, cones, and other neural elements.

PATIENT TEACHING
- Make sure the patient is oriented to his environment.
- Explain safety measures to prevent injury.
- Emphasize the importance of frequent hand washing and avoiding rubbing the eyes.
- If vision loss is progressive or permanent, refer the patient to appropraite social service agencies for assistance with adaptation and equipment.
- Discuss underlying disorder, diagnostic tests, and treatment plan.

Visual blurring

◆ Refers to the loss of visual acuity with indistinct visual details

HISTORY

◆ Ask about eye pain, trauma, sudden vision loss, or discharge.
◆ Find out about the onset of visual blurring.
◆ Ask about recent accidents or injuries.
◆ Obtain a medical and drug history.

PHYSICAL ASSESSMENT

◆ Inspect the eye; note lid edema, drainage, conjunctival or scleral redness, an irregularly shaped iris, and excessive blinking.
◆ Assess for pupillary changes.
◆ Test visual acuity in both eyes.
◆ Assess neurologic status and level of consciousness (LOC).

CAUSES

MEDICAL
Brain tumor
◆ Visual blurring occurs with decreased LOC, headache, apathy, behavioral changes, memory loss, decreased attention span, dizziness, and confusion.
◆ Related findings include aphasia, seizures, ataxia, and signs of hormonal imbalance.
◆ Later findings include vomiting, increased systolic blood pressure, widened pulse pressure, and decorticate posture.

Cataract
◆ Gradual blurring with halo vision (an early sign), visual glare in bright light, progressive vision loss, and a gray pupil that turns milky white occur with a cataract.

Concussion
◆ Blurred, double, or temporary vision loss occurs with a concussion.
◆ Related findings include changes in LOC and behavior.

Conjunctivitis
◆ Visual blurring occurs with photophobia, pain, burning, tearing, itching, and a feeling of fullness around the eyes.
◆ Redness near the fornices (brilliant red suggests a bacterial cause; milky red, an allergic cause) and drainage (copious, mucopurulent, and flaky in bacterial conjunctivitis; stringy in allergic conjunctivitis) occur.
◆ With viral conjunctivitis, copious tearing, minimal exudate, and an enlarged preauricular lymph node occur.

Corneal abrasions
◆ Visual blurring with severe eye pain occurs with corneal abrasions.
◆ Other findings include photophobia, redness, and excessive tearing.

Diabetic retinopathy
◆ Retinal edema and hemorrhage produce gradual blurring, which may progress to blindness.
◆ Loss of central vision and color vision may occur.

Eye tumor
◆ If the macula is involved, blurring may be the first symptom.
◆ Other findings include varying visual field losses.

Glaucoma
◆ With acute angle-closure glaucoma, an ocular emergency, visual blurring and severe pain begin suddenly in one eye.
◆ Other acute findings include halo vision; a moderately dilated, nonreactive pupil; conjunctival injection; a cloudy cornea; and decreased visual acuity.
◆ With chronic angle-closure glaucoma, transient visual blurring and halo vision may precede pain and blindness.

Hypertension
◆ Visual blurring and a constant morning headache occur with hypertension.
◆ With a diastolic blood pressure over 120 mm Hg, a severe throbbing headache occurs.
◆ Other findings include restlessness, confusion, nausea, vomiting, seizures, and decreased LOC.

Hyphema
◆ Visual blurring from blunt eye trauma with hemorrhage into the anterior chamber causes moderate pain, diffuse conjunctival injection, visible blood in the anterior chamber, ecchymoses, eyelid edema, and a hard eye.

Iritis
◆ Sudden blurring, moderate to severe eye pain, photophobia, conjunctival injection, and a constricted pupil occur with iritis.

Macular degeneration (dry form)
◆ Initially, painless visual blurring or dimming, especially noticeable with reading and worsens at night.
◆ Other findings include blind spots and progressive loss of central vision.

Macular degeneration (wet form)
◆ Blurring with darkened vision occurs in the affected eye.
◆ A blind spot occurs in the visual field with distorted straight lines and eventual loss of central vision.

Migraine headache
◆ Migraine headache is characterized by blurring and paroxysmal attacks of a severe, throbbing, headache.
◆ Nausea, vomiting, sensitivity to light and noise, and sensory or visual auras may also occur.

Multiple sclerosis
◆ In the early stage, blurred vision, diplopia, and paresthesia occur.
◆ In later stages, nystagmus, muscle weakness, paralysis, spasticity, hyperreflexia, intention tremor, and ataxic gait occur.
◆ Other findings include urinary frequency, urgency, and incontinence.

Optic neuritis
◆ An acute attack of blurring and vision loss from inflammation, degeneration, or demyelinization of the optic nerve occur with this disorder.
◆ Scotomas and eye pain occur.
◆ Hyperemia of the optic disk, large vein distention, blurred disk margins, and filling of the physiologic cup are revealed upon ophthalmoscopic examination.

Retinal detachment
◆ Sudden visual blurring may be the first symptom, followed by visual floaters and recurring light flashes.
◆ Progressive detachment increases vision loss.

Retinal vein occlusion (central)
◆ Gradual visual blurring and varying degrees of vision loss occur in one eye.

Stroke
◆ Brief attacks of visual blurring occur before or with a stroke.
◆ Associated findings include decreased LOC, contralateral hemiplegia, dysarthria, dysphagia, ataxia, unilateral sensory loss, agnosia, aphasia, homonymous hemianopsia, diplopia, disorientation, and apraxia.
◆ Other findings include urine retention or incontinence, constipation, personality changes, emotional lability, and seizures.

Temporal arteritis
◆ Sudden blurred vision with vision loss and a throbbing headache occur.
◆ Early findings include malaise, anorexia, weight loss, weakness, low-grade fever, and generalized muscle aches.
◆ Later findings include confusion; disorientation; swollen, nodular, tender temporal arteries; and erythema of overlying skin.

Uveitis (posterior)
◆ Blurred vision, conjunctival injection, visual floaters, pain, and photophobia occur with this disorder.

Vitreous hemorrhage
◆ Sudden visual blurring and varying vision loss occur in one eye.
◆ Associated findings include visual floaters or dark streaks and partial vision with a reddish haze.

OTHER
Drugs
◆ Anticholinergics, antihistamines, clomiphene, cycloplegics, guanethidine, phenothiazines, phenylbutazone, reserpine, or thiazide diuretics can cause visual blurring.

NURSING CONSIDERATIONS
◆ Prepare the patient for diagnostic tests.
◆ Initiate safety measures to prevent injury.
◆ Provide emotional support as needed.

PEDIATRIC TIPS
◆ Blurring may stem from congenital syphilis or cataracts, refractive errors, eye injuries or infections, and increased intracranial pressure.

PATIENT TEACHING
◆ Teach the patient to instill eyedrops properly.
◆ Explain the need for orientation to his environment.
◆ Instruct the patient in safety measures.
◆ Discuss underlying disorder.

Visual floaters

OVERVIEW

◆ Are characterized by particles of blood or cellular debris that move about in the vitreous
◆ Appear as spots or dots as they enter the visual field
◆ Commonly signal retinal detachment, an ocular emergency, with sudden onset
◆ May be chronic and occur normally in elderly or myopic patients

ACTION STAT! *Sudden onset of visual floaters may signal retinal detachment. Ask the patient if he also sees flashing lights or spots in the affected eye. Is he experiencing a curtainlike loss of vision? If so, notify an ophthalmologist immediately and restrict his eye movements until the diagnosis is made.*

HISTORY

◆ Obtain a drug and allergy history.
◆ Ask about nearsightedness (a predisposing factor), use of corrective lenses, eye trauma, or other eye disorders.
◆ Ask about a history of granulomatous disease, diabetes mellitus, or hypertension, which may have predisposed him to retinal detachment, vitreous hemorrhage, or uveitis.

PHYSICAL ASSESSMENT

◆ Inspect the eyes for signs of injury, such as bruising or edema, and determine the patient's visual acuity. (See *Testing visual acuity,* page 589.)

CAUSES

MEDICAL

Retinal detachment

◆ Floaters and light flashes appear suddenly in the portion of the visual field where the retina is detached from the choroid.
◆ As the retina detaches further (a painless process), the patient develops gradual vision loss, likened to a cloud or curtain falling in front of the eyes.
◆ Ophthalmoscopic examination reveals a gray, opaque, detached retina with an indefinite margin. Retinal vessels appear almost black.

Uveitis (posterior)

◆ This disorder may cause visual floaters accompanied by gradual eye pain, photophobia, blurred vision, and conjunctival injection.

Vitreous hemorrhage

◆ Rupture of the retinal vessels produces a shower of red or black dots or a red haze across the visual field.
◆ Vision suddenly becomes blurred in the affected eye, and visual acuity may be greatly reduced.

NURSING CONSIDERATIONS

◆ Encourage bed rest and provide a calm environment.
◆ Depending on the cause of the floaters, the patient may require eye patches, surgery, or a corticosteroid or other drug therapy. If bilateral eye patches are necessary—as in retinal detachment—ensure the patient's safety.
◆ Identify yourself when you approach the patient, and orient him to time frequently.
◆ Provide sensory stimulation, such as a radio or compact disc player.
◆ Place pillows or towels behind the patient's head to maintain the appropriate position for the patient.
◆ Warn him not to touch or rub his eyes and to avoid straining or sudden movements.

PEDIATRIC TIPS

◆ Visual floaters in children usually follow a traumatic injury that causes retinal detachment or vitreous hemorrhage.
◆ They may also result from vitreous debris, a benign congenital condition with no other signs or symptoms.

GERIATRIC TIPS

◆ Elderly patients may experience increased myopia caused by lens changes.

PATIENT TEACHING

◆ Teach the patient and his family about underlying diagnosis and treatment plan.
◆ Explain all hospital procedures and tests.
◆ Teach the patient about prescribed medications.

Vomiting

OVERVIEW

- Refers to the forceful expulsion of gastric contents through the mouth
- Occurs as a coordinated sequence of abdominal muscle contractions and reverse esophageal peristalsis
- Is characteristically preceded by nausea (see *Managing a dehydration emergency*)

HISTORY

- Ask about the onset, duration, and intensity of vomiting. (See *Identifying causes of vomiting*.)
- Determine aggravating or alleviating factors.
- Ask about nausea, abdominal pain, anorexia, weight loss, changes in bowel habits, excessive belching or flatus, and bloating or fullness.
- Obtain a medical history, including GI, endocrine, and metabolic disorders; infections; and cancer, including chemotherapy and radiation therapy.
- Ask about current drug use and alcohol consumption.
- Find out if pregnancy is possible.

PHYSICAL ASSESSMENT

- Inspect the abdomen for distention.
- Auscultate for bowel sounds and bruits.
- Palpate for rigidity and tenderness, and test for rebound tenderness.
- Palpate and percuss the liver for enlargement.
- Assess buccal mucosa and skin turgor for sufficient hydration.

ACTION STAT!

Managing a dehydration emergency

SIGNS AND SYMPTOMS

- Decreased skin turgor
- Decreased urination
- Dry eyes and few tears when crying
- Dry mouth and mucous membranes
- Increased thirst
- Irritability
- Listlessness, low energy level
- Sunken cheeks, eyes, possibly abdomen, fontanel (in infants)
- Weakness or light-headedness

ACTIONS

- Notify physician.
- Institute I.V. fluid replacement therapy.
- Draw blood for electrolytes, renal studies, liver function tests, and complete blood count.
- Assess vital signs frequently until stable.
- Administer prescribed antiemetic (such as droperidol, granisetron, metoclopramide, ondansetron, or prochlorperazine depending on source of vomiting and effectiveness).
- Offer supportive care while patient is vomiting.
- Provide meticulous mouth care after episodes.

TOP TECHNIQUE

Identifying causes of vomiting

When you collect a sample of the patient's vomitus, observe it carefully for clues to the underlying disorder. Here's what vomitus may indicate:

BILE-STAINED (GREENISH) VOMITUS

Obstruction below the pylorus, as from a duodenal lesion

BLOODY VOMITUS

Upper GI bleeding (if bright red may result from gastritis or a peptic ulcer; if dark red, from esophageal or gastric varices)

BROWN VOMITUS WITH A FECAL ODOR

Intestinal obstruction or infarction

BURNING, BITTER-TASTING VOMITUS

Excessive hydrochloric acid in gastric contents

COFFEE-GROUND VOMITUS

Digested blood from slowly bleeding gastric or duodenal lesion

UNDIGESTED FOOD

Gastric outlet obstruction, as from a gastric tumor or ulcer

MEDICAL

Adrenal insufficiency
- Vomiting, nausea, anorexia, and diarrhea commonly occur with adrenal insufficiency.
- Other findings include weakness; fatigue; weight loss; bronze skin; orthostatic hypotension; and a weak, irregular pulse.

Anthrax (GI)
- Vomiting occurs with a loss of appetite, nausea, and a fever after eating contaminated food.
- GI anthrax may progress to abdominal pain, severe bloody diarrhea, and hematemesis.

Appendicitis
- Vomiting and nausea occur after or with abdominal pain.
- Vague epigastric or periumbilical discomfort occurs and rapidly progresses to severe, stabbing pain in the right-lower-quadrant.
- A positive McBurney's sign—severe pain and tenderness on palpation about 2″ (5 cm) from the right anterior superior spine of the ilium, on a line between that spine and the umbilicus—may also occur.
- Related findings include abdominal rigidity and tenderness, anorexia, constipation or diarrhea, cutaneous hyperalgesia, fever, tachycardia, and malaise.

Bulimia
- Polyphagia that alternates with self-induced vomiting, fasting, or diarrhea are classic findings.
- Anorexia, a morbid fear of obesity, and calloused knuckles (from self-induced vomiting) are signs and symptoms of the disorder.

Cholecystitis (acute)
- Nausea and mild vomiting after severe right-upper-quadrant pain that may radiate to the back or shoulders occur with acute cholecystitis.
- Related findings include abdominal tenderness and, possibly, rigidity and distention, fever, and diaphoresis.

Cholelithiasis
- Nausea and vomiting with severe unlocalized right-upper-quadrant or epigastric pain after ingestion of fatty foods occur with cholelithiasis.
- Other findings include abdominal tenderness and guarding, flatulence, belching, epigastric burning, pyrosis, tachycardia, and restlessness.

Cholera
- Cholera causes vomiting with abrupt watery diarrhea.
- Thirst, weakness, muscle cramps, decreased skin turgor, oliguria, tachycardia, and hypotension from severe water and electrolyte loss may also occur.

Cirrhosis
- In the early stage, nausea and vomiting, anorexia, aching abdominal pain, and constipation or diarrhea occur.
- In later stages, jaundice, hepatomegaly, and abdominal distention occur.

Ectopic pregnancy
- In this life-threatening disorder, ectopic pregnancy causes vomiting, nausea, vaginal bleeding, and lower abdominal pain.
- A tender abdominal mass and a 1- to 2-month history of amenorrhea is characteristic of this disorder.

Electrolyte imbalances
- Nausea and vomiting frequently occur along with arrhythmias, tremors, seizures, anorexia, malaise, and weakness.

Escherichia coli *0157:H7*
- Vomiting occus with watery or bloody diarrhea, nausea, fever, and abdominal cramps.
- Acute renal failure may occur in children younger than 5 and elderly patients.

Food poisoning
- Commonly, vomiting, diarrhea, severe and cramping abdominal pain, prostration, and fever occur.

Gastritis
- Commonly, nausea and vomiting of mucus or blood occur with gastritis.
- Other findings include epigastric pain, belching, and fever.

Gastroenteritis
- Nausea, vomiting (often of undigested food), diarrhea, and abdominal cramping occur with gastroenteritis.
- Associated findings include fever, malaise, hyperactive bowel sounds, and abdominal pain and tenderness.

Gestational hypertension
- Nausea and vomiting occurs with rapid weight gain, epigastric pain, edema, elevated blood pressure, oliguria, severe frontal headache, and blurred or double vision.

Heart failure
- Nausea and vomiting occur especially with right-sided heart failure.
- Tachycardia, ventricular gallop, fatigue, dyspnea, crackles, peripheral edema, and neck vein distention may also occur.

Hepatitis
- In the early stage, nausea and vomiting, fatigue, myalgia, arthralgia, headache, photophobia, anorexia, pharyngitis, cough, and fever occur.

Hyperemesis gravidarum
- Unremitting nausea and vomiting lasting beyond the first trimester occurs with this disorder.
- Undigested food, mucus, and small amounts of bile in the vomitus occur early in the disorder; later, a coffee-ground appearance occurs.
- Other findings include weight loss, headache, and delirium.

Increased intracranial pressure
- Projectile vomiting not preceded by nausea occurs with ICP.

(continued)

- Decreased level of consciousness (LOC), and Cushing's triad (bradycardia, hypertension, and respiratory pattern changes) may also occur.
- Other findings include headache, widened pulse pressure, impaired motor movement, vision disturbances, pupillary changes, and papilledema.

Intestinal obstruction
- Commonly, nausea and vomiting (bilious or fecal) occur with intestinal obstruction.
- Usually episodic and colicky abdominal pain occurs, possibly becoming severe and steady.
- Constipation occurs early in large intestinal obstruction and late in small intestinal obstruction.
- Obstipation occurs in complete obstruction.
- High-pitched and hyperactive bowel sounds occur in partial obstruction and hypoactive or absent bowel sounds in complete obstruction.

Labyrinthitis
- Nausea, vomiting, severe vertigo, progressive hearing loss, nystagmus and, possibly, otorrhea occur with labyrinthitis.

Listeriosis
- After ingesting food contaminated with *Listeria monocytogenes*, vomiting, fever, abdominal pain, myalgias, nausea, and diarrhea occur.

Ménière's disease
- Sudden, brief, recurrent attacks of nausea and vomiting, dizziness, vertigo, hearing loss, tinnitus, and nystagmus occur with this disease.

Mesenteric artery ischemia
- In this life-threatening disorder, mesenteric artery ischemia causes nausea and vomiting and severe, cramping abdominal pain, especially after meals.
- Associated findings include diarrhea or constipation, abdominal tenderness and bloating, anorexia, weight loss, and abdominal bruits.

Mesenteric venous thrombosis
- Nausea, vomiting, and abdominal pain with diarrhea or constipation, abdominal distention, hematemesis, and melena occur with mesenteric venous thrombosis.

Metabolic acidosis
- Nausea, vomiting, anorexia, diarrhea, Kussmaul's respirations, and decreased LOC occur with this disorder.

Migraine headache
- Premonitory nausea and vomiting occur with a migraine headache.
- Other findings include fatigue, photophobia, light flashes, increased noise sensitivity and, possibly, partial vision loss and paresthesia.

Motion sickness
- Nausea and vomiting with headache, vertigo, dizziness, fatigue, diaphoresis, and dyspnea are signs and symptoms of motion sickness.

Myocardial infarction
- Nausea and vomiting may occur with an MI, but the main symptom is severe substernal chest pain, which may radiate to the left arm, jaw, or neck.
- Dyspnea, pallor, clammy skin, diaphoresis, and restlessness may occur.

Pancreatitis (acute)
- In the early stage, vomiting usually precedes nausea.
- Other findings include steady and severe epigastric or left-upper-quadrant pain may radiate to the back, abdominal tenderness and rigidity, hypoactive bowel sounds, anorexia, and fever.
- In severe cases, tachycardia, restlessness, hypotension, skin mottling, and cold, sweaty extremities may occur.

Peptic ulcer
- Nausea and vomiting may follow sharp, burning or gnawing epigastric pain.

- Pain occurs especially when the stomach is empty or after ingestion of alcohol, caffeine, or aspirin.
- Hematemesis or melena may also occur.

Peritonitis
- Nausea and vomiting usually occur with acute abdominal pain.
- Related findings include high fever with chills; tachycardia; hypoactive or absent bowel sounds; abdominal distention, rigidity, and tenderness; weakness; pale, cold skin; diaphoresis; hypotension; signs of dehydration; and shallow respirations.

Q fever
- In this rickettsial infection, vomiting with fever, chills, severe headache, malaise, chest pain, nausea, and diarrhea occur.

Rhabdomyolysis
- Vomiting along with muscle weakness or pain, fever, nausea, malaise, and dark urine occur.

Thyrotoxicosis
- Nausea and vomiting occur with the classic findings of severe anxiety, heat intolerance, weight loss despite increased appetite, diaphoresis, diarrhea, tremors, tachycardia, and palpitations.
- Other findings include exophthalmos, ventricular or atrial gallop, and an enlarged thyroid.

Ulcerative colitis
- Vomiting, nausea, and anorexia with the common sign of recurrent diarrhea with blood, pus, and mucus occur with ulcerative colitis.
- Related findings include fever, chills, and weight loss.

Volvulus
- Vomiting with rapid, marked abdominal distention and sudden, severe abdominal pain occur.
- Twisting of intestine at least 180 degrees in its mesentery leads to blood vessel compression and ischemia.

- In adults, volvulus is common in the sigmoid bowel; in children, the small bowel.
- It can also occur in the stomach or cecum.

OTHER
Drugs
- Anesthetics, antibiotics, antineoplastics, chloride replacements, estrogens, ferrous sulfate, levodopa (Sinemet), opiates, oral potassium, quinidine sulfate, and sulfasalazine (Asulfidine) may cause vomiting.
- Overdoses of cardiac glycosides and theophylline may also cause vomiting.
- Syrup of ipecac may be used to induce vomiting for overdoses.

Radiation and surgery
- Radiation therapy can cause vomiting if it disrupts the gastric mucosa.
- Commonly, postoperative nausea and vomiting occurs, especially after abdominal surgery.

NURSING CONSIDERATIONS

- Draw blood to determine electrolyte and acid-base balance.
- Position the patient to prevent aspiration of vomitus.
- Monitor vital signs and intake and output.
- Maintain hydration by giving sips of water or ice chips if tolerated or by I.V. fluids if patient is hospitalized.
- Give drugs for pain promptly. If possible, give these by injection or suppository.
- If an opioid is used, monitor bowel sounds, flatus, and bowel movements.

PEDIATRIC TIPS
- In a neonate, pyloric obstruction may cause projectile vomiting; Hirschsprung's disease may cause fecal vomiting.
- Intussusception may lead to vomiting of bile and fecal matter.
- Infants and young children are susceptible to dehydration—a medical emergency—if vomiting persists for 2 days without the ability to retain fluids.

GERIATRIC TIPS
- Rule out intestinal ischemia first because it's especially common in elderly patients.
- Debilitated and undernourished patients are more susceptible to dehydration.

PATIENT TEACHING

- Explain deep-breathing techniques to postoperative patients.
- Discuss how to replace fluid losses.
- Teach the patient to adjust his diet by starting with clear liquids and advancing to a bland diet.
- Discuss underlying disorder, diagnostic tests, and treatment plan.

Vulvar lesions

- Occur as cutaneous lumps, nodules, papules, vesicles, or ulcers that appear on the vulva

HISTORY

- Ask about the onset of vulvar lesions.
- Inquire about associated findings, such as swelling, pain, or discharge.
- Question the patient about sexual activity and the potential for sexually transmitted disease (STD) exposure.

PHYSICAL ASSESSMENT

- Examine the lesion and obtain cultures. (See *Recognizing common vulvar lesions.*)
- Examine the rest of the skin for rashes and lesions.

TOP TECHNIQUE

Recognizing common vulvar lesions

Various disorders can cause vulvar lesions. For example, sexually transmitted diseases account for most vulvar lesions in premenopausal women, whereas vulvar tumors and cysts account for most lesions in women ages 50 to 70. These illustrations will help you recognize some of the most common vulvar lesions.

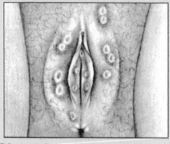

Primary genital herpes produces multiple ulcerated lesions surrounded by red halos.

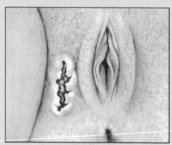

Basal cell carcinoma can produce an ulcerated lesion with raised, poorly rolled edges.

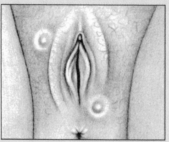

Primary syphilis produces chancres that appear as ulcerated lesions with raised borders.

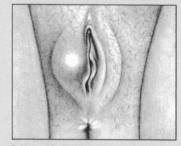

Epidermal inclusion cysts produce a round lump that usually appears on the labia majora.

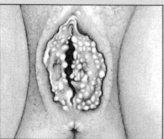

Squamous cell carcinoma can produce a large, granulomatous-appearing ulcer.

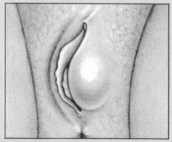

Bartholin's duct cysts produce a tense, nontender, palpable lump that usually appears on the labia minora.

CAUSES

MEDICAL
Basal cell carcinoma
- Tumor is nodular and has a central ulcer and a raised, poorly rolled border.
- Pruritus, bleeding, discharge, and a burning sensation may occur.

Benign cysts
- Epidermal inclusion cysts (usually round) appear on labia majora.
- Bartholin's duct cysts are usually tense, and nontender and on one side of the posterior labia minora.
- Bartholin's abscess causes gradual pain and tenderness.

Genital warts
- Painless red and pink swellings occur on vulva, vagina, and cervix.
- Other findings include pruritus, erythema, and a profuse, mucopurulent, vaginal discharge.

Gonorrhea
- Vulvar lesions, usually confined to Bartholin's glands, occur with pruritus, a burning sensation, pain, and a green-yellow vaginal discharge, but most patients are asymptomatic.
- Other findings include dysuria, urinary incontinence, severe pelvic and lower abdominal pain, and vaginal redness, swelling, bleeding, and vulvar engorgement.

Herpes simplex (genital)
- Fluid-filled vesicles appear on cervix and, possibly, on the vulva, labia, perianal skin, or vagina.
- Initially painless, vesicles may rupture and develop into extensive, shallow, painful ulcers, with redness and edema, and tender inguinal lymph nodes.
- Other findings include fever, malaise, and dysuria.

Molluscum contagiosum
- Raised vulvar papules are 1 to 2 mm in diameter and pearly or flesh-colored with umbilicated centers and white cores.

Pediculosis pubis
- Erythematous vulvar papules occur with pruritus and irritation.
- Adult pubic lice and nits are visible on pubic hair.

Squamous cell carcinoma
- Invasive carcinoma may produce vulvar pruritus, pain, and a lump.
- Carcinoma in situ produces a vulvar lesion that may be white or red, raised, well defined, moist, crusted, and isolated.

Squamous cell hyperplasia
- Vulvar lesions may be well delineated or poorly defined; localized or extensive; and red, brown, white, or both red and white.
- Intense pruritus, possibly with vulvar pain, intense burning, and dyspareunia, is the cardinal symptom.

Syphilis
- Papules with indurated, raised edges and clear bases on the vulva, vagina, or cervix occur 10 to 90 days after initial contact.
- Findings include a maculopapular, pustular, or nodular rash; headache; malaise; anorexia; weight loss; fever; nausea; vomiting; lymphadenopathy; and a sore throat.

Viral disease (systemic)
- Varicella, measles, and other systemic viral diseases may produce vulvar lesions.

NURSING CONSIDERATIONS
- Give a systemic antibiotic, an antiviral, a topical corticosteroid, a topical testosterone, or an antipruritic, as prescribed.
- Provide emotional support.

PEDIATRIC TIPS
- Vulvar lesions in children may result from congenital syphilis or gonorrhea; assess for sexual abuse.

GERIATRIC TIPS
- Vulvar dystrophies and neoplasia occur more frequently with advancing age.

PATIENT TEACHING
- Explain that sitz baths may make the patient more comfortable.
- Provide instruction in safer sex practices.
- Discuss underlying disorder and treatment plan.

Weight gain, excessive

OVERVIEW

- Refers to ingested calories that exceed body requirements for energy, resulting in increased adipose tissue storage
- May also occur when fluid retention causes edema

HISTORY

- Ask about previous pattern of weight gain and loss.
- Find out about a family history of obesity, thyroid disease, or diabetes mellitus.
- Note eating and activity patterns.
- Determine exercise habits.
- Ask about vision disturbances, hoarseness, paresthesia, increased urination and thirst, impotence, or menstrual irregularities.
- Take a drug history.

PHYSICAL ASSESSMENT

- Note mental status, memory, and response time.
- Measure skin-fold thickness. (See *Evaluating nutritional status*.)
- Note fat distribution and the presence of edema.
- Note overall nutritional status.
- Inspect for other abnormalities, such as abnormal body hair distribution or hair loss and dry skin.
- Take vital signs.
- Determine body mass index and waist circumference.

 TOP TECHNIQUE

Evaluating nutritional status

If your patient gains or loses excessive weight, you can help assess his nutritional status by measuring his skin-fold thickness and midarm circumference and by calculating his midarm muscle circumference. Skin-fold measurement reflects adipose tissue mass (subcutaneous fat accounts for about 50% of the body's adipose tissue). Midarm measurement reflects both skeletal muscle and adipose tissue mass.

Use the steps described here to gather these measurements. Then express them as a percentage of standard measurements by using this formula:

$$\frac{\text{actual measurement}}{\text{standard measurement}} \times 100 = \underline{\qquad}\%$$

Standard anthropometric measurements vary according to the patient's age and sex and can be found in a chart of normal anthropometric values. The abridged chart below lists standard arm measurements for adult men and women.

TEST	STANDARD	
Triceps skin fold	Men	12.5 mm
	Women	16.5 mm
Midarm circumference	Men	29.3 mm
	Women	28.5 mm
Midarm muscle circumference	Men	25.3 mm
	Women	23.2 mm

A triceps or subscapular skin-fold measurement below 60% of the standard value indicates severe depletion of fat reserves; measurement between 60% and 90% indicates moderate to mild depletion; and above 90% indicates significant fat reserves. A midarm circumference of less than 90% of the standard value indicates caloric deprivation; greater than 90% indicates adequate or ample muscle and fat. A midarm muscle circumference of less than 90% indicates protein depletion; greater than 90% indicates adequate or ample protein reserves.

To measure the triceps skin fold, locate the midpoint of the patient's upper arm, using a non-stretch tape measure and mark it with a felt-tip pen. Then grasp the skin with your thumb and forefinger about 1 cm above the midpoint. Place the calipers at the midpoint and squeeze them for about 3 seconds. Record the measurement registered at the handle gauge to the nearest 0.5 mm. Take two more readings and average the three.

To measure the subscapular skin fold, use your thumb and forefinger to grasp the skin just below the angle of the scapula, in line with the natural cleavage of the skin. Apply the calipers and proceed as you would when measuring the triceps skin fold. Both subscapular and triceps skin-fold measurements are reliable measurements of fat loss or gain during hospitalization.

To measure midarm circumference, return to the midpoint you marked on the patient's upper arm. Then use a tape measure to determine the arm circumference at this point. This measurement reflects both skeletal muscle and adipose tissue mass and helps evaluate protein and calorie reserves. To calculate midarm muscle circumference, multiply the triceps skin-fold thickness (in centimeters) by 3.143, and subtract this figure from the midarm circumference. Midarm muscle circumference reflects muscle mass alone, providing a more sensitive index of protein reserves.

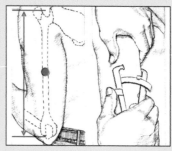

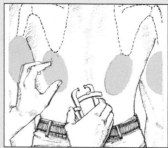

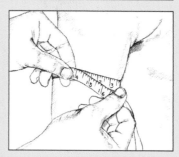

CAUSES

MEDICAL
Acromegaly
- Moderate weight gain occurs with coarsened facial features, projecting jaw, enlarged hands and feet, increased sweating, oily skin, deep voice, back and joint pain, lethargy, sleepiness, and heat intolerance.
- Hirsutism may occur occasionally.

Diabetes mellitus
- Increased appetite may lead to weight gain, although weight loss may also occur.
- Other findings include fatigue, polydipsia, polyuria, polyphagia, nocturia, weakness, and somnolence.

Gestational hypertension
- Rapid weight gain with nausea and vomiting, epigastric pain, elevated blood pressure, and blurred or double vision occur with this disorder.

Heart failure
- Weight gain from edema occurs.
- Associated findings include paroxysmal nocturnal dyspnea, tachypnea, nausea, orthopnea, and fatigue.

Hypercortisolism
- Excessive weight gain, usually over the trunk and the back of the neck (buffalo hump), occurs with hypercortisolism.
- Related findings include slender extremities, moon face, weakness, purple striae, emotional lability, and increased susceptibility to infection.
- In men, gynecomastia occurs.
- In women, hirsutism, acne, and menstrual irregularities occur.

Hyperinsulinism
- Increased appetite leads to weight gain.
- Emotional lability, indigestion, weakness, diaphoresis, tachycardia, vision disturbances, and syncope may also occur.

Hypogonadism
- Weight gain is common.
- Prepubertal hypogonadism cause eunuchoid body proportions with relatively sparse facial and body hair and a high-pitched voice.
- Postpubertal hypogonadism causes loss of libido, impotence, and infertility.

Hypothyroidism
- Weight gain occurs despite anorexia.
- Other signs and symptoms include fatigue; cold intolerance; constipation; menorrhagia; slowed intellectual and motor activity; dry, pale, cool skin; dry, sparse hair; and thick, brittle nails.
- Other possible findings include myalgia, hoarseness, hypoactive deep tendon reflexes, bradycardia, and abdominal distention.
- Eventually, a dull facial expression with periorbital edema occurs.

Nephrotic syndrome
- Weight gain results from edema.
- In severe cases, anasarca develops— increasing body weight as much as 50%.
- Related findings include abdominal distention, orthostatic hypotension, and lethargy.

Pancreatic islet cell tumor
- Excessive hunger leads to weight gain.
- Other findings include emotional lability, weakness, malaise, fatigue, restlessness, diaphoresis, palpitations, tachycardia, vision disturbances, and syncope.

OTHER
Drugs
- Corticosteroids, phenothiazines, and tricyclic antidepressants (from fluid retention and increased appetite) can cause excessive weight gain.
- Cyproheptadine hydrochloride (from increased appetite), hormonal contraceptives (from fluid retention), and lithium (Eskalith) (from hypothyroidism) may all cause excessive weight gain.

NURSING CONSIDERATIONS

- Psychological counseling may be necessary.
- If the patient is obese or has a cardiopulmonary disorder, exercises should be monitored closely.
- Prepare the patient for studies to rule out possible secondary causes that include serum thyroid function studies, lipid level, glucose level, and dexamethasone suppression testing.

PEDIATRIC TIPS
- Weight gain can result from an endocrine disorder or from inactivity caused by Prader-Willi syndrome, Down syndrome, Werdnig-Hoffmann disease, muscular dystrophy, and cerebral palsy.
- Other causes include poor eating habits, sedentary recreation, and emotional problems.

GERIATRIC TIPS
- Normal weight increases with age, but shouldn't exceed 15% over normal body weight.
- Aerobic and muscle-building exercises are beneficial for longevity as well as weight control.

PATIENT TEACHING

- Discuss underlying disorder, if present.
- Emphasize the importance of weight control.
- Explain the importance of behavior modification and dietary compliance.
- Provide guidance in appropriate exercise.

Weight loss, excessive

OVERVIEW

◆ Occurs with decreased food intake, decreased food absorption, increased metabolic requirements, or a combination of these

HISTORY

◆ Take a diet history, noting use of diet pills and laxatives.
◆ Question the patient about why he isn't eating properly, if applicable.
◆ Ask about previous weight and if weight loss is intentional.
◆ Note sources of anxiety or depression.
◆ Ask about changes in bowel habits, nausea, vomiting, abdominal pain, excessive thirst, excessive urination, or heat intolerance.

PHYSICAL ASSESSMENT

◆ Check height and weight.
◆ Take vital signs and note general appearance.
◆ Examine the skin for turgor and abnormal pigmentation.
◆ Look for signs of infection or irritation on the roof of the mouth; note hyperpigmentation of the buccal mucosa.
◆ Check the eyes for exophthalmos and the neck for swelling.
◆ Evaluate breath sounds.
◆ Inspect the abdomen for wasting; palpate for masses, tenderness, and an enlarged liver.

CAUSES

MEDICAL
Adrenal insufficiency
◆ Weight loss, anorexia, weakness, fatigue, irritability, syncope, nausea, vomiting, abdominal pain, and diarrhea or constipation occur with this disorder.
◆ Other findings include hyperpigmentation at the joints, belt line, palmar creases, lips, gums, tongue, and buccal mucosa.

Anorexia nervosa
◆ Self-imposed weight loss of 10% to 50% of premorbid weight characterizes this disorder.
◆ Findings include a morbid fear of becoming fat, skeletal muscle atrophy, loss of fatty tissue, hypotension, constipation, dental caries, susceptibility to infection, blotchy or sallow skin, cold intolerance, hairiness on the face and body, dryness or loss of scalp hair, and amenorrhea.
◆ Other related findings include dehydration or metabolic acidosis or alkalosis from self-induced vomiting or use of laxatives and diuretics.

Cancer
◆ Weight loss occurs with findings specific to the tumor, including fatigue, pain, nausea, vomiting, anorexia, abnormal bleeding, or a palpable mass.

Crohn's disease
◆ Weight loss occurs with chronic cramping, abdominal pain, and anorexia.
◆ Associated findings include diarrhea, nausea, fever, tachycardia, abdominal tenderness and guarding, hyperactive bowel sounds, and abdominal distention.

Cryptosporidiosis
◆ Weight loss occurs with profuse watery diarrhea, abdominal cramping, flatulence, anorexia, malaise, fever, nausea, vomiting, and myalgia.

Depression
◆ Excessive weight loss or gain occurs with insomnia or hypersomnia, anorexia, apathy, fatigue, suicidal thoughts, and feelings of worthlessness.

Diabetes mellitus
◆ Weight loss occurs despite increased appetite.
◆ Other findings include polydipsia, polyuria, weakness, fatigue, and blurred vision.

Esophagitis
◆ Avoidance of eating and weight loss from painful inflammation of the esophagus occur with esophagitis.
◆ Associated findings include intense pain in the mouth and anterior chest with hypersalivation, dysphagia, tachypnea, and hematemesis.

Gastroenteritis
◆ Malabsorption and dehydration cause sudden weight loss in acute viral infections or gradual weight loss in parasitic infections.
◆ Other findings include poor skin turgor, dry mucous membranes, tachycardia, hypotension, diarrhea, abdominal pain and tenderness, hyperactive bowel sounds, nausea, vomiting, fever, and malaise.

Herpes simplex (type 1)
◆ Painful fluid-filled blisters in and around mouth make eating painful, causing decreased food intake and weight loss.
◆ Fever and pharyngitis may also occur.

Leukemia
◆ Acute form causes progressive weight loss; severe prostration; high fever; swollen, bleeding gums; and bleeding tendencies.
◆ Chronic form causes progressive weight loss, malaise, fatigue, pallor, enlarged spleen, bleeding tendencies, anemia, skin eruptions, anorexia, and fever.

Lymphoma
◆ Gradual weight loss occurs.
◆ Other findings include fever, fatigue, night sweats, malaise, hepatosplenomegaly, and lymphadenopathy.

Pulmonary tuberculosis
◆ Weight loss occurs with fatigue, weakness, anorexia, night sweats, and low-grade fever.
◆ A cough with bloody or mucopurulent sputum, dyspnea, and pleuritic chest pain may also occur.

Stomatitis
◆ Weight loss occurs from the inability to eat caused by inflammation of the oral mucosa (usually red, swollen, and ulcerated).
◆ Related findings include fever, increased salivation, malaise, mouth pain, anorexia, and swollen, bleeding gums.

Thyrotoxicosis
◆ Increased metabolism causes weight loss.
◆ Other characteristic findings include nervousness, heat intolerance, diarrhea, increased appetite, palpitations, tachycardia, diaphoresis, fine tremor, an enlarged thyroid, and exophthalmos.

Ulcerative colitis
◆ Weight loss is a late sign.
◆ Bloody diarrhea with pus or mucus is an initial characteristic sign.
◆ Weakness, crampy lower abdominal pain, tenesmus, anorexia, low-grade fever, and nausea and vomiting may also occur.

OTHER
Drugs
◆ Amphetamines and inappropriate dosage of thyroid preparations commonly lead to weight loss.
◆ Chemotherapeutics cause stomatitis, which, when severe, causes weight loss.
◆ Laxative abuse may cause a malabsorptive state that leads to weight loss.

Surgery
◆ Intestinal and stomach surgeries that remove or bypass portions of the digestive tract may cause weight loss due to decreased absorption or intake capacity.

NURSING CONSIDERATIONS
◆ Take daily calorie counts and weigh the patient weekly.
◆ Consult a nutritionist to determine an appropriate diet with adequate calories.
◆ Administer hyperalimentation or tube feedings to maintain nutrition.

PEDIATRIC TIPS
◆ In infants, weight loss may be from failure-to-thrive syndrome.
◆ In children, severe weight loss may be the first indication of diabetes mellitus.

GERIATRIC TIPS
◆ Some elderly patients experience mild, gradual weight loss from changes in body composition.
◆ Rapid, unintentional weight loss is highly predictive of morbidity and mortality in elderly patients.
◆ Other causes include tooth loss, difficulty chewing, social isolation, and alcoholism.

PATIENT TEACHING
◆ Provide guidance in proper diet and keeping a food diary.
◆ Instruct the patient in good oral hygiene.
◆ Provide a referral to nutritional and psychological counseling, if appropriate.
◆ Discuss underlying disorder and treatment plan.

Wheezing

OVERVIEW

- Is characterized by adventitious breath sounds with a high-pitched, musical, squealing, creaking, or groaning quality
- Caused by air flowing at a high velocity through a narrowed airway
- Also known as *sibilant rhonchi*
- Can't be cleared by coughing

 ACTION STAT! *Examine the degree of respiratory distress. Take other vital signs, and note hypotension or hypertension, decreased oxygen saturation, and an irregular, weak, rapid, or slow pulse. Help the patient relax, give humidified oxygen, and encourage slow, deep breathing. Have emergency resuscitation equipment readily available. Supply nebulization treatments with bronchodilators. Insert an I.V. catheter for drug administration, such as diuretics, steroids, bronchodilators, and sedatives. Perform the abdominal thrust maneuver for airway obstruction. (See When wheezing stops.)*

ACTION STAT!

When wheezing stops

If you no longer hear wheezing in a patient having an acute asthma attack, the attack may be far from over. When bronchospasm and mucosal swelling become severe, little air can move through the airways. As a result, wheezing stops.

If all the assessment criteria—labored breathing, prolonged expiratory time, and accessory muscle use—point to acute bronchial obstruction (a medical emergency), maintain the patient's airway and give oxygen and medications as ordered to relieve the obstruction. The patient may begin to wheeze again when the airways open more.

HISTORY

- Ask what triggers the wheezing.
- Ask about smoking habits.
- Find out about the onset, productivity, and frequency of coughing; obtain a description of any sputum.
- Inquire about a history of asthma, allergies, cancer, or pulmonary or cardiac disorders.
- Find out about recent surgery, illness, or trauma, or changes in appetite, weight, exercise tolerance, or sleep patterns.
- Take a drug history.
- Ask about exposure to irritants and toxic fumes.

PHYSICAL ASSESSMENT

- Examine the nose and mouth for congestion, drainage, or signs of infection.
- If coughing produces sputum, obtain a sample for examination.
- Check for cyanosis, pallor, clamminess, masses, tenderness, swelling, distended neck veins, and enlarged lymph nodes.
- Inspect the chest for abnormal configuration and asymmetrical motion.
- Determine if the trachea is midline.
- Auscultate for crackles, rhonchi, or pleural friction rubs.
- Percuss for dullness or hyperresonance.
- Auscultate for heart and breath sounds.

CAUSES

MEDICAL
Anaphylaxis
- Tracheal edema or bronchospasm can result in severe wheezing and stridor.
- Initial findings include fright, weakness, sneezing, dyspnea, nasal pruritus, urticaria, erythema, angioedema, and signs of respiratory distress.
- Other findings include nasal edema and congestion; profuse, watery rhi-

norrhea; chest or throat tightness; and dysphagia.
- Arrhythmias and hypotension may also result.

Aspiration of a foreign body
- Partial obstruction produces sudden onset of wheezing and possibly stridor; a dry, paroxysmal cough; gagging; and hoarseness.
- Other findings include tachycardia, dyspnea, decreased breath sounds, and possibly cyanosis.
- Fever, pain, and swelling may be produced by a retained foreign body.

Aspiration pneumonitis
- Wheezing with tachypnea, marked dyspnea, cyanosis, tachycardia, fever, productive (eventually purulent) cough, and pink, frothy sputum occur with this disorder.

Asthma
- Wheezing heard at the mouth during expiration is an initial and classic sign.
- An initially dry cough later becomes productive with thick mucus.
- Other findings include apprehension, prolonged expiration, intercostal and supraclavicular retractions, rhonchi, accessory muscle use, nasal flaring, and tachypnea.
- Tachycardia, diaphoresis, and flushing or cyanosis may also occur.

Bronchial adenoma
- Severe wheezing with chronic cough and recurring hemoptysis occurs.
- In later stages, symptoms of airway obstruction occur.

Bronchiectasis
- Excessive mucus causes intermittent and localized or diffuse wheezing.
- A copious, foul-smelling, mucopurulent cough is a classic finding and is accompanied by hemoptysis, rhonchi, and coarse crackles.
- Weight loss, fatigue, weakness, exertional dyspnea, fever, malaise, and late-stage clubbing may also occur.

Bronchiolitis

◆ An upper respiratory infection causes inflammation and partial obstruction of the bronchioles that produce wheezing.
◆ Other findings include excessive mucus production, crackles, cough, dyspnea, tachypnea, nasal flaring, and retraction.

Bronchitis (chronic)

◆ Wheezing varies in severity, location, and intensity.
◆ Findings include prolonged expiration, coarse crackles, scattered rhonchi, and a hacking cough that later becomes productive.
◆ Other findings include dyspnea, accessory muscle use, barrel chest, tachypnea, clubbing, edema, weight gain, and cyanosis.

Bronchogenic carcinoma

◆ Obstruction may cause localized wheezing.
◆ Typical findings include a productive cough, dyspnea, hemoptysis (initially blood-tinged sputum, possibly leading to massive hemorrhage), anorexia, and weight loss.

Chemical pneumonitis (acute)

◆ Mucosal injury causes increased secretions and edema, leading to wheezing, dyspnea, orthopnea, crackles, malaise, fever, and a productive cough with purulent sputum.
◆ Signs of conjunctivitis, pharyngitis, laryngitis, and rhinitis may also occur.

Emphysema

◆ Mild to moderate wheezing occur.
◆ Other findings include dyspnea, malaise, tachypnea, diminished breath sounds, peripheral cyanosis, pursed-lip breathing, accessory muscle use, barrel chest, a chronic productive cough, clubbing, anorexia, and malaise.

Inhalation injury

◆ Wheezing occurs after initial findings of hoarseness and coughing, singed nasal hairs, orofacial burns, and soot-stained sputum.

◆ In later stages, crackles, rhonchi, and respiratory distress occur.

Pneumothorax (tension)

◆ In this life-threatening disorder, tension pneumothorax causes wheezing, dyspnea, tachycardia, tachypnea, and sudden, severe, sharp chest pain (often one-sided).
◆ Other findings include a dry cough, cyanosis, accessory muscle use, asymmetrical chest wall movement, anxiety, and restlessness.

Pulmonary coccidioidomycosis

◆ Wheezing and rhonchi occur with cough, fever, chills, pleuritic chest pain, headache, weakness, fatigue, sore throat, backache, malaise, anorexia, and an itchy, macular rash.

Pulmonary edema

◆ In this life-threatening disorder, pulmonary edema causes wheezing with coughing, exertional and paroxysmal nocturnal dyspnea and, later, orthopnea.
◆ Other findings include tachycardia, tachypnea, crackles, and a diastolic gallop.
◆ In severe pulmonary edema, labored respirations; a productive cough and frothy, bloody sputum; arrhythmias; and shock may occur.

Pulmonary tuberculosis

◆ Fibrosis causes wheezing in the late stages.
◆ Common findings include a mild to severe productive cough with pleuritic chest pain and fine crackles, night sweats, anorexia, weight loss, fever, malaise, dyspnea, and fatigue.

Thyroid goiter

◆ Wheezing, dysphagia, and respiratory difficulty are caused by a compressed airway due to thyroid goiter.
◆ Other findings include swollen and distended neck.

Tracheobronchitis

◆ Wheezing, rhonchi, and moist or coarse crackles may be auscultated.

◆ Related findings include a cough, fever, sudden chills, muscle and back pain, and substernal tightness.

NURSING CONSIDERATIONS

◆ Place the patient in semi-Fowler's position to ease breathing.
◆ Perform pulmonary physiotherapy as necessary.
◆ Give an antibiotic to treat infection, a bronchodilator to relieve bronchospasm and maintain patent airways, a steroid to reduce inflammation, and a mucolytic or expectorant to increase the flow of secretions, as prescribed.
◆ Provide humidification to thin secretions.

PEDIATRIC TIPS

◆ Primary causes of wheezing in children include bronchospasm, mucosal edema, and accumulation of secretions, which may occur with such disorders as cystic fibrosis, aspiration of a foreign body, acute bronchiolitis, and pulmonary hemosiderosis.
◆ Children are especially susceptible to wheezing because their small airways allow rapid obstruction.

PATIENT TEACHING

◆ Tell the patient how to promote drainage and prevent pooling of secretions, if needed.
◆ Explain deep-breathing and coughing techniques.
◆ Emphasize the importance of increasing fluid intake.
◆ Provide information about taking prescribed drugs.
◆ Discuss infection control techniques, as appropriate.
◆ Explain underlying disorder, diagnostic studies, and treatment plan.

Selected references

ACC Atlas of Pathophysiology, 2nd ed. Philadelphia: Lippincott Williams & Wilkins, 2005.

Aydinok, Y., et al. "Menorrhagia Due to Abnormalities of the Platelet Function: Evaluation of Two Young Patients," *Pediatrics International* 49(1):106-8, February 2007.

Backer, J.H. "The Symptom Experience of Patients with Parkinson's Disease," *Journal of Neuroscience Nursing* 38(1):51-7, February 2006.

Banning, M. "Chronic Obstructive Pulmonary Disease: Clinical Signs and Infections," *British Journal of Nursing* 15(16):874-80, September 2006.

Bogart, L.M., et al. "Symptoms of Interstitial Cystitis, Painful Bladder Syndrome, and Similar Diseases in Women: A Systematic Review," *Journal of Urology* 177(2):450-6, February 2007.

deFreitas, G.R., and Andre, C. "Absence of the Babinski Sign in Brain Death: A Prospective Study of 144 Cases," *Journal of Neurology* 252(1):106-7, January 2005.

Diagnostic and Statistical Manual of Mental Disorders, 4th ed. Text Revision (DSMV-IV-TR). Washington, D.C.: American Psychiatric Publishing, 2000.

Diseases: A Nursing Process Approach to Excellent Care, 4th ed. Philadelphia: Lippincott Williams & Wilkins, 2006.

Harrell, J.S., et al. "Changing Our Future: Obesity and the Metabolic Syndrome in Children and Adolescents," *Journal of Cardiovascular Nursing* 21(4):322-30, July-August 2006.

Kasper, D.L., et al. *Harrison's Principles of Internal Medicine,* 16th ed. New York: McGraw-Hill Book Co., 2005.

Kisiel, M. "Nursing Observations: Knowledge to Help Prevent Critical Illness," *British Journal of Nursing* 15(19):1052-6, October-November 2006.

Kovar, M., et al. "Diagnosing and Treating Benign Paroxysmal Positional Vertigo," *Journal of Gerontological Nursing* 32(12):22-7, December 2006.

Lindberg, C.E. "The Experience of Physical Symptoms Among Women Living with HIV," *Nursing Clinics of North America* 41(3):395-408, vi, September 2006.

Lippincott Manual of Nursing Practice Series: Alarming Signs & Symptoms. Philadelphia: Lippincott Williams & Wilkins, 2007.

Lorenz, K.A., et al. "Quality Measures for Symptoms and Advance Care Planning in Cancer: A Systematic Review," *Journal of Clinical Oncology* 24(30):4933-8, October 2006.

Meechan, G.T., et al. "Who Is Not Reassured Following Benign Diagnosis of Breast Symptoms?" *Psychooncology* 14(3):239-46, March 2005.

Merkley, K. "Vulvovaginitis and Vaginal Discharge in the Pediatric Patient," *Journal of Emergency Nursing* 31(4):400-2, August 2005.

Motl, R.W., et al. "Symptoms, Self-Efficacy, and Physical Activity Among Individuals with Multiple Sclerosis," *Research in Nursing & Health* 29(6):597-606, December 2006.

Nettina, S.M. *Lippincott Manual of Nursing Practice,* 8th ed. Philadelphia: Lippincott Williams & Wilkins, 2005.

Nurse's Quick Check: Signs & Symptoms. Philadelphia: Lippincott Williams & Wilkins, 2006.

Nursing2007 Drug Handbook, 27th ed. Philadelphia: Lippincott Williams & Wilkins, 2007.

Posey, A.D. "Symptom Perception: A Concept Exploration," *Nursing Forum* 41(3):113-24, July-September 2006.

Professional Guide to Signs & Symptoms, 5th ed. Philadelphia: Lippincott Williams & Wilkins, 2007.

Rotegard, A.K., et al. "Mapping Nurses' Natural Language to Oncology Patients' Symptom Expressions," *Studies in Health Technology and Informatics* 122:987-8, 2006.

Savoy, N.B. "Differentiating Stridor in Children at Triage: It's Not Always Croup," *Journal of Emergency Nursing* 31(5):503-5, October 2005.

Signs & Symptoms: A 2-in-1 Reference for Nurses. Philadelphia: Lippincott Williams & Wilkins, 2005.

Stevenson, S.B. "Is It Just a Seizure?" *Journal of Pediatric Health Care* 20(5):336-7, 361-4, September-October 2006.

Steward-Amidei, C. "The Newest Vital Sign?" *Journal of Neuroscience Nursing* 38(5):335, October 2006.

Tengvall, O.M., et al. "Differences in Pain Patterns for Infected and Noninfected Patients with Burn Injuries," *Pain Management Nursing* 7(4):176-82, December 2006.

Thompson, H.J., and Bourbonniere, M. "Traumatic Injury in the Older Adult from Head to Toe," *Critical Care Nursing Clinics of North America* 18(3):419-31, September 2006.

Thompson, J. "Psychological and Physical Etiologies of Heart Palpitations," *Nurse Practitioner* 31(2):14-7, 19-23, February 2006.

Tosti, A., et al. "Alopecia Areata During Treatment with Biologic Agents," *Archives of Dermatology* 142(12):1653-4, December 2006.

Treger, I., et al. "Orthostatic Hypotension and Cerebral Blood Flow Velocity in the Rehabilitation of Stroke Patients," *International Journal of Rehabilitation Research* 29(4):339-42, December 2006.

Wang, C.S., et al. "Does This Dyspneic Patient in the Emergency Department Have Congestive Heart Failure?" *JAMA* 294(15):1944-56, October 2005.

Weiss, J.N., et al. "From Pulses to Pulseless: The Saga of Cardiac Alternans," *Circulation Research* 98(10)1244-53, May 2006.

Welch, E. "Headache," *Nursing Standard* 19(24):45-52, February-March 2005.

Williams, P.D., et al. "Symptom Monitoring and Dependent Care During Cancer Treatment in Children: Pilot Study," *Cancer Nursing* 29(3):188-197, May-June 2006.

Index

i refers to an illustration; t refers to a table.

i refers to an illustration; t refers to a table.

i refers to an illustration; t refers to a table.

i refers to an illustration; t refers to a table.

i refers to an illustration; t refers to a table.

i refers to an illustration; t refers to a table.

i refers to an illustration; t refers to a table.

i refers to an illustration; t refers to a table.

Endocarditis
  chills in, 120-121
  clubbing in, 127
  diaphoresis in, 170
  Janeway's lesions in, 321
  Osler's nodes in, 423
  splenomegaly in, 540
Endocrine disorders
  erectile dysfunction in, 213
  impotence in, 314
Endometrial cancer, postmenopausal
    vaginal bleeding in, 581
Endometrial hyperplasia, post-
    menopausal vaginal bleeding
    in, 581
Endometrial polyps
  metrorrhagia in, 360
  postmenopausal vaginal bleeding
    in, 581
Endometriosis
  abdominal pain in, 7
  dysmenorrhea in, 184
  dyspareunia in, 186
  menorrhagia in, 358
  metrorrhagia in, 361
Endometritis
  metrorrhagia in, 361
  vaginal discharge in, 582
Endophthalmitis, vision loss in, 589
Endotracheal intubation, emergency,
    assisting with, 544i
Enterobiasis, pruritus in, 460
Enuresis, 208-209
  helping child to overcome, 209
Envenomation
  arm edema in 203
  leg edema in, 206
Epididymal cysts, scrotal swelling
    in, 522
Epididymitis, scrotal swelling in, 522
Epidural hemorrhage
  decreased level of consciousness
    in, 337
  headache in, 275
  muscle spasticity in, 378-379
Epiglottiditis
  barking cough in, 141
  costal and sternal respirations in, 511
  stridor in, 545
Epilepsy. See Seizures.

Episcleritis
  conjunctival injection in, 132
  increased tearing in, 555
Episiotomy, dyspareunia in, 186
Epistaxis, 210-211
  controlling, with nasal packing, 211i
Erectile dysfunction, 212-213
Erysipelas
  butterfly rash in, 103
  erythema in, 215
  peau d'orange in, 443
Erythema, 214-217
  drugs associated with, 216i
  rare causes of, 216
Erythema migrans, papular rash in, 431
Erythema multiforme
  mouth lesions in, 366
  vesicular rash in, 586
Erythroplakia, mouth lesions in, 367
Escherichia coli O157:H7 infection
  abdominal pain in, 7
  diarrhea in, 172
  fever in, 234
  nausea in, 392
  vomiting in, 597
Esophageal achalasia, nonproductive
    cough in, 143
Esophageal cancer
  dysphagia in, 190
  halitosis in, 270
  hematemesis in, 287
  melena in, 356
  pyrosis in, 494
Esophageal diverticula
  dysphagia in, 190
  nonproductive cough in, 143
  pyrosis in, 494
Esophageal obstruction by foreign
    body, dysphagia in, 190
Esophageal occlusion, nonproductive
    cough in, 143
Esophageal rupture, hematemesis
    in, 287
Esophageal spasm
  chest pain in, 116
  dysphagia in, 190
Esophageal stricture, dysphagia in, 190
Esophageal tumor, drooling in, 180
Esophageal varices
  hematemesis in, 287
  hematochezia in, 289
  melena in, 356

Esophagitis
  dysphagia in, 190
  excessive weight loss in, 604
  nonproductive cough in, 143
Esophagus, ruptured, subcutaneous
    crepitation in, 153
Eustachian tube patency, tinnitus in,
    560-561
Exfoliative dermatitis, alopecia in, 16
Exophthalmos, 218-219
  unilateral, detecting, 218i
Extensor plantar reflex. *See* Babinski's
    reflex.
External ear canal tumor, hearing loss
    in, 279
Extraocular muscles, testing, 174i
Eye, external, examining, 222i
Eye abrasion
  conjunctival injection in, 132
  increased tearing in, 554
Eye discharge, 220-221
  assessing source of, 220i
Eye pain, 222-223
Eye tumor, visual blurring in, 592

F

Face, major nerve pathways of, 224i
Facial nerve paralysis, decreased saliva-
    tion in, 518-519
Facial pain, 224-225
Facial palsy, masklike facies in, 350
Facial trauma, facial edema in, 205
Fasciculations, 226-227
Fat emboli, purpura in, 490
Fatigue, 228-229
Fat necrosis
  breast dimpling in, 82
  breast pain in, 87
Febrile disorders
  bounding pulse in, 471
  tachycardia in, 549
  tachypnea in, 550
  widened pulse pressure in, 475
Fecal incontinence, 230-231
Fetor hepaticus, 232-233
Fever, 234-235
  chills and, 120i
  development of, 234i
Fibrocystic breast disease
  breast nodule in, 85
  breast pain in, 87
  nipple discharge in, 397

i refers to an illustration; t refers to a table.

i refers to an illustration; t refers to a table.

i refers to an illustration; t refers to a table.

Hemothorax, asymmetrical chest
expansion in, 113
Hepatic abscess, chills in, 120
Hepatic disease. *See also specific type.*
erythema in, 215
purpura in, 490
Hepatic encephalopathy
agitation in, 14
apraxia in, 41
asterixis in, 44
athetosis in, 48
decerebrate posture in, 159
fetor hepaticus in, 233
generalized tonic-clonic seizures
in, 528
halitosis in, 271
hyperactive deep tendon reflexes
in, 163
Hepatic failure, scissors gait in, 252
Hepatic porphyria, constipation in,
134-135
Hepatitis
abdominal pain in, 8
anorexia in, 27
clay-colored stools in, 543
dyspepsia in, 189
epistaxis in, 210
hepatomegaly in, 296
jaundice in, 324
nausea in, 392
splenomegaly in, 540
taste abnormalities in, 553
vomiting in, 597
Hepatobiliary disease, pruritus in, 460
Hepatocerebral degeneration, ataxia
in, 47
Hepatomegaly, 296-297
abdominal mass in, 5
Hernia
chest pain in, 116
dyspepsia in, 189
pyrosis in, 495
scrotal swelling in, 522
tracheal deviation in, 562
Herniated disk
fasciculations in, 227
footdrop in, 244
Kernig's sign in, 333
muscle atrophy in, 372
muscle weakness in, 380, 382
neck pain in, 394

Herniated disk *(continued)*
paresthesia in, 438
steppage gait in, 256
Herpes simplex
excessive weight loss in, 605
mouth lesions in, 366-367
throat pain in, 557
vaginal discharge in, 583
vesicular rash in, 586-587
vulvar lesions in, 601
Herpes simplex encephalitis, amnesia
in, 20
Herpes zoster
abdominal pain in, 8
chest pain in, 116
earache in, 199
eye discharge in, 221
eye pain in, 223
facial edema in, 205
facial pain in, 225
increased tearing in, 555
mouth lesions in, 367
nipple discharge in, 397
paresthesia in, 438
pruritus in, 460
sluggish pupils in, 486
vertigo in, 584
vesicular rash in, 587
vision loss in, 590
Hiccups, 298-299
pathophysiology of, 298i
High cardiac output states, pulsus
biferiens in, 481
Hip pain, causes of, 334
Hirsutism, 300-301
Histoplasmosis, splenomegaly in, 540
Hoarseness, 302-303
Hodgkin's disease
alopecia in, 16
chills in, 120
diaphoresis in, 169
lymphadenopathy in, 347
muscle weakness in, 382
neck pain in, 394
nonproductive cough in, 144
pruritus in, 460
Homans' sign, 304-305
eliciting, 304i
Hordeolum
eye pain in, 223
facial edema in, 205
Horner's syndrome, miosis in, 362

Human immunodeficiency virus infection, papular rash in, 431. *See
also* Acquired immunodeficiency
syndrome.
Huntington's disease
athetosis in, 48
chorea in, 123
dystonia in, 195
muscle flaccidity in, 374
Hydrocele, scrotal swelling in, 522
Hydronephrosis, abdominal mass in, 5
Hyperaldosteronism, orthostatic hypotension in, 418
Hypercalcemia
constipation in, 135
polydipsia in, 452
polyuria in, 457
Hypercalcemic nephropathy, nocturia
in, 400
Hypercapnia, tremors in, 564-565
Hypercortisolism. *See also* Cushing's
syndrome.
buffalo hump in, 101
excessive weight gain in, 603
fatigue in, 228
moon facies in, 365
muscle atrophy in, 372
muscle weakness in, 382
purple striae in, 489
signs of, 100i
Hyperemesis gravidarum
nausea in, 392
vomiting in, 597
Hyperinsulinism, excessive weight gain
in, 603
Hypernatremia, decreased level of
consciousness in, 338
Hyperosmolar hyperglycemic non-
ketotic syndrome
decreased level of consciousness
in, 338
tachycardia in, 549
tachypnea in, 551
Hyperpigmentation, 306-309
Hyperpnea, 310-311
managing, 310
Hyperprolactinemia, hirsutism in, 300
Hypersensitivity pneumonitis, nonproductive cough in, 144
Hypersensitivity reaction, agitation
in, 14
Hypersplenism, splenomegaly in, 541

i refers to an illustration; t refers to a table.

i refers to an illustration; t refers to a table.

i refers to an illustration; t refers to a table.

i refers to an illustration; t refers to a table.

Muscle trauma, muscle spasms in, 377
Muscle weakness, 380-383
Muscular dystrophy
  shallow respirations in, 505
  waddling gait in, 259
Myasthenia gravis
  asymmetrical chest expansion in, 113
  diplopia in, 175
  dysarthria in, 183
  dysphagia in, 191
  dyspnea in, 193
  fatigue in, 229
  footdrop in, 244-245
  gag reflex abnormalities in, 247
  masklike facies in, 350
  muscle weakness in, 382
  ocular deviation in, 407
  paralysis in, 435
  ptosis in, 465
  shallow respirations in, 505
Mydriasis, 384-385
Myeloproliferative disorder, purpura
    in, 490
Myocardial infarction
  anxiety in, 33
  arm pain in, 43
  atrial gallop in, 261
  blood pressure decrease in, 66
  blood pressure increase in, 70
  bradycardia in, 79
  chest pain in, 116
  diaphoresis in, 170
  dyspnea in, 193
  fatigue in, 229
  jaw pain in, 326
  nausea in, 393
  tachycardia in, 549
  vomiting in, 598
Myoclonus, 386-387
Myotonic dystrophy
  alopecia in, 17
  drooling in, 180
  ptosis in, 465
  sluggish pupils in, 487
Myringitis, otorrhea in, 424-425
Myxedema
  facial edema in, 205
  generalized edema in, 201
Myxedema crisis, decreased level of
    consciousness in, 338

N

Narcolepsy, fatigue in, 229
Nasal deformities, nasal obstruction
    in, 390
Nasal flaring, 388-389
Nasal fracture
  epistaxis in, 210
  nasal obstruction in, 390
Nasal obstruction, 390-391
Nasal polyps
  anosmia in, 29
  nasal obstruction in, 390
Nasal/sinus tumors, rhinorrhea in, 512
Nasal speculum, how to use, 512i
Nasal tumors, nasal obstruction in, 390
Nasopharyngeal tumors, nasal obstruc-
    tion in, 390
Nausea, 392-393
Neck pain, 394-395
Neck sprain, neck pain in, 394-395
Negative oculocephalic reflex. *See* Doll's
    eye reflex.
Neoplasms. *See also* Cancer.
  anosmia in, 29
  arm pain in, 43
  fever in, 234-235
Nephritis, hematuria in, 290
Nephropathy, obstructive, hematuria
    in, 290
Nephrotic syndrome
  abdominal distention in, 3
  excessive weight gain in, 603
  facial edema in, 205
  generalized edema in, 201
  leg edema in, 207
Nervous system disorders, anhidrosis
    in, 25
Neurofibromatosis
  café-au-lait spots in, 105
  generalized tonic-clonic seizures
    in, 528
  simple partial seizures in, 531
Neurogenic claudication, intermittent
    claudication in, 319
Neurogenic shock, blood pressure
    decrease in, 66
Neuromuscular failure, apnea in, 37
Neuropathy, miosis in, 363
Neurosyphilis, paralysis in, 435
Nipple discharge, 396-397
  eliciting, 396i

Nipple inversion, differentiating, from
    retraction, 398i
Nipple retraction, 398-399
  differentiating, from inversion, 398i
Nocturia, 400-401
Nocturnal myoclonus, insomnia in, 316
Non-Hodgkin's lymphoma, lym-
    phadenopathy in, 347
Nosebleed. *See* Epistaxis.
Nuchal rigidity, 402-403
Nutritional deficiencies
  confusion in, 131
  purpura in, 490
Nutritional status, evaluating, 602i
Nystagmus, 404-405
  assessing, 404i

O

Obesity
  buffalo hump in, 101
  hepatomegaly in, 297
  pyrosis in, 495
  shallow respirations in, 505
Obsessive-compulsive disorder, anxiety
    in, 33
Obstructive uropathy, flank pain
    in, 236-237
Occipital lobe lesion, hemianopsia
    in, 293
Occlusive vascular disease, leg pain
    in, 335
Ocular deviation, 406-407
Ocular lacerations, conjunctival injec-
    tion in, 133
Ocular muscle dystrophy, ptosis in, 465
Ocular trauma
  nonreactive pupils in, 485
  ptosis in, 465
  vision loss in, 590
Ocular tumors, conjunctival injection
    in, 133
Oculomotor nerve palsy
  mydriasis in, 385
  nonreactive pupils in, 485
Oligomenorrhea, 408-409
Oliguria, 410-413
  development of, 411i
Olivopontocerebellar degeneration,
    dysarthria in, 183
Opisthotonos, 414-415
  as sign of meningeal irritation, 415i

---

i refers to an illustration; t refers to a table.

i refers to an illustration; t refers to a table.

---

i refers to an illustration; t refers to a table.

i refers to an illustration; t refers to a table.

i refers to an illustration; t refers to a table.

i refers to an illustration; t refers to a table.

---

i refers to an illustration; t refers to a table.

i refers to an illustration; t refers to a table.

---

i refers to an illustration; t refers to a table.